Recent Advances in Anti-Cancer Drug Discovery

Recent Advances in Anti-Cancer Drug Discovery

Editor: Niko Jonas

AMERICAN
MEDICAL PUBLISHERS
www.americanmedicalpublishers.com

AMERICAN
MEDICAL PUBLISHERS
www.americanmedicalpublishers.com

Cataloging-in-Publication Data

Recent advances in anti-cancer drug discovery / edited by Niko Jonas.
p. cm.
Includes bibliographical references and index.
ISBN 979-8-88740-421-9
1. Antineoplastic agents. 2. Drugs--Design. 3. Cancer--Chemotherapy. 4. Pharmaceutical chemistry.
5. Biopharmaceutics. 6. Pharmacognosy. I. Jonas, Niko.
RS431.A64 R43 2023
615.798--dc23

American Medical Publishers,
41 Flatbush Avenue,
1st Floor, New York,
NY 11217, USA

ISBN 979-8-88740-421-9 (Hardback)

Contents

Contents

Preface

Cancer is a life threatening disease and it can be treated with anti-cancer drugs. These drugs have been developed over the years, from natural substances primarily from minerals and green plants to chemically manufactured chemotherapeutic agents. New drug discovery is a time-consuming, difficult, challenging and costly process. Computer-aided drug discovery (CADD) has grown as a promising and potent technique for designing drugs that are quicker, less expensive and more successful. Recent developments in computational technologies for drug discovery have illustrated a major and remarkable impact on the design of anti-cancer drugs. These developments have also yielded useful insights into the field of cancer therapy. A few categories of drugs effective in the treatment of cancer include hormone therapies, steroids, immunotherapy or biological therapies, general chemotherapeutic drugs, and bisphosphonates. This book contains some path-breaking studies on anti-cancer drug discovery. From theories to research to practical applications, case studies related to all contemporary topics of relevance to this field have been included herein. This book will serve as a reference to a broad spectrum of readers.

This book is a comprehensive compilation of works of different researchers from varied parts of the world. It includes valuable experiences of the researchers with the sole objective of providing the readers (learners) with a proper knowledge of the concerned field. This book will be beneficial in evoking inspiration and enhancing the knowledge of the interested readers.

In the end, I would like to extend my heartiest thanks to the authors who worked with great determination on their chapters. I also appreciate the publisher's support in the course of the book. I would also like to deeply acknowledge my family who stood by me as a source of inspiration during the project.

Editor

1

Nasal Drug Delivery of Anticancer Drugs for the Treatment of Glioblastoma: Preclinical and Clinical Trials

Franciele Aline Bruinsmann [1,2,†], Gustavo Richter Vaz [2,3,†], Aline de Cristo Soares Alves [1], Tanira Aguirre [4], Adriana Raffin Pohlmann [1,5], Silvia Stanisçuaski Guterres [1] and Fabio Sonvico [2,*]

1 Programa de Pós-Graduação em Ciências Farmacêuticas, Universidade Federal do Rio Grande do Sul, Porto Alegre 90610-000, Brazil; fbruinsmann@gmail.com (F.A.B.); alves.alinecs@yahoo.com.br (A.d.C.S.A.); adriana.pohlmann@ufrgs.br (A.R.P.); silvia.guterres@ufrgs.br (S.S.G.)

2 Food and Drug Department, University of Parma, Parco Area delle Scienze 27/a, 43124 Parma, Italy; richtervaz@gmail.com

3 Laboratório de Nanotecnologia Aplicada à Saúde, Programa de Pós-Graduação em Ciências da Saúde, Universidade Federal do Rio Grande, Rio Grande, RS 96210-900, Brazil

4 Programa de Pós-Graduação em Biociências, Universidade Federal de Ciências da Saúde de Porto Alegre, Porto Alegre, RS 900500-170, Brazil; tanira@ufcspa.edu.br

5 Departamento de Química Orgânica, Instituto de Química, Universidade Federal do Rio Grande do Sul, Porto Alegre 91501-970, Brazil

* Correspondence: fabio.sonvico@unipr.it;

† These Authors contributed equally to this work.

Abstract: Glioblastoma (GBM) is the most lethal form of brain tumor, being characterized by the rapid growth and invasion of the surrounding tissue. The current standard treatment for glioblastoma is surgery, followed by radiotherapy and concurrent chemotherapy, typically with temozolomide. Although extensive research has been carried out over the past years to develop a more effective therapeutic strategy for the treatment of GBM, efforts have not provided major improvements in terms of the overall survival of patients. Consequently, new therapeutic approaches are urgently needed. Overcoming the blood–brain barrier (BBB) is a major challenge in the development of therapies for central nervous system (CNS) disorders. In this context, the intranasal route of drug administration has been proposed as a non-invasive alternative route for directly targeting the CNS. This route of drug administration bypasses the BBB and reduces the systemic side effects. Recently, several formulations have been developed for further enhancing nose-to-brain transport, mainly with the use of nano-sized and nanostructured drug delivery systems. The focus of this review is to provide an overview of the strategies that have been developed for delivering anticancer compounds for the treatment of GBM while using nasal administration. In particular, the specific properties of nanomedicines proposed for nose-to-brain delivery will be critically evaluated. The preclinical and clinical data considered supporting the idea that nasal delivery of anticancer drugs may represent a breakthrough advancement in the fight against GBM.

Keywords: nasal delivery; glioblastoma multiforme; drug delivery; nanoparticles; nose-to-brain delivery; pre-clinical studies; clinical evaluation

---

1. Introduction

Malignant brain tumors are devastating diseases with high morbidity and mortality in adults. In children, they represent the second leading cause of cancer related deaths [1,2]. Glioblastoma multiforme (GBM) is the most common and the most lethal malignant primary brain tumor in adults. Moreover, GBM shows a recurrence rate of higher than 90%, even after multimodal treatment that combines surgery and chemotherapy [3]. The World Health Organization (WHO) classifies GBM as Grade IV, which is the highest in CNS tumors classification, based on the level of malignancy. Indeed, GBM is the most invasive and aggressive type of glial tumors. Primary GBMs, i.e., which arise without a known precursor, are the most common form of GBM (~90%), and they tend to be more aggressive and generally affect older patients. Alternatively, secondary GBMs develop slowly through progression from a lower-grade astrocytic tumor (WHO Grade II or III). These tumors are more frequent in younger patients and they are characterized by a significantly more favorable prognosis. Histologically, primary and secondary GBMs are indistinguishable, but they differ in their genetic and epigenetic profiles [4,5]. It is estimated that GBM has an incidence of 3.21 cases per 100,000 persons in the United States [6], with median survival time of around 7–15 months from the time of diagnosis [7]. The incidence rates of glioblastoma increase with age, with the highest rates in individuals aged between 75 and 84 years [6]. Patient survival at five years form diagnosis is lower than 5% [8]. The etiology of GBM is complex and it has not been fully elucidated, but a mix of genetic and environmental factors is the most likely cause of the disease [9].

GBM is a tumor that is extremely challenging to treat due to its highly invasive nature. Current treatments are based on maximal surgical resection, followed by radiotherapy and adjuvant chemotherapy [10]. Temozolomide (TMZ) is the standard chemotherapeutic agent for the treatment of GBM. This second-generation imidazotetrazinone derivative exerts its anticancer effect through DNA methylation [11]. TMZ is, in fact, a prodrug, which is spontaneously hydrolyzed at physiological pH to its alkylating metabolite 3-methyl-(triazen-1-yl)-imidazole-4-carboxamide (MTIC) [11]. TMZ is orally administered and it leads to fewer side effects when compared with other chemotherapeutic agents parenterally administered [12]. Notwithstanding, its clinical effectiveness remains limited, since tumors rapidly develop resistance to the treatment [13]. In addition, several GBM cases are intrinsically resistant to TMZ, even during initial treatments. This inherent resistance is a consequence of various defense mechanisms, such as the expression of multi-drug resistance proteins and DNA repair systems impairment [14]. The extensive and complete surgical resection of GBM represents the most effective way to increase the survival of GBM patients [15]. However, the surgical intervention is difficult and, in most cases, less than 90% of the tumor can be removed [16]. In fact, these tumors exhibit a high degree of invasiveness and are often localized in important functional areas of the brain, including areas that are involved in the control of speech, motor functions, and senses [17]. Furthermore, the blood–brain barrier (BBB) limits the passage of molecules, including many anticancer drugs, from the bloodstream into the brain [18]. As a consequence of the restrictive nature of the BBB combined with the low brain permeability to most drugs, high doses have to be administered to obtain therapeutic concentrations in the brain. Although several strategies have been proposed to overcome these obstacles (e.g., oncolytic viruses, targeted therapies, immunotherapy, vaccines, etc.), brain delivery of therapeutic molecules against glioblastoma remains a challenge [19].

Nose-to-brain delivery has been proposed as a non-invasive approach to directly access the brain through bypassing the BBB. It is actively investigated as an alternative administration route for the delivery of pharmaceutically active molecules that are potentially useful in a number of CNS disorders. In particular, the intranasal delivery route could represent a major breakthrough in the treatment of GBM, since it offers an effective drug delivery approach for a number of innovative therapeutic strategies (Figure 1).

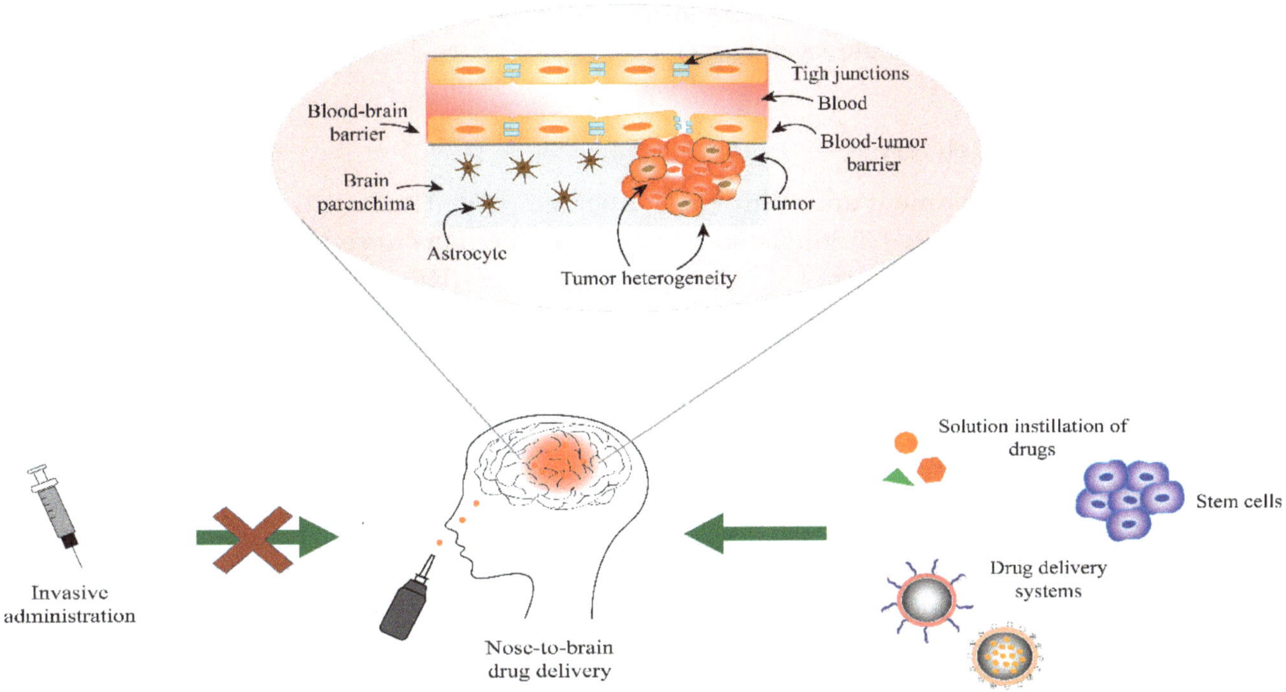

Figure 1. Obstacles and opportunities in the nose to brain drug delivery approaches for the treatment of glioblastoma multiforme (GBM).

2. Blood-Brain and Blood-Tumor Barriers (BBB/BTB)

The BBB protects the CNS by exhibiting a highly selective permeability to substances that are present in blood in order to preserve brain homeostasis and ensure the correct neuronal functioning of the brain. The BBB is a cellular barrier and its properties are mainly due to the presence of tight junctions (TJ) between the endothelial cells of brain capillaries and the involvement of surrounding cells, i.e., adjoining pericytes, astrocytes, and microglia [20,21]. The BBB selectively ensures the supply of essential nutrients and oxygen into the CNS, while also preventing the passage of macromolecules as well as of undesirable toxic or infectious agents, thus providing an adequate brain homeostasis [22,23]. Along with these defensive functions, the BBB also prevents the entry of xenobiotic drugs from the blood into the brain. The BBB is only normally permeable to small and lipophilic molecules, with a molecular weight (Mw) lower than 400–500 Da [24]. In addition, the LogP that is required for an efficient transport across the BBB is estimated to be in the range of 1.5 and 2.7 [25]. Low hydrogen-bonding potential is another important drug characteristic to ensure access to the CNS [26].

In brain tumors, the microenviroment differs from that of the healthy brain, since the morphology, function, and organization of BBB are affected. The result of this alteration is the formation of the so-called blood-tumor barrier (BTB) [27–29]. In high-grade gliomas, as in glioblastoma, the BTB is made from existing and newly formed blood vessels that contribute to the delivery of nutrients and oxygen to the tumor and facilitate glioma cell migration to other parts of the brain [27,30]. The tumor expansion creates hypoxic areas that trigger the overexpression of vascular endothelial growth factor (VEGF) and, consequently, the promotion of neoangiogenesis [31]. The neovascularization process commonly leads to the formation of abnormal vessels that are then able to sustain the high metabolic activity of the tumor cells. The increased fenestration or loss of tight junctions between endothelial cells characterizes these vessels. Furthermore, these new vascular endothelial cells are overexpressing caveolae, have increased pinocytotic activity, and are rich in mitochondria [31–33]. Nevertheless, the BTB presents continuous fenestrated vessels with a defined pore size, which precludes the entrance of hydrophilic compounds and large molecules to the brain tumor [30,34]. As a consequence, most of the antitumor agents are not delivered to the brain tumors due to the presence of BTB [30,34]. The permeability of the BTB can increase as the brain tumor progresses to the late development stages, since an impairment of the BBB/BTB often occurs along with an intensification of the enhanced permeability and retention (EPR) effect, which results in a tendency of large molecules and particles in the nanoscale to accumulate at the brain tumor site [32,34].

3. Nose-to-Brain Drug Delivery

The choice of the treatment and, ultimately, average patient survival, depend on the glioma type, size, location, and grade [35,36]. In some cases, the median survival can be extended by the addition of adjuvant chemotherapy (TMZ) to the radiotherapy (RT) [37,38]. Stupp et al. found that the median survival of patients receiving TMZ in addition to RT was 14.6 months when compared with 12.1 months among those who were assigned to RT alone [39]. However, despite the benefits, treatment with TMZ can entail some severe side effects, such as nausea, vomiting, lymphopenia, neutropenia, thrombocytopenia, fatigue, disturbed sleep, and depression [40–42]. Furthermore, the risk of neurocognitive impairment is increased when RT is administered to the whole brain and even more when the chemotherapy is associated to RT [43–45].

Approaches to overcome the physiological barriers and limitations to access the human CNS include the exploitation of ways that are suitable for the direct administration of the drug to the brain. This can be done by intraventricular, intrathecal, or nasal administration [46]. The intrathecal administration requires some risky surgical procedures and the drugs administered can present limited distribution throughout the brain parenchyma and cerebrospinal fluid (CSF). A better distribution into the CSF can be obtained by intraventricular administration, but this type of administration requires the implant of drug release controlling reservoirs. Furthermore, some severe side effects can occur when drugs are intrathecally and intraventricularly administrated, including meningitis, arachnoiditis, and focal neurologic injury. Moreover, these approaches will result in the potential increase of drug-related toxicities because of the restricted volume of distribution if CSF flow abnormalities are present [47,48]. As a consequence, these invasive brain administration approaches appear to only be applicable to a limited number of selected patients.

The intranasal route of administration is able to bypass the BBB and it appears to be an alternative route for the delivery of drugs to the CNS. In fact, several evidences have been provided in the scientific literature supporting the claim that drugs can reach the CNS after administration into the nasal cavity [49–51]. It is essential to understand the mechanisms of transport of the compounds, the anatomy of the nervous system, and the pathophysiology of the disease, as well as several experimental parameters, in order to design a formulation that allows access to the CNS through the intranasal route efficiently [52]. In the next paragraphs, the anatomical organization of the nasal cavity will be briefly discussed, focusing on the structures that are necessary for understanding nose-to-brain transport, since excellent descriptions can be found in many review papers and textbooks [53].

Anatomically, the nose presents two cavities limited by a septal and a lateral wall dominated by the turbinates, structures that are responsible for the temperature regulation and humidification of the inspired air [54]. The innervation of the human nasal cavity can be divided into sensory and olfactory nerves. The sensory innervation consists of the first and second divisions of the trigeminal nerve (ophthalmic nerve and maxillary nerve), while the olfactory innervation is ascribed to the olfactory nerve [55,56]. The nasal cavity can be divided into three regions: the vestibular region, the respiratory region, and the olfactory region. The vestibular region, which is located in the frontal part of the nasal cavity, is followed by the respiratory region that presents approximately 130 cm^2 of area, and it is characterized by the sensory/trigeminal innervation. In humans, this is the largest region and it can reach up to 80–90% of the nasal cavity [57]. The respiratory epithelium is responsible for covering the nasal conchae, i.e., bone projections of the lateral walls of the nasal cavity and also the paranasal sinuses, i.e., cavities in the facial bones that communicate with the nasal cavity [58]. The last region of the nasal cavity is the olfactory region, which, in humans, represents approximately 10% of the nasal cavity surface area. This region is located in the upper part of the nasal fossa, below the lamina cribrosa (or cribriform plate) of the ethmoid bone and it is innervated by the olfactory nerve [54,59,60]. Olfactory cells are bipolar unmyelinated neurons that present dendrites with terminations protruding above the surface of the nasal mucosa interspaced between the supporting cells and an axon extending through the connective tissue towards the olfactory bulb located in the CNS [61]. The constant replacement of olfactory receptor neurons makes the olfactory mucosa relatively "leaky", allowing for the nose-to-brain transport [62]. The molecular weight and the hydrophilic/lipophilic nature of the drug directly influence the absorption of the drugs through the nasal route. Poor bioavailability after nasal administration is generally observed for drugs with a molecular weight greater than 1 kDa [63]. Lipophilic compounds presenting a molecular weight lower than 1 kDa in some cases present bioavailability close to 100%, i.e., similar to drug exposure obtained after intravenous administration [64].

Mucociliary clearance takes place after the administration into the nasal cavity of a formulation, generally starting from the vestibular region [65]. The formulation is then moved to the posterior region of the nasal cavity in the direction of the respiratory and olfactory regions. The transport to the brain of the drug or of the formulation itself can happen via five different pathways: the olfactory nerve, the trigeminal nerve, the lymphatic, the CSF, and the vascular pathway. The nose-to-brain transport can occur via a single route or through a combination of pathways mentioned above, depending of the nature of the drug, the characteristics of the formulation and the physiological conditions [66]. The substances can then move towards lamina propria and the brain by two different mechanisms, the intracellular and the extracellular transport mechanisms. Once at the lamina propria, the substances follow the perineural channels that are created by a glial cell type, the olfactory ensheathing cells, which cover the non-myelinated axons, cross the cribriform plate, and enter into the CSF and olfactory bulb (Figure 2).

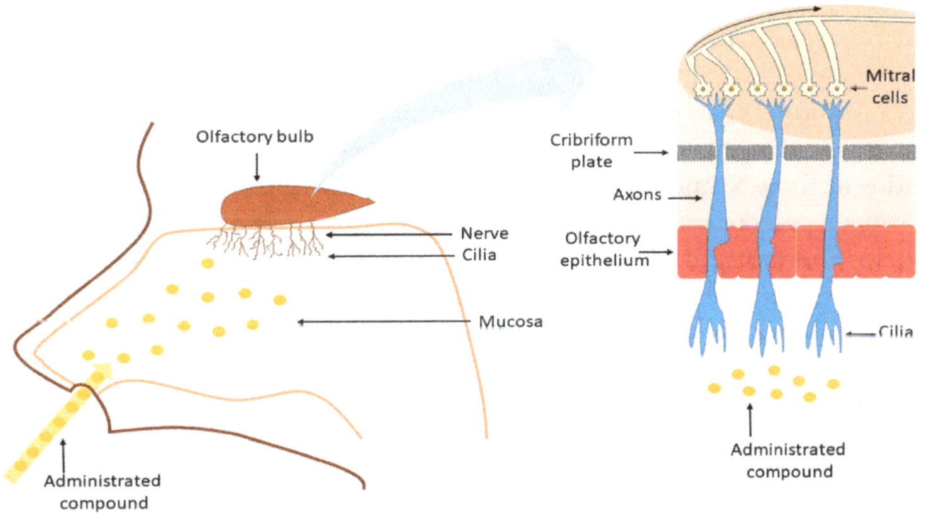

Figure 2. Structures involved in nose-to-brain transport by the olfactory pathway.

From the CSF, the substances are then distributed throughout the brain via bulk flow after being mixed with the interstitial fluid. They are also rapidly distributed throughout the CNS via perivascular transport [52,67].

The olfactory nerve pathway exploits the unique position of olfactory receptor neurons located in the olfactory mucosa, being a direct connection between CNS and the external environment [23,68]. The permeation of the compounds to the CNS occurs along or within the neurons present at the olfactory epithelium through the olfactory pathway [69]. In the case of intraneuronal axonal transport, the compounds are internalized in the olfactory epithelial neurons and then conveyed to the olfactory bulb, thus enabling the compounds to be further distributed to the rest of the brain [70]. In the intracellular form of transport, generally preferred by substances with a hydrodynamic radius above 20 nm, permeation can happen through endocytosis by sensory olfactory neurons and subsequent intraneuronal transport to the olfactory bulb, or through transcellular transport to the cells of the lamina propria [49,71]. However, the intraneuronal axonal transport is usually quite slow, with the times of delivery to the CNS ranging from hours to several days. The paracellular transport involves the absorption of the compounds across the nasal epithelium and the extracellular diffusion associated with bundles of nerves with consequent migration to the cranial compartment [72]. In fact, the perineural spaces of the cranial nerves, as in the case of the olfactory and trigeminal nerves, seem to allow for communication with the CSF of the subarachnoid space, which allows a rapid access route for the molecules absorbed across the nasal mucosa to reach the CNS [70]. The direct nose-to-brain transport can also occur by the trigeminal nerve, which innervates the respiratory and olfactory epithelia of the nasal cavity and allows the access of compounds to the caudal and rostral sections of the brain after intranasal administration [73,74]. However, it is important to point out that it is not generally possible to determine a specific/exclusive way that molecules/peptides access the CNS after the nasal administration, because this access can occur simultaneously by multiple pathways [66]. In fact, in conjunction with these pathways, other mechanisms can also provide access to the CNS from the nasal cavity, such as the nasal and the brain lymphatic systems that connect to the CSF and CNS interstitial spaces drainage by bulk flow mechanisms through perivascular channels surrounding blood vessels [66,75]. Another mode for the penetration of compounds into the CNS from the nasal respiratory region is through an indirect way via the vascular pathway. In fact, nasal blood vessels present continuous but fenestrated endothelia that enable the small molecule passage and the delivery to the brain by distribution across the BBB [74,76].

Despite the numerous advantages, nose-to-brain drug delivery can be limited as a result of some aspects that are related to the intranasal administration, such as low bioavailability of peptides and proteins due to enzymatic degradation, high clearance from the nasal cavity due to mucociliary transport, and other restrictions determined by the anatomy of the nasal cavity, such as small administration volume, limited surface area of the olfactory mucosa, mucus barrier, etc. In terms of enzymatic degradation, it can occur in the lumen of the nasal cavity or during transit across the epithelial barriers due to the presence of exo-peptidases, such as mono- and diaminopeptidases, which can cleave peptides at their N and C terminal and endo-peptidases that can attack internal peptide bonds [77]. The mucus present in the upper respiratory region acts as a physical and chemical barrier that entraps particles and molecules. The mucus is then drained from the nasal cavity into the pharynx through ciliary movement to be swallowed or expectorated [58]. Despite these limitations, Quintana and collaborators [78] reported results from a clinical trial that investigated the intranasal delivery of oxytocin (OT) to 16 male health adults. The treatment groups were divided in: two different doses of intranasal OT, i.e., eight and 24 IU; one IU intravenous OT and placebo with a period of at least six days between treatments to prevent potential carryover and/or administration-related effects. The blood samples were collected to determine the peripheral levels of OT, cross-reactive vasopressin (AVP), and cortisol. All of the treatments produced similar plasma OT increases when compared with placebo. However, the behavioral data that were obtained by emotional expression evaluation suggested that OT delivered intranasally while using a Breath Powered bi-directional device (Optinose, Oslo, Norway) reached the brain and influenced social cognition, whereas IV administered OT, which similarly increased plasma OT concentration, did not. The data from this study supported a direct nose-to-brain effect, independent of blood absorption, for low-dose (8 IU) OT [78].

4. Drugs for GBM Treatment Administered Intranasally

Several studies have been conducted to determine the best treatment of GBM via the intranasal approach, while using monotherapy or drug combinations, including natural and/or synthetic compounds. The studies that were conducted with this purpose of developing an effective way to treat this aggressive brain tumor are summarized below.

Natural compounds, such as curcumin (CC), a polyphenolic extracted from the rhizomes of the *Curcuma longa* that presents anti-oxidant and anti-inflammatory characteristics, are interesting in the treatment of cancer and neurodegenerative disorders and they have been proposed for the treatment of GBM. The anticancer activity of CC has been attributed to the ability of the compound to reduce the expression of E3 ubiquitin ligase NEDD4, a neuronal precursor that is responsible for substrate recognition implicated in cancer development, and the inhibition of Notch1 and pAKT cancer cells signaling pathways, leading to glioma cell growth inhibition, apoptosis, and the suppression of migration and invasion [79,80]. Mukherjee and collaborators [81] used the intranasal route to deliver CC coupled to a glioblastoma specific antibody (CD68 Ab). The targeted CC-CD68 Ab conjugate was intranasally administered to mice in which glioma GL261 cells were implanted in the brain. Ten days after GL261 cells implantation, male adults C57BL/6 mice had CC-CD68 Ab solution in PBS intranasally administered every 72 h, while another group of animals received a solution of a commercially available lipid-complexed form of CC, i.e., Curcumin Phytosome (CCP), by intraperitoneal injection every 72 h. The intranasal delivery of CC-CD68 Ab conjugate and the intraperitoneal injection of CCP both caused GL261 brain tumor remission in 50% of mice, which confirmed that the CD68 Ab could be delivered to the brain via the intranasal route and confirming that CD68 Ab presented a targeted therapeutic effect after intranasal delivery. Furthermore, 70% of the animals that received CC-CD68 Ab intranasal and 60% of those treated intraperitoneal with CCP were still alive at day 90, while all of the control group animals, i.e., vehicle-treated mice, were already dead at that time. In the same study, a marked induction and activation of microglial NF-kB and STAT1 transcription factors were also observed. The transcription factors function together to cause the induction of nitric oxide synthase (iNOS) and, consequently, tumor regression. Therefore, the findings in this study indicate that intranasally delivered CC targeted conjugates can directly kill GBM cells and also repolarize tumor-associated microglial cells (TAMs) to the tumoricidal state [81].

Another natural compound, anthranoid 4,5-dihydroxyanthraquinone-2-carboxylic acid, which is also known as rhein, exhibits anti-inflammatory, anti-oxidant, anti-fibrosis, neuroprotective, and anti-tumor activities [82,83]. The anti-tumor activity of rhein is attributed to the inhibition of MAPK, PI3K-AKT, and HIF-1 signaling pathways and the down-regulation of VEGF signaling pathway [83,84]. Blacher and colleagues [85], aiming at demonstrating that the inhibition of the ectoenzyme CD38 in tumor microenvironment can attenuate glioma progression, conducted a study while using a syngeneic mouse glioma progression model. The animals, C57BL/6J wild-type (WT) and CD38-deficient C57BL/6J (CD38-/-) mice, were pretreated with vehicle or rhein by nasal administration. After 24 h, the glioma cells (GL261) were intracranially injected into the brains of the mice and the administration of vehicle or rhein was carried three times per week over 22 days. The researchers found that the rhein is capable of inhibiting the CD38 enzymatic activity, which reduces the microglia activation that support the progression of the tumor. In fact, the intranasal administration of rhein to WT mice significantly inhibited glioma progression, suggesting that CD38 is a therapeutic target in the tumor microenvironment and that small-molecule inhibitors of CD38 may serve as a useful approach for treating glioma. Furthermore, computed tomography (CT) images of the mice brains showed that the WT and Cd38-/- mice treated intranasally with rhein had the volume of the tumor reduced. However, this effect was significantly higher in WT mice when compared to Cd38-/- (reduction of 74 and 19% on day 22, respectively), demonstrating that rhein inhibits glioma progression and that this effect is mainly CD38 dependent. With this study, it was possible to conclude that the intranasal administration is an effective drug delivery route to the CNS and that the rhein has therapeutic potential for treating glioblastoma [85]. These data additionally support the possibility of brain access from the nasal cavity and demonstrate that the compounds can be directed to the CNS to be effective in the treatment of GBM, even in monotherapy.

Nevertheless, other studies explored the use of compounds in combination. The study that was performed by Shingaki and coworkers evaluated the direct brain uptake from the nasal cavity of a model drug, 5-fluorouracil (5-FU), and whether the inhibition of CSF secretion by choroid plexus could lead to increased drug concentration in the brain [86]. 5-FU is a fluoropyrimidine that is widely used in the treatment of malignant tumors, such as breast, skin, colorectal, and neck [87]. This uracil pyrimidine analog is an antimetabolite drug that can inhibit the thymidylate synthase enzyme and perform a mis-incorporation of fluoronucleotides into RNA and DNA, which leads to cytotoxicity and cell death [88–90]. In this study, 5-FU was intravenously infused or nasally perfused in the presence and absence of intravenous administration of acetazolamide (AZA) in male Wistar rats. In groups of co-treatment, AZA (25 mg/kg) was injected 15 min. before starting the nasal perfusion of 5-FU. AZA is an inhibitor of the secretion of CSF by choroid plexus epithelial cells. In these cells, the CSF secretion is linked to the active transport of Na^+ ions and AZA significantly decreases the activity of the Na/K ATPase [91]. The study demonstrated that the intravenous administration of AZA was able to enhance the CSF concentration of nasally administered 5-FU by 200–300% when compared to that obtained by 5-FU nasal perfusion without pre-treatment with AZA. AZA enhancement of nose-to-brain drug transport was obtained by decreasing the CSF secretion from the choroid plexus and, thus, sustaining the concentration of the nasally applied drug in the CSF [86]. These results demonstrated that 5-FU is capable of accessing the brain through nasal administration. It was concluded that the co-administration of active compounds to treat neurological diseases with drugs that can decrease CSF secretion from the choroid plexus could be an interesting alternative to the treatment of diseases into the brain, like GBM, since an enhancement of the concentrations of the active compounds in the brain is obtained.

In another study, the same group reported a similar effect on the nasal administration of methotrexate (MTX) in male Wistar rats [92]. MTX is a folic acid antagonist that inhibits enzyme dihydrofolate reductase, having a therapeutic effect on a wide range of cancer types [93]. MTX presents a low penetration across the BBB, which limits its therapeutic use for GBM treatment by the oral route [94]. In the study, MTX was nasally administrated while using sodium carboxymethyl cellulose (CMC) to enhance the nasal residence time of the formulation, and AZA was orally administrated 30 min. before the nasal administration of MTX as a co-therapy. The brain uptakes of tritium labelled MTX after intranasal administration of a formulation containing CMC and after intraperitoneal administration were evaluated by blood samples and analysis of the cerebral cortex. MTX was administered for five days with the interval of two days between each treatment to evaluate the results after repeated administrations. The results showed that the amount of MTX quantified in CSF was higher than in the plasma 15 min. after intranasal administration, which indicated significant direct transport of MTX from the nasal cavity to the CSF. In contrast, a higher concentration was obtained in plasma when compared to those obtained in the CSF after intraperitoneal administration. At the same time, the effect of oral administration of AZA 30 min. before the nasal administration of MTX was evaluated and it was found that the co-treatment increased the concentration of MTX in CSF by 195% [92]. The study demonstrated that the intranasal administration is a promising route of the administration of drugs directed towards brain diseases and that AZA can enhance the amount of MTX in the CSF, which is in agreement with the results that were obtained with 5-FU [86,92].

In another study, MTX was loaded in chitosan microspheres that were designed for nasal administration. The microspheres were produced by spray-drying technique while using chitosan with different molecular weights to promote the nose-to-brain delivery of the MTX. The animals received MTX by the intravenous injection or MTX was intranasally administered while using a drug solution or MTX-loaded chitosan microspheres. The study demonstrated a higher concentration of MTX in rat brain tissues after intranasal administration of the MTX-loaded chitosan microspheres when compared to the MTX solution, while MTX could not be detected in rat brain sections after the intravenous administration. The fact that MTX-loaded chitosan microspheres showed a higher nose-to-brain transport, when compared to MTX aqueous solution after nasal administration, was attributed to the presence of chitosan. Indeed, chitosan is considered to be a safe mucoadhesive polymer that could effectively improve the nose-to-brain transport of a hydrophilic drug, like MTX, through intranasal administration [95].

Another study proposed the nasal delivery of temozolomide (TMZ) [96]. TMZ is efficiently absorbed after oral administration and it is available in capsules. Additionally, TMZ has shown good penetration across the BBB and a tolerable toxicity profile [97]. However, the increase in survival for the multimodal treatment with TMZ and radiotherapy is only 2.5 months when compared with radiotherapy alone and existing studies suggest that 60–75% of patients with GBM present no clinical benefit from treatment with TMZ [98]. Based on these data, a rat model bearing orthotopic C6 glioma xenografts was used to study the therapeutic effect of the intranasal administration of TMZ to exploit the brain-targeting properties of this delivery route. In fact, the intranasal administration of TMZ was proposed to limit the systemic exposure to the drug and thus reduce the toxic effects on healthy organs. The animals were treated with saline solution or with TMZ by three different administration routes, intravenous, oral, or intranasal, and the tumor size, rat survival time, and pathological changes were observed during the 40 days of the experiment. Magnetic resonance imaging showed a significant reduction in the volume of glioma xenografts in the intranasal TMZ group when compared to all of the other groups, including controls ($p < 0.05$). Analysis of proliferating cell nuclear antigen (PCNA) and tumor cell apoptosis that were obtained by immunohistochemistry and terminal deoxynucleotidyl transferase dUTP nick end labelling (TUNEL) assay demonstrated that the animals that were treated by the intranasal route presented the lowest expression of PCNA and the highest tumor cell apoptosis rate. The median survival time of the C6 glioma-bearing rats was also significantly longer in the intranasal TMZ group when compared to the other three groups. The control animals that were treated with saline solution survived 20 days, the animals treated with TMZ orally administered survived 21.5 days, animals receiving TMZ intravenously survived 19 days, while animals that were treated with TMZ intranasally survived 31 days [96]. The results presented in this study suggest that the intranasal TMZ administration can suppress the growth of C6 glioma in vivo and it might serve as an effective strategy for glioma treatment.

Intranasal administration in nude mice xenograft models carrying human glioblastoma tumors generated from the human glioma stem cell lines TG16, TG1N, and TG20 by Pineda and co-authors also tested a solution of TMZ in dimethyl sulfoxide (DMSO) [99]. The human glioma cell lines TG16, TG1N, and TG20 were administered by intrastriatal injection to ten-week-old female Swiss nu/nu mice. One month after the graft, the anesthetized mice intranasally received 10 μL of TMZ or vehicle; this procedure was repeated three times a week for two weeks. The TMZ administered intranasally delayed tumor growth and significantly extended the lifespan of the mice engrafted with TG16 and TG1N cells, but presented no effects on the tumors generated by TG20 cells that are resistant to TMZ in vitro. The presented results demonstrated that the intranasal route should be further considered as an option for TMZ delivery into the brain to treat intrastriatal brain tumors [99].

The studies that are reviewed above collectively demonstrate that the intranasal administration of anticancer drugs can induce benefits in the treatment of GBM and the intranasal route of administration might allow for direct access of the drugs to the brain serving as an effective strategy for glioblastoma treatment. However, meaningful comparative studies between intranasal and other administration routes (oral or parenteral) should be always duly conducted to conclusively highlight the potential clinical benefits of using the nose-to-brain delivery over more traditional but well-established administration routes.

Clinical Trials on the Use of Intranasal Perillyl Alcohol for Glioblastoma Treatment

Perillyl alcohol (POH) is a natural compound that belongs to the group of hydroxylated monoterpenes found in many essential oils (peppermint, spearmint, cherries, and others) [100]. The amphipathic character of POH makes it readily soluble in biological membranes and it has been found to be capable of interacting with the lipid bilayers of gliomas cells, leading to effective POH delivery into these cells [101]. A post translational Ras inhibition effect has been suggested by some studies as the main mechanism of anticancer action of POH but not observed in others. Thus, the action of POH is often described as pleiotropic, affecting multiple cell growth regulation processes [102].

Thirteen clinical studies were conducted while using orally delivered POH to cancer patients (ovarian, prostate, breast, colorectal, and pancreatic cancers) to establish the safety and efficacy of this molecule [103]. POH was dosed in capsules along with soybean oil, and the dose regimen included dozens of capsules per day per patient. However, no significant therapeutic response was observed, and the trials were halted before reaching Phase 3 clinical trials. In subsequent studies, the focus was shifted to the use of the intranasal route for the delivery for POH. Here we will briefly summarize the results of the clinical trials that were conducted on GBM patients, although an excellent review has been recently published on this specific topic [102].

To date, POH is the only therapeutic agent that is intended for cancer treatment employing the intranasal route that reached clinical trials Phases 1 and 2. It should be noted that these studies use an inhalation protocol, which might not solely involve the nose-to-brain delivery mechanism. Clinical trials have consistently showed the safety and tolerability of POH administered by the nasal route for up to eight years in addition to positive therapeutic responses in some cases [102,104,105]. The first clinical trial that was carried out in Brazil enrolled 37 patients with recurrent malignant glioma, including 29 with glioblastoma aging from 38 to 62 years old. POH was administered by inhalation four times a day at a concentration of 0.3% *v/v* to deliver a total daily dose of 220 mg. After six months, 14 patients with GBM showed partial response (one patient) or stable disease parameters (13 patients), suggesting some antitumor activity for POH [106]. A following study included 141 patients with recurrent glioblastoma divided into a treatment group, which included 83 patients with recurrent primary GBM and six with secondary GBM receiving POH and a control group with 52 patients receiving supportive care. The treatment consisted of the inhalation of POH four times per day to reach a total daily dose of 440 mg. The results showed a significant increase in survival between the POH treated groups over control group, between patients with secondary GBM over patients with primary GBM and between patients with tumor with deeper localization (thalamus, basal ganglia) over those with tumor at the lobar region. Subsequently, a four-year study with a cohort of 198 patients with recurrent malignant glioma (151 with primary GBM and 38 with secondary GBM) was conducted while again using a protocol of inhalation of POH four times a day, but adopting a higher dosing compared to previous studies (533.6 mg/day). Patients with secondary GBM had a significant increase in survival time when compared to patients with primary GBM, confirming the results of the previous studies, but, most importantly, 19% of patients that were enrolled in this trial remained in clinical remission after four years under exclusive POH inhalation treatment [104]. Santos and colleagues recently reported a study that combined the inhalation of POH (55 mg four times per day) with a ketogenic diet (KD) for three months. In the context of cancer therapy, some authors argue that the KD is viewed as a metabolic therapy and it consists of a high-fat, low-carbohydrate with adequate amounts of protein, promoting a specific metabolic state that is characterized by increased ketone body levels and low glucose levels in the blood [102]. The data showed that the 88% of patients that followed this treatment showed partial responses and stable disease parameters at the end of the study [107].

Encouraged by the positive results that were observed in the clinical trials performed in Brazil, a synthetic GMP grade POH (NEO100) is now under Phase 1/2A clinical trials in the U.S.A. sponsored by Neonc Technologies, Inc. (NCT02704858) [103]. These studies started in 2016 and are still recruiting patients with recurrent glioblastoma. The treatment protocol will follow that adopted in previous trials, with a regimen of POH being inhaled four times a day over a period of six months. Four dosing levels will be studied: 96 mg, 144 mg, 192 mg, and 288 mg per inhalation in order to determine the maximum tolerated dose (MTD). A total of 25 patients will be treated at the MTD and pharmacokinetic studies will be conducted during Phase 1 at the first dosing and after the first dose of the third cycle [103]. The study is expected to be concluded in October 2020 and no partial results were made available to date.

5. Drug Delivery Systems for Nose-to-Brain Delivery in Glioblastoma Therapy

Several therapies that apply novel drug delivery systems are under investigation for the treatment of GBM. Recently, nanoparticles (NP) have received significant attention due to the several advantages that they offer over conventional therapy, such as, for example, their ability in some cases to carry drugs across the BBB [34,108]. Furthermore, these systems offer controlled drug release, which potentially allow for a decrease in the frequency of administrations [109]. Moreover, nanoparticles are expected to improve the drug physicochemical stability and increase the biological availability [110,111].

The application of NP for the direct enhancement of drug delivery from the nasal cavity to the brain demonstrates great potential. The encapsulation of drugs into NP can overcome some of the problems related to intranasal administration (e.g., the poor capacity of penetration through the nasal mucosa, the rapid mucociliary clearance, and the enzymatic degradation), and thus enhance nose-to-brain drug delivery [112]. The small diameter of the NP also allows for them to be more effectively transcellularly transported to the brain [61]. Besides, NP may offer improved drug delivery to the brain, since they can prevent extracellular transport by P-glycoprotein (P-gp) efflux proteins localized in the olfactory epithelium and the endothelial cells that surround the olfactory bulb [113,114]. Additionally, the nanocarriers may also have their surface functionalized with specific ligands to transport agents even more effectively through the BBB [115]. Chitosan nanoparticles, polymeric nanoparticles, liposomes, solid lipid nanoparticles, nanoemulsions, micelles, and nanoplexes, among others, are the NP that have been mainly studied for nose-to-brain delivery. Table 1 summarizes the main features of the NP specifically designed for GBM therapy by the intranasal route in recent years and under pre-clinical stages of development.

Table 1. Characteristics and pre-clinical findings in the last 10 years using nanocarriers administered by the intranasal route for GBM therapy.

Drug	Type of Nanocarrier	Surface Modification	Preparation Method	Size (nm)	Zeta Potential (mV)	In Vivo Model	Ref.
Bevacizumab	Polymeric NPs(PLGA)	-	Emulsification-evaporation	185.0 ± 3.0	~−2	U-87-luc mice	[116]
Ecto-5′-nucleotidase (CD73)	Nanoemulsion	-	Microfluidization	262.7 ± 12.8	+3.5 ± 3.0	C6 rat glioma	[117]
Teriflunomide	Microemulsion	-	Progressive aqueous phase titration	22.81 ± 0.48	−22.62 ± 1.1	-	[118]
Melatonin	Polymeric NPs(PCL)	-	Nanoprecipitation	166.7 ± 6.3	−34.0 ± 5.2	-	[119]
Temozolomide	Polymeric NPs(PLGA)	Anti-EPHA3	Emulsion-solvent evaporation	125 to 146	−21 to + 23	C6 rat glioma	[120]
Kaempferol	Nanoemulsion	Chitosan	High-pressure homogenization	180.53 ± 4.90 (coated) 145.07 ± 4.91 (uncoated)	+26.09 ± 2.67 (coated) −18.10 ± 2.55 (uncoated)	-	[121]
Temozolomide	Nanoemulsion	-	High-pressure homogenization	134 nm	−13.11	-	[122]
Farnesylthiosalicylic acid	Hybrid nanoparticles	-	Emulsion sonication	164.3 ± 10.3	−12.0 ± 1.3	RG2 rat glioma	[123]
Curcumin	Microemulsion	-	Oil titration method	<20	~+10	-	[124]
Curcumin	Nanostructured Lipid Carriers	-	High pressure homogenization	146.8	−21.4 ± 1.87	-	[125]
siRNA	Chitosan nanoparticles	-	Ionic gelation	141 ± 5	+32	GL261 tumor bearing mice	[126]
siRNA siRNA + TMZ or immunotherapy	Chitosan nanoparticles	-	Ionic gelation	141	+32	GL261 tumor bearing mice	[127]
Methotrexate	Polymeric nanodispersion(PLA)	-	Emulsion/Solvent evaporation	351 ± 13.4	+25.1 ± 1.2	-	[128]
Carboplatin	Polymericnanoparticles(PCL)	-	Double emulsion/solvent evaporation	311.6 ± 4.7	−16.3 ± 3.7	-	[129]
BMP4 plasmid DNA	Polymeric nanoparticles(PBAE)	-	Self-assembly	218 ± 7	+17 ± 1	U87 rat glioma	[130]
Camptothecin	Polymer micelles(MPEG-PCL)	Tat	Self-assembly	88.5 ± 20.2	+10.4 ± 2.84	C6 rat glioma	[131]
siRaf-1/Camptothecin	Polymer micelles(MPEG-PCL)	Tat	Self-assembly	60 to 200	−2.86 to 15.9	C6 rat glioma	[132]

Abbreviations: PLGA, Poly(lactic-co-glycolic acid); PCL, Poly(ε-caprolactone); PLA, Poly(lactic acid); PBAE, Poly(beta-amino ester); MPEG-PCL, Methoxy[poly(ethylene glycol)]-b-[poly(ε-caprolactone)] amphiphilic block copolymers.

5.1. Polymer-based NP

Polymeric NP are an extremely versatile formulation approach and have demonstrated great potential in drug delivery. Recently, some authors proposed melatonin-loaded poly(ε-caprolactone) (PCL) nanoparticles (MLT-NP) for intranasal administration in the treatment of GBM [119]. Melatonin (MLT) is an indolic hormone that is synthesized and secreted by the pineal gland, acting in the regulation of the circadian cycle [133]. Synthetic MLT is marketed as a dietary supplement. Therefore, MLT is not officially approved by the FDA for any specific therapeutic indication. However, there are several studies that show its action as antioxidant, antitumor, immune system modulator, and neuroprotective agent [134,135]. However, its short half-life, low oral bioavailability, poor solubility, and extensive first-pass metabolism that limit the drug's ability to reach therapeutic concentrations limit its therapeutic use [136]. MLT-NP were characterized by an average size of 166.7 ± 6.3 nm and 51% encapsulation efficiency (EE), and showed a controlled release of MLT (71.2% release in 48 h). The formulation demonstrated strong activity against the U-87 MG glioblastoma cell line, which resulted in an IC_{50} ~2500-fold lower than that of the free MLT. Moreover, selective cytotoxicity effects of MLT-NP towards the tumor cell line were demonstrated, since, at low doses of MLT-NP, no cytotoxic effect was observed against MRC-5 human pulmonary fibroblasts. Fluorescence tomography images evidenced a rapid and direct translocation of the NP from the nasal cavity to the brain after the nasal administration of MLT-NP to rats. The in vivo pharmacokinetic study was conducted on male Wistar rat and the result showed a significant increase in the brain uptake of the MLT when MLT-NP were administered. Moreover, 0.5 h after administration, the percentage of administered MLT-NP in the brain was ~9- and ~18-fold higher than that of obtained using an MLT suspension administered intranasally and orally, respectively [119].

In a similar study, another group developed a polymeric NP formulation of carboplatin while using the biodegradable polymer poly(ε-caprolactone) [129]. Carboplatin (CPt) is an antineoplastic drug that belongs to the class of platinum-based alkylating agents and is approved for the treatment of various forms of cancer. However, the development of resistance, systemic toxicity, and rapid blood clearance are common problems that are related to CPt use in clinical practice [137]. CPt is available as a solution (Paraplatin®, Bristol-Meyers Squibb) for intravenous administration. Polyvinyl alcohol (PVA) was selected as the emulsifying agent for the production of the polymeric NP, as it provides the nanocarriers with lower particle size and enhances the maximal EE, while at the same time reducing particle aggregation. The in vitro drug release studies showed that the drug was released from the NP with a biphasic pattern characterized by an initial burst, followed by a prolonged sustained release due to a non-Fickian diffusion. Permeation studies across sheep nasal mucosa provided data similar to the in vitro release studies. In vitro cytotoxicity towards LN229 human GBM cells showed enhanced cytotoxicity by CPt-loaded NP only for long incubation times (96 h). In situ nasal perfusion studies that were conducted in Wistar rats with two CPt-loaded PCL NP containing different amounts of PVA demonstrated that both of the formulations showed progressive nasal absorption of CPt over time. Indeed, nanoencapsulated CPt showed better nasal absorption when compared to the free drug, as indicated by the smaller amount of CPt detected in the perfusate after intranasal administration [129].

GBM is characterized as a highly vascularized tumor as a consequence of the overexpression of endothelial growth factor (VEGF) [138]. Bevacizumab (BCZ; Avastin®, Roche), an anti-VEGF monoclonal antibody, was approved by the FDA (2009) to be used as a single agent in the treatment of patients with recurrent GBM [139]. However, BCZ failed to improve overall patient survival rates in some clinical studies [140,141]. Sousa and collaborators developed BCZ-loaded PLGA NP with the objective of improving BCZ bioavailability and targeting the drug efficiently to the brain [116]. BCZ-loaded PLGA NP (185.0 ± 3.0 nm with slightly negative charge) and control (Avastin®) were intranasally administered to CD-1 mice for seven days. The in vivo pharmacokinetic study demonstrated a significant increase of BCZ concentration in the brain, with 5400 ± 2313 ng/g brain tissues and 1346 ± 391 ng/g brain tissues for PLGA NP and control, respectively. The amount of BCZ that was found in blood and off-target organs (lung and liver) was insignificant in the case of

PLGA NP formulation. On the other hand, BCZ was found in the blood, lung, and liver after intranasal administration of Avastin® control. Thus, the improvement offered by nose-to-brain delivery might be an alternative for decreasing the systemic side effects of BCZ. The authors examined the efficacy of the nanoformulation in a nude mice orthotopic GBM model while using bioluminescence and VEGF quantification. Upon nasal administration once a week for 14 days, the BCZ-loaded PLGA NP showed a significantly higher anti-angiogenic effect as compared to Avastin® intranasally administered. However, in terms of tumor growth, no statistical difference was observed between the treatments. The authors attributed these results to the previously reported slow release profile of BCZ from PLGA NP [142]. They also suggested that another in vivo model should be used to increase the number of administrations and evaluate tumor growth for a longer time [116].

Another group worked on lipid-PEG-PLGA hybrid nanoparticles (HNP) for intranasal delivery of farnesylthiosalicylic acid (FTA) with the aim of increasing the brain-targeting efficacy [123]. FTA, which is also known as salirasib, is a synthetic derivative of salicylic acid. FTA is a potent and specific inhibitor of Ras proteins, which are found in most malignant tumors [143]. However, FTA presents poor oral bioavailability and it is not able to cross the BBB at effective concentrations [144]. HNP were produced by the emulsion sonication method and it showed a particle size of around 160 nm and negative surface charge (−12 mV). The in vitro cytotoxicity after 24 h showed that the hybrid nanocarriers significantly decreased rat glioma-2 (RG2) cells viability of ~60%, as compared to only ~13% obtained while using free FTA treatment. Furthermore, cytotoxicity studies towards healthy cells evaluated using L929 mouse fibroblasts evidenced a significant toxic effect for free drug treatment, whereas FTA-loaded HNP did not show significant toxicity. For the in vivo studies, the RG2 cells were unilaterally implanted into the right *striatum* of female Wistar rats. After 10 days, glioma bearing rats received a single dose intravenous treatment or five repeated doses intranasally of FTA-loaded HNP (500 μM/20 μL). Free FTA and blank HNP were used as controls. The data obtained by magnetic resonance imaging (MRI) showed that tumor area decreased by 57.3% and 31.0% when compared to the controls for the single intravenous and repeated intranasal doses of HNP, respectively. In fact, intravenous and intranasal administrations of free drug and blank nanocarriers both had no significant effect in vivo. After a treatment period of five days, the intranasal administration of the nanocarrier achieved a significant decrease of 55.7% in tumor area, which was similar to that observed by intravenous administration of the same formulation (Figure 3A). This result was corroborated by the in vivo distribution studies that indicated that the percentage of the FTA dose reaching the brain was similar after intranasal and intravenous administration of HNP (Figure 3B). However, the highest accumulation of NP was detected in the olfactory bulb after intranasal administration, whereas following intravenous administration the nanocarrier caused a high accumulation of FTA in the spleen and liver (Figure 3B) [123].

Recently, several researchers have proposed the inclusion of nanoformulations within mucoadhesive gelling systems for nasal administration to enhance the nasal residence time and reduce the mucociliary clearance [145,146]. For example, Jain and collaborators developed an innovative MTX formulation for GBM by encapsulating the drug into polymeric PLA NP (MTX-NP) and including poloxamer 188 in combination with Carbopol 934 in the formulation to obtain a thermosensitive hydrogel [128]. It was demonstrated that the MTX-NP formulation mucoadhesion correlates with the amount of Carbopol 934 included while using a mucoadhesiveness testing apparatus. In vivo studies that were carried out using male Wistar rats indicated that the combination of the in situ gelling system and NP resulted in an increase of MTX in the brain when compared to data that were obtained with the MTX solution. The pharmacokinetic parameters demonstrated an increase in area under the plasma concentration–time curve (AUC) for the drug when administered through the nasal route when compared to the administration through the intravenous route. Moreover, PLA MTX-NP enhanced the maximum drug concentration (C_{max}) and AUC 1.5 times as compared to the control MTX solution that was administered by the nasal route [128].

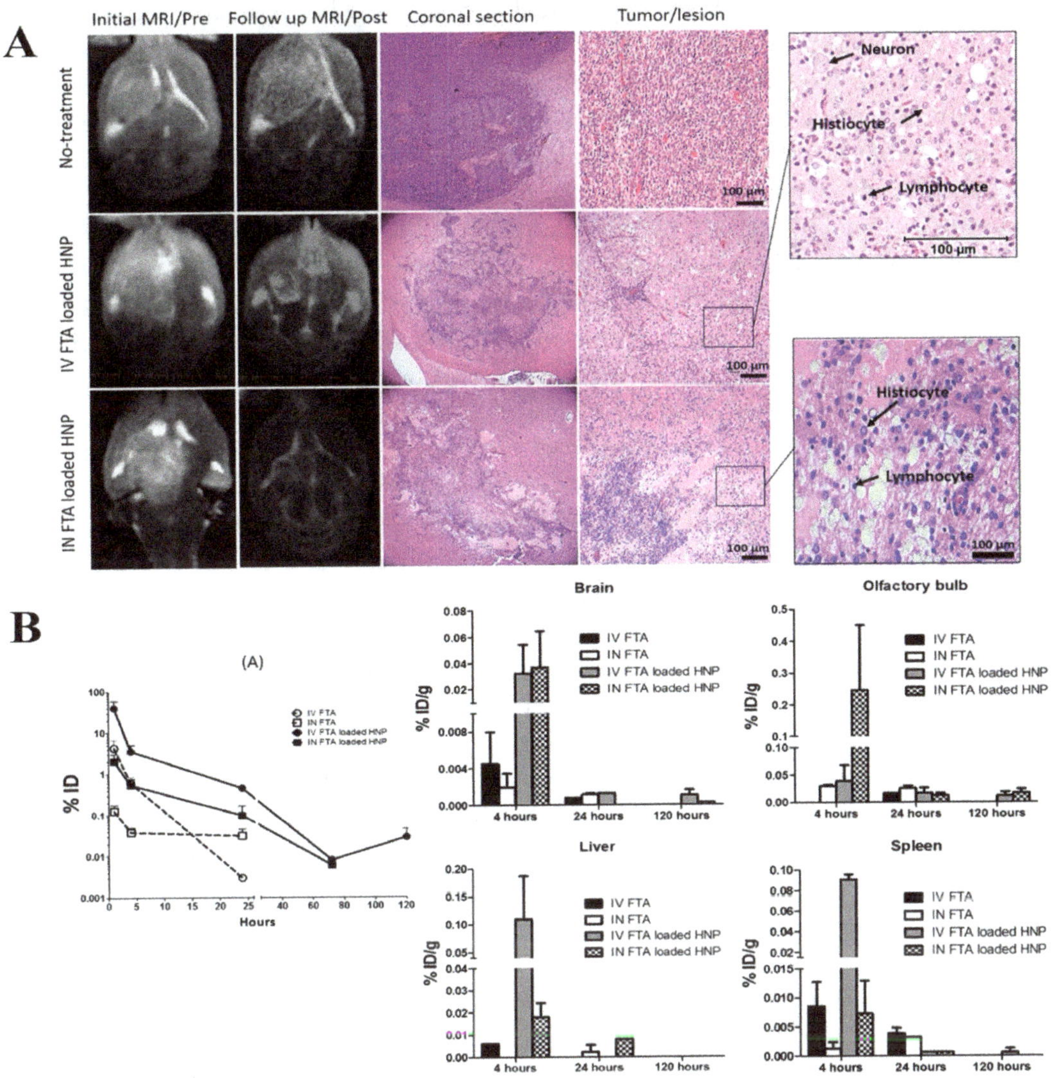

Figure 3. Initial/pre-treatment and follow up/post-treatment MRI images of rat brains from non-treated animals or after treatments with IV or IN farnesylthiosalicylic acid (FTA) loaded hybrid nanoparticles (HNP) formulations and their corresponding coronal brain sections stained with hematoxylin and eosin (Panel A). In the coronal brain sections, the upper panels show a dense tumor area in the right *striatum* of non-treated rats, whereas the middle and lower panels show cellular re-organization of tumor cells after treatment with IV or IN administered FTA-loaded HNP, respectively. Presence of inflammatory response is shown by the abundant presence of histiocytes and lymphocytes. Biodistribution study of the formulations in healthy rats (Panel B). (**A**) Plasma FTA concentration *versus* time profile for the four treatment formulations. (**B**) Distribution of FTA in brain, olfactory bulb, liverm and spleen of healthy rats after 4, 24, and 120 h post-administration (reproduced with permission from [123]).

5.2. Lipid-Based NP

The encapsulation of drugs into nanocarriers has enhanced the therapeutic potential of a wide variety of molecules in view of the treatment of GBM. Among several bioactive compounds, many researchers have shown interest in the nanoencapsulation of curcumin. In fact, NP are able to overcome a number of limitations that are related to this natural compound, such as low solubility, low oral bioavailability, and low capacity to cross the BBB [147,148].

In this context, Madane and Mahajan developed a nanostructured lipid carrier (NLC) system for curcumin (CC) while using hot high-pressure homogenization [124]. CC showed a biphasic release pattern from NLC formulations, initially showing a burst release of approximately 25%, followed by a sustained release up to 24 h. Moreover, an ex vivo permeability study that was carried out using

Franz diffusion cells showed greater drug permeability across sheep nasal mucosa of CC that were formulated in the NLC system when compared to the free drug suspension. The in vitro cytotoxicity studies using the human astrocytoma-glioblastoma cell line U-373 MG showed IC_{50} values of 9.8 ng/mL for the nanoformulation and 13.6 ng/mL for the positive control (adrenomycin), demonstrating the potential effectiveness of CC-NLCs against glioblastoma. Biodistribution studies in Wistar rats showed a higher drug concentration in the animal brain after intranasal administration of CC-NLCs than free drug suspension (C_{max} was 5.4321 ± 2.098 ng/g with t_{max} 180 min. and 8.6201 ± 8.182 ng/g with t_{max} 120 min. for the free drug and for CC-loaded NLC, respectively) [124].

In another study, Shinde et al. investigated the brain bioavailability and efficacy in vitro of CC-loaded microemulsions (ME) after nasal and intravenous administration in rats [125]. The proposed drug delivery system consisted of microemulsion formulated with CC and docosahexaenoic acid (DHA), which, in addition to improving the CC bioavailability, also has antitumor effects of its own. In fact, the results of in vitro cytotoxicity studies showed a synergistic effect of CC with DHA that was formulated in a ME against the human U-87 MG glioblastoma cell line. Indeed, the IC_{50} value was 3.7 ± 0.2 ng/mL for CC-loaded DHA-ME, 502.7 ± 24.6 ng/mL for CC-ME, while it was 747.8 ± 53.0 ng/mL for a simple CC solution, thus confirming the synergistic anticancer effect of CC and DHA in the ME. It was suggested by the authors that the anticancer activity of DHA could be due to its natural affinity to the neuronal cells and DHA capacity to induce lipid peroxidation. Moreover, the combination of CC with DHA and its subsequent encapsulation in ME increased the distribution to the brain after intravenous and intranasal administration in healthy rats. CC brain concentrations following intranasal administration were strikingly higher when compared to intravenous administration, especially in the case of the MEs. In particular, the brain targeting efficiency (DTE) and direct transport percentage (DTP) that were calculated for the CC-loaded DHA-ME were 1,615% and 97%, respectively [125].

On a similar note, Gadhave and his team worked on ME and mucoadhesive hydrogel (MME) for the intranasal delivery of teriflunomide (TFM) with the aim of increasing the brain delivery of TFM [118]. TFM is a selective and reversible inhibitor of the mitochondrial enzyme dihydroorotate dehydrogenase that is necessary for the de novo synthesis of pyrimidine nucleotides [149]. The FDA approved the TFM in September 2012 for the treatment of adults with multiple sclerosis and it is available as a tablet for oral administration (Aubagio®, Sanofi-Aventis). However, it has been reported that the oral administration of TFM should be performed with caution due to the high risk of severe liver injury [150]. Recent studies have demonstrated the potential of TFM as an antitumor agent in breast cancer [151], prostate cancer [152], and lung cancer [153]. The development and optimization of TFM-MME were performed while using a Box-Behnken design of experiments. The optimized formulations were formulated by using the mixture of mucoadhesive agents HPMC K4M (0.3%) and Poloxamer 407 (17%). In the cytotoxicity assay that was carried out in the human U-87 MG glioblastoma cell line, the authors used carmustine as positive control. After 48 h of treatment, the cell viability was reduced to 38.5% and 37.8% at 160 μg/mL for carmustine and TFM-MME, respectively, which indicated that the cytotoxicity profiles against glioma cells were comparable. The in vivo biodistribution study in Swiss Albino mice was assessed by gamma scintigraphy via ^{99m}Tc labeling of the particles. The TFM-MME formulation showed enhanced brain accumulation (C_{max} 0.62% RA/g) with a DTPof 99.2% and a DTE of 359% when compared with the intravenous administration of TFM-ME. However, the in vitro and in vivo studies did not include the free TFM controls as comparators with the proposed ME. The in vivo safety of TFM-ME and TFM-MME was evaluated in toxicological studies that were carried out while using male Wistar rats receiving daily administrations of the two formulations for 28 days. TFM-MME formulation did not reflect any changes in liver or kidney biomarkers, hematology, and histopathological examination at low and medium doses. The study still needs more robust in vitro and in vivo investigations to demonstrate the efficacy of the TFM-ME and TFM-MME for treatment of GBM, although these formulations were demonstrated to be safe for nasal administration [118].

Colombo and collaborators investigated the brain biodistribution and antitumor efficacy of nanoemulsions containing kaempferol (KPF) that were prepared by high-pressure homogenization with and without chitosan [121]. KPF is a natural flavonol that is found in several species of edible plants (berries, broccoli, apples, grapes, cabbage, and beans) and medicinal plants (*Ginkgo biloba*, *Rosmarinus officinalis*, *Aloe vera*, *Centella asiatica*, and *Hypericum perforatum*) [154]. This compound has shown antioxidant, anti-inflammatory, and anti-tumor activities [155]. Despite its excellent properties, it is a substance with low aqueous solubility and low oral bioavailability [156]. As a consequence, the FDA does not approve KPF and there are no pharmaceutical formulations that are available in the market containing this natural compound. However, when formulated in a nanoemulsion coated with chitosan, the amount of KPF permeating across pig nasal mucosa in ex vivo diffusion studies while using Franz diffusion cells significantly increased. Furthermore, during in vitro experiments, the formulation that was coated with chitosan reduced C6 glioma cell viability through the induction of apoptosis to a greater extent than either unencapsulated KPF or a chitosan-free nanoemulsion loaded with KPF. The IC_{50} values of the formulation that was coated with chitosan was about 20-fold smaller than free KPF. In vivo studies in Wistar rats indicated a significant increase in brain uptake after intranasal administration in comparison to the control KPF solution. The formulation that was coated with chitosan significantly enhanced the amount of drug reaching the brain. The KPF brain concentration that was detected after nasal administration of chitosan coated KPF-loaded nanoemulsion was, in fact, 5- and 4.5-fold higher than that obtained using the free drug solution and KPF-loaded nanoemulsion without chitosan, respectively. The increased KPF concentration in the brain was not only attributed to the intranasal administration, but also to the mucoadhesive properties and efficient permeation enhancement provided by chitosan [157,158].

Khan and collaborators proposed another approach based on lipid nanostructures [122], who developed nano-lipid chitosan hydrogel formulations for the nose-to-brain delivery of TMZ. The formulations were prepared by high-pressure homogenization while using vitamin E, as the lipid and Gelucire® 44/14, polysorbate 80, and Transcutol® as surfactants. Afterwards, the nano-lipid formulations were dispersed in chitosan (1.0% *w*/*v*) and converted to a hydrogel. The optimized formulation (size 134 nm, −13.11 mV, EE% 88.45) was able to control the TMZ release (60% release in 24 h) and increase the TMZ permeability of the TMZ by 2.5 times across nasal mucosa. Along with this, the formulation increased the in vitro cytotoxicity of TMZ towards the C6 glioma cell line. In vivo studies in Wistar rats showed an increased DTE of 326% and a DTP of 93% after intranasal administration of chitosan gel formulation containing the TMZ-loaded nano-lipids in comparison to the intranasal administration of nano-lipid formulation as a control (DTE, 113.36% and DTP, 71.74%) [122].

Recently, Azambuja and co-workers developed cationic nanoemulsions (NE) to deliver CD73 small interfering RNA (siRNA CD73) for GBM treatment through the intranasal route [117]. Ecto-5′-nucleotidase (CD73) regulates the extracellular adenosine monophosphate (AMP) and adenosine levels, which have been described as proliferation and drug resistance factors [159,160]. Moreover, CD73 is overexpressed in GBM cells and its inhibition impairs tumor progression [161]. The cationic nanoemulsions were manufactured by microfluidization while using lecithin, medium chain triglycerides, and 1,2-dioleoyl-sn-glycero-3-trimethylammonium propane (DOTAP). The NE-siRNA CD73 were prepared by the adsorption of siRNA to blank formulations (ζ-potential +32 mV) while using different theoretical ratios of cationic lipids to siRNA. In vitro studies using rat C6 glioma cells demonstrated that the NE-siRNA CD73 efficiently decrease cell viability after 48 h of treatment. On the other hand, NE-siRNA scramble that was used as control did not induce any alteration in C6 glioma cell viability. Additionally, cytotoxicity studies showed that the formulation was safe and it did not produce any toxicity in rat primary astrocyte cultures. Interestingly, it was demonstrated that tumor cells took up NE-siRNA CD73, both in vitro and in vivo, which resulted in CD73 knockdown. The in vivo results in glioblastoma-bearing rats demonstrated that NE-siRNA CD73 treatment by intranasal administration significantly decreased the glioma growth by 60% when compared to the control groups (untreated and NE-siRNA scramble). Furthermore, neither NE-siRNA CD73 nor NE-siRNA scramble treatment induced systemic toxicities to glioblastoma-implanted rats [117].

5.3. Polysaccharide NP

Galectin 1 (Gal-1) is a protein that is over-expressed in GBM and is highly associated with tumor progression [162]. The knockdown of Gal-1 using siRNA administration has shown promising results in GBM. Van Woensel and collaborators recently developed chitosan nanoparticles that were loaded with a Gal-1 siRNA for nasal delivery to treat GBM [126]. Gal-1 siRNA loaded chitosan NPs were spontaneously formed by direct complexation due the electric interaction of positively charged chitosan and negatively charged siRNA, which resulted in the successful encapsulation of the siRNA in the nanoparticles and protecting them from ribonucleases (RNases). The NP strongly adhered to the nasal mucosa and the siRNAs were detectable up to 8 h after administration, while the free siRNA only showed weak mucoadhesion. This was attributed to the mucoadhesive properties of chitosan that allowed the nanoparticles to overcome mucociliary clearance and improve the retention time in the nasal cavity [158]. In addition, the encapsulated siRNAs were effectively delivered to the glioma cells from the nasal cavity, since a strong reduction in Gal-1 expression was observed. There was also a reduction in the vascular diameter of the tumor microenvironment in the GL261mice brain tumor model [126].

In a subsequent study, the same group showed that Gal-1 knockdown obtained through nasal administration of chitosan nanoparticles that were loaded with a Gal-1 siRNA displays synergistic effects with TMZ oral treatment and immunotherapy with dendritic cell (DC) vaccination or programmed cell death protein-1 (PD-1) blockade via intraperitoneal administration, suggesting the possibility of combination therapy. The intranasal delivery of Gal-1 siRNA induced a remarkable switch in the tumor micro-environment cellular composition, which reduced macrophage polarization from M1 (pro-inflammatory) to M2 (anti-inflammatory) and inhibited the recruitment of monocytic myeloid derived suppressor cells during GBM progression. Furthermore, the results demonstrated that the median survival increased from 32 days in TMZ treated mice, to 53 days in mice that were orally and nasally treated with TMZ with chitosan nanoparticles loaded with a Gal-1 siRNA. The prophylactic vaccination model showed that the combining DC vaccine with chitosan nanoparticles that were loaded with a Gal-1 siRNA intranasally administered also increased the median survival to 53 days. Similarly, the concomitant intranasal administration of chitosan nanoparticles loaded with a Gal-1 siRNA improved the therapeutic effect of anti-PD-1 antibodies, and increased the median survival to 51.5 days when compared to the control groups (17.5 and 30 days for untreated mice and anti-PD-1 antibodies alone, respectively) [127].

5.4. Targeted NP

The functionalization of the surface of nanocarriers with targeting moieties is one strategy for improving brain tumor accumulation of drug delivery systems. Ephrin type-A receptor 3 (EPHA3) is a membrane-associated receptor that is overexpressed in the stroma and vasculature of gliomas [163]. Chu and co-authors developed PLGA NP functionalized with anti-EPHA3 antibodies for direct nose-to-brain delivery of temozolomide butyl ester (TBE) [120]. Nanoparticles that were loaded with TMZ were prepared by emulsion-solvent evaporation method and subsequently coated with N-trimethylated chitosan (TMC) and their surface functionalized with anti-EPHA3 antibodies. The drug release studies showed a sustained release of TMZ from the nanoparticles by up to 48 h. The results of a cytotoxicity assay on the C6 cells and of nanoparticles cellular uptake demonstrated that anti-EPHA3 functionalization could enhance GBM targeting increasing the cytotoxic effect of the drug. Furthermore, the fluorescence distribution and anti-glioma efficacy in glioma-bearing rats confirmed that the enhanced antitumoral effects were attributed to the nanoparticles surface modification. Anti-EPHA3 functionalized nanoparticles increased the median animal survival by 1.37-folds when compared to the non-targeted nanoparticles. Overall, the author concluded that anti-EPHA3 modified PLGA NP might potentially serve as a nose-to-brain drug carrier for the treatment of GBM [120].

Kanazawa et al. performed a comparative study between methoxy[poly(ethylene glycol)]-*b*-[poly(ε-caprolactone)] (MPEG-PCL) polymer micelles and the trans-activator of transcription (TAT) peptide-modified MPEG-PCL micelles [164]. TAT is a cell-penetrating peptide (CPP) that is derived from human immunodeficiency virus type 1 (HIV-1) containing a protein transduction domain that can induce endocytosis [165]. Polymer micelles were prepared by self-assembly exploiting the amphiphilic properties of the block copolymer. The use of micelles that were modified with TAT and loaded with a model drug, i.e., coumarin, showed an enhancement of direct intranasal brain delivery. Furthermore, the effect of particle size (100, 200, 300, and 600 nm) was investigated on brain distribution after the intranasal administration to glioma C6 cells-bearing rats. The coumarin concentrations in the brain administered with 100 nm micelles were significantly higher than in rat brain that was administered with 600 nm. Interestingly, the drug concentrations in the left side of the brain were higher than those in the right non-inoculated side [164].

Camptothecin (CPT) was encapsulated in TAT-modified micelles and administered by the intranasal route in rats in a later study from the same group. CPT, a quinolone alkaloid, is an inhibitor of the nuclear enzyme DNA-topoisomerase I, which relieves the DNA torsional strain by inducing reversible single-stranded breaks. This naturally occurring alkaloid is extracted from the bark of the Chinese tree, *Camptotheca acuminata* [166]. Even though CPT has shown interesting antitumor activity, its clinical use is limited by extremely low solubility, poor stability, and systemic toxicity. In fact, CPT was discontinued during Phase II trials in 1972 although the initial clinical trials had shown strong antitumor activity. CPT caused severe and unpredictable adverse effects, including myelosuppression, vomiting, diarrhea, and severe hemorrhagic cystic disease [167]. An in vitro cytotoxicity study in rat C6 glioma cells indicated that the CPT-loaded MPEG-PCL-TAT micelles showed higher cytotoxicity than CPT-loaded MPEG-PCL micelles. In vivo, when compared to unmodified micelles, TAT-modified micelles significantly increased the median survival time of rats bearing intracranial glioma tumors. Furthermore, body weight was significantly reduced when compared to untreated rats after seven days of nasal treatment with a simple CPT solution, which indicated severe systemic toxicity. In contrast, CPT-loaded MPEG-PCL or CPT-loaded MPEG-PCL-TAT did not cause significant changes in total body weight, which suggested that micellar formulations were effective in reducing the systemic toxicity of the drug [131].

This approach has also been studied to improve the co-administration of anticancer drugs and siRNA to the brain [132]. MPEG-PCL-TAT micelles were loaded with anti-rat Raf-1 siRNA (siRaf-1) and CPT and then evaluated for their brain uptake efficiency on a C6 glioma model (Figure 4A). When compared to intravenous delivery, intranasal delivered MPEG-PCL-TAT loaded with siRaf-1 significantly enhanced the nucleic acid concentration in rats brain (Figure 4C). As shown in Figure 4B and D, significant inhibition of tumor growth in vitro and in vivo was demonstrated. This was attributed to the combined effects of the CPT and the Raf-1 gene silencing of siRaf-1 in glioma tissues [132].

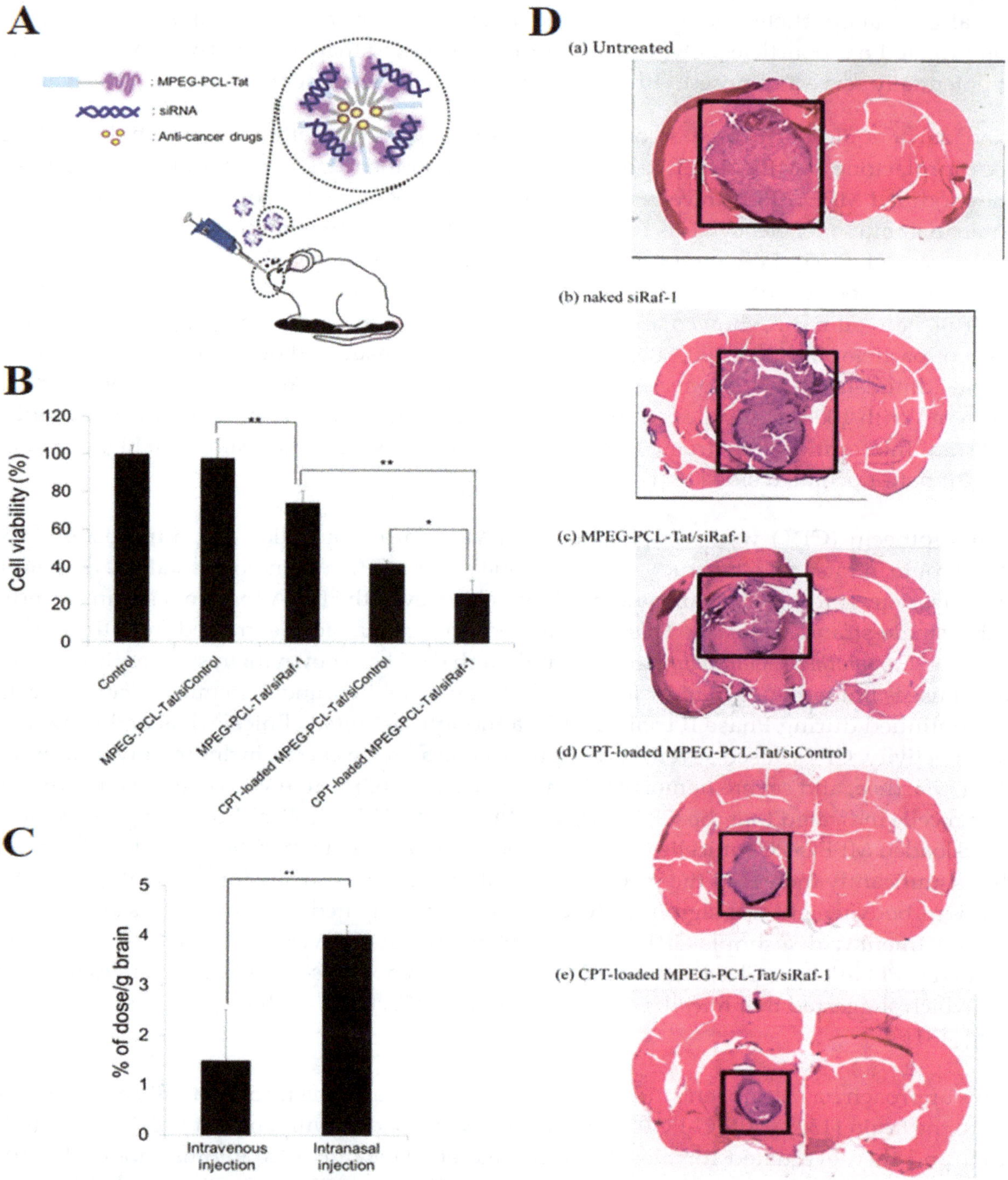

Figure 4. In vitro and in vivo efficacy of cell-penetrating peptide-modified micelles. (**A**) Illustrative model for camptothecin (CPT)-loaded MPEG-PCL-Tat/siRaf-1. (**B**) In vitro cytotoxicity (WST-8 assay) in C6 glioma cells transfected with CPT-loaded MPEG-PCL-Tat/siRaf-1 complexes. (**C**) Distribution of siRNA in brain tissue after intravenous or intranasal administration of MPEG-PCL-Tat/siRNA complex. Rats were killed after the administration of siRNA/MPEG-PCL-Tat complex (20 μg as siRNA), and each brain was enucleated. (**D**) Images of HE-stained brain tissue in intracranial C6 glioma-bearing rats after intranasal administration of siRaf-1 complexed with camptothecin-loaded micelles. After 2 weeks, tissues were taken from untreated rats (**a**) and rats treated with naked siRaf-1 (**b**), MPEG-PCL-Tat/siRaf-1 complex (**c**), CPT-loaded MPEG-PCL-Tat/siControl (**d**), and CPT-loaded MPEG-PCL-Tat/siRaf-1 (**e**) (* $p < 0.05$, ** $p < 0.01$) (adapted with permission from [132].

6. Stem Cells for Treatment of GBM

Stem cells have been proposed in recent years for glioma therapy [168–171]. These cells have a tropism for brain tumoral tissue, a minimum tropism for normal neural cells, and the capability to cross the BBB [172–176]. Stem cells can be derived from multipotent stem cells, such as mesenchymal stem cells (MSCs) and neuronal stem cells (NSCs) [176]. MSCs are hematopoietic stem cells and they can be isolated from different tissue sources, making them easier to isolate than NSCs [177,178]. MSCs have the ability to self-renewal, to differentiate in specific functional cellular and immune-compatible nature [176]. MSCs established from adipose tissue [179], human dermis [180], and human umbilical cordon [181] can inhibit tumor cells proliferation through the secretion of a tumor suppressor soluble molecule, the dickkopf-1 (DKK-1). The authors observed an antitumoral effect through the inhibition of glioma cells migration, invasion, proliferation, and survival in a study with normal rat embryonic NSCs. Interestingly, the levels of mutant p53, serine/threonine kinase AKT phosphorylation, and extracellular signal-regulated protein kinases (ERK1/2), all of the pathways related to GBM uncontrolled growth, evasion of apoptosis, and enhanced tumor invasion were decreased [182].

The intranasal route is considered to be an interesting approach to administer stem cells. A study of Reitz and co-workers focused on the nasal delivery of neural stem/progenitor cells (NSPCs) to target brain tumors [183]. Intracerebral human (U87 and NCE-G55T2) and murine (syngenic Gl261) glioma cell-based glioblastoma models were used to evaluate the specific accumulation in mice brain of the NSPCs. The NSPCs intranasal administration was initiated ten days after glioma cells injection. The histological analysis performed five days after the start of the treatment demonstrated the presence of NSPCs in peritumoral and intratumoral areas of brain. The absence of NSPCs in the brains of animals belonging to the control group confirmed the NSPCs tropism for the tumor. The distribution study showed that the cells entered in the brain tumor area 6 h post-administration. The migration initially occurred (within 24 h) via the olfactory pathway, while the cells migrated later via the microvasculature of nasal mucosa [183]. In a different study, it was demonstrated that the nose-to-brain migration of MSCs that were delivered into the nasal cavity occurred via the olfactory and trigeminal pathways [184].

Stem cells have also been proposed as carriers to deliver cytotoxic agents with the intent to exploit their tropism towards brain tumors. Dey and co-workers evaluated the ability of NSCs to carry the oncolytic virus (OV) CRAd-S-pK7 by intranasal administration [185]. CRAd-S-pK7 virus selectively infects tumor cells [186] and the stem cells were able to efficiently deliver OV in various models of glioma [187–189]. In this study, NSCs were genetically modified without changes in their phenotype to improve their tropism towards tumor signaling. In two mice models of malignant glioma (GBM43 and GBM6 intracranial xenografts), the administration of NSCs by intranasal route extended the survival of CRAd-S-pK7 viruses in glioma tissue. This result was attributed to an efficient migration of modified NSCs to the brain tissue and the successful delivery of CRAd-S-pK7 to the tumor site. In addition, the authors were able to verify an extension of animal survival when treated with NSCs carrying the OV in association with radiotherapy (median survival benefit of five days) [185].

In another study, Balyasnikova and co-workers demonstrated that MSCs expressing TNF-related apoptosis-inducing ligand (TRAIL) were able to reach the tumoral tissue and improve the median survival of the irradiated mice with intracranial U87 glioma xenografts in comparison to the non-irradiated and irradiated control mice [190]. TRAIL is an anticancer protein that is expressed and secreted by several stem cells. Additionally, it selectively promotes apoptosis in glioma cells with minimal effects on healthy cells [177]. The authors also verified the rapid MSCs delivery via the nasal cavity, with the detection of MSCs in the animal brains already within 2 h after administration and their subsequent infiltration in the intracranial tumors.

The stem cells approach for GBM treatment has also been combined with nanotechnology. Mangraviti and co-workers developed a system that combined polymeric nanoparticles and human adipose tissue derived MSCs to deliver bone morphogenetic protein 4 (BMP4) and evaluated the antitumor effect in a primary malignant glioma model [130]. Polymeric NP of poly(beta-amino ester)s (PBAE) were determined to be a good option for the transfection of MSCs due to their favorable physicochemical characteristics: hydrodynamic diameter next to 220 nm, polydispersity index lower than 0.2, and positive zeta potential. Thus, MSCs were transfected with polymeric nanoparticles to express BMP4 and subsequently administered via an intranasal route in rats. The treatment with BMP4 expressing MSCs significantly improved the survival of tumor bearing animals: 60% of treated rats survived up to 16 days after treatment with a 21.4% increase in median survival time over the control group animals [130].

7. Conclusions

GBM is a devastating brain disease with an extremely poor prognosis. Usually, the oral route of administration is considered to be the most convenient for patients. However, for the pharmacological treatment of GBM, it is essential for drugs to reach the brain in their bioactive form. Yet, the therapeutic agent has to overcome several biological barriers when orally administered, such as enzymatic degradation, first-pass metabolism, and BBB. At the moment, TMZ is the chemotherapy agent most used clinically in the treatment of GBM and it is orally administered. In the treatment of GBM, the intranasal route of administration and, more specifically, nose-to brain delivery, potentially presents several advantages over the oral and parenteral route for administering anticancer drugs. In this review, we reported that different therapeutic agents (small organic molecules, biotech compounds, stem cells) are under investigation for GBM treatment exploiting intranasal delivery. In terms of delivery systems, drugs that are entrapped into nanostructured carriers (nanoemulsions, microemulsions, and polymeric and lipid nanoparticles) have been designed and investigated to enhance nose-to-brain delivery. Some of these innovative formulations present surface modified nanocarriers that are able to target receptors and proteins overexpressed in GBM cells facilitating the specific drug delivery to the tumor cells. Nevertheless, most studies are currently only in a pre-clinical phase of development, where promising results remain based on animal models. Overall, the data that were obtained in pre-clinical models suggested a better biodistribution and an improved therapeutic effect of anticancer compounds after intranasal delivery. In addition, long-term clinical studies that were carried in humans with POH demonstrated patient compliance and promising results in selected GBM patients while using this route of delivery. Although there are still a restricted number of studies specifically focused on the intranasal delivery of anticancer compounds to treat GBM, this strategy has the potential to be clinically used for both innovative new drugs and drugs already in use, and may lead to new therapeutic options for GBM patients in the near future.

References

1. Leece, R.; Xu, J.; Ostrom, Q.T.; Chen, Y.; Kruchko, C.; Barnholtz-Sloan, J.S. Global incidence of malignant brain and other central nervous system tumors by histology, 2003–2007. *Neuro Oncol.* **2017**, *19*, 1553–1564. [CrossRef] [PubMed]
2. Izycka-Swieszewska, E.; Bien, E.; Stefanowicz, J.; Szurowska, E.; Szutowicz-Zielinska, E.; Koczkowska, M.; Sigorski, D.; Kloc, W.; Rogowski, W.; Adamkiewicz-Drozynska, E. Malignant gliomas as second neoplasms in pediatric cancer survivors: Neuropathological study. *BioMed Res. Int.* **2018**, *2018*, 4596812. [CrossRef] [PubMed]

3. Morsy, A.A.; Ng, W.H. Re-do craniotomy for recurrent glioblastoma. *CNS Oncol.* **2015**, *4*, 55–57. [CrossRef] [PubMed]
4. Ohgaki, H.; Kleihues, P. The definition of primary and secondary glioblastoma. *Clin. Cancer Res.* **2013**, *19*, 764–772. [CrossRef] [PubMed]
5. Wilson, T.A.; Karajannis, M.A.; Harter, D.H. Glioblastoma multiforme: State of the art and future therapeutics. *Surg. Neurol. Int.* **2014**, *5*, 64. [PubMed]
6. Ostrom, Q.T.; Gittleman, H.; Truitt, G.; Boscia, A.; Kruchko, C.; Barnholtz-Sloan, J.S. CBTRUS Statistical Report: Primary Brain and Other Central Nervous System Tumors Diagnosed in the United States in 2011–2015. *Neuro Oncol.* **2018**, *20*, iv1–iv86. [CrossRef]
7. Ozdemir-Kaynak, E.; Qutub, A.A.; Yesil-Celiktas, O. Advances in glioblastoma multiforme treatment: New models for nanoparticle therapy. *Front. Physiol.* **2018**, *19*, 170. [CrossRef]
8. Thakkar, J.P.; Dolecek, T.A.; Horbinski, C.; Ostrom, Q.T.; Lightner, D.D.; Barnholtz-Sloan, J.S.; Villano, J.L. Epidemiologic and molecular prognostic review of glioblastoma. *Cancer Epidemiol. Prev. Biomark.* **2014**, *23*, 1985–1996. [CrossRef]
9. Song, W.; Ruder, A.M.; Hu, L.; Li, Y.; Ni, R.; Shao, W.; Kaslow, R.A.; Butler, M.; Tang, J. Genetic epidemiology of glioblastoma multiforme: Confirmatory and new findings from analyses of human leukocyte antigen alleles and motifs. *PLoS ONE* **2009**, *4*, e7157. [CrossRef]
10. Han, S.J.; Englot, D.J.; Birk, H.; Molinaro, A.M.; Chang, S.M.; Clarke, J.L.; Prados, M.D.; Taylor, J.W.; Berger, M.S.; Butowski, N.A. Incidence rates of glioblastoma increase, with rates highest in individuals age 75 to 84 years. *Neurosurgery* **2015**, *62*, 160–165. [CrossRef]
11. Wang, H.; Cai, S.; Ernstberger, A.; Bailey, B.J.; Wang, M.Z.; Cai, W.; Goebel, W.S.; Czader, M.B.; Crean, C.; Suvannasankha, A.; et al. Temozolomide-mediated DNA methylation in human myeloid precursor cells: Differential involvement of intrinsic and extrinsic apoptotic pathways. *Clin. Cancer Res.* **2013**, *19*, 2699–2709. [CrossRef] [PubMed]
12. Xu, W.; Li, T.; Gao, L.; Zheng, J.; Shao, A.; Zhang, J. Efficacy and safety of long-term therapy for high-grade glioma with temozolomide: A meta-analysis. *Oncotarget* **2017**, *8*, 51758–51765. [CrossRef] [PubMed]
13. Tiek, D.M.; Rone, J.D.; Graham, G.T.; Pannkuk, E.L.; Haddad, B.R.; Riggins, R.B. Alterations in cell motility, proliferation, and metabolism in novel models of acquired temozolomide resistant glioblastoma. *Sci. Rep.* **2018**, *8*, 7222. [CrossRef] [PubMed]
14. Syro, L.V.; Rotondo, F.; Camargo, M.; Ortiz, L.D.; Serna, C.A.; Kovacs, K. Temozolomide and pituitary tumors: Current understanding, unresolved issues, and future directions. *Front. Endocrinol.* **2018**, *9*, 318. [CrossRef] [PubMed]
15. Li, Y.M.; Suki, D.; Hess, K.; Sawaya, R. The influence of maximum safe resection of glioblastoma on survival in 1229 patients: Can we do better than gross-total resection? *J. Neurosurg.* **2016**, *124*, 977–988. [CrossRef] [PubMed]
16. Pirzkall, A.; McGue, C.; Saraswathy, S.; Cha, S.; Liu, R.; Vandenberg, S.; Lamborn, K.R.; Berger, M.S.; Chang, S.M.; Nelson, S.J. Tumor regrowth between surgery and initiation of adjuvant therapy in patients with newly diagnosed glioblastoma. *Neuro Oncol.* **2009**, *11*, 842–852. [CrossRef] [PubMed]
17. Davis, M.E. Glioblastoma: Overview of disease and treatment. *Clin. J. Oncol. Nurs.* **2016**, *20*, S2–S8. [CrossRef]
18. Harder, B.G.; Blomquist, M.R.; Wang, J.; Kim, A.J.; Woodworth, G.F.; Winkles, J.A.; Loftus, J.C.; Tran, N.L. Developments in blood-brain barrier penetrance and drug repurposing for improved treatment of glioblastoma. *Front. Oncol.* **2018**, *8*, 462. [CrossRef]
19. Paolillo, M.; Boselli, C.; Schinelli, S. Glioblastoma under siege: An overview of current therapeutic strategies. *Brain Sci.* **2018**, *8*, 15. [CrossRef]
20. Guo, J.; Schlich, M.; Cryan, J.F.; O'Driscoll, C.M. Targeted drug delivery via folate receptors for the treatment of brain cancer: Can the promise deliver? *J. Pharm. Sci.* **2017**, *106*, 3413–3420. [CrossRef]
21. Greene, C.; Campbell, M. Tight junction modulation of the blood brain barrier: CNS delivery of small molecules. *Tissue Barriers* **2016**, *4*, e1138017. [CrossRef] [PubMed]
22. Burgo, L.S.; Hernández, R.M.; Orive, G.; Pedraz, J.L. Nanotherapeutic approaches for brain cancer management. *Nanomedicine* **2014**, *10*, 905–919. [CrossRef] [PubMed]
23. Illum, L. Transport of drugs from the nasal cavity to the central nervous system. *Eur. J. Pharm. Sci.* **2000**, *11*, 1–18. [CrossRef]

24. Mc Carthy, D.J.; Malhotra, M.; O'Mahony, A.M.; Cryan, J.F.; O'Driscoll, C.M. Nanoparticles and the blood-brain barrier: Advancing from in-vitro models towards therapeutic significance. *Pharm. Res.* **2015**, *32*, 1161–1185. [CrossRef]
25. Pajouhesh, H.; Lenz, G.R. Medicinal chemical properties of successful central nervous system drugs. *NeuroRx* **2005**, *2*, 541–553. [CrossRef]
26. Warren, K.E. Beyond the blood:brain barrier: The importance of central nervous system (CNS) pharmacokinetics for the treatment of CNS tumors, including diffuse intrinsic pontine glioma. *Front. Oncol.* **2018**, *8*, 239. [CrossRef]
27. Van Tellingen, O.; Yetkin-Arik, B.; de Gooijer, M.C.; Wesseling, P.; Wurdinger, T.; de Vries, H.E. Overcoming the blood-brain tumor barrier for effective glioblastoma treatment. *Drug Resist Updates* **2015**, *19*, 1–12. [CrossRef]
28. Li, M.; Deng, H.; Peng, H.; Wang, Q. Functional nanoparticles in targeting glioma diagnosis and therapies. *J. Nanosci. Nanotechnol.* **2014**, *14*, 415–432. [CrossRef]
29. Chacko, A.M.; Li, C.; Pryma, D.A.; Brem, S.; Coukos, G.; Muzykantov, V. Targeted delivery of antibody-based therapeutic and imaging agents to CNS tumors: Crossing the blood-brain barrier divide. *Expert Opin. Drug Deliv.* **2013**, *10*, 907–926. [CrossRef]
30. Meng, J.; Agrahari, V.; Youm, I. Advances in targeted drug delivery approaches for the central nervous system tumors: The inspiration of nanobiotechnology. *J. Neuroimmune Pharmacol.* **2017**, *12*, 84–98. [CrossRef]
31. Ganipineni, L.P.; Danhier, F.; Préat, V. Drug delivery challenges and future of chemotherapeutic nanomedicine for glioblastoma treatment. *J. Control. Release* **2018**, *281*, 42–57. [CrossRef] [PubMed]
32. Li, M.; Luo, Z.; Xia, Z.; Shen, X.; Cai, K. Time-sequenced drug delivery approaches towards effective chemotherapeutic treatment of glioma. *Mater. Horiz.* **2017**, *4*, 977. [CrossRef]
33. Lyday, R.W.; Etters, A.M.; Kim, C.; Magana, F.; Pontipiedra, G.M.; Singh, N.K.M.; Kadavakollu, S. PDE5 inhibitors offer novel mechanisms in combination and solo cancer therapy. *Curr. Cancer Ther. Rev.* **2017**, *13*, 107–119. [CrossRef]
34. Liu, Y.; Lu, W. Recent advances in brain tumor-targeted nano-drug delivery systems. *Expert Opin. Drug Deliv.* **2012**, *9*, 671–686. [CrossRef]
35. Larjavaara, S.; Mäntylä, R.; Salminen, T.; Haapasalo, H.; Raitanen, J.; Jääskeläinen, J.; Auvinen, A. Incidence of gliomas by anatomic location. *Neuro Oncol.* **2007**, *9*, 319–325. [CrossRef]
36. Hadziahmetovic, M.; Shirai, K.; Chakravarti, A. Recent advancements in multimodality treatment of gliomas. *Future Oncol.* **2011**, *7*, 1169–1183. [CrossRef]
37. Buckner, J.C.; Shaw, E.G.; Pugh, S.L.; Chakravarti, A.; Gilbert, M.R.; Barger, G.R.; Coons, S.; Ricci, P.; Bullard, D.; Brown, P.D.; et al. Radiation plus procarbazine, CCNU, and vincristine in low-grade glioma. *N. Engl. J. Med.* **2016**, *374*, 1344–1355. [CrossRef]
38. Cairncross, G.; Wang, M.; Shaw, E.; Jenkins, R.; Brachman, D.; Buckner, J.; Fink, K.; Souhami, L.; Laperriere, N.; Curran, W.; et al. Phase III trial of chemoradiotherapy for anaplastic oligodendroglioma: Long-term results of RTOG 9402. *J. Clin. Oncol.* **2013**, *31*, 337–343. [CrossRef]
39. Stupp, R.; Mason, W.P.; Van den Bent, M.J.; Weller, M.; Fisher, B.; Taphoorn, M.J.; Belanger, K.; Brandes, A.A.; Marosi, C.; Bogdahn, U.; et al. Radiotherapy plus concomitant and adjuvant temozolomide for glioblastoma. *N. Engl. J. Med.* **2005**, *352*, 987–996. [CrossRef]
40. Weller, M.; van den Bent, M.; Hopkins, K.; Tonn, J.C.; Stupp, R.; Falini, A.; Cohen-Jonathan-Moyal, E.; Frappaz, D.; Henriksson, R.; Balana, C.; et al. EANO guideline for the diagnosis and treatment of anaplastic gliomas and glioblastoma. *Lancet Oncol.* **2014**, *15*, e395–e403. [CrossRef]
41. Stupp, R.; Brada, M.; van den Bent, M.J.; Tonn, J.C.; Pentheroudakis, G.; ESMO Guidelines Working Group. High-grade glioma: ESMO Clinical Practice Guidelines for diagnosis, treatment and follow-up. *Ann. Oncol.* **2014**, *25* (Suppl. 3), 93–101. [CrossRef] [PubMed]
42. Armstrong, T.S.; Shade, M.Y.; Breton, G.; Gilbert, M.R.; Mahajan, A.; Scheurer, M.E.; Vera, E.; Berger, A.M. Sleep-wake disturbance in patients with brain tumors. *Neuro Oncol.* **2017**, *19*, 323–335. [CrossRef] [PubMed]
43. Taphoorn, M.J.; Heimans, J.J.; van der Veen, E.A.; Karim, A.B. Endocrine functions in long-term survivors of low-grade supratentorial glioma treated with radiation therapy. *J. Neurooncol.* **1995**, *2*, 97–102. [CrossRef] [PubMed]

44. Gregor, A.; Cull, A.; Traynor, E.; Stewart, M.; Lander, F.; Love, S. Neuropsychometric evaluation of long-term survivors of adult brain tumours: Relationship with tumour and treatment parameters. *Radiother. Oncol.* **1996**, *41*, 55–59. [CrossRef]
45. Surma-aho, O.; Niemela, M.; Vilkki, J.; Kouri, M.; Brander, A.; Salonen, O.; Paetau, A.; Kallio, M.; Pyykkönen, J.; Jääskeläinen, J. Adverse long-term effects of brain radiotherapy in adult low-grade glioma patients. *Neurology* **2001**, *56*, 1285–1290. [CrossRef] [PubMed]
46. Hersh, D.S.; Wadajkar, A.S.; Roberts, N.; Perez, J.G.; Connolly, N.P.; Frenkel, V.; Winkles, J.A.; Woodworth, G.F.; Kim, A.J. Evolving Drug Delivery Strategies to Overcome the Blood Brain Barrier. *Curr. Pharm. Des.* **2016**, *22*, 1177–1193. [CrossRef]
47. Grossman, S.A.; Trump, D.L.; Chen, D.C.; Thompson, G.; Camargo, E.E. Cerebrospinal fluid flow abnormalities in patients with neoplastic meningi tis. An evaluation using 111indium-DTPA ventriculography. *Am. J. Med.* **1982**, *73*, 641–647. [CrossRef]
48. Blakeley, J. Drug delivery to brain tumors. *Curr. Neurol. Neurosci. Rep.* **2008**, *8*, 235–241. [CrossRef]
49. Lochhead, J.J.; Thorne, R.G. Intranasal delivery of biologics to the central nervous system. *Adv. Drug Deliv. Rev.* **2012**, *64*, 614–628. [CrossRef]
50. Chapman, C.D.; Frey, W.H.; Craft, S.; Danielyan, L.; Hallschmid, M.; Schioth, H.B.; Benedict, C. Intranasal treatment of central nervous system dysfunction in humans. *Pharm. Res.* **2013**, *30*, 2475–2484. [CrossRef]
51. Chauhan, M.B.; Chauhan, N.B. Brain Uptake of Neurotherapeutics after Intranasal versus Intraperitoneal Delivery in Mice. *J. Neurol. Neurosurg.* **2015**, *2*, 9. [CrossRef]
52. Dhuria, S.V.; Hanson, L.R.; Frey, W.H., II. Intranasal Delivery to the Central Nervous System: Mechanisms and Experimental Considerations. *J. Pharm. Sci.* **2010**, *99*, 1654–1673. [CrossRef] [PubMed]
53. Lledo, P.M.; Gheusi, G.; Vincent, J.D. Information processing in the mammalian olfactory system. *Physiol. Rev.* **2005**, *85*, 281–317. [CrossRef] [PubMed]
54. Dahl, R.; Mygind, N. Anatomy, physiology and function of the nasal cavities in health and disease. *Adv. Drug Deliv. Rev.* **1998**, *29*, 3–12.
55. Geurkink, N. Nasal anatomy, physiology and function. *J. Allergy Clin. Immunol.* **1983**, *72*, 123–128. [CrossRef]
56. Watelet, J.B.; Van Cauwenberge, P. Applied anatomy and physiology of the nose and paranasal sinuses. *Allergy* **1999**, *57*, 14–25. [CrossRef]
57. Jafek, B.W. Ultrastructure of human nasal mucosa. *Laryngoscope* **1983**, *93*, 1576–1599. [CrossRef]
58. Junqueira, L.C.; Carneiro, J. *Biologia Celular e Molecular*, 9th ed.; Guanabara Koogan: Rio de Janeiro, Brazil, 2012; pp. 337–338.
59. Leopold, D.A. The relationship between nasal anatomy and human olfaction. *Laryngoscope* **1988**, *98*, 1232–1238. [CrossRef]
60. Gizurarson, S. Anatomical and histological factors affecting intranasal drug and vaccine delivery. *Curr. Drug Deliv.* **2012**, *9*, 566–582. [CrossRef]
61. Mistry, A.; Stolnik, S.; Illum, L. Nanoparticles for direct nose-to-brain delivery of drugs. *Int. J. Pharm.* **2009**, *379*, 146–157. [CrossRef]
62. Caggiano, M.; Kauer, J.S.; Hunter, D.D. Globose basal cells are neuronal progenitors in the olfactory epithelium: A lineage analysis using a replication-incompetent retrovirus. *Neuron* **1994**, *13*, 339–352. [CrossRef]
63. Arora, P.; Sharma, S.; Garg, S. Permeability issues in nasal drug delivery. *Drug Discov. Today* **2002**, *7*, 967–975. [CrossRef]
64. Pires, A.; Fortuna, A.; Alves, G.; Falcão, A. Intranasal Drug Delivery: How, Why and What for? *J. Pharm. Sci.* **2009**, *12*, 288–311. [CrossRef] [PubMed]
65. Vyas, T.K.; Babbar, A.K.; Sharma, R.K.; Singh, S.; Misra, A. Intranasal mucoadhesive microemulsions of clonazepam: Preliminary studies on brain targeting. *J. Pharm. Sci.* **2006**, *95*, 570–580. [CrossRef] [PubMed]
66. Gomez, D.; Martinez, J.A.; Hanson, L.R.; Frey, W.H., II; Toth, C.C. Intranasal treatment of neurodegenerative diseases and stroke. *Front. Biosci.* **2012**, *4*, 74–89. [CrossRef]
67. Einer-Jensen, N.; Hunter, R. Counter-current transfer in reproductive biology. *Reproduction* **2005**, *129*, 9–18. [CrossRef]
68. Charlton, S.; Jones, N.S.; Davis, S.S.; Illum, L. Distribution and clearance of bioadhesive formulations from the olfactory region in man: Effect of polymer type and nasal delivery device. *Eur. J. Pharm. Sci.* **2007**, *30*, 295–302. [CrossRef]

69. Crowe, T.P.; Greenlee, M.H.W.; Kanthasamy, A.G.; Hsu, W.H. Mechanism of intranasal drug delivery directly to the brain. *Life Sci.* **2018**, *195*, 44–52. [CrossRef]
70. Illum, L. Is nose-to-brain transport of drugs in man a reality? *J. Pharm. Pharmacol.* **2004**, *56*, 3–17. [CrossRef]
71. Conner, S.D.; Schmid, S.L. Regulated portals of entry into the cell. *Nature* **2003**, *422*, 37–44. [CrossRef]
72. Jansson, B.; Björk, E. Visualization of In Vivo Olfactory Uptake and Transfer Using Fluorescein Dextran. *J. Drug Target.* **2002**, *10*, 379–386. [CrossRef] [PubMed]
73. Schaefer, M.L.; Böttger, B.; Silver, W.L.; Finger, T.E. Trigeminal collaterals in the nasal epithelium and olfactory bulb: A potential route for direct modulation of olfactory information by trigeminal stimuli. *J. Comp. Neurol.* **2002**, *444*, 221–226. [CrossRef] [PubMed]
74. Lochhead, J.J.; Wolak, D.J.; Pizzo, M.E.; Thorne, R.G. Rapid transport within cerebral perivascular spaces underlies widespread tracer distribution in the brain after intranasal administration. *J. Cereb. Blood Flow Metab.* **2015**, *35*, 371–381. [CrossRef] [PubMed]
75. Groothuis, D.R.; Vavra, M.W.; Schlageter, K.E.; Kang, E.W.; Itskovich, A.C.; Hertzler, S.; Allen, C.V.; Lipton, H.L. Efflux of drugs and solutes from brain: The interactive roles of diffusional transcapillary transport, bulk flow and capillary transportes. *J. Cereb. Blood Flow Metab.* **2007**, *27*, 43–56. [CrossRef] [PubMed]
76. Grevers, G.; Herrmann, U. Fenestrated endothelia in vessels of the nasal mucosa. An electron-microscopic study in the rabbit. *Arch. Otorhinolaryngol.* **1987**, *244*, 55–60. [CrossRef] [PubMed]
77. Lee, V.H. Enzymatic barriers to peptide and protein absorption. *Crit. Rev. Ther. Drug Carr. Syst.* **1988**, *5*, 69–97. [CrossRef]
78. Quintana, D.S.; Westlye, L.T.; Rustan, Ø.G.; Tesli, N.; Poppy, C.L.; Smevik, H.; Tesli, M.; Røine, M.; Mahmoud, R.A.; Smerud, K.T.; et al. Low-dose oxytocin delivered intranasally with Breath Powered device affects social-cognitive behavior: A randomized four-way crossover trial with nasal cavity dimension assessment. *Transl. Psychiatry* **2015**, *5*, e602. [CrossRef]
79. Wang, X.; Deng, J.; Yuan, J.; Tang, X.; Wang, Y.; Chen, H.; Liu, Y.; Zhou, L. Curcumin exerts its tumor suppressive function via inhibition of NEDD4 oncoprotein in glioma cancer cells. *Int. J. Oncol.* **2017**, *51*, 467–477. [CrossRef]
80. Nasr, M. Development of an optimized hyaluronic acid-based lipidic nanoemulsion co-encapsulating two polyphenols for nose to brain delivery. *Drug Deliv.* **2016**, *23*, 1444–1452. [CrossRef]
81. Mukherjee, S.; Baidoo, J.; Fried, A.; Atwi, D.; Dolai, S.; Boockvar, J.; Symons, M.; Ruggieri, R.; Raja, K.; Banerjee, P. Curcumin changes the polarity of tumor-associated microglia and eliminates glioblastoma. *Int. J. Cancer* **2016**, *139*, 2838–2849. [CrossRef]
82. Zhou, Y.X.; Xia, W.; Yue, W.; Peng, C.; Rahman, K.; Zhang, H. Rhein: A Review of Pharmacological Activities. *Evid. Based Complement. Altern. Med.* **2015**, *2015*, 578107. [CrossRef] [PubMed]
83. Sun, H.; Luo, G.; Chen, D.; Xiang, Z.A. Comprehensive and System Review for the Pharmacological Mechanism of Action of Rhein, an Active Anthraquinone Ingredient. *Front. Pharmacol.* **2016**, *7*, 247. [CrossRef] [PubMed]
84. Cong, X.D.; Ding, M.J.; Dai, D.Z.; Wu, Y.; Zhang, Y.; Dai, Y. ER stress, P66shc, and P-Akt/Akt mediate adjuvant-induced inflammation, which is blunted by argirein, a supermolecule and rhein in rats. *Inflammation* **2012**, *35*, 1031–1040. [CrossRef] [PubMed]
85. Blacher, E.; Baruch, B.B.; Levy, A.; Geva, N.; Green, K.D.; Garneau-Tsodikova, S.; Fridman, M.; Stein, R. Inhibition of glioma progression by a newly discovered CD38 inhibitor. *Int. J. Cancer* **2015**, *136*, 1422–1433. [CrossRef] [PubMed]
86. Shingaki, T.; Hidalgo, I.J.; Furubayashi, T.; Katsumi, H.; Sakane, T.; Yamamoto, A.; Yamashita, S. The transnasal delivery of 5-fluorouracil to the rat brain is enhanced by acetazolamide (the inhibitor of the secretion of cerebrospinal fluid). *Int. J. Pharm.* **2009**, *377*, 85–91. [CrossRef]
87. Van Kuilenburg, A.B.P. Dihydropyrimidine dehydrogenase and the efficacy and toxicity of 5-fluorouracil. *Eur. J. Cancer* **2004**, *40*, 939–950. [CrossRef]
88. Diasio, R.B.; Harris, B.E. Clinical pharmacology of 5-fluorouracil. *Clin. Pharmacokinet.* **1989**, *16*, 215–237. [CrossRef]
89. Silva, P. *Farmacologia*, 8th ed.; Guanabara Koogan: Rio de Janeiro, Brazil, 2010; pp. 1064–1071.
90. Longley, D.B.; Harkin, D.P.; Johnston, P.G. 5-Flurouracil: Mechanisms of action and clinical strategies. *Nat. Rev. Cancer* **2003**, *3*, 330–338. [CrossRef]

91. Uldall, M.; Botfield, H.; Jansen-Olesen, I.; Sinclair, A.; Jensen, R. Acetazolamide lowers intracranial pressure and modulates the cerebrospinal fluid secretion pathway in healthy rats. *Neurosci. Lett.* **2017**, *645*, 33–39. [CrossRef]
92. Shingaki, T.; Inoue, D.; Furubayashi, T.; Sakane, T.; Katsumi, H.; Yamamoto, A.; Yamashita, S. Transnasal Delivery of Methotrexate to Brain Tumors in Rats: A New Strategy for Brain Tumor Chemotherapy. *Mol. Pharm.* **2010**, *7*, 1561–1568. [CrossRef]
93. Hagner, N.; Joerger, M. Cancer chemotherapy: Targeting folic acid synthesis. *Cancer Manag. Res.* **2010**, *2*, 293–301. [PubMed]
94. Abolmaali, S.S.; Tamaddon, A.M.; Dinarvand, R. A review of therapeutic challenges and achievements of methotrexate delivery systems for treatment of cancer and rheumatoid arthritis. *Cancer Chemother. Pharmacol.* **2013**, *71*, 1115–1130. [CrossRef] [PubMed]
95. Sun, Y.; Shi, K.; Wan, F.; Cui, F. Methotrexate-loaded microspheres for nose to brain delivery: In vitro/in vivo evaluation. *J. Drug Deliv. Sci. Technol.* **2012**, *22*, 167–174. [CrossRef]
96. Li, Y.; Gao, Y.; Liu, G.; Zhou, X.; Wang, Y.; Wang, Y.; Ma, L. Intranasal administration of temozolomide for brain-targeting delivery: Therapeutic effect on glioma in rats. *Nan Fang Yi Ke Da Xue Xue Bao* **2014**, *34*, 631–635.
97. Baker, S.D.; Wirth, M.; Statkevich, P. Absorption, metabolism and excretion of 14C-temozolomide following oral administration to patients with advanced cancer. *Clin. Cancer Res.* **1999**, *5*, 309–317.
98. Mrugala, M.M.; Chamberlain, M.C. Mechanisms of Disease: Temozolomide and glioblastoma-look to the future. *Nat. Clin. Pract. Oncol.* **2008**, *5*, 476–486. [CrossRef]
99. Pineda, J.R.; Jeitany, M.; Andrieux, A.; Junier, M.P.; Chneiweiss, H.; Boussin, F.D. Intranasal Administration of Temozolomide Delayed the Development of Brain Tumors Initiated by Human Glioma Stem-Like Cell in Nude Mice. *Cancer Sci. Ther.* **2017**, *9*, 374–378.
100. Chen, T.C.; Fonseca, C.O.; Schönthal, A.H. Preclinical development and clinical use of perillyl alcohol for chemoprevention and cancer therapy. *Am. J. Cancer Res.* **2015**, *5*, 1580–1593.
101. da Fonseca, C.O.; Khandelia, H.; Salazar, M.D.A.; Schönthal, A.H.; Meireles, O.C.; Quirico-Santos, T. Perillyl alcohol: Dynamic interactions with the lipid bilayer and implications for long-term inhalational chemotherapy for gliomas. *Surg. Neurol. Int.* **2016**, *7*, 1–11. [CrossRef]
102. Chen, T.C.; da Fonseca, C.O.; Schönthal, A.H. Intranasal Perillyl Alcohol for Glioma Therapy: Molecular Mechanisms and Clinical Development. *Int. J. Mol. Sci.* **2018**, *19*, 3905. [CrossRef]
103. ClinicalTrials.gov. Available online: https://clinicaltrials.gov/ct2/show/NCT02704858 (accessed on 22 September 2019).
104. da Fonseca, C.O.; Simão, M.; Lins, I.R.; Caetano, R.O.; Futuro, D.; Quirico-Santos, T. Efficacy of monoterpene perillyl alcohol upon survival rate of patients with recurrent glioblastoma. *J. Cancer. Res. Clin. Oncol.* **2011**, *137*, 287–293. [CrossRef] [PubMed]
105. da Fonseca, C.O.; Teixeira, R.M.; Silva, J.C.; De Saldanha, D.A.; Gama Fischer, J.; Meirelles, O.C.; Landeiro, J.A.; Quirico-Santos, T. Long-term outcome in patients with recurrent malignant glioma treated with Perillyl alcohol inhalation. *Anticancer Res.* **2013**, *33*, 5625–5631. [PubMed]
106. da Fonseca, C.O.; Schwartsmann, G.; Fischer, J.; Nagel, J.; Futuro, D.; Quirico-Santos, T.; Gattass, C.R. Preliminary results from a phase I/II study of perillyl alcohol intranasal administration in adults with recurrent malignant gliomas. *Surg. Neurol.* **2008**, *70*, 259–266. [CrossRef] [PubMed]
107. Santos, J.G.; Da Cruz, W.M.S.; Schönthal, A.H.; Salazar, M.D.; Fontes, C.A.P.; Quirico-Santos, T.; Da Fonseca, C.O. Efficacy of a ketogenic diet with concomitant intranasal perillyl alcohol as a novel strategy for the therapy of recurrent glioblastoma. *Oncol. Lett.* **2018**, *15*, 1263–1270. [CrossRef]
108. Bernardi, A.; Braganhol, E.; Jäger, E.; Figueiró, F.; Edelweiss, M.I.; Pohlmann, A.R.; Guterres, S.S.; Battastini, A.M. Indomethacin-loaded nanocapsules treatment reduces in vivo glioblastoma growth in a rat glioma model. *Cancer Lett.* **2009**, *281*, 53–63. [CrossRef]
109. Saludas, L.; Pascual-Gil, S.; Roli, F.; Garbayo, E.; Blanco-Prieto, M.J. Heart tissue repair and cardioprotection using drug delivery systems. *Maturitas* **2018**, *110*, 1–9. [CrossRef]
110. Pohlmann, A.R.; Fonseca, F.N.; Paese, K.; Detoni, C.B.; Coradini, K.; Beck, R.C.; Guterres, S.S. Poly(e-caprolactone) microcapsules and nanocapsules in drug delivery. *Expert Opin. Drug Deliv.* **2013**, *10*, 623–638. [CrossRef]

111. Frank, L.A.; Contri, R.V.; Beck, R.C.; Pohlmann, A.R.; Guterres, S.S. Improving drug biological effects by encapsulation into polymeric nanocapsules. *Wiley Interdiscip. Rev. Nanomed. Nanobiotechnol.* **2015**, *7*, 623–639. [CrossRef]
112. Comfort, C.; Garrastazu, G.; Pozzoli, M.; Sonvico, F. Opportunities and challenges for the nasal administration of nanoemulsions. *Curr. Top. Med. Chem.* **2015**, *15*, 356–368. [CrossRef]
113. Graff, C.L.; Pollack, G.M. Functional evidence for P-glycoprotein at the nose-brain barrier. *Pharm. Res.* **2005**, *22*, 86–93. [CrossRef]
114. Pires, P.C.; Santos, A.O. Nanosystems in nose-to-brain drug delivery: A review of non-clinical brain targeting studies. *J. Control. Release* **2018**, *270*, 89–100. [CrossRef] [PubMed]
115. Sonvico, F.; Clementino, A.; Buttini, F.; Colombo, G.; Pescina, S.; Guterres, S.S.; Pohlmann, A.R.; Nicoli, S. Surface-Modified Nanocarriers for Nose-to-Brain Delivery: From Bioadhesion to Targeting. *Pharmaceutics* **2018**, *10*, 34. [CrossRef] [PubMed]
116. Sousa, F.; Dhaliwal, H.K.; Gattacceca, F.; Sarmento, B.; Amiji, M.M. Enhanced anti-angiogenic effects of bevacizumab in glioblastoma treatment upon intranasal administration in polymeric nanoparticles. *J. Control. Release* **2019**, *309*, 37–47. [CrossRef] [PubMed]
117. Azambuja, J.; Schuh, R.S.; Michels, L.R.; Gelsleichter, N.E.; Beckenkamp, L.R.; Iser, I.C.; Lenz, G.S.; de Oliveira, F.H.; Venturin, G.; Greggio, S.; et al. Nasal Administration of Cationic Nanoemulsions as CD73-siRNA Delivery System for Glioblastoma Treatment: A New Therapeutical Approach. *Mol. Neurobiol.* **2019**, *56*, 1–15. [CrossRef]
118. Gadhavea, D.; Gorain, B.; Tagalpallewar, A.; Kokare, C. Intranasal teriflunomide microemulsion: An improved chemotherapeutic approach in glioblastoma. *J. Drug Deliv. Sci. Technol.* **2019**, *51*, 276–289. [CrossRef]
119. de Oliveira Junior, E.R.; Nascimento, T.L.; Salomão, M.A.; da Silva, A.C.G.; Valadares, M.C.; Lima, E.M. Increased Nose-to-Brain Delivery of Melatonin Mediated by Polycaprolactone Nanoparticles for the Treatment of Glioblastoma. *Pharm. Res.* **2019**, *36*, 131. [CrossRef]
120. Chu, L.; Aiping, W.; Ni, L.; Yan, X.; Song, Y.; Zhao, M.; Sun, K.; Mu, H.; Liu, S.; Wu, Z.; et al. Nose-to-brain delivery of temozolomide-loaded PLGA nanoparticles functionalized with anti-EPHA3 for glioblastoma targeting. *Drug Deliv.* **2018**, *25*, 1634–1641. [CrossRef]
121. Colombo, M.; Figueiró, F.; de Fraga Dias, A.; Teixeira, H.F.; Battastini, A.M.O.; Koester, L.S. Kaempferol-loaded mucoadhesive nanoemulsion for intranasal administration reduces glioma growth in vitro. *Int. J. Pharm.* **2018**, *543*, 214–223. [CrossRef]
122. Khan, A.; Aqil, M.; Imam, S.S.; Ahad, A.; Sultana, Y.; Ali, A.; Khan, K. Temozolomide loaded nano lipid based chitosan hydrogel for nose to brain delivery: Characterization, nasal absorption, histopathology and cell line study. *Int. J. Biol. Macromol.* **2018**, *116*, 1260–1267. [CrossRef]
123. Sekerdag, E.; Lüle, S.; Bozdağ Pehlivan, S.; Öztürk, N.; Kara, A.; Kaffashi, A.; Vural, I.; Işıkay, I.; Yavuz, B.; Oguz, K.K.; et al. A potential non-invasive glioblastoma treatment: Nose-to-brain delivery of farnesylthiosalicylic acid incorporated hybrid nanoparticles. *J. Control. Release* **2017**, *261*, 187–198. [CrossRef]
124. Shinde, R.L.; Devarajan, P.V. Docosahexaenoic acid-mediated, targeted and sustained brain delivery of curcumin microemulsion. *Drug Deliv.* **2017**, *24*, 152–161. [CrossRef] [PubMed]
125. Madane, R.G.; Mahajan, H.S. Curcumin-loaded nanostructured lipid carriers (NLCs) for nasal administration: Design, characterization, and in vivo study. *Drug Deliv.* **2016**, *23*, 1326–1334. [PubMed]
126. Van Woensel, M.; Wauthoz, N.; Rosière, R.; Mathieu, V.; Kiss, R.; Lefranc, F.; Steelant, B.; Dilissen, E.; Van Gool, S.W.; Mathivet, T.; et al. Development of siRNA-loaded chitosan nanoparticles targeting Galectin-1 for the treatment of glioblastoma multiforme via intranasal administration. *J. Control. Release* **2016**, *227*, 71–81. [CrossRef] [PubMed]
127. Van Woensel, M.; Mathivet, T.; Wauthoz, N.; Rosière, R.; Garg, A.D.; Agostinis, P.; Mathieu, V.; Kiss, R.; Lefranc, F.; Boon, L.; et al. Sensitization of glioblastoma tumor micro-environment to chemo- and immunotherapy by Galectin-1 intranasal knock-down strategy. *Sci. Rep.* **2017**, *7*, 1217. [CrossRef]
128. Jain, D.S.; Bajaj, A.N.; Athawale, R.B.; Shikhande, S.S.; Pandey, A.; Goel, P.N.; Gude, R.P.; Patil, S.; Raut, P. Thermosensitive PLA based nanodispersion for targeting brain tumor via intranasal route. *Mater. Sci. Eng. C Mater. Biol. Appl.* **2016**, *63*, 411–421. [CrossRef]
129. Alex, A.T.; Joseph, A.; Shavi, G.; Rao, J.V.; Udupa, N. Development and evaluation of carboplatin-loaded PCL nanoparticles for intranasal delivery. *Drug Deliv.* **2016**, *23*, 2144–2153. [CrossRef]

130. Mangraviti, A.; Tzeng, S.Y.; Gullotti, D.; Kozielski, K.L.; Kim, J.E.; Seng, M.; Abbadi, S.; Schiapparelli, P.; Sarabia-Estrada, R.; Vescovi, A.; et al. Non-virally engineered human adipose mesenchymal stem cells produce BMP4, target brain tumors, and extend survival. *Biomaterials* **2016**, *100*, 53–66. [CrossRef]
131. Taki, H.; Kanazawa, T.; Akiyama, F.; Takashima, Y.; Okada, H. Intranasal Delivery of Camptothecin-Loaded Tat-Modified Nanomicells for Treatment of Intracranial Brain Tumors. *Pharmaceuticals* **2012**, *5*, 1092–1102. [CrossRef]
132. Kanazawa, T.; Morisaki, K.; Suzuki, S.; Takashima, Y. Prolongation of life in rats with malignant glioma by intranasal siRNA/drug codelivery to the brain with cell-penetrating peptide-modified micelles. *Mol. Pharm.* **2014**, *11*, 1471–1478. [CrossRef]
133. Zawilska, J.; Skene, D.; Arendt, J. Physiology and pharmacology of melatonin in relation to biological rhythms. *Pharmacol. Rep.* **2009**, *61*, 383–410. [CrossRef]
134. Kostoglou-Athanassiou, I. Therapeutic applications of melatonin. *Ther. Adv. Endocrinol. Metab.* **2013**, *4*, 13–24. [CrossRef] [PubMed]
135. Menéndez-Menéndez, J.; Martínez-Campa, C. Melatonin: An Anti-Tumor Agent in Hormone-Dependent Cancers. *Int. J. Endocrinol.* **2018**, *2018*, 3271948. [CrossRef] [PubMed]
136. Yadav, S.K.; Srivastava, A.K.; Dev, A.; Kaundal, B.; Choudhury, S.R.; Karmakar, S. Nanomelatonin triggers superior anticancer functionality in a human malignant glioblastoma cell line. *Nanotechnology* **2017**, *28*, 365102. [CrossRef] [PubMed]
137. Hamelers, I.H.; Van Loenen, E.; Staffhorst, R.W.; De Kruijff, B.; de Kroon, A.I. Carboplatin nanocapsules: A highly cytotoxic, phospholipid-based formulation of carboplatin. *Mol. Cancer Ther.* **2006**, *5*, 2007–2012. [CrossRef] [PubMed]
138. Huang, W.J.; Chen, W.W.; Zhang, X. Glioblastoma multiforme: Effect of hypoxia and hypoxia inducible factors on therapeutic approaches. *Oncol. Lett.* **2016**, *12*, 2283–2288. [CrossRef] [PubMed]
139. Wick, W.; Weller, M.; Van den Bent, M.; Stupp, R. Bevacizumab and recurrent malignant gliomas: A European perspective. *J. Clin. Oncol.* **2010**, *28*, e188–e189. [CrossRef]
140. Chinot, O.L.; Wick, W.; Mason, W.; Henriksson, R.; Saran, F.; Nishikawa, R.; Carpentier, A.F.; Hoang-Xuan, K.; Kavan, P.; Cernea, D.; et al. Bevacizumab plus radiotherapy-temozolomide for newly diagnosed glioblastoma. *N. Engl. J. Med.* **2014**, *370*, 709–722. [CrossRef]
141. Gilbert, M.R.; Dignam, J.J.; Armstrong, T.S.; Wefel, J.S.; Blumenthal, D.T.; Vogelbaum, M.A.; Colman, H.; Chakravarti, A.; Pugh, S.; Won, M.; et al. A randomized trial of bevacizumab for newly diagnosed glioblastoma. *N. Engl. J. Med.* **2014**, *370*, 699–708. [CrossRef]
142. Sousa, F.; Cruz, A.; Fonte, P.; Pinto, I.M.; Neves-Petersen, M.T.; Sarmento, B. A new paradigm for Antiangiogenic therapy through controlled release of bevacizumab from PLGA nanoparticles. *Sci. Rep.* **2017**, *7*, 3736. [CrossRef]
143. Rotblat, B.; Ehrlich, M.; Haklai, R.; Kloog, Y. The Ras inhibitor farnesylthiosalicylic acid (Salirasib) disrupts the spatiotemporal localization of active Ras: A potential treatment for cancer. *Methods Enzymol.* **2008**, *439*, 467–489.
144. Goldberg, L.; Haklai, R.; Bauer, V.; Heiss, A.; Kloog, Y. New derivatives of farnesylthiosalicylic acid (salirasib) for cancer treatment: Farnesylthiosalicylamide inhibits tumor growth in nude mice models. *J. Med. Chem.* **2009**, *52*, 197–205. [CrossRef] [PubMed]
145. Ugwoke, M.I.; Verbeke, N.; Kinget, R. The biopharmaceutical aspects of nasal mucoadhesive drug delivery. *J. Pharm. Pharmacol.* **2001**, *53*, 3–21. [CrossRef] [PubMed]
146. Kaur, P.; Garg, T.; Rath, G.; Goyal, A.K. In situ nasal gel drug delivery: A novel approach for brain targeting through the mucosal membrane. *Artif. Cells Nanomed. Biotechnol.* **2016**, *44*, 1167–1176. [CrossRef] [PubMed]
147. Liu, W.; Zhai, Y.; Heng, X.; Che, F.Y.; Chen, W.; Sun, D.; Zhai, G. Oral bioavailability of curcumin: Problems and advancements. *J. Drug Target.* **2016**, *24*, 694–702. [CrossRef] [PubMed]
148. Agrawal, M.; Saraf, S.; Saraf, S.; Antimisiaris, S.G.; Chougule, M.B.; Shoyele, S.A.; Alexander, A. Nose-to-brain drug delivery: An update on clinical challenges and progress towards approval of anti-Alzheimer drugs. *J. Control. Release* **2018**, *281*, 139–177. [CrossRef] [PubMed]
149. Bar-Or, A.; Pachner, A.; Menguy-Vacheron, F.; Kaplan, J.; Wiendl, H. Teriflunomide and its mechanism of action in multiple sclerosis. *Drugs* **2014**, *74*, 659–674. [CrossRef]
150. Xuan, J.; Ren, Z.; Qing, T.; Couch, L.; Shi, L.; Tolleson, W.H.; Guo, L. Mitochondrial dysfunction induced by leflunomide and its active metabolite. *Toxicology* **2018**, *396–397*, 33–45. [CrossRef]

151. Huang, O.; Zhang, W.; Zhi, Q.; Xue, X.; Liu, H.; Shen, D.; Geng, M.; Xie, Z.; Jiang, M. Teriflunomide, an immunomodulatory drug, exerts anticancer activity in triple negative breast cancer cells. *Exp. Biol. Med.* **2015**, *240*, 426–437. [CrossRef]
152. Hail, N., Jr.; Chen, P.; Bushman, L.R. Teriflunomide (Leflunomide) Promotes Cytostatic, Antioxidant, and Apoptotic Effects in Transformed Prostate Epithelial Cells: Evidence Supporting a Role for Teriflunomide in Prostate Cancer Chemoprevention. *Neoplasia* **2010**, *12*, 464–475. [CrossRef]
153. Jiang, L.; Zhang, W.; Li, W.; Ling, C.; Jiang, M. Anti-inflammatory drug, leflunomide and its metabolite teriflunomide inhibit NSCLC proliferation in vivo and in vitro. *Toxicol. Lett.* **2018**, *282*, 154–165. [CrossRef]
154. Calderón-Montaño, J.M.; Burgos-Morón, E.; Pérez-Guerrero, C.; López-Lázaro, M. A review on the dietary flavonoid kaempferol. *Mini Rev. Med. Chem.* **2011**, *11*, 298–340. [CrossRef] [PubMed]
155. Rajendran, P.; Rengarajan, T.; Nandakumar, N.; Palaniswami, R.; Nishigaki, Y.; Nishigaki, I. Kaempferol, a potential cytostatic and cure for inflammatory disorders. *Eur. J. Med. Chem.* **2014**, *86*, 103–112. [CrossRef] [PubMed]
156. Chen, Z.P.; Sun, J.; Chen, H.X.; Xiao, Y.Y.; Liu, D.; Chen, J.; Cai, H.; Cai, B.C. Comparative pharmacokinetics and bioavailability studies of quercetin, kaempferol and isorhamnetin after oral administration of Ginkgo biloba extracts, Ginkgo biloba extract phospholipid complexes and Ginkgo biloba extract solid dispersions in rats. *Fitoterapia* **2010**, *81*, 1045–1052. [CrossRef] [PubMed]
157. Vllasaliu, D.; Exposito-Harris, R.; Heras, A.; Casettari, L.; Garnett, M.; Illum, L.; Stolnik, S. Tight junction modulation by chitosan nanoparticles: Comparison with chitosan solution. *Int. J. Pharm.* **2010**, *400*, 183–193. [CrossRef]
158. Casettari, L.; Illum, L. Chitosan in nasal delivery systems for therapeutic drugs. *J. Control. Release* **2014**, *190*, 189–200. [CrossRef] [PubMed]
159. Ujházy, P.; Berleth, E.S.; Pietkiewicz, J.M.; Kitano, H.; Skaar, J.R.; Ehrke, M.J.; Mihich, E. Evidence for the involvement of ecto-5′-nucleotidase (CD73) in drug resistance. *Int. J. Cancer* **1996**, *68*, 493–500. [CrossRef]
160. Bavaresco, L.; Bernardi, A.; Braganhol, E.; Cappellari, A.R.; Rockenbach, L.; Farias, P.F.; Wink, M.R.; Cañedo, A.D.; Battastini, A.M.O. The role of ecto-5′-nucleotidase in glioma cell line proliferation. *Mol. Cell Biochem.* **2008**, *319*, 61–68. [CrossRef]
161. Wink, M.R.; Lenz, G.; Braganhol, E.; Tamajusuku, A.S.; Schwartsmann, G.; Sarkis, J.J.; Battastini, A.M. Altered extracellular ATP, ADP and AMP catabolism in glioma cell lines. *Cancer Lett.* **2003**, *198*, 211–218. [CrossRef]
162. Toussaint, L.G., 3rd; Nilson, A.E.; Goble, J.M.; Ballman, K.V.; James, C.D.; Lefranc, F.; Kiss, R.; Uhm, J.H. Galectin-1, a gene preferentially expressed at the tumor margin, promotes glioblastoma cell invasion. *Mol. Cancer* **2012**, *11*, 32. [CrossRef]
163. Janes, P.W.; Slape, C.I.; Farnsworth, R.H.; Atapattu, L.; Scott, A.M.; Vail, M.E. EphA3 biology and cancer. *Growth Factors* **2014**, *32*, 176–189. [CrossRef]
164. Kanazawa, T.; Taki, H.; Tanaka, K.; Takashima, Y.; Okada, H. Cell-Penetrating Peptide-Modified Block Copolymer Micelles Promote Direct Brain Delivery via Intranasal Administration. *Pharm. Res.* **2011**, *28*, 2130–2139. [CrossRef]
165. Pescina, S.; Ostacolo, C.; Gomez-Monterrey, I.M.; Sala, M.; Bertamino, A.; Sonvico, F.; Padula, C.; Santi, P.; Bianchera, A.; Nicoli, S. Cell penetrating peptides in ocular delivery: State of the art. *J. Control. Release* **2018**, *284*, 84–102. [CrossRef]
166. Li, F.; Jiang, T.; Li, Q.; Ling, X. Camptothecin (CPT) and its derivatives are known to target topoisomerase I (Top1) as their mechanism of action: Did we miss something in CPT analogue molecular targets for treating human disease such as cancer? *Am. J. Cancer Res.* **2017**, *7*, 2350–2394. [PubMed]
167. Martino, E.; Della Volpe, S.; Terribile, E.; Benetti, E.; Sakaj, M.; Centamore, A.; Sala, A.; Collina, S. The long story of camptothecin: From traditional medicine to drugs. *Bioorgan. Med. Chem. Lett.* **2017**, *27*, 701–707. [CrossRef] [PubMed]
168. Lee, D.H.; Ahn, Y.; Kim, S.U.; Wang, K.C.; Cho, B.K.; Phi, J.H.; Park, I.H.; Black, P.M.; Carroll, R.S.; Lee, J.; et al. Targeting rat brainstem glioma using human neural stem cells and human mesenchymal stem cells. *Clin. Cancer Res.* **2009**, *15*, 4925–4934. [CrossRef]
169. Nakamizo, A.; Marini, F.; Amano, T.; Khan, A.; Studeny, M.; Gumin, J.; Chen, J.; Hentschel, S.; Vecil, G.; Dembinski, J.; et al. Human bone marrow-derived mesenchymal stem cells in the treatment of gliomas. *Cancer Res.* **2005**, *65*, 3307–3318. [CrossRef]

170. Barish, M.E.; Herrmann, K.; Tang, Y.; Herculian, S.A.; Metz, M.; Aramburo, S.; Tirughana, R.; Gutova, M.; Annala, A.; Moats, R.A.; et al. Human neural stem cell biodistribution and predicted tumor coverage by a diffusible therapeutic in a mouse glioma model. *Stem Cells Transl. Med.* **2017**, *6*, 1522–1532. [CrossRef]
171. Gutova, M.; Flores, L.; Adhikarla, V.; Tsaturyan, L.; Tirughana, R.; Aramburo, S.; Metz, M.; Gonzaga, J.; Annala, A.; Synold, T.W.; et al. Quantitative evaluation of intraventricular delivery of therapeutic neural stem cells to orthotopic glioma. *Front. Oncol.* **2019**, *9*, 68. [CrossRef]
172. Klopp, A.H.; Spaeth, E.L.; Dembinski, J.L.; Woodward, W.A.; Munshi, A.; Meyn, R.E.; Cox, J.D.; Andreeff, M.; Marini, F.C. Tumor irradiation increases the recruitment of circulating mesenchymal stem cells into the tumor microenvironment. *Cancer Res.* **2007**, *67*, 11687–11695. [CrossRef]
173. Karp, J.M.; Leng Teo, G.S. Mesenchymal stem cell homing: The devil is in the details. *Cell Stem Cell.* **2009**, *4*, 206–216. [CrossRef]
174. Aboody, K.S.; Najbauer, J.; Metz, M.Z.; D'Apuzzo, M.; Gutova, M.; Annala, A.J.; Synold, T.W.; Couture, L.A.; Blanchard, S.; Moats, R.A.; et al. Neural stem cell-mediated enzyme/prodrug therapy for glioma: Preclinical studies. *Sci. Transl. Med.* **2013**, *5*, 184ra59. [CrossRef] [PubMed]
175. Cao, M.; Mao, J.; Duan, X.; Lu, L.; Zhang, F.; Lin, B.; Chen, M.; Zheng, C.; Zhang, X.; Shen, J. In vivo tracking of the tropism of mesenchymal stem cells to malignant gliomas using reporter gene-based MR imaging. *Int. J. Cancer* **2018**, *142*, 1033–1046. [CrossRef] [PubMed]
176. Li, M.; Sun, S.; Dangelmajer, S.; Zhang, Q.; Wang, J.; Hu, F.; Dong, F.; Kahlert, U.D.; Zhu, M.; Lei, T. Exploiting tumor-intrinsic signals to induce mesenchymal stem cell-mediated suicide gene therapy to fight malignant glioma. *Stem Cell Res. Ther.* **2019**, *10*, 88. [CrossRef] [PubMed]
177. Young, J.S.; Morshed, R.A.; Kim, J.W.; Balyasnikova, I.V.; Ahmed, A.U.; Lesniak, M.S. Advances in stem cells, induced pluripotent stem cells, and engineered cells: Delivery vehicles for anti-glioma therapy. *Expert Opin. Drug Deliv.* **2014**, *11*, 1733–1746. [CrossRef]
178. Bexell, D.; Svensson, A.; Bengzon, J. Stem cell-based therapy for malignant glioma. *Cancer Treat. Rev.* **2013**, *39*, 358–365. [CrossRef]
179. Zhu, Y.; Sun, Z.; Han, Q.; Liao, L.; Wang, J.; Bian, C.; Li, J.; Yan, X.; Liu, Y.; Shao, C.; et al. Human mesenchymal stem cells inhibit cancer cell proliferation by secreting DKK1. *Leukemia* **2009**, *23*, 925–933. [CrossRef]
180. Qiao, L.; Xu, Z.L.; Zhao, T.J.; Ye, L.H.; Zhang, X.D. DKK1 secreted by mesenchymal stem cells inhibits growth of breast cancer cells via depression of Wnt signaling. *Cancer Lett.* **2008**, *269*, 67–77. [CrossRef]
181. Ma, S.; Liang, S.; Jiao, H.; Chi, L.; Shi, X.; Tian, Y.; Yang, B.; Guan, F. Human umbilical cord mesenchymal stem cells inhibit C6 glioma growth via secretion of dickkopf-1 (DKK1). *Mol. Cell Biochem.* **2014**, *385*, 277–286. [CrossRef]
182. An, J.; Yan, H.; Li, X.; Tan, R.; Chen, X.; Zhang, Z.; Liu, Y.; Zhang, P.; Lu, H.; Liu, Y. The inhibiting effect of neural stem cells on proliferation and invasion of glioma cells. *Oncotarget* **2017**, *8*, 76949–76960. [CrossRef]
183. Reitz, M.; Demestre, M.; Sedlacik, J.; Meissner, H.; Fiehler, J.; Kim, S.U.; Westphal, M.; Schmidt, N.O. Intranasal delivery of neural stem/progenitor cells: A noninvasive passage to target intracerebral glioma. *Stem Cells Transl. Med.* **2012**, *1*, 866–873. [CrossRef]
184. Danielyan, L.; Schäfer, R.; von Ameln-Mayerhofer, A.; Buadze, M.; Geisler, J.; Klopfer, T.; Klopfer, T.; Burkhardt, U.; Proksch, B.; Verleysdonk, S.; et al. Intranasal delivery of cells to the brain. *Eur. J. Cell Biol.* **2009**, *88*, 315–324. [CrossRef] [PubMed]
185. Dey, M.; Yu, D.; Kanojia, D.; Li, G.; Sukhanova, M.; Spencer, D.A.; Pituch, K.C.; Zhang, L.; Han, Y.; Ahmed, A.U.; et al. Intranasal oncolytic virotherapy with CXCR4-enhanced stem cells extends survival in mouse model of glioma. *Stem Cell Rep.* **2016**, *7*, 471–482. [CrossRef] [PubMed]
186. Ulasov, I.V.; Zhu, Z.B.; Tyler, M.A.; Han, Y.; Rivera, A.A.; Khramtsov, A.; Curiel, D.T.; Lesniak, M.S. Survivin-driven and fiber-modified oncolytic adenovirus exhibits potent antitumor activity in established intracranial glioma. *Hum. Gene Ther.* **2007**, *18*, 589–602. [CrossRef] [PubMed]
187. Ahmed, A.U.; Tyler, M.A.; Thaci, B.; Alexiades, N.G.; Han, Y.; Ulasov, I.V.; Lesniak, M.S. A comparative study of neural and mesenchymal stem cell-based carriers for oncolytic adenovirus in a model of malignant glioma. *Mol. Pharm.* **2011**, *8*, 1559–1572. [CrossRef]
188. Ahmed, A.U.; Thaci, B.; Tobias, A.L.; Auffinger, B.; Zhang, L.; Cheng, Y.; Kim, C.K.; Yunis, C.; Han, Y.; Alexiades, N.G.; et al. A preclinical evaluation of neural stem cell-based cell carrier for targeted antiglioma oncolytic virotherapy. *J. Natl. Cancer Inst.* **2013**, *105*, 968–977. [CrossRef]

189. Morshed, R.A.; Gutova, M.; Juliano, J.; Barish, M.E.; Hawkins-Daarud, A.; Oganesyan, D.; Vazgen, K.; Yang, T.; Annala, A.; Ahmed, A.U.; et al. Analysis of glioblastoma tumor coverage by oncolytic virus-loaded neural stem cells using MRI based tracking and histological reconstruction. *Cancer Gene Ther.* **2015**, *22*, 55–61. [CrossRef]
190. Balyasnikova, I.V.; Prasol, M.S.; Ferguson, S.D.; Han, Y.; Ahmed, A.U.; Gutova, M.; Tobias, A.L.; Mustafi, D.; Rincón, E.; Zhang, L.; et al. Intranasal delivery of mesenchymal stem cells significantly extends survival of irradiated mice with experimental brain tumors. *Mol. Ther.* **2014**, *22*, 140–148. [CrossRef]

2

Mitocanic Di- and Triterpenoid Rhodamine B Conjugates

Sophie Hoenke [1], Immo Serbian [1], Hans-Peter Deigner [2] and René Csuk [1,*]

1 Organic Chemistry, Martin-Luther University Halle-Wittenberg, Kurt-Mothes Street 2, D-06120 Halle, Germany; sophie.hoenke@chemie.uni-halle.de (S.H.); immo.serbian@chemie.uni-halle.de (I.S.)
2 Medical and Life Science Faculty, Institute of Precision Medicine, Furtwangen University, Jakob–Kienzle–Street 17, D-78054 Villigen–Schwenningen, Germany; dei@hs-furtwangen.de
* Correspondence: rene.csuk@chemie.uni-halle.de;

Academic Editor: José Antonio Lupiáñez

Abstract: The combination of the "correct" triterpenoid, the "correct" spacer and rhodamine B (**RhoB**) seems to be decisive for the ability of the conjugate to accumulate in mitochondria. So far, several triterpenoid rhodamine B conjugates have been prepared and screened for their cytotoxic activity. To obtain cytotoxic compounds with EC_{50} values in a low nano-molar range combined with good tumor/non-tumor selectivity, the Rho B unit has to be attached via an amine spacer to the terpenoid skeleton. To avoid spirolactamization, secondary amines have to be used. First results indicate that a homopiperazinyl spacer is superior to a piperazinyl spacer. Hybrids derived from maslinic acid or tormentic acid are superior to those from oleanolic, ursolic, glycyrrhetinic or euscaphic acid. Thus, a tormentic acid-derived **RhoB** conjugate **32**, holding a homopiperazinyl spacer can be regarded, at present, as the most promising candidate for further biological studies.

Keywords: triterpenoic acid; maslinic acid; tormentic acid; betulinic acid; oleanolic acid; rhodamine B; cytotoxicity

1. Introduction

Cancer remains one of the leading causes of death worldwide, and the incidence is increasing. Cancer is the second-leading cause of death globally, accounting for 9.6 million deaths in 2018 [1]. It is expected that in 2030, 21 million people worldwide will suffer from cancer [2]. Tremendous progress, however, has been made in the treatment of individual cancers [3–6]. This is due, on one hand, to improved early detection and prophylaxis and, on the other, to the development of highly efficient drugs in a wide range of different substance classes. Thus, the probability of premature death from cancer per year decreased from 8.3% in the year 2000 to 6.9% in 2015. It is expected to be as low as 5.3% in 2030, saving approximately 1.1 million lives per year [7].

Both proteins and small molecules have proven their worth in therapy and are in use in the clinic. However, low-molecular-weight drugs often bear the stigma of reduced selectivity in which the cytotoxic drug not only targets cancerous cells, but it also damages healthy tissue. This increases serious side effects and stress symptoms in patients, including nausea, heart or brain damage, impairments to the central nervous system and damage to cells of the inner ear; losses of fertility, hearing and hair have also been noted [8].

These serious side effects and impairments limit the use and acceptance of a drug, as they reduce patient compliance due to a significantly reduced quality of life. This not only endangers the chances of successful therapy, but it often also leads to discontinuation of the therapy [9,10].

Since the problems of reconversion of cancer cells into normal cells ("reprogramming", for example, of terminally differentiated cancer cells into cancer cells of benign phenotypes) [11] have only remotely been solved today, cancer cells have to be removed either by surgery or destroyed by radiation or chemotherapy. Cell death by chemotherapy can be induced in many different ways [12–17], but the mitochondria play a major role in the life or death of a cell. Thus, agents that target mitochondria and induce a controlled cell death, so called "mitocans", have received increased attention in recent years [17–38]. This seems even more significant inasmuch as cancer cells are closely linked to dysregulated apoptosis of the cells; as a consequence, drug resistance of the cancer cells can develop [39].

Mitocans (as well as other cytotoxic agents) are often able to induce apoptosis; however, the death of a cell, irrespective of whether this cell is malignant, is not random at all. Triggering of controlled cell death is always preferable to an unselective rupture of membranes following the application of extreme but locally applied heat, freeze–thaw cycles or steep osmotic gradients. Controlled cell death can be triggered on a cellular level from nuclear, reticular, cytoskeletal, lysosomal, membrane or, most important, mitochondrial origins [16].

Usually, the cells in a living organism closely cooperate, and cells are constantly in an equilibrium between life and death. Triggering programmed cell death routines removes damaged, infected and out-of-control cells from the organism. The problem arises from the latter cells, since most cancer cells do not respond to extrinsic apoptotic triggers. Thus, mitochondria present a target of emerging interest for cancer therapy as they can trigger apoptosis through an intrinsic pathway. Apoptosis usually starts with loss of mitochondrial membrane potential, followed by the release of cytochrome c and activation of caspase 3 [40]. Furthermore, permeabilization of the outer mitochondrial membrane and the release of cytochrome c are required in many cell death stimuli [41]. This release of cytochrome c can be regarded as a "point of no return" finally leading to the death of the cell. This highlights the importance of mitochondrial compartmentation and explains the devastating effect following permeabilization of the mitochondrial membrane [42–44]. In addition to membrane permeabilization, the opening of the mitochondrial permeability transition pore is also considered an important event resulting in mitochondrial depolarization and the release of apoptotic factors [29].

In recent years, triterpenes have repeatedly and increasingly entered the focus of scientific interest. Extensive studies on their apoptotic and cytotoxic properties have been performed. A major concern in dealing with cancer is the MDR (multiple drug resistance) phenotype [39]. These cancer cells overexpress ATP-dependent transporters that eject toxic compounds from the cell before they cause harm to the cell. Some triterpenes are known inhibitors of the efflux pump MDR1, but they are also known to downregulate the transcription factor NF-κB. For cancer, it is widely accepted [45] that NF-κB promotes tumor migration and tumor proliferation.

2. Results

Mitochondrial membranes of malignant cells hold an increased membrane potential compared to non–malignant cells [46]. This effect fosters the accumulation of cationic molecules [17,47,48], hence inducing high selectivity for mitocans holding a (more or less) lipophilic cation such as a rhodamine scaffold. The same effect applies for triphenylphosphonium cations [49–57] and to a small extent for quaternary ammonium ions [58–60], zwitterionic *N*-oxides [60,61] and triterpenes substituted with BODIPYs [62–66] or a safirinium moiety [67]. However, the presence of a cationic center is not alone decisive for achieving high cytotoxic effects [60].

Rhodamine B (**RhoB**) seems to be a privileged scaffold. This fluorescent dye, also known as rhodamine 610, C.I. Pigment violet 1, basic violet 10, and C.I. 45170 [68], was invented in 1888 ("Tetraethyl-rhodamine") by M. Cérésole [69,70], and since then it has been widely used in biology, biotechnology and as a biosensor [71,72]. **RhoB** exists in an equilibrium [73–77] between an "open" positively charged form A (Figure 1) that is fluorescent and a "closed", non–fluorescent form B. Under acidic conditions, pink-colored A dominates, while colorless B dominates under basic conditions. Further, in less polar organic solvents, the zwitterionic form C undergoes a rapid reversible conversion to B [78–81].

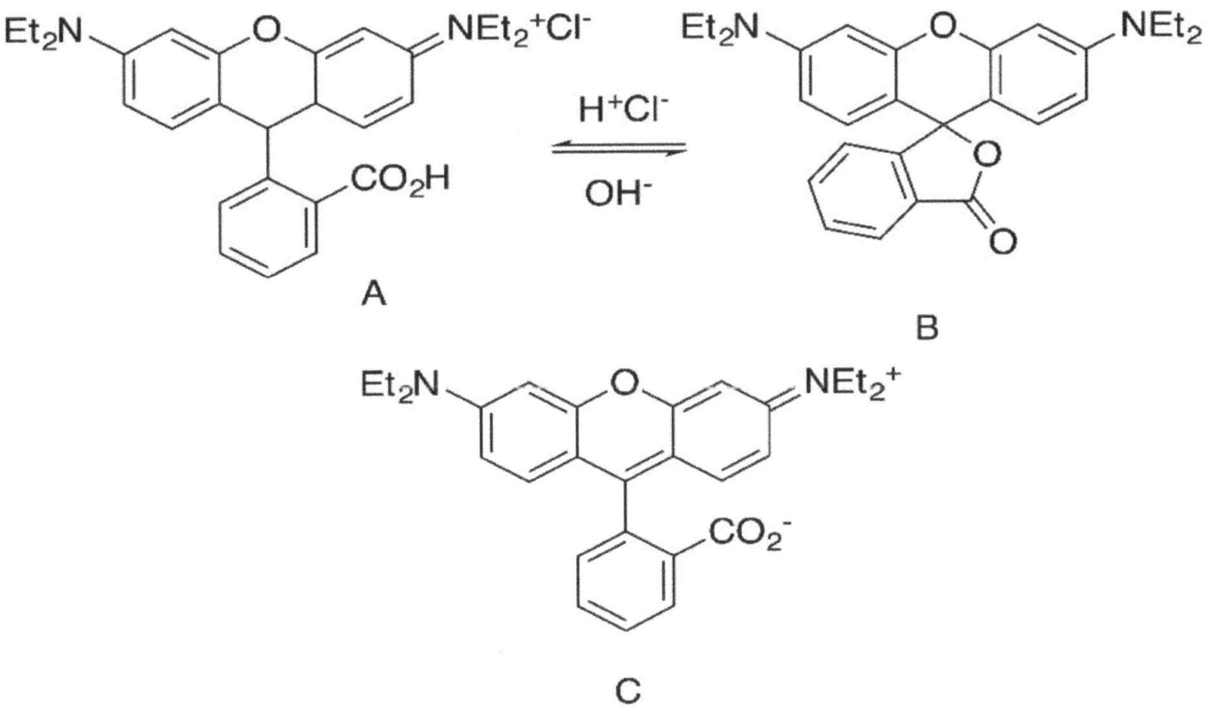

Figure 1. Structure of Rhodamine B (**Rho**B) in its "open" form **A**, "closed" lactone form **B** and the zwitterion **C**.

RhoB is suspected to be carcinogenic [82–85]. The LD_{50} value for orally administered RhoB in rats is >500 mg/kg, and an older report classified **RhoB** (as well as Rho6G) as possibly carcinogenic in rats [85]. **RhoB**, however, seems not to be mutagenic in Chinese hamster ovary cells [86], but it presents a genotoxic hazard for mammalian organisms [87]. As far as the **RhoB**–triterpene conjugates are concerned, two types of compounds have been accessed so far: triterpenes with a **RhoB** moiety directly attached to the skeleton of the triterpene, and compounds wherein these two units are separated by a suitable spacer.

To date, hybrid molecules have been prepared from oleanolic acid (**OA**, Figure 2), ursolic acid (**UA**), glycyrrhetinic acid (**GA**), betulinic acid (**BA**), maslinic acid (**MA**), augustic acid (**AU**), 11-keto-β-boswellic acid (**KBA**), asiatic acid (**AA**), tormentic acid (**TA**) and euscaphic acid (**EA**).

By means of suitable double-staining experiments, it could be shown that these hybrids are actually effective as mitocans [88], and preliminary molecular modeling studies suggest these compounds might target the mitochondrial NADH dehydrogenase and mitochondrial succinate dehydrogenase [89]. Both enzymes are part of the mitochondrial electron transport chain; this also suggests an increased production of reactive oxygen species (ROS). An increased production of ROS would lead to an oxidative damage of the cell and trigger apoptosis through an intrinsic pathway. Therefore, the integrity of the **RhoB** basic structure seems to be of crucial importance. It has been shown that derivatives from the triphenylmethane dye malachite green still exhibit increased cytotoxicity as compared to their parent compounds [90]. The cytotoxicity, however, of these hybrids was much lower than those observed for the **RhoB** derivatives (vide infra).

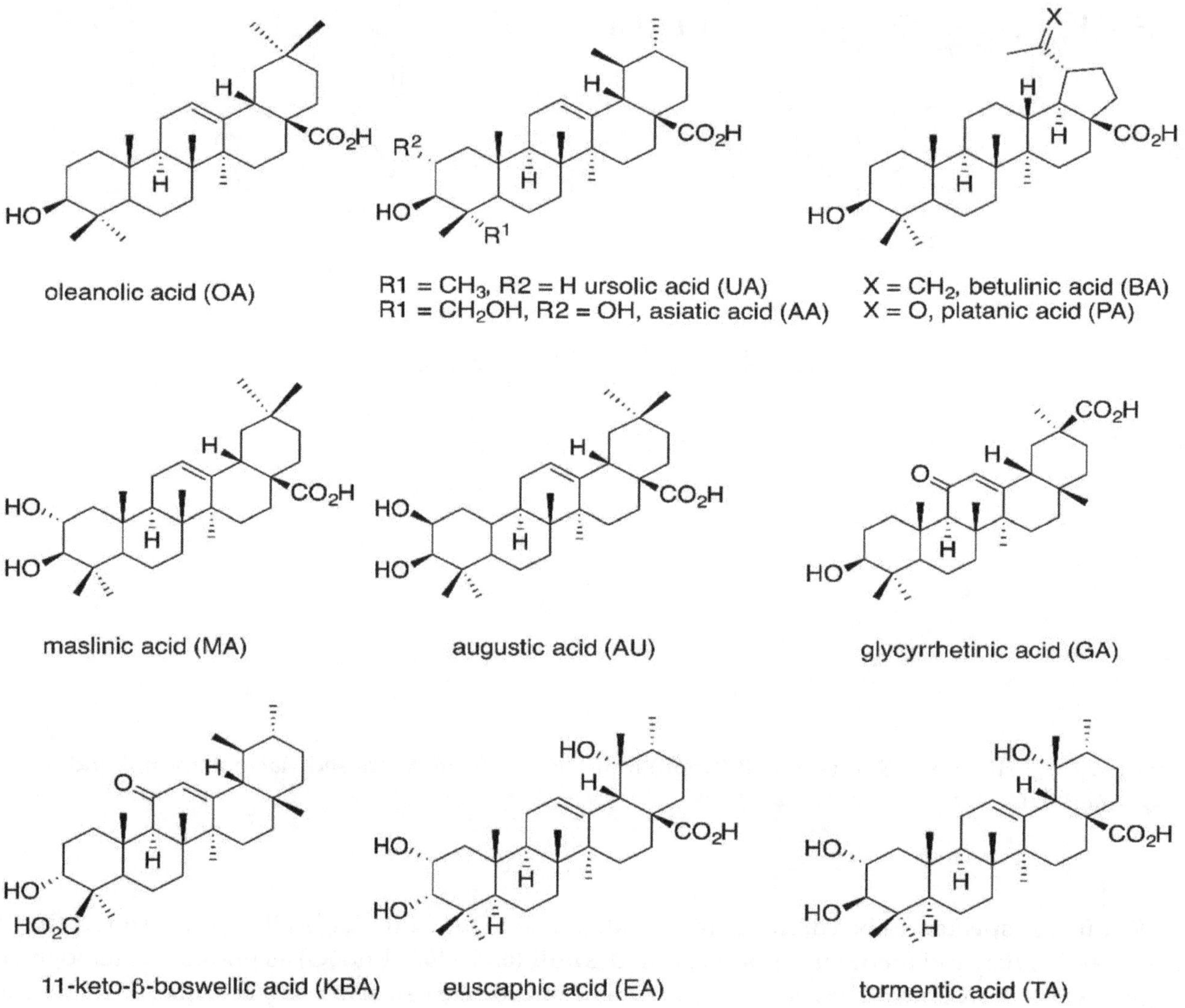

Figure 2. Structure of some important pentacyclic triterpenoic acids.

The triterpenoid skeleton is equally important. Here, too, it was shown that "simple" RhoB conjugates **1–9** (Figure 3) also had lower cytotoxicity than the corresponding triterpenoid analogs, but their tumor cell/non-tumor cell selectivity was also diminished (Table 1) [91].

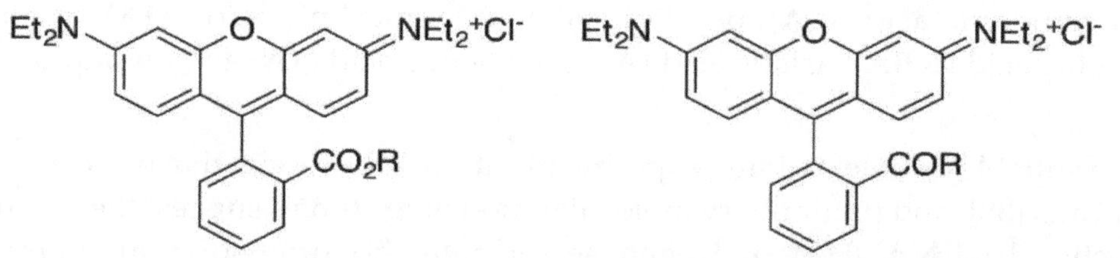

Esters:

1 R = ethyl
2 R = hexyl
3 R = eicosyl

Amides:

4 R = morpholinyl
5 R = thiomorpholinyl
6 R = 2,2-dimethyl-morpholinyl
7 R = N-methylpiperazinyl
8 R = N,N-diethylamino
9 R = piperazinyl

Figure 3. Structures of "simple" **RhoB** conjugates **1–9**.

Table 1. Cytotoxicity of selected "simple" **RhoB** conjugates.

Compound	A375	HT29	MCF-7	A2780	FaDu	NIH 3T3
RhoB	>30	>30	>30	>30	>30	>30
1	0.38	0.41	0.23	0.21	0.30	0.96
2	0.19	0.19	0.14	0.17	0.15	0.32
3	>30	>30	>30	>30	>30	>30
4	7.09	5.46	1.54	1.66	4.53	>30
5	1.79	1.54	0.44	0.52	1.12	5.09
6	3.05	1.74	0.49	0.70	1.52	7.92
7	16.05	17.34	3.74	3.62	11.78	>30
8	1.03	0.54	0.32	0.27	0.64	3.27
9	>30	>30	17.80	26.40	>30	>30

EC_{50} in μM from SRB assays; cut-off 30 μM.

Of special interest seems the morpholinyl derivative **4** inasmuch as this compound held the highest selectivity of this series with respect to MCF-7 carcinoma cells (S = ($EC_{50, NIH 3T3}$ / $EC_{50, MCF-7}$) > 19.5) and A2780 ovarian cancer cells (S = ($EC_{50, NIH 3T3}$ / $EC_{50, A27807}$) > 18.1) [90].

The highest cytotoxicity was observed for the hexyl ester **2** (EC_{50} = 0.15–0.19 μM) for the different tumor cell lines. Interestingly, an eicosyl ester **3** with a lipophilicity similar to that of triterpenoids did not show even moderate cytotoxicity [90], while hydroxycinnamic acid rhodamine B conjugates displayed good cytotoxicity in the low μM range [92].

The importance of the presence of a triterpenoid backbone is also evident from studies concerning RhoB steroid conjugates (Figure 4) [93]. In these studies, the reaction of the steroids cholesterol, testosterone, prednisone and abiraterone with an activated **RhoB** chloride furnished ester conjugates holding low EC_{50} values (SRB assays with several human tumor cell lines, Table 2). Thus, a testosterone conjugate **10** held EC_{50} = 60 nm for MCF-7 cells, but acted by necrosis (20%, A2780 cells). A prednisone conjugate **11** was less cytotoxic (0.2 μM for MCF-7 cells) but acted in A2780 cells mainly by apoptosis (48%) and late apoptosis (14%). In addition, this compound showed a higher selectivity for the A2780 tumor cells (S = 73) than for NIH 3T3 fibroblasts. For comparison, an abiratone conjugate **12** was less cytotoxic and also less selective [93].

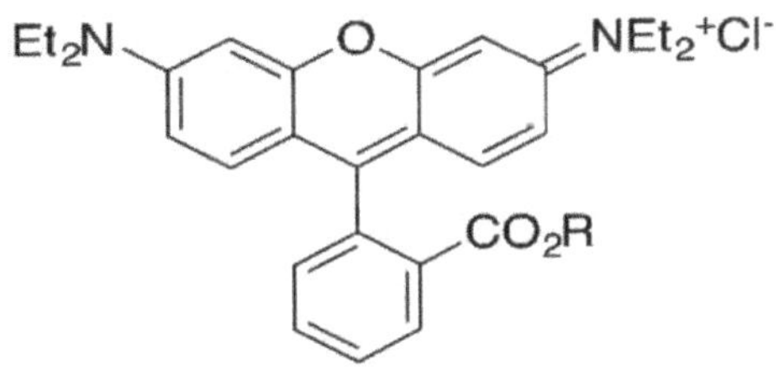

R = testosterone (10) or prednisone (11) or abiratone (12)

Figure 4. RhoB steroid conjugates from the esterification of RhoB with testosterone (→ **10**), prednisone (→ **11**) or abiratone (→ **12**), respectively.

Table 2. Cytotoxicity of selected steroidal **RhoB** conjugates.

Compound	A375	HT29	MCF-7	A2780	FaDu	NIH 3T3
10	0.16	0.12	0.06	0.08	0.26	0.25
11	0.11	0.64	0.21	0.31	0.40	1.81
12	0.22	0.21	0.23	0.13	0.24	0.37

EC_{50} in μM from SRB assays.

A closer look at the cell cycle by FACS (with A2780 cells) showed a decrease of the G1 and G2/M peak with an increase of cells in the S phase. For cells treated with **11**, the S phase peak and the subG1/apoptosis peak increased significantly. However, for all compounds the selectivity between tumor cells and non-malignant fibroblasts NIH 3T3 was small and never exceeded 7.3 (**11**, for MCF-7 cells) [93].

A similar behavior was observed for dehydroabietylamine (DHAA) derivatives **13–16** (Figure 5, Table 3). These products were easily obtained from dehydroabietylamine by the microwave-assisted multicomponent Ugi reaction using paraformaldehyde, an isocyanide and **RhoB** with yields between 47 and 50% [94].

Table 3. Cytotoxicity of selected **DHAA**-derived **RhoB** conjugates.

Compound	A375	HT29	MCF-7	A2780	FaDu	NIH 3T3
13	3.2	0.18	0.10	0.37	0.23	0.28
14	0.23	0.32	0.16	0.57	0.35	0.41
15	0.20	0.28	0.12	0.66	0.32	0.44
16a/16b	>30	>30	>30	>30	>30	>30

EC_{50} in µM from SRB assays.

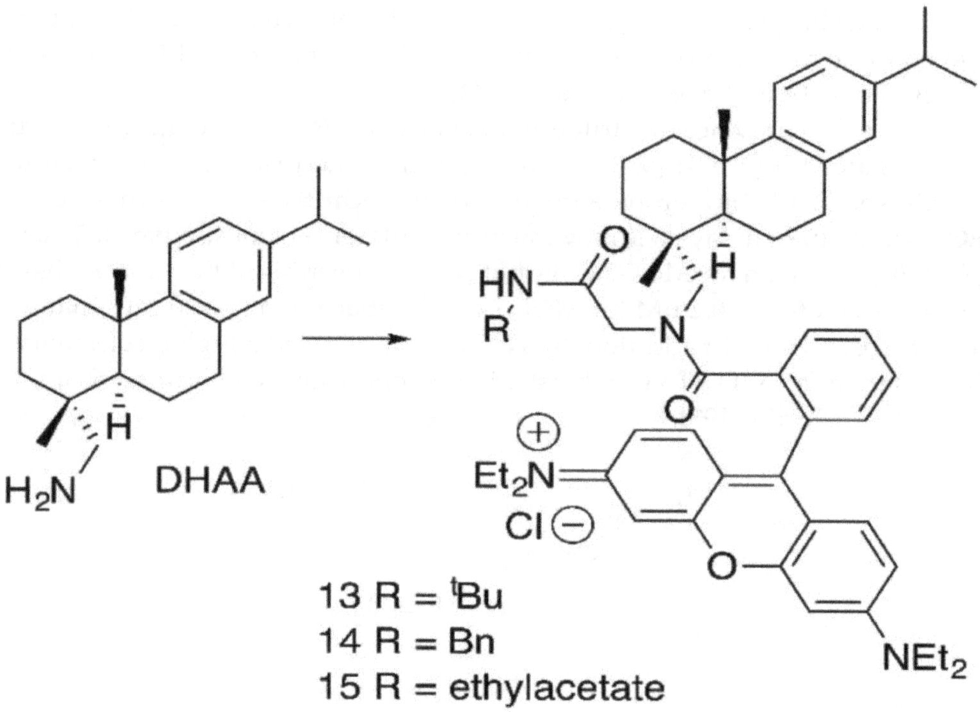

Figure 5. Dehydroabiethylamine (**DHAA**)-derived **RhoB** conjugates **13–15** obtained by Ugi-multi component reactions.

Although the cytotoxicity of these compounds was good, their pharmacological potential was restricted by low selectivity values. Interestingly enough, products **16a/16b** (Figure 6), having been obtained from a simple Schotten–Baumann reaction with **DHAA** and **RhoB,** were not cytotoxic at all [94]. As mentioned above, **RhoB** conjugates derived from primary amines are able to form intramolecular non-fluorescent spirolactams (here **16a**). From a photo-induced ring opening reaction, **16b** was obtained from **16a** very quickly within 10 s of irradiation either with visible light or with UV light (λ = 254 or 366 nm). This equilibrium is also strongly influenced by changes in temperature, and at room temperature **16a** dominates the equilibrium [94].

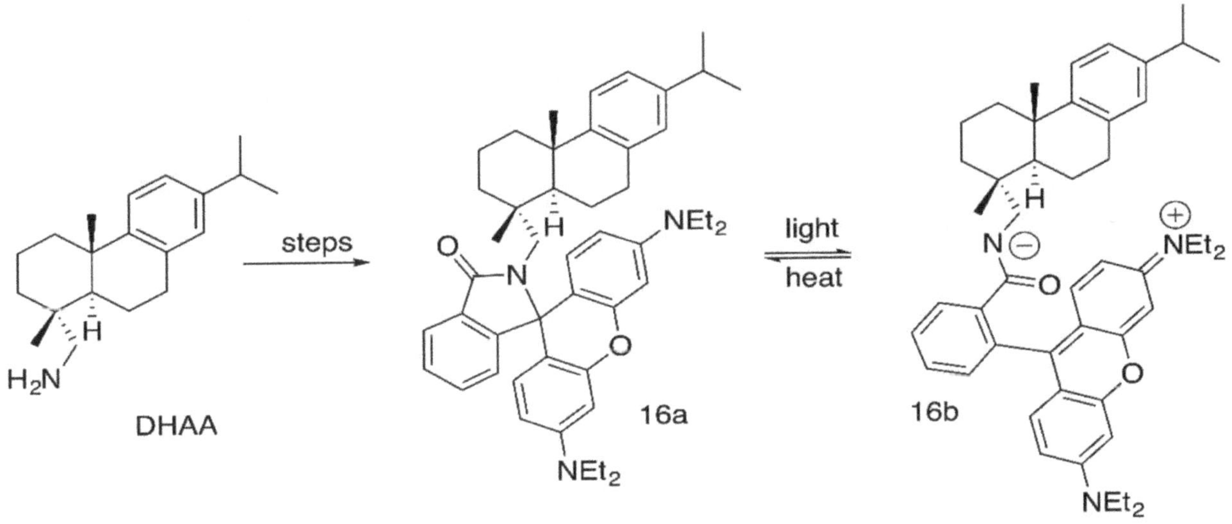

Figure 6. Synthesis of **DHAA**-derived **RhoB** conjugates **16a/16b** and their equilibrium.

As far as the triterpene **RhoB** conjugates are concerned, the **RhoB** moiety can be attached to the triterpenoid scaffold either directly (e.g., in form of a triterpene **RhoB** ester) or with the aid of a suitable spacer. Pentacyclic triterpenoic acids (Figure 2) holding an **RhoB** moiety without an extra spacer have been prepared by esterification of **UA, OA, GA** and **BA** with **RhoB**, respectively, (Figure 7) [95].

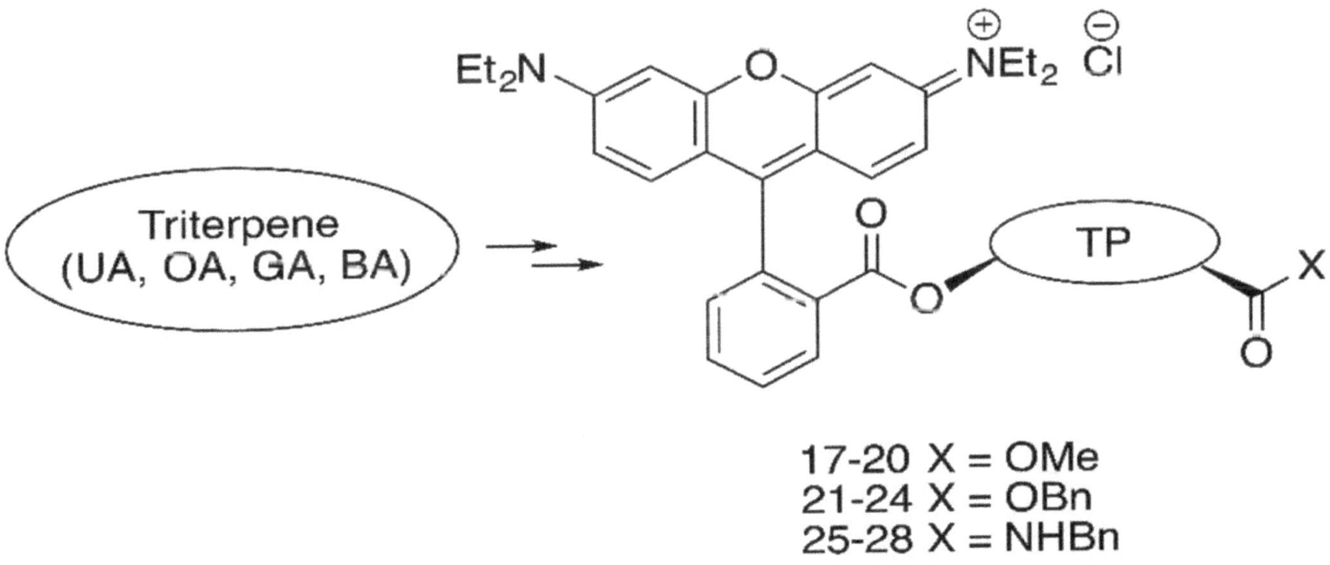

Figure 7. Un-spacered **UA-, OA-, GA-** and **BA**-derived esters **17–24** and amides **25–28.**

All of these compounds had EC_{50} values between 0.02 and 15.8 μM (Table 4); thereby, the cytotoxicity of benzyl esters **21–24** was lower than the cytotoxicity of the methyl esters **17–20,** while the benzyl amides **25–28** were the most cytotoxic compounds of this series. The presence of a benzyl ester group as in **21–24** seems to be disadvantageous, while the opposite is true for the benzyl amides **25–28**. Compound **27** was the most cytotoxic compound (EC_{50} = 0.02–0.08 μM), but it was not selective for human tumor cells. Extra staining experiments showed this compound to be accumulated in the mitochondria of A2780 cells and to act mainly by apoptosis [95].

Table 4. Cytotoxicity of un-spacered esters **UA-**, **OA-**, **GA-** and **BA**-derived esters **17–24** and amides **25–28**.

Compound	TP	R	FaDu	A2780	HT29	MCF-7	SW1736	NIH 3T3
17	UA	OMe	1.96	1.75	1.85	1.83	1.72	1.84
18	OA	OMe	1.99	1.14	2.75	2.31	1.76	2.63
19	GA	OMe	0.19	0.08	0.15	0.18	0.15	0.20
20	BA	OMe	1.29	0.42	0.61	0.81	0.74	1.77
21	UA	OBn	15.79	10.10	11.41	13.75	12.66	15.42
22	OA	OBn	9.12	3.35	8.90	9.40	9.05	11.25
23	GA	OBn	1.54	0.90	1.42	1.47	1.13	1.28
24	BA	OBn	7.59	3.36	5.33	5.05	6.43	8.04
25	UA	NBn	0.44	0.34	0.45	0.30	0.24	0.37
26	OA	NBn	0.50	0.32	0.46	0.36	0.27	0.40
27	GA	NBn	0.06	0.02	0.06	0.04	0.04	0.08
28	BA	NBn	0.54	0.31	0.53	0.47	0.45	0.54

EC_{50} in μM from SRB assays.

Noteworthy in this context is the higher cytotoxicity of the glycyrrhetinic acid derivatives as compared to analogs derived from **OA**, **UA** or **BA**. Extensions in the design of these compounds led to the synthesis of triterpene conjugates with further modifications in the backbone (→ tormentic acid (**TA**) and euscaphic acid (**EA**)) as well as to changes in the ring size of the heterocyclic spacer between the backbone of the triterpene and the **RhoB** moiety (Figure 8).

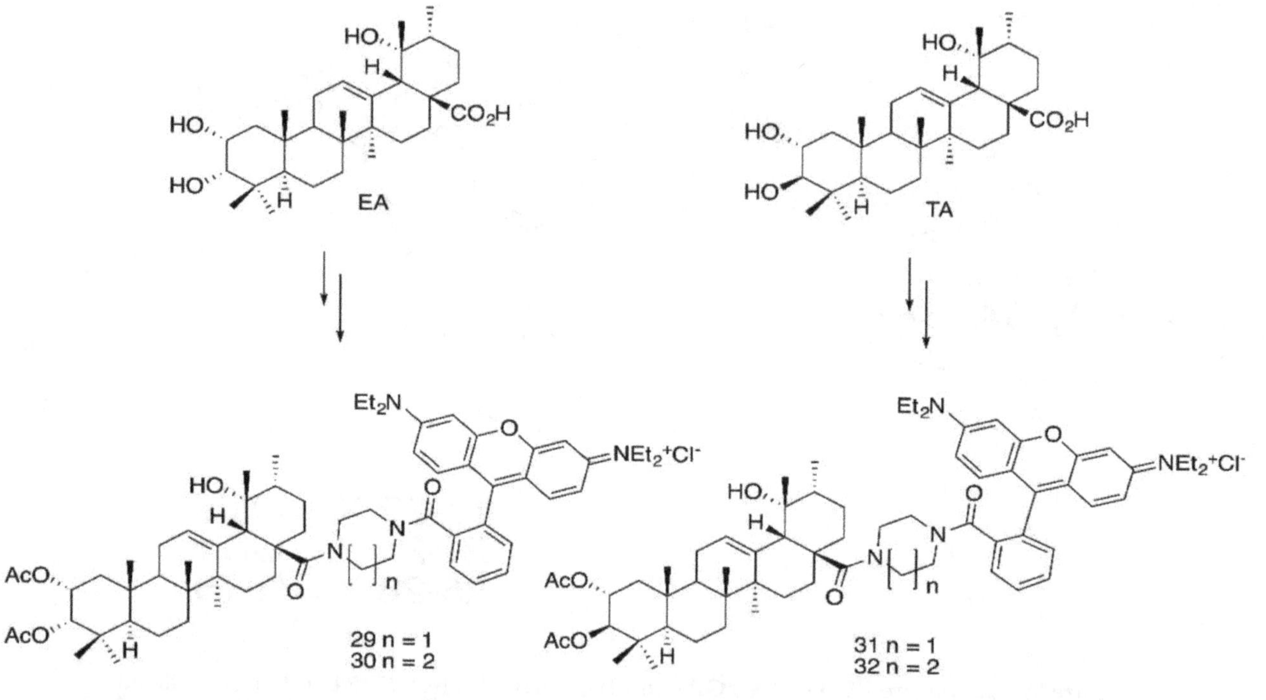

Figure 8. Synthesis of euscaphic (**EA**)- or tormentic acid (**TA**)-derived **RhoB** conjugates **29–32**.

The significantly higher cytotoxicity (Table 5) of **TA**-derived **32** seems particularly noteworthy when comparing the different spacers: Thereby, the presence of a homopiperazinyl spacer [96] (as in **32**) proved to be clearly superior to the piperazinyl moiety (as in **31**). A similar trend was also noted for **EA**-derived compounds **29** and **30**. On the other hand, **TA**-derived compounds were more cytotoxic than the corresponding **EA** derivatives. Interestingly, the absolute configuration at C–2 and C–3 in **TA** corresponds exactly to the configuration found in maslinic acid (**MA**). Several **MA** derivatives (for example [97,98], a diacetylated benzylamide **EM2**, Figure 9) were of higher cytotoxicity and better selectivity than their corresponding **OA** or **UA** derivatives.

Table 5. Cytotoxicity of euscaphic (**EA**)- or tormentic acid (**TA**)-derived **RhoB** conjugates **29–32**, asiatic acid (**AA**)-derived **33** and maslinic acid (**MA**)-derived amide **EM2**.

Compound	A375	HT29	MCF-7	A2780	FaDu	NIH 3T3
29	0.19	0,19	0.094	0.066	0.074	0.21
30	0.012	0.012	0.022	0.004	0.004	0.164
31	0.14	0.16	0.0084	0.037	0.041	0.25
32	0.06	0.005	0.008	0.001	0.001	0.19
33	n.d.	0.017	0.012	0.008	n.d.	0.178
EM2	n.d.	4.70	7.70	0.50	n.d.	33.8

EC_{50} in μM from SRB assays.

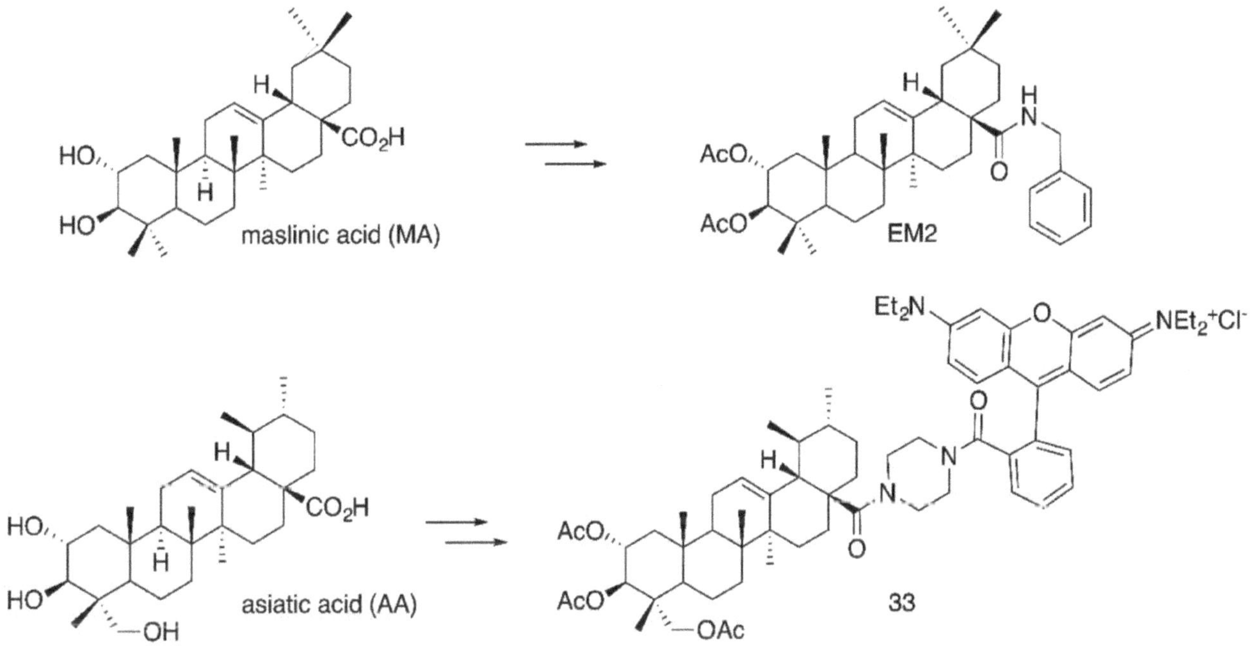

Figure 9. Synthesis of maslinic acid (**MA**)-derived **EM2** holding the same absolute configuration of hydroxyl groups in ring A as asiatic acid (**AA**)-derived conjugate **33**.

The same configuration is found in asiatic acid (**AA**). Again, its acetylated piperazinyl-rhodamine B conjugate **33** was most cytotoxic to many human tumor cell lines, being accumulated in the mitochondria, and it also acted as a mitocan [99]. However, for this compound an unusual non-linear rate of growth was detected for some human tumor cell lines (e.g., colorectal carcinoma HT29 and melanoma 518A2). In a bimodal manner at two different concentrations the tumor cells were killed, a phenomenon that might be due to an accelerated recovery of the mitochondrial membrane potential or due to a modulation of the mitochondrial permeability pores. However, at present a concentration-triggered activation of a metabolizing enzyme cannot completely be ruled out [99].

A graphical comparison of all derivatives (using the target line A2780 as an example) is given in Figure 10 including a comparison of tumor cell/non-tumor cell selectivity (A2780 vs. NIH 3T3) of all compounds.

From Figure 10 the high potential of compound **32** (selectivity for A2780 or FaDu cells, ca. 190) becomes clearly visible, making this compound an interesting drug for advanced testing and biological screening.

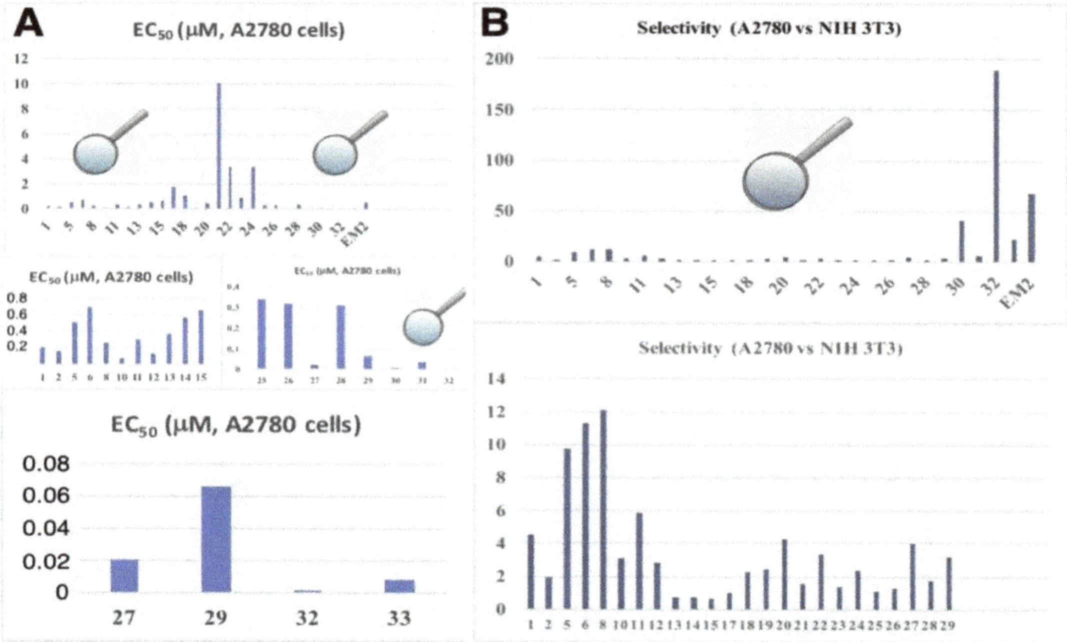

Figure 10. Graphical representation of the cytotoxicity of all compounds (EC_{50} in µM) for the cell line A2780 (**A**) combined with a comparison of tumor cell/non-tumor cell selectivity (A2780 vs. NIH 3T3, selectivity = ($EC_{50,\ NIH3T3}/EC_{50,\ A2780}$)) of all compounds (**B**).

3. Conclusions

OA-derived **RhoB** conjugates appear to be superior to analog **UA**-derived compounds in the majority of cases with respect to their cytotoxicity. Although **AKBA**-derived derivatives have good cytotoxicity properties, they were found to be less cytotoxic compared to other triterpene carboxylic acid derivatives, but they often showed better tumor cell/non-tumor cell selectivity. So far, the best cytotoxicity properties have been found for **MA-**, **EA-** and **TA-**derived derivatives. These allowed the transition to compounds of nano-molar activity, while many other triterpene carboxylic acid derivatives were cytotoxic only on a micro-molar concentration range. **MA-** derived derivatives seem to be approximately equivalent to **EA**-derived compounds. They are currently only surpassed in many tumor cell lines only by the analogous derivatives from **TA**. From results available so far, it can be concluded that compounds holding a homopiperazinyl spacer are superior to those with a piperazinyl spacer. This underlines the importance of the spacer for obtaining good cytotoxicity properties. Replacement of the secondary amide derived spacer by a primary amine like ethylenediamine has invariably led to **RhoB** conjugates of insignificant cytotoxicity (EC_{50} > 30 µM) due to the formation of a spirolactam holding no positive charge in the RhoB part.

However, the presence of a distal cation is not sufficient to obtain compounds with excellent cytotoxicity, as has been shown for several quaternary ammonium compounds or compounds where the **RhoB** part has been replaced by, for example, malachite green, a BODIPY residue or a safirinium group. In addition, the latter compounds do not act as mitocans, since their primary target is the endoplasmic reticulum.

A statement on the extent to which the replacement of the **RhoB** group with another rhodamine has a positive effect on biological activity cannot be made at present. The cytotoxic properties of these compounds, other spacers and other triterpene carboxylic acids are currently the subject of further investigation. The combination of the "correct" parent structure, the "correct" spacer and the "correct" **RhoB** seems to be decisive for the ability of the conjugate to accumulate in mitochondria. So far, a tormentic acid acid-derived **RhoB** conjugate **32** holding a homopiperazinyl spacer can be regarded as the most promising candidate for further biological studies. At present, no extended investigations have been carried out on the precise mode of action of these molecules.

Author Contributions: Conceptualization, R.C. and H.-P.D.; validation, S.H., I.S. and R.C.; investigation, S.H.; writing—original draft preparation, R.C. writing—review and editing, R.C., S.H., I.S., H.-P.D. All authors have read and agreed to the published version of the manuscript.

Acknowledgments: We like to thank all members of our groups for their continuing support and skillful work in the laboratories.

References

1. Available online: https://www.who.int/health-topics/cancer-tab=tab_1 (accessed on 20 October 2020).
2. Bray, F.; Jemal, A.; Grey, N.; Ferlay, J.; Forman, D. Global cancer transitions according to the Human Development Index (2008–2030): A population-based study. *Lancet Oncol.* **2012**, *13*, 790–801. [CrossRef]
3. Siegel, R.L.; Mph, K.D.M.; Sauer, A.G.; Fedewa, S.A.; Butterly, L.F.; Anderson, J.C.; Cercek, A.; Smith, R.A.; Jemal, A. Colorectal cancer statistics, 2020. *CA: A Cancer J. Clin.* **2020**, *70*, 145–164. [CrossRef] [PubMed]
4. Markham, M.J.; Wachter, K.; Agarwal, N.; Bertagnolli, M.M.; Chang, S.M.; Dale, W.; Diefenbach, C.S.M.; Rodriguez-Galindo, C.; George, D.J.; Gilligan, T.D.; et al. Clinical Cancer Advances 2020: Annual Report on Progress Against Cancer From the American Society of Clinical Oncology. *J. Clin. Oncol.* **2020**, *38*, 1081. [CrossRef] [PubMed]
5. Oostveen, M.; Pritchard-Jones, K. Pharmacotherapeutic Management of Wilms Tumor: An Update. *Pediatr. Drugs* **2019**, *21*, 1–13. [CrossRef]
6. Di Paolo, A.; Arrigoni, E.; Luci, G.; Cucchiara, F.; Danesi, R.; Galimberti, S. Precision Medicine in Lymphoma by Innovative Instrumental Platforms. *Front. Oncol.* **2019**, *9*, 1417. [CrossRef]
7. Available online: https://www.paho.org/hq/index.php?option=com_docman&view=download&category_slug=4-cancer-country-profiles-2020&alias=51561-global-cancer-profile-2020&Itemid=270&lang=fr (accessed on 20 October 2020).
8. Green, D.R. Cancer and Apoptosis: Who Is Built to Last? *Cancer Cell* **2017**, *31*, 2–4. [CrossRef]
9. Pretta, A.; Trevisi, E.; Bregni, G.; Deleporte, A.; Hendlisz, A.; Sclafani, F. Treatment compliance in early-stage anal cancer. *Ann. Oncol.* **2020**, *31*, 1282–1284. [CrossRef]
10. Muzumder, S.; Srikantia, N.; Vashishta, G.D.; Udayashankar, A.H.; Raj, J.M.; Sebastian, M.G.J.; Kainthaje, P.B. Compliance, toxicity and efficacy in weekly versus 3-weekly cisplatin concurrent chemoradiation in locally advanced head and neck cancer. *J. Radiother. Pr.* **2018**, *18*, 21–25. [CrossRef]
11. Gong, L.; Yan, Q.; Zhang, Y.; Fang, X.; Liu, B.; Guan, X.-Y. Cancer cell reprogramming: A promising therapy converting malignancy to benignity. *Cancer Commun.* **2019**, *39*, 1–13. [CrossRef]
12. Fuchs, Y.; Steller, H. Live to die another way: Modes of programmed cell death and the signals emanating from dying cells. *Nat. Rev. Mol. Cell Biol.* **2015**, *16*, 329–344. [CrossRef]
13. Wang, C.X.; Youle, R.J. The Role of Mitochondria in Apoptosis. *Annu. Rev. Genet.* **2009**, *43*, 95–118. [CrossRef] [PubMed]
14. Johnstone, R.W.; Ruefli, A.A.; Lowe, S.W. Apoptosis: A link between cancer genetics and chemotherapy. *Cell* **2002**, *108*, 153–164. [CrossRef]
15. Fiers, W.; Beyaert, R.; Declercq, W.; Vandenabeele, P. More than one way to die: Apoptosis, necrosis and reactive oxygen damage. *Oncogene* **1999**, *18*, 7719–7730. [CrossRef] [PubMed]
16. Galluzzi, L.; Pedro, J.M.B.-S.; Kroemer, G. Organelle-specific initiation of cell death. *Nat. Cell Biol.* **2014**, *16*, 728–736. [CrossRef] [PubMed]
17. Bing, Y.; Dong, L.; Neuzil, J. Mitochondria: An intriguing target for killing tumour-initiating cells. *Mitochondrion* **2016**, *26*, 86–93. [CrossRef]
18. Pei, J.; Panina, S.B.; Kirienko, N.V. An Automated Differential Nuclear Staining Assay for Accurate Determination of Mitocan Cytotoxicity. *J. Vis. Exp.* **2020**, *159*, e61295. [CrossRef]
19. Panina, S.B.; Pei, J.; Baran, N.; Konopleva, M.; Kirienko, N.V. Utilizing Synergistic Potential of Mitochondria-Targeting Drugs for Leukemia Therapy. *Front. Oncol.* **2020**, *10*, 435. [CrossRef]
20. Ralph, S.J.; Neuzil, J. Mitochondria as Targets for Cancer Therapy. In *Mitochondria and Cancer*; Costello, L., Singh, K., Eds.; Springer: New York, NY, USA, 2009; pp. 211–249.

21. Ralph, S.J.; Rodríguez-Enríquez, S.; Neuzil, J.; Moreno-Sánchez, R. Bioenergetic pathways in tumor mitochondria as targets for cancer therapy and the importance of the ROS-induced apoptotic trigger. *Mol. Asp. Med.* **2010**, *31*, 29–59. [CrossRef]
22. Ralph, S.J.; Rodríguez-Enríquez, S.; Neuzil, J.; Saavedra, E.; Moreno-Sánchez, R. The causes of cancer revisited: "Mitochondrial malignancy" and ROS-induced oncogenic transformation – Why mitochondria are targets for cancer therapy. *Mol. Asp. Med.* **2010**, *31*, 145–170. [CrossRef] [PubMed]
23. Chiu, H.Y.; Tay, E.X.Y.; Ong, D.S.T.; Taneja, R. Mitochondrial Dysfunction at the Center of Cancer Therapy. *Antioxidants Redox Signal.* **2020**, *32*, 309–330. [CrossRef]
24. Singh, Y.; Viswanadham, K.K.D.R.; Pawar, V.K.; Meher, J.; Jajoriya, A.K.; Omer, A.; Jaiswal, S.; Dewangan, J.; Bora, H.K.; Singh, P.; et al. Induction of Mitochondrial Cell Death and Reversal of Anticancer Drug Resistance via Nanocarriers Composed of a Triphenylphosphonium Derivative of Tocopheryl Polyethylene Glycol Succinate. *Mol. Pharm.* **2019**, *16*, 3744–3759. [CrossRef] [PubMed]
25. Nguyen, C.; Pandey, S. Exploiting Mitochondrial Vulnerabilities to Trigger Apoptosis Selectively in Cancer Cells. *Cancers* **2019**, *11*, 916. [CrossRef] [PubMed]
26. Olivas-Aguirre, M.; Pottosin, I.; Dobrovinskaya, O. Mitochondria as emerging targets for therapies against T cell acute lymphoblastic leukemia. *J. Leukoc. Biol.* **2019**, *105*, 935–946. [CrossRef]
27. Sassi, N.; Biasutto, L.; Mattarei, A.; Carraro, M.; Giorgio, V.; Citta, A.; Bernardi, P.; Garbisa, S.; Szabò, I.; Paradisi, C.; et al. Cytotoxicity of a mitochondriotropic quercetin derivative: Mechanisms. *Biochim. et Biophys. Acta (BBA) - Gen. Subj.* **2012**, *1817*, 1095–1106. [CrossRef] [PubMed]
28. Sassi, N.; Mattarei, A.; Azzolini, M.; Bernardi, P.; Szabò, I.; Paradisi, C.; Zoratti, M.; Biasutto, L. Mitochondria-targeted resveratrol derivatives act as cytotoxic pro-oxidants. *Curr. Pharm. Des.* **2014**, *20*, 172–179. [CrossRef]
29. Chen, G.; Wang, F.; Trachootham, D.; Huang, P. Preferential killing of cancer cells with mitochondrial dysfunction by natural compounds. *Mitochondrion* **2010**, *10*, 614–625. [CrossRef]
30. Guzman-Villanueva, D.; Weissig, V. Mitochondria-Targeted Agents: Mitochondriotropics, Mitochondriotoxics, and Mitocans. *Muscarinic Receptors* **2016**, *240*, 423–438. [CrossRef]
31. Rohlena, J.; Dong, L.-F.; Neuzil, J. Targeting the mitochondrial electron transport chain complexes for the induction of apoptosis and cancer treatment. *Curr. Pharm. Biotechnol.* **2013**, *14*, 377–389. [CrossRef]
32. Rohlena, J.; Dong, L.; Ralph, S.J.; Neuzil, J. Anticancer Drugs Targeting the Mitochondrial Electron Transport Chain. *Antioxidants Redox Signal.* **2011**, *15*, 2951–2974. [CrossRef]
33. Kornblihtt, L.I.; Carreras, M.C.A.; Blanco, G. Targeting Mitophagy in Combined Therapies of Haematological Malignancies. *Autophagy Curr. Trends Cell. Physiol. Pathol.* **2016**, *19*, 411–431. [CrossRef]
34. Neuzil, J.; Dong, L.-F.; Rohlena, J.; Truksa, J.; Ralph, S.J. Classification of mitocans, anti-cancer drugs acting on mitochondria. *Mitochondrion* **2013**, *13*, 199–208. [CrossRef] [PubMed]
35. Neuzil, J.; Dyason, J.C.; Freeman, R.; Dong, L.; Prochazka, L.; Wang, X.-F.; Scheffler, I.; Ralph, S.J. Mitocans as anti-cancer agents targeting mitochondria: Lessons from studies with vitamin E analogues, inhibitors of complex II. *J. Bioenerg. Biomembr.* **2007**, *39*, 65–72. [CrossRef] [PubMed]
36. Neuzil, J.; Wang, X.-F.; Dong, L.-F.; Low, P.; Ralph, S.J. Molecular mechanism of 'mitocan'-induced apoptosis in cancer cells epitomizes the multiple roles of reactive oxygen species and Bcl-2 family proteins. *FEBS Lett.* **2006**, *580*, 5125–5129. [CrossRef] [PubMed]
37. Morrison, B.J.; Andera, L.; Reynolds, B.A.; Ralph, S.J.; Neuzil, J. Future use of mitocans against tumour-initiating cells? *Mol. Nutr. Food Res.* **2009**, *53*, 147–153. [CrossRef] [PubMed]
38. Hahn, T.; Polanczyk, M.J.; Borodovsky, A.; Ramanathapuram, L.V.; Akporiaye, E.T.; Ralph, S.J. Use of anti-cancer drugs, mitocans, to enhance the immune responses against tumors. *Curr. Pharm. Biotechnol.* **2013**, *14*, 357–376. [CrossRef] [PubMed]
39. Amaral, L.; Spengler, G.; Molnar, J. Identification of Important Compounds Isolated from Natural Sources that Have Activity Against Multidrug-resistant Cancer Cell Lines: Effects on Proliferation, Apoptotic Mechanism and the Efflux Pump Responsible for Multi-resistance Phenotype. *Anticancer. Res.* **2016**, *36*, 5665–5672. [CrossRef]
40. Abdelmageed, N.; Morad, S.A.; Elghoneimy, A.A.; Syrovets, T.; Simmet, T.; El-Zorba, H.; El-Banna, H.A.; Cabot, M.; Abdel-Aziz, M.I. Oleanolic acid methyl ester, a novel cytotoxic mitocan, induces cell cycle arrest and ROS-Mediated cell death in castration-resistant prostate cancer PC-3 cells. *Biomed. Pharmacother.* **2017**, *96*, 417–425. [CrossRef]

41. Bhola, P.D.; Letai, A. Mitochondria—Judges and Executioners of Cell Death Sentences. *Mol. Cell* **2016**, *61*, 695–704. [CrossRef]
42. Jacotot, E.E.; Ferri, K.K.; El Hamel, C.C.; Brenner, C.C.; Druillennec, S.S.; Hoebeke, J.; Rustin, P.P.; Métivier, D.D.; Lenoir, C.C.; Geuskens, M.; et al. Control of Mitochondrial Membrane Permeabilization by Adenine Nucleotide Translocator Interacting with HIV-1 Viral Protein R and Bcl-2. *J. Exp. Med.* **2001**, *193*, 509–520. [CrossRef]
43. Zamzami, N.; Kroemer, G. The mitochondrion in apoptosis: How Pandora's box opens. *Nat. Rev. Mol. Cell Biol.* **2001**, *2*, 67–71. [CrossRef]
44. Zamzami, N.; Maisse, C.; Métivier, D.; Kroemer, G. Chapter 8 Measurement of membrane permeability and permeability transition of mitochondria. *Echinoderms Part B* **2001**, *65*, 147–158. [CrossRef]
45. Yang, H.; Dou, Q.P. Targeting apoptosis pathway with natural terpenoids: Implications for treatment of breast and prostate cancer. *Curr. Drug Targets* **2010**, *11*, 733–744. [CrossRef] [PubMed]
46. Fulda, S.; Kroemer, G. Mitochondria as Therapeutic Targets for the Treatment of Malignant Disease. *Antioxidants Redox Signal.* **2011**, *15*, 2937–2949. [CrossRef] [PubMed]
47. Serafim, T.L.; Carvalho, F.S.; Pereira, G.; Greene, A.; Perkins, E.; Holy, J.; Krasutsky, D.A.; Kolomitsyna, O.N.; Krasutsky, P.A.; Oliveira, P.J. Lupane triterpenoids as mitocans against breast cancer cells. *Eur. J. Clin. Invest.* **2013**, *43*, 48–49.
48. Serafim, T.L.; Carvalho, F.S.; Bernardo, T.C.; Pereira, G.C.; Perkins, E.; Holy, J.; Krasutsky, D.A.; Kolomitsyna, O.N.; Krasutsky, P.A.; Oliveira, P.J. New derivatives of lupine triterpenoids disturb breast cancer mitochondria and induce cell death. *Bioorg. Med. Chem.* **2014**, *22*, 6270–6287. [CrossRef] [PubMed]
49. Grymel, M.; Zawojak, M.; Adamek, J. Triphenylphosphonium Analogues of Betulin and Betulinic Acid with Biological Activity: A Comprehensive Review. *J. Nat. Prod.* **2019**, *82*, 1719–1730. [CrossRef]
50. Kolevzon, N.; Kuflik, U.; Shmuel, M.; Benhamron, S.; Ringel, I.; Yavin, E. Multiple Triphenylphosphonium Cations as a Platform for the Delivery of a Pro-Apoptotic Peptide. *Pharm. Res.* **2011**, *28*, 2780–2789. [CrossRef]
51. Spivak, A.Y.; Nedopekina, D.A.; Khalitova, R.R.; Gubaidullin, R.; Odinokov, V.N.; Bel'Skii, Y.P.; Bel'Skaya, N.V.; Khazanov, V.A. Triphenylphosphonium cations of betulinic acid derivatives: Synthesis and antitumor activity. *Med. Chem. Res.* **2017**, *26*, 518–531. [CrossRef]
52. Akhmetova, V.R.; Nedopekina, D.A.; Shakurova, E.R.; Khalitova, R.R.; Gubaidullin, R.R.; Odinokov, V.N.; Dzhemilev, U.M.; Bel'Skii, Y.P.; Bel'Skaya, N.V.; Stankevich, S.A.; et al. Synthesis of lupane triterpenoids with triphenylphosphonium substituents and studies of their antitumor activity. *Russ. Chem. Bull.* **2013**, *62*, 188–198. [CrossRef]
53. Huang, H.; Wu, H.; Huang, Y.; Zhang, S.; Lam, Y.-W.; Ao, N. Antitumor activity and antitumor mechanism of triphenylphosphonium chitosan against liver carcinoma. *J. Mater. Res.* **2018**, *33*, 2586–2597. [CrossRef]
54. Strobykina, I.Y.; Andreeva, O.V.; Belenok, M.G.; Semenova, M.N.; Semenov, V.V.; Chuprov-Netochin, R.N.; Sapunova, A.S.; Voloshina, A.D.; Dobrynin, A.B.; Semenov, V.E.; et al. Triphenylphosphonium conjugates of 1,2,3-triazolyl nucleoside analogues. Synthesis and cytotoxicity evaluation. *Med. Chem. Res.* **2020**, *29*, 1–15. [CrossRef]
55. Jara, J.A.; Castro-Castillo, V.; Saavedra-Olavarría, J.; Peredo, L.; Pavanni, M.; Jaña, F.; Letelier, M.E.; Parra, E.; Becker, M.I.; Morello, A.; et al. Antiproliferative and Uncoupling Effects of Delocalized, Lipophilic, Cationic Gallic Acid Derivatives on Cancer Cell Lines. Validation in Vivo in Singenic Mice. *J. Med. Chem.* **2014**, *57*, 2440–2454. [CrossRef] [PubMed]
56. Kafkova, A.; Trnka, J. Mitochondria-targeted compounds in the treatment of cancer. *Neoplasma* **2020**, *67*, 450–460. [CrossRef] [PubMed]
57. Ye, Y.; Zhang, T.; Yuan, H.; Li, D.; Lou, H.; Fan, P. Mitochondria-Targeted Lupane Triterpenoid Derivatives and Their Selective Apoptosis-Inducing Anticancer Mechanisms. *J. Med. Chem.* **2017**, *60*, 6353–6363. [CrossRef]
58. Sarek, J.; Biedermann, D.; Eignerova, B.; Hajduch, M. Synthesis and Evaluation of Biological Activity of the Quaternary Ammonium Salts of Lupane-, Oleanane-, and Ursane-Type Acids. *Synthesis* **2010**, *22*, 3839–3848. [CrossRef]
59. Kataev, V.E.; Strobykina, I.Y.; Zakharova, L.Y. Quaternary ammonium derivatives of natural terpenoids. Synthesis and properties. *Russ. Chem. Bull.* **2014**, *63*, 1884–1900. [CrossRef]
60. Brandes, B.; Koch, L.; Hoenke, S.; Deigner, H.-P.; Csuk, R. The presence of a cationic center is not alone decisive for the cytotoxicity of triterpene carboxylic acid amides. *Steroids* **2020**, *163*, 108713. [CrossRef]

61. Perreault, M.; Maltais, R.; Dutour, R.; Poirier, D. Explorative study on the anticancer activity, selectivity and metabolic stability of related analogs of aminosteroid RM-133. *Steroids* **2016**, *115*, 105–113. [CrossRef]
62. Brandes, B.; Hoenke, S.; Fischer, L.; Csuk, R. Design, synthesis and cytotoxicity of BODIPY FL labelled triterpenoids. *Eur. J. Med. Chem.* **2020**, *185*, 111858. [CrossRef]
63. Barut, B.; Çoban, Ö.; Özgür, Y.C.; Baş, H.; Sari, S.; Biyiklioglu, Z.; Demirbaş, Ü.; Özel, A. Synthesis, DNA interaction, in vitro/in silico topoisomerase II inhibition and photodynamic therapy activities of two cationic BODIPY derivatives. *Dye. Pigment.* **2020**, *174*, 108072. [CrossRef]
64. Barut, B.; Özgür, Y.C.; Sari, S.; Çoban, Ö.; Keleş, T.; Biyiklioglu, Z.; Abudayyak, M.; Demirbaş, Ü.; Özel, A. Novel water soluble BODIPY compounds: Synthesis, photochemical, DNA interaction, topoisomerases inhibition and photodynamic activity properties. *Eur. J. Med. Chem.* **2019**, *183*, 11685. [CrossRef] [PubMed]
65. Taki, S.; Ardestani, M.S. Novel nanosized AS1411-chitosan-BODIPY conjugate for molecular fluorescent imaging. *Int. J. Nanomed.* **2019**, *14*, 3543–3555. [CrossRef] [PubMed]
66. Li, M.; Li, X.; Cao, Z.; Wu, Y.; Chen, J.-A.; Gao, J.; Wang, Z.; Guo, W.; Gu, X. Mitochondria-targeting BODIPY-loaded micelles as novel class of photosensitizer for photodynamic therapy. *Eur. J. Med. Chem.* **2018**, *157*, 599–609. [CrossRef] [PubMed]
67. Kraft, O.; Kozubek, M.; Hoenke, S.; Serbian, I.; Major, D.; Csuk, R. Cytotoxic triterpenoid–safirinium conjugates target the endoplasmic reticulum. *Eur. J. Med. Chem.* **2020**, 112920. [CrossRef] [PubMed]
68. Cooksey, C. Quirks of dye nomenclature. 5. Rhodamines. *Biotech. Histochem.* **2015**, *91*, 1–6. [CrossRef]
69. Ceresole, M. Rhodamin Dye. U.S. Patent 516589 A 18940313, 13 March 1894.
70. Ceresole, M. Red Dyestuff. U.S. Patent 456081 18910714, 14 July 1891.
71. Kim, H.N.; Lee, M.H.; Kim, H.J.; Kim, J.S.; Yoon, J. A new trend in rhodamine-based chemosensors: Application of spirolactam ring-opening to sensing ions. *Chem. Soc. Rev.* **2008**, *37*, 1465–1472. [CrossRef]
72. Wang, D.; Wang, Z.; Li, Y.; Song, Y.; Song, Y.; Zhang, M.; Yu, H. A single rhodamine spirolactam probe for localization and pH monitoring of mitochondrion/lysosome in living cells. *New J. Chem.* **2018**, *42*, 11102–11108. [CrossRef]
73. Adamovich, L.P.; Mel'nik, V.V.; McHedlov-Petrosyan, N.O. Rhodamine B equilibriums in water-salt solutions. *Zh. Fiz. Khim.* **1979**, *53*, 356–359.
74. Hinckley, D.A.; Seybold, P.G. Thermodynamics of the rhodamine B lactone zwitterion equilibrium: An undergraduate laboratory experiment. *J. Chem. Educ.* **1987**, *64*, 362. [CrossRef]
75. Ramart-Lucas, P. Structure of rhodamine from its absorption spectrum. *Compt. Rend.* **1938**, *207*, 1416–1418.
76. Ramette, R.W.; Blackburn, T.R. Specific effects of cations on rhodamine B equilibriums. *J. Phys. Chem.* **1958**, *62*, 1601–1603. [CrossRef]
77. Ramette, R.W.; Sandell, E.B. Rhodamine B equilibriums. *J. Am. Chem. Soc.* **1956**, *78*, 4872–4878. [CrossRef]
78. Hinckley, D.A.; Seybold, P.G.; Borris, D.P. Solvatochromism and thermochromism of rhodamine solutions. *Spectrochim. Acta Part A Mol. Spectrosc.* **1986**, *42*, 747–754. [CrossRef]
79. Beija, M.; Afonso, C.A.M.; Martinho, J.M.G. Synthesis and applications of Rhodamine derivatives as fluorescent probes. *Chem. Soc. Rev.* **2009**, *38*, 2410–2433. [CrossRef]
80. Arbeloa, F.L.; Estevez, M.J.T. Photophysics of rhodamines: Molecular structure and solvent effects. *J. Phys. Chem.* **1991**, *95*, 2203–2208. [CrossRef]
81. Arbeloa, T.L.; Estévez, M.T.; López-Arbeloa, F.; Aguirresacona, I.U.; Arbeloa, I.L. Luminescence properties of rhodamines in water/ethanol mixtures. *J. Lumin* **1991**, *48*, 400–404. [CrossRef]
82. Milvy, P.; Kay, K. Mutagenicity of 19 major graphic arts and printing dyes. *J. Toxicol. Environ. Heal. Part A* **1978**, *4*, 31–36. [CrossRef]
83. Smart, P.L. A review of the toxicity of twelve fluorescent dyes used for water tracing. *NSS Bull.* **1984**, *46*, 21–33.
84. Umeda, M. Experimental production of sarcoma in rats by injection of rhodamine B. I. *Gann* **1952**, *43*, 120–122.
85. Umeda, M. Experimental study of xanthene dyes as carcinogenic agents. *Gann* **1956**, *47*, 51–78.
86. Nestmann, E.R.; Douglas, G.R.I.; Matula, T.E.; Grant, C.; Kowbel, D.J. Mutagenic activity of rhodamine dyes and their impurities as detected by mutation induction in Salmonella and DNA damage in Chinese hamster ovary cells. *Cancer Res.* **1979**, *39*, 4412–4417. [PubMed]
87. Elliott, G.S.; Mason, R.W.; Edwards, I.R. Studies on the pharmacokinetics and mutagenic potential of rhodamine b. *J. Toxicol. Clin. Toxicol.* **1990**, *28*, 45–59. [CrossRef] [PubMed]

88. Sommerwerk, S.; Heller, L.; Kerzig, C.; Kramell, A.E.; Csuk, R. Rhodamine B conjugates of triterpenoic acids are cytotoxic mitocans even at nanomolar concentrations. *Eur. J. Med. Chem.* **2017**, *127*, 1–9. [CrossRef] [PubMed]
89. Macasoi, I.; Mioc, M.; Vaduva, D.B.; Ghiulai, R.; Mioc, A.; Soica, C.; Muntean, D.; Dumitrascu, V. In silico Evaluation of the Antiproliferative Mithocondrial Targeted Mechanism of Action of Some Pentacyclic Triterpene Derivatives. *Rev. Chim.* **2019**, *69*, 3361–3363. [CrossRef]
90. Friedrich, S.; Serbian, I.; Hoenke, S.; Wolfram, R.K.; Csuk, R. Synthesis and cytotoxic evaluation of malachite green derived oleanolic and ursolic acid piperazineamides. *Med. Chem. Res.* **2020**, *29*, 926–933. [CrossRef]
91. Serbian, I.; Hoenke, S.; Kraft, O.; Csuk, R. Ester and amide derivatives of rhodamine B exert cytotoxic effects on different human tumor cell lines. *Med. Chem. Res.* **2020**, *29*, 1655–1661. [CrossRef]
92. Kozubek, M.; Serbian, I.; Hoenke, S.; Kraft, O.; Csuk, R. Synthesis and cytotoxic evaluation of hydroxycinnamic acid rhodamine B conjugates. *Results Chem.* **2020**, *2*, 100057. [CrossRef]
93. Serbian, I.; Hoenke, S.; Csuk, R. Synthesis of some steroidal mitocans of nanomolar cytotoxicity acting by apoptosis. *Eur. J. Med. Chem.* **2020**, *199*, 112425. [CrossRef]
94. Wiemann, J.; Fischer, L.; Kessler, J.; Ströhl, D.; Csuk, R. Ugi Multicomponent-reaction: Syntheses of cytotoxic dehydroabietylamine derivatives. *Bioorganic Chem.* **2018**, *81*, 567–576. [CrossRef]
95. Wolfram, R.K.; Heller, L.; Csuk, R. Targeting mitochondria: Esters of rhodamine B with triterpenoids are mitocanic triggers of apoptosis. *Eur. J. Med. Chem.* **2018**, *152*, 21–30. [CrossRef]
96. Wolfram, R.K.; Fischer, L.; Kluge, R.; Ströhl, D.; Al-Harrasi, A.; Csuk, R. Homopiperazine-rhodamine B adducts of triterpenoic acids are strong mitocans. *Eur. J. Med. Chem.* **2018**, *155*, 869–879. [CrossRef]
97. Siewert, B.; Pianowski, E.; Obernauer, A.; Csuk, R. Towards cytotoxic and selective derivatives of maslinic acid. *Bioorg. Med. Chem.* **2014**, *22*, 594–615. [CrossRef]
98. Sommerwerk, S.; Heller, L.; Kuhfs, J.; Csuk, R. Urea derivates of ursolic, oleanolic and maslinic acid induce apoptosis and are selective cytotoxic for several human tumor cell lines. *Eur. J. Med. Chem.* **2016**, *119*, 1–16. [CrossRef]
99. Kahnt, M.; Wiemann, J.; Fischer, L.; Sommerwerk, S.; Csuk, R. Transformation of asiatic acid into a mitocanic, bimodal-acting rhodamine B conjugate of nanomolar cytotoxicity. *Eur. J. Med. Chem.* **2018**, *159*, 143–148. [CrossRef] [PubMed]

3

Synthesis and Evaluation of Novel 2*H*-Benzo[*e*]-[1,2,4]thiadiazine 1,1-Dioxide Derivatives as PI3Kδ Inhibitors

Ya-Ping Gong †, Long-Qian Tang †, Tong-Shen Liu and Zhao-Peng Liu *

Department of Medicinal Chemistry, Key Laboratory of Chemical Biology (Ministry of Education), School of Pharmaceutical Sciences, Shandong University, Jinan 250012, China; 201614474@mail.sdu.edu.cn (Y.-P.G.); lqtang.student@sina.com (L.-Q.T.); jshrlts@163.com (T.-S.L.)

* Correspondence: liuzhaop@sdu.edu.cn;

† Ya-Ping Gong and Long-Qian Tang contributed equally to this work.

Academic Editor: Qiao-Hong Chen

Abstract: In previous work, we applied the rotation-limiting strategy and introduced a substituent at the 3-position of the pyrazolo [3,4-*d*]pyrimidin-4-amine as the affinity element to interact with the deeper hydrophobic pocket, discovered a series of novel quinazolinones as potent PI3Kδ inhibitors. Among them, the indole derivative **3** is one of the most selective PI3Kδ inhibitors and the 3,4-dimethoxyphenyl derivative **4** is a potent and selective dual PI3Kδ/γ inhibitor. In this study, we replaced the carbonyl group in the quinazolinone core with a sulfonyl group, designed a series of novel 2*H*-benzo[*e*][1,2,4]thiadiazine 1,1-dioxide derivatives as PI3Kδ inhibitors. After the reduction of nitro group in *N*-(2,6-dimethylphenyl)-2-nitrobenzenesulfonamide **5** and *N*-(2,6-dimethylphenyl)-2-nitro-5-fluorobenzenesulfonamide **6**, the resulting 2-aminobenzenesulfonamides were reacted with trimethyl orthoacetate to give the 3-methyl-2*H*-benzo[*e*][1,2,4]thiadiazine 1,1-dioxide derivatives. After bromination of the 3-methyl group, the nucleophilic substitution with the 3-iodo-1*H*-pyrazolo[3,4-*d*]pyrimidin-4-amine provided the respective iodide derivatives, which were further reacted with a series of arylboronic acids via Suzuki coupling to furnish the 2*H*-benzo[*e*][1,2,4]thiadiazine 1,1-dioxide derivatives **15a–J** and **16a–d**. In agreement with the quinazolinone derivatives, the introduction of a 5-indolyl or 3,4-dimethoxyphenyl at the affinity pocket generated the most potent analogues **15a** and **15b** with the IC_{50} values of 217 to 266 nM, respectively. In comparison with the quinazolinone lead compounds **3** and **4**, these 2*H*-benzo[*e*][1,2,4]thiadiazine 1,1-dioxide derivatives exhibited much decreased PI3Kδ inhibitory potency, but maintained the high selectivity over other PI3K isoforms. Unlike the quinazolinone lead compound **4** that was a dual PI3Kδ/γ inhibitor, the benzthiadiazine 1,1-dioxide **15b** with the same 3,4-dimethoxyphenyl moiety was more than 21-fold selective over PI3Kγ. Moreover, the introducing of a fluorine atom at the 7-position of the 2*H*-benzo[*e*][1,2,4]thiadiazine 1,1-dioxide core, in general, was not favored for the PI3Kδ inhibitory activity. In agreement with their high PI3Kδ selectivity, **15a** and **15b** significantly inhibited the SU-DHL-6 cell proliferation.

Keywords: PI3Ks; PI3Kδ inhibitors; 2*H*-benzo[*e*][1,2,4]thiadiazine 1,1-dioxide; anticancer; anticancer agents

---

1. Introduction

Phosphoinositide 3-kinases (PI3Ks) are a family of lipid kinases that regulate numerous biological functions, including cell growth, proliferation, differentiation, motility, and intracellular trafficking, through the phosphorylation of the phosphatidylinositol 4,5-bisphosphate (PIP2) to generate the lipid second messenger phosphatidylinositol 3,4,5-trisphosphate (PIP3) [1–3]. There are three classes of the PI3K enzyme, of which class I PI3Ks are the mostly studied and further divided into subgroups IA (PI3Kα, PI3Kβ, and PI3Kδ) and IB (PI3Kγ) based on the signaling pathways and the regulatory proteins to which they bind [4,5]. The class IA PI3K isoforms mediate the signal transduction from receptor tyrosine kinases [6], while the IB isoform PI3Kγ is principally activated by G-protein coupled receptors [7]. PI3Kα and PI3Kβ are ubiquitously expressed, while PI3Kδ and PI3Kγ are dominantly expressed in leukocytes [8–10]. All the class I PI3K isoforms are implicated in cancer [11–16]. There are also mounting evidences that support a therapeutic role for inhibition of PI3Kα in diabetes [17,18], PI3Kβ in thrombosis [19,20], PI3Kδ and PI3Kγ in both rheumatoid arthritis and asthma [21–24], PI3Kδ in activated PI3Kδ syndrome (APDS) [25–27], and PI3Kγ in idiopathic pulmonary fibrosis [28]. Therefore, the development of PI3K isoform selective inhibitors is a promising therapeutic strategy for the treatment of these PI3Ks-related diseases. The selective PI3Kδ inhibitor idelalisib (Figure 1) is approved by FDA for follicular lymphoma (FL) and small lymphocytic lymphoma (SLL) and for chronic lymphocytic leukemia (CLL) in combination with rituximab [29,30]. The dual PI3Kδ/γ inhibitor duvelisib (Figure 1) is approved for adult patients with relapsed or refractory CLL or SLL, and relapsed or refractory FL after at least two prior systemic therapies [31]. However, in the clinical application of idelalisib, infectious and autoimmune toxicities were observed, and the unique toxicities are associated with inhibition of different isoforms of the PI3K enzyme [32]. To improve the isoform selectivity of the quinazolinone-based PI3Kδ inhibitors, in previous work, we introduced a pyrazolo [3,4-*d*]pyrimidin-4-amine moiety as the hinge region binding group, a substituent at the 3-position of the pyrazolo[3,4-*d*]pyrimidine core as the affinity element to interact with the deeper hydrophobic pocket, and a 2,6-dimethylphenyl to limit the free rotation of the 3-phenyl in idelalisib, discovered the indole derivative **3** as one of the most selective PI3Kδ inhibitors (IC_{50} = 8.6 nM) with more than 3630-fold, 390-fold and 40-fold selective for PI3Kδ over PI3Kα, β and γ, and the 3,4-dimethoxyphenyl derivative **4** as a potent and selective dual PI3Kδ/γ inhibitor (IC_{50} = 8.4 nM for PI3Kδ, IC_{50} = 62 nM for PI3Kγ) with more than 1400-fold, 820-fold selective for PI3Kδ over PI3Kα and PI3Kβ [33]. Considering the importance of sulfonamides in drug discovery [34–36], we replaced the carbonyl group in the quinazolinone core, and reported here the synthesis and preliminary evaluation of 2*H*-benzo[*e*][1,2,4]thiadiazine 1,1-dioxide derivatives as PI3Kδ inhibitors.

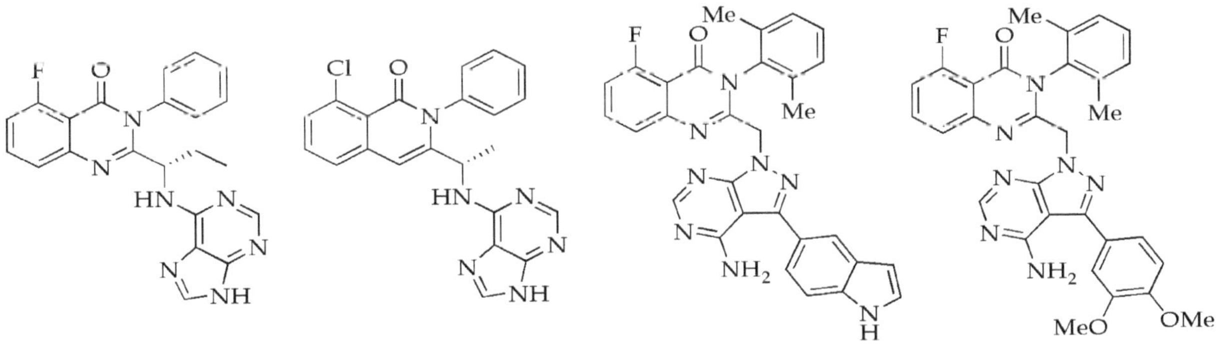

1 (Idelalisib) 2 (Duvelisib) 3 4

Figure 1. Selective PI3Kδ and dual PI3Kδ/γ inhibitors.

2. Results and Discussion

2.1. Chemistry

All the new 2*H*-benzo[*e*][1,2,4]thiadiazine 1,1-dioxide derivatives were prepared following a general synthetic route shown in Scheme 1. The 2-nitrobenzene-1-sulfonamides **5** and **6** were readily prepared according to the reported method by the reaction of 2-nitrobenzene-1-sulfonyl chloride or 5-fluoro-2-nitrobenzene-1-sulfonyl chloride with 2,6-dimethylbenzenamine in methanol and water solution in the presence of CH_3COONa under refluxing conditions [37]. Reduction of the nitro group to amine was carried out using hydrazine monohydrate in the presence of ferric chloride and activated charcoal in methanol under reflux conditions in excellent yields (95% and 99%). The resulting 2-aminobenzenesulfonamides **7** and **8** were reacted with trimethyl orthoacetate to give the corresponding 3-methyl-2*H*-benzo[*e*][1,2,4]thiadiazine 1,1-dioxide derivatives **9** and **10** in 51% and 40%, respectively. In the bromination of the allyl methyl group using *N*-bromosuccinimide (NBS), the main compounds were found to be the dibrominated products. Therefore, compounds **9** and **10** were reacted with only 0.5 equivalent of NBS in glacial acetic acid to give the monobrominated derivatives **11** and **12** in moderate yields (79% and 72% based on NBS). Nucleophilic substitution of **11** and **12** with 3-iodo-1*H*-pyrazolo[3,4-*d*]pyrimidin-4-amine, which was readily prepared from 5-amino-1*H*-pyrazole-4-carbonitrile in two steps by the known procedures [38], resulted in the iodides **13** and **14** in 86 and 58% yields, respectively. Finally, the incorporation of the affinity elements was achieved through the Suzuki coupling of **13** and **14** with the appropriate boronic acid in dioxane and water catalyzed by $Pd(PPh_3)_4$ under refluxing conditions, and the target 2*H*-benzo[*e*][1,2,4]thiadiazine 1,1-dioxide derivatives **15a–J** and **16a–d** were obtained in 34–91% and 51–84% yields. The structures of these 2*H*-benzo[*e*][1,2,4]thiadiazine 1,1-dioxide derivatives were characterized by ^{1}H-nuclear magnetic resonance (NMR) and ^{13}C-NMR (please refer to the Supplementary Materials).

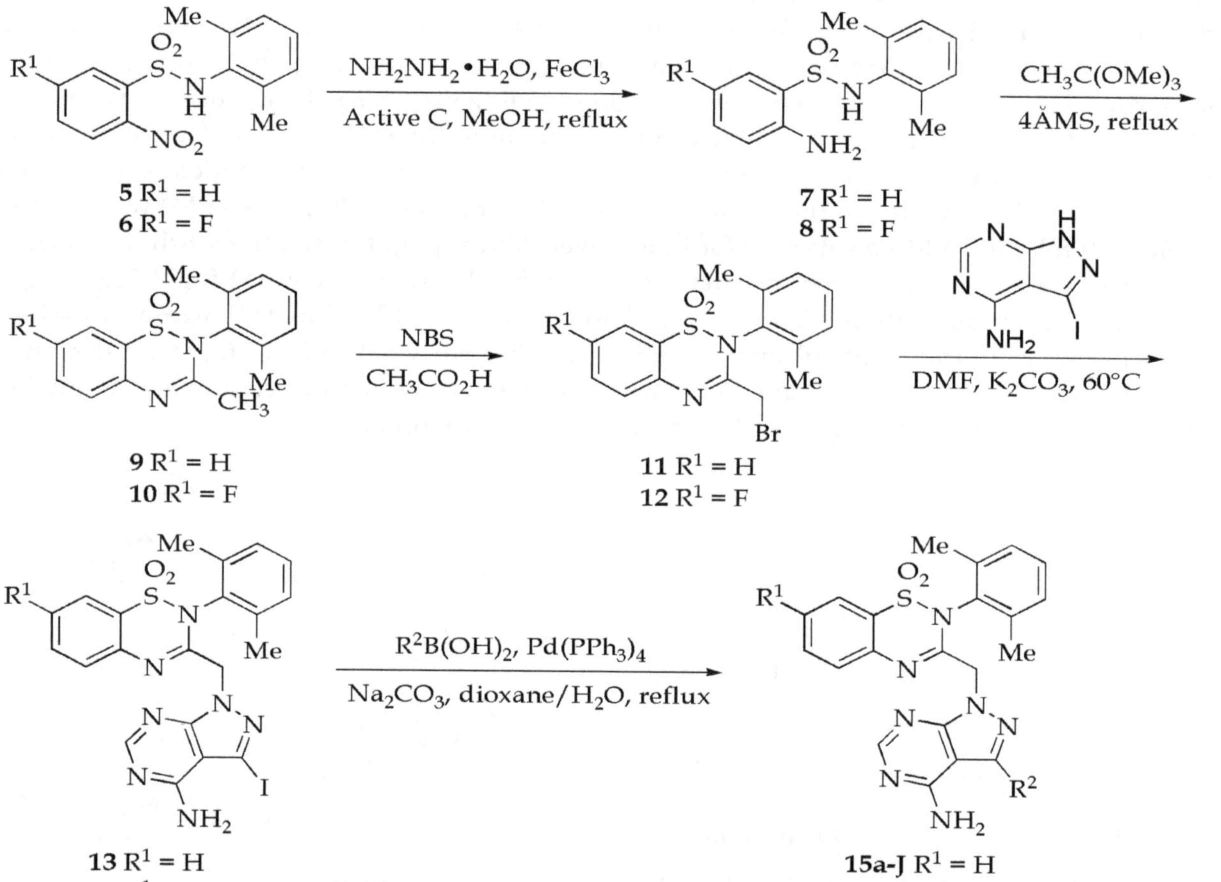

Scheme 1. Synthesis of 2*H*-benzo[*e*][1,2,4]thiadiazine 1,1-dioxide derivatives.

2.2. *PI3Kδ Inhibitory Activity and Isoform Selectivity*

Compounds **15a–J** were first tested for their inhibitory activity against PI3Kδ using the ADP-Glo luminescent assay [39], using a pan-PI3K inhibitor PI-103 as a positive control [40]. As shown in Table 1, the substitution at the 3-position of the pyrazolo[3,4-d]pyrimidine with 5-indolyl or 3,4-dimethoxyphenyl led to the relative potent analogues **15a** and **15b** with IC_{50} values of 217 to 266 nM, respectively. The 6-methoxypyridin-3-yl derivative **15d** exhibited moderate PI3Kδ inhibitory activity (IC_{50} = 498 nM), whereas the 3-fluoro-4-methoxyphenyl analogue **15c** only had marginal activity. In comparison with **15b**, the substitution of the 3,4-dimethoxypheny group for 2,3-dihydrobenzo[*b*][1,4]dioxin-6-yl (**15e**), benzo[*d*][1,3]dioxol-5-yl (**15f**), 4-methoxyphenyl (**15g**), 3-methoxyphenyl (**15h**), 4-(trifluoromethoxy)phenyl (**15i**), and phenyl (**15j**) was not tolerated, indicating the subtle requirements at the affinity pocket of PI3Kδ.

Table 1. PI3Kδ inhibitory activity of **15a–j** and **16a–d**.

Compd.	Structure	R	IC_{50} (nM) [a]
15a		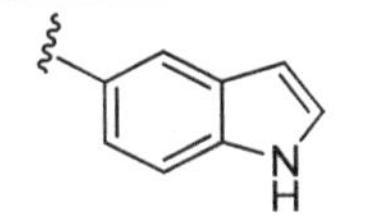	217 ± 28
15b		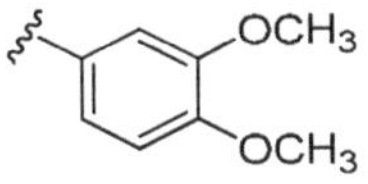	266 ± 31
15c		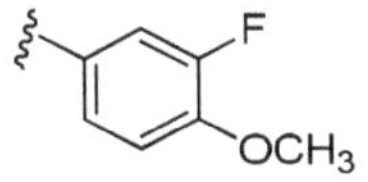	980 ± 45
15d		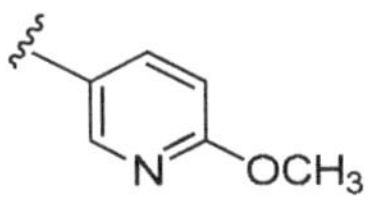	498 ± 33
15e	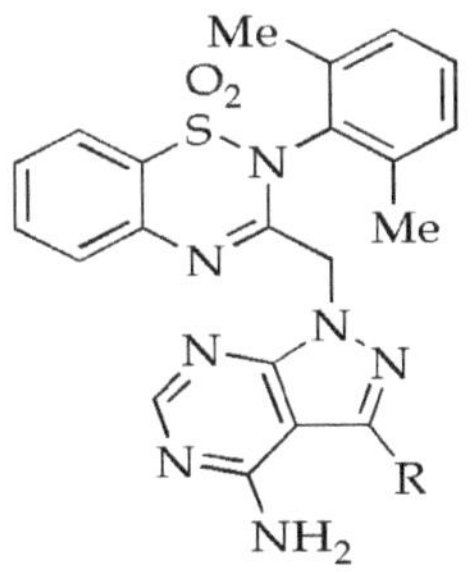	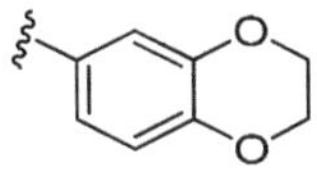	>1000
15f		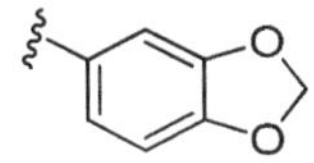	>1000
15g		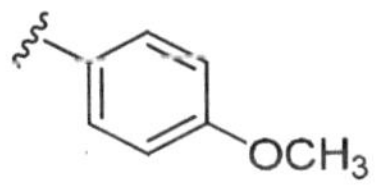	>1000
15h		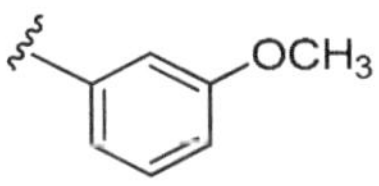	>1000
15i		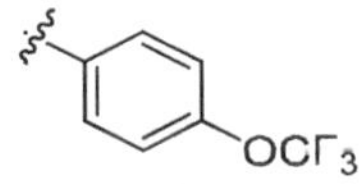	>1000
15j		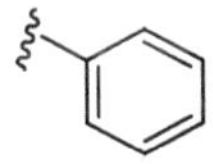	>1000
16a		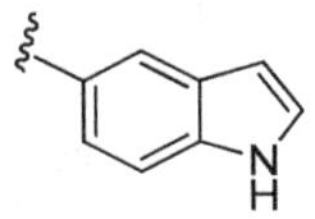	>1000
16b	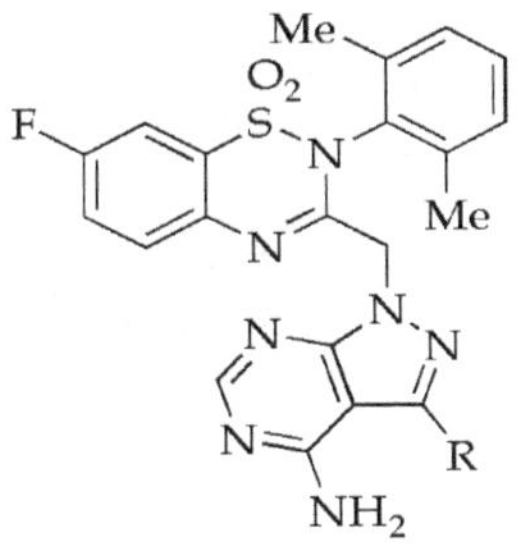	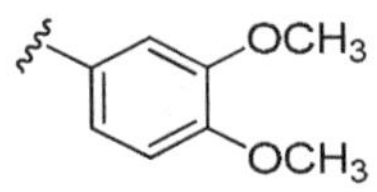	518 ± 62
16c		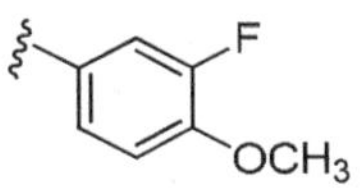	824 ± 76
16d		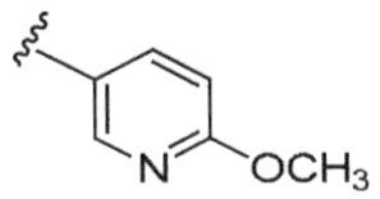	823 ± 69
	PI-103		1.6 ± 0.1

[a] The IC_{50} values are shown as the mean ± SD from two separate experiments.

In order to increase the inhibitory activity of compound **15a–d**, a fluorine atom was introduced at the 7-position of the 2*H*-benzo[*e*][1,2,4]thiadiazine 1,1-dioxide, and compounds **16a–d** were prepared and evaluated for their PI3Kδ inhibitory activity. In comparison with **15a**, the fluorinated compound **16a** lost its activity (Table 1), and compounds **16b** and **16d** showed almost 2-fold decrease in potency. In contrast, compound **16c** with a 3-fluoro-4-methoxyphenyl moiety at the affinity pocket showed a slight increase in potency.

Compared with the leading quinazolinone derivatives **3** and **4**, these 2*H*-benzo[*e*][1,2,4]-thiadiazine 1,1-dioxide derivatives **15a–j** and **16a–d** showed much decreased PI3Kδ inhibitory activity. However, the most potent derivatives **15a** and **15b** proved to be selective PI3Kδ inhibitors (Table 2). The indole derivative **15a** showed significantly lower potency against other three isoforms of class I PI3K and was more than 140-fold selective for PI3Kδ over PI3Kα, β and γ. The 3,4-dimethoxyphenyl derivative **15b** was more than 60-fold, 90-fold and 20-fold selective for PI3Kδ over PI3Kα, PI3Kβ, and PI3Kγ, respectively. In comparison with the lead **4**, **15b** was more selective over PI3Kγ (21-fold vs. 7-fold).

Table 2. The isoform selectivity and SU-DHL-6 cell growth inhibitory activity of **15a** and **15b**.

Compound	IC_{50} (nM) [a]				GI_{50} (μM) [a]
	PI3Kα	**PI3Kβ**	**PI3Kδ**	**PI3Kγ**	**SU-DHL-6**
15a	>50,000	30596 ± 875	217 ± 28	>50,000	2.13 ± 0.09
15b	16364 ± 768	24189 ± 495	266 ± 31	5838 ± 135	2.50 ± 0.11
PI-103	6.5 ± 0.7	23 ± 1.6	1.6 ± 0.1	78 ± 4.3	0.039 ± 0.011 [b]

[a] The IC_{50} or GI_{50} values are shown as the mean ± SD from two separate experiments; [b] CAL-101 was the positive control.

2.3. SU-DHL-6 Cell Growth Inhibitory Activity

The selective PI3Kδ inhibitors **15a** and **15b** were further evaluated for their antiproliferative activity against human B-cell SU-DHL-6. **15a** and **15b** significantly inhibited SU-DHL-6 cell proliferation with the GI_{50} of 2.13 and 2.50 μM, respectively (Table 2), which were in consistent with their PI3Kδ inhibitory potency.

2.4. Molecular Modeling Study

Molecular docking studies were conducted on the new discovered selective PI3Kδ inhibitors **15a** and **15b**. As shown in Figure 2, the pyrazolo[3,4-d]pyrimidine portion in both compounds **15a** and **15b** forms hydrogen bonds with Glu826 and Val828 in the hinge region.

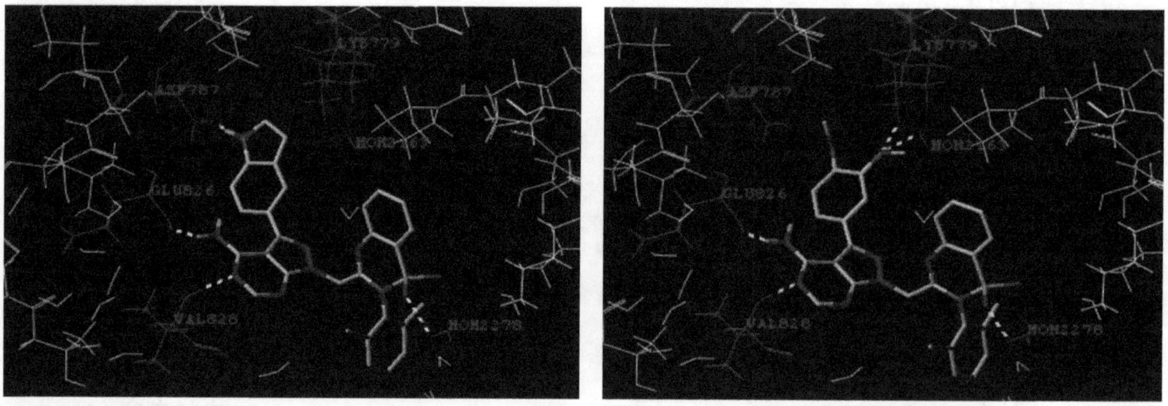

Figure 2. Molecular docking studies of **15a** (left) and **15b** (right).

Both inhibitors bind to the PI3Kδ isoform in an 'induced fit' conformation in which the 2*H*-benzo[*e*][1,2,4]thiadiazine 1,1-dioxide moiety is sandwiched between Trp760 and Met752 as these residues move apart to create the specificity pocket. The indol-5-yl (**15a**) in the specificity pocket forms an additional hydrogen bond with Asp787. Like the carbonyl oxygen in **3** and **4**, one sulfonyl oxygen in both **15a** and **15b** acts as hydrogen bond acceptor from the H_2O2278. In compound **15b**, only the 3-methoxy group forms hydrogen bonding with Lys779, while in lead **4**, the 3-methoxy interacts with Tyr813 and Asp911, the 4-methoxy interacts with Lys779 [33]. These differences may contribute its less potency against PI3Kδ than **4**. In comparison with **3** and **4**, the lack of a 8-fluorine at the 2*H*-benzo[*e*][1,2,4]thiadiazine 1,1-dioxide core in **15a** and **15b** may also be related to their lower PI3Kδ inhibitory activity.

3. Materials and Methods

3.1. General Chemical Experimental Procedures

^{1}H- and ^{13}C-NMR spectra were recorded on a Bruker-600 NMR spectrometer (Brucker Co., Ltd., Zurich, Switzerland). All spectra were recorded at room temperature for DMSO or $CDCl_3$ solutions. High resolution mass spectra (HRMS) were obtained on a 6520 QTOF instrument (Agilent Technologies Inc., Santa Clara, CA, USA by electrospray ionization (ESI). Melting points were determined on an X-6 micromelting point apparatus (Beijing Tech. Co., Ltd., Beijing, China) without corrections. Column chromatography was performed on silica gel (200–300 mesh). All reactions involving oxygen- or moisture sensitive compounds were carried out under a dry N_2 atmosphere using anhydrous solvents. Unless otherwise noted, reagents were added by syringe.

2-Amino-N-(2,6-dimethylphenyl)benzenesulfonamide (**7**)

To a stirred solution of *N*-(2,6-dimethylphenyl)-2-nitrobenzenesulfonamide (**5**, 19.4 g, 63.3 mmol) in methanol (200 mL), ferric chloride (5.1 g, 19 mmol) and activated charcoal (6.5 g) was added and refluxed for 30 min. 80% Hydrazine monohydrate (31.7 g, 633 mmol) was then added dropwise and refluxed for 5 h. After filtration, the filtrate was concentrated and the residue was dissolved in EtOAc (200 mL), washed with brine, dried over anhydrous Na_2SO_4. After filtration and evaporation, the residue was purified by silica gel chromatography (EtOAc/hexane = 1:3) to give **7** (16.5 g, 95%) as a white solid, m.p. 144–146 °C; lit. [41] m.p. 144–145 °C.

2-Amino-N-(2,6-dimethylphenyl)-5-fluorobenzenesulfonamide (**8**)

According to the procedures described for the synthesis of **7**, compound **8** were obtained as a colorless solid (16 g) in 99% yield, m.p. 185–186 °C; ^{1}H-NMR (DMSO-d_6) δ 9.44 (s, 1H, SO_2NH), 7.21 (td, J = 9.0, 3.0 Hz, 1H, Ar-H), 7.07 (td, J = 8.4, 1.5 Hz, 1H, Ar-H), 7.01 (d, J = 7.8 Hz, 2H, Ar-H), 6.97 (dd, J = 8.4, 3.0 Hz, 1H, Ar-H), 6.85 (dd, J = 9.0, 4.8 Hz, 1H, Ar-H), 5.85 (s, 2H, NH_2), 2.04 (s, 6H, 2,6-$(CH_3)_2$); MS (ESI) calcd. for $C_{14}H_{14}FN_2O_2S$ $[M-H]^-$: 293.1, found: 293.3.

2-(2,6-Dimethylphenyl)-3-methy-2H-benzo[e][1,2,4]thiadiazine 1,1-dioxide (**9**)

A mixture of **7** (5 g, 18.1 mmol), trimethyl orthoacetate (50 mL) and 4Ă molecular sieve (10 g) was refluxed for 10 h. After cooling to room temp., the mixture was concentrated and the residue was dissolved in EtOAc (200 mL), washed with brine, dried over anhydrous Na_2SO_4. After filtration and evaporation, the residue was purified by silica gel chromatography (EtOAc/hexane = 1:5) to give **9** (2.8 g, 51%) as a white solid, m.p. 162–163 °C; ^{1}H-NMR ($CDCl_3$) δ 7.89 (d, J = 7.8 Hz, 1H, Ar-H), 7.70 (td, J = 8.4, 1.2 Hz, 1H, Ar-H), 7.60 (d, J = 8.4 Hz, 1H, Ar-H), 7.47 (td, J = 7.8, 1.2 Hz, 1H, Ar-H), 7.21 (t, J = 7.2 Hz, 1H, Ar-H), 7.18 (d, J = 7.8 Hz, 2H, Ar-H), 2.22 (s, 6H, 2,6-$(CH_3)_2$), 2.11 (s, 3H, 3-CH_3); ^{13}C-NMR ($CDCl_3$) δ 154.34, 142.55, 138.58, 133.51, 132.59, 129.99, 129.27, 127.65, 127.23, 126.90, 121.01, 23.38, 18.62; MS (ESI) *m/z* calcd. for $C_{16}H_{17}N_2O_2S$ $[M+H]^+$ 301.1, found 301.0.

2-(2,6-Dimethylphenyl)-7-fluoro-3-methy-2H-benzo[e][1,2,4]thiadiazine 1,1-dioxide (**10**)

According to the procedures described for the synthesis of **9**, compound **10** were obtained as a colorless solid (6.9 g) in 40% yield, m.p. 150–151 °C; ^{1}H-NMR (DMSO-d_6) δ 7.89 (dt, J = 7.2, 1.5 Hz,

1H, Ar-H), 7.73 (dd, J = 7.2, 1.2 Hz, 2H, Ar-H), 7.36 (t, J = 7.2 Hz, 1H, Ar-H), 7.29 (d, J = 7.8 Hz, 2H, Ar-H), 2.13 (s, 6H, 2,6-$(CH_3)_2$), 2.06 (s, 3H, 3-CH_3); ^{13}C-NMR (DMSO-d_6) δ 160.28 (d, J_{C-F} = 249.2 Hz), 154.02, 139.26 (d, J_{C-F} = 3.0 Hz), 138.59, 132.62, 130.88 (d, J_{C-F} = 7.6 Hz), 130.66, 129.79, 127.96 (d, J_{C-F} = 9.1 Hz), 122.58 (d, J_{C-F} = 24.2 Hz), 107.95 (d, J_{C-F} = 27.2 Hz), 23.25, 18.47; MS (ESI) *m/z* calcd. for $C_{16}H_{16}FN_2O_2S$ $[M + H]^+$ 319.1, found 319.0.

3-Bromomethyl-2-(2,6-dimethylphenyl)-2H-benzo[e][1,2,4]thiadiazine 1,1-dioxide (**11**)

Compound **9** (1.0 g, 3.3 mmol) was dissolved in glacial acetic acid (10 mL), and then NBS (0.3 g, 1.65 mmol) was added. After the mixture was stirred at room temperature for 0.5 h, distilled water (50 mL) was added. The mixture was extracted by dichloromethane, washed with brine, dried over anhydrous Na_2SO_4. After filtration and evaporation, the residue was purified by silica gel chromatography (EtOAc/hexane = 1:10) to give **11** (0.5 g) with a conversion yield of 79% as a white solid, m.p. 150–151°C; ^{1}H-NMR ($CDCl_3$) δ 7.90 (dd, J = 7.8, 1.2 Hz, 1H, Ar-H), 7.75 (td, J = 8.4, 1.2 Hz, 1H, Ar-H), 7.69 (dd, J = 7.8, 0.6 Hz, 1H, Ar-H), 7.55 (td, J = 8.4, 1.2 Hz, 1H, Ar-H), 7.29 (t, J = 7.8 Hz, 1H, Ar-H), 7.19 (d, J = 7.8 Hz, 2H, Ar-H), 3.97 (s, 2H, CH_2Br), 2.24 (s, 6H, 2,6-$(CH_3)_2$); ^{13}C-NMR ($CDCl_3$) δ 151.86, 142.16, 138.89, 133.69, 132.14, 130.36, 129.51, 128.37, 128.25, 127.79, 121.00, 28.91, 18.95; MS (ESI) *m/z* calcd. for $C_{16}H_{16}BrN_2O_2S$ $[M + H]^+$ 379.0 and 381.0, found 381.3 and 383.4.

3-Bromomethyl-2-(2,6-dimethylphenyl)-7-fluoro-2H-benzo[e][1,2,4]thiadiazine 1,1-dioxide (**12**)

According to the procedures described for the synthesis of **11**, compound **12** were obtained as a colorless solid (0.65 g) in 72% conversion yield, m.p. 185–186 °C; ^{1}H-NMR (DMSO-d_6) δ 7.95 (dd, J = 8.4, 3.0 Hz, 1H, Ar-H), 7.84 (dd, J = 10.8, 5.4 Hz, 1H, Ar-H), 7.79 (td, J = 10.8, 3.0 Hz, 1H, Ar-H), 7.37 (t, J = 8.4 Hz, 1H, Ar-H), 7.29 (d, J = 9.0 Hz, 2H, Ar-H), 4.10 (s, 2H, CH_2Br), 2.14 (s, 6H, 2,6-$(CH_3)_2$); ^{13}C-NMR (DMSO-d_6) δ 161.21 (d, J_{C-F} = 250.6 Hz), 151.77, 138.82, 132.20, 131.54 (d, J_{C-F} = 9.1 Hz), 130.94, 129.97, 129.28, 128.60 (d, J_{C-F} = 9.1 Hz), 122.87 (d, J_{C-F} = 24.2 Hz), 108.32 (d, J_{C-F} = 25.7 Hz), 30.02, 18.72; MS (ESI) *m/z* calcd.for $C_{16}H_{15}BrFN_2O_2S$ $[M + H]^+$ 397.0 and 399.0, found 397.2 and 399.1.

3-((4-Amino-3-iodo-1H-pyrazolo[3,4-d]pyrimidin-1-yl)methyl)-2-(2,6-dimethylphenyl)-2H-benzo[e]-[1,2,4]thiadiazine 1,1-dioxide (**13**)

To a solution of **11** (1.1 g, 2.9 mmol) and 3-iodo-1*H*-pyrazolo[3,4-d]pyrimidin-4-amine (1.1 g, 4.4 mmol) in DMF (8 mL), K_2CO_3 (0.8 g, 5.8 mmol) was added. After stirring at 60 °C for 5 h, the mixture was poured into water (100 mL), extracted by EtOAc. The organic layer was washed with brine, dried over anhydrous Na_2SO_4. After filtration and evaporation, the residue was purified by silica gel chromatography (EtOAc/hexane = 1:10) to give **13** (1.4 g, 86%) as a white solid, m.p. 242–243 °C; ^{1}H-NMR (DMSO-d_6) δ 8.07 (s, 1H, Ar-H), 7.94 (dd, J = 7.8, 1.2 Hz, 1H, Ar-H), 7.80 (td, J = 7.8, 1.2 Hz, 1H, Ar-H), 7.65 (td, J = 7.8, 1.2 Hz, 1H, Ar-H), 7.43 (d, J = 7.8 Hz, 1H, Ar-H), 7.25 (t, J = 7.2 Hz, 1H, Ar-H), 7.17 (d, J= 7.2 Hz, 2H, Ar-H), 5.12 (s, 2H, NCH_2), 2.07 (s, 6H, 2,6-$(CH_3)_2$); ^{13}C-NMR ($CDCl_3$) δ 162.77, 161.35, 159.35, 156.17, 146.35, 143.45, 139.66, 136.44, 135.32, 134.48, 133.91, 133.26, 132.44, 108.30, 95.82, 60.13, 54.33, 23.17; MS (ESI) *m/z* calcd. for $C_{21}H_{19}IN_7O_2S$ $[M + H]^+$ 560.0, found 560.2.

3-((4-Amino-3-iodo-1H-pyrazolo[3,4-d]pyrimidin-1-yl)methyl)-2-(2,6-dimethylphenyl)-7-fluoro-2H-benzo-[e][1,2,4]thiadiazine 1,1-dioxide (**14**)

Following the procedures described for the synthesis of **13**, compound **14** were obtained as a white solid (1.6 g) in 58% yield, m.p. 243–244 °C; ^{1}H-NMR (DMSO-d_6) δ 8.08 (s, 1H, Ar-H), 7.92 (dd, J = 11.4, 4.2 Hz, 1H, Ar-H), 7.68 (td, J = 13.2, 4.2 Hz, 1H, Ar-H), 7.54 (dd, J = 13.2, 7.2 Hz, 1H, Ar-H), 7.26 (dd, J = 13.2, 10.2 Hz, 1H, Ar-H), 7.17 (d, J = 11.4 Hz, 2H, Ar-H), 5.13 (s, 2H, NCH_2), 2.06 (s, 6H, 2,6-$(CH_3)_2$); ^{13}C-NMR (DMSO-d_6) δ 160.89 (d, J_{C-F} = 250.7 Hz), 158.02, 156.61, 154.57, 150.89, 138.69, 131.55, 131.46 (d, J_{C-F} = 7.6 Hz), 130.64, 129.76, 128.54 (d, J_{C-F} = 7.6 Hz), 122.71 (d, J_{C-F} = 22.7 Hz), 108.28 (d, J_{C-F} = 25.7 Hz), 103.55, 91.13, 79.59, 49.55, 18.40; MS (ESI) *m/z* calcd. for $C_{21}H_{18}FIN_7O_2S$ $[M + H]^+$ 578.0, found 578.0.

3-((4-Amino-3-(1H-indol-5-yl)-1H-pyrazolo[3,4-d]pyrimidin-1-yl)methyl)-2-(2,6-dimethylphenyl)-2H-benzo[e][1,2,4]thiadiazine 1,1-dioxide (**15a**)

To a solution of **13** (180 mg, 0.30 mmol) in dioxane (4 mL) and distilled water (1.5 mL) was added 1*H*-indol-5-ylboronic acid (88 mg, 0.55 mmol), sodium carbonate anhydrous (103 mg, 0.97 mmol) and $Pd(PPh_3)_4$ (12 mg, 0.03 mmol). The mixture was degassed with N_2, and refluxed for 4 h. After cooling to room temperature, EtOAc (50 mL) and distilled water (10 mL) were added, and the organic layer was washed brine, dried over Na_2SO_4. After filtration and evaporation, the residue was purified by silica gel chromatography (EtOAc/hexane = 1:1) to give **15a** (161 mg, 91%) as a white solid, m.p. 216–217 °C; ^{1}H-NMR ($CDCl_3$) δ 11.32 (s, 1H, NH), 8.09 (s, 1H, Ar-H), 7.95 (dd, *J* = 7.8, 1.2 Hz, 1H, Ar-H), 7.81 (td, *J* = 7.8, 1.2 Hz, 2H, Ar-H), 7.65 (td, *J* = 7.8, 0.6 Hz, 1H, Ar-H), 7.57 (d, *J* = 8.4 Hz, 1H, Ar-H), 7.52 (d, *J* = 7.8 Hz, 1H, Ar-H), 7.45 (t, *J* = 3.0 Hz, 1H, Ar-H), 7.38 (dd, *J* = 8.4, 1.8 Hz, 1H, Ar-H), 7.25 (t, *J* = 7.8 Hz, 1H, Ar-H), 7.15 (d, *J* = 7.8 Hz, 2H, Ar-H), 6.55 (t, *J* = 8.4, 1.8 Hz, 1H, Ar-H), 5.20 (s, 2H, NCH_2), 2.04 (s, 6H, 2,6-$(CH_3)_2$); ^{13}C-NMR (CDCl3) δ 158.53, 156.22, 155.43, 152.04, 146.79, 141.79, 138.70, 136.53, 134.86, 131.96, 130.48, 129.70, 129.09, 128.51, 128.47, 127.83, 127.04, 123.90, 121.76, 121.20, 120.52, 112.68, 102.22, 97.86, 49.61, 18.35; HRMS (ESI) *m/z* calcd. for $C_{29}H_{25}N_8O_2S$ $[M + H]^+$ 549.1816, found 549.1829.

3-((4-Amino-3-(3,4-dimethoxyphenyl)-1H-pyrazolo[3,4-d]pyrimidin-1-yl)methyl)-2-(2,6-dimethylphenyl)-2H-benzo[e][1,2,4]thiadiazine 1,1-dioxide (**15b**)

According to the procedures described for the synthesis of **15a**, compound **15b** were obtained as a white solid (61 mg) in 75% yield, m.p. 220–222 °C; ^{1}H-NMR (DMSO-d_6) δ 8.31 (s, 1H, NH), 8.09 (s, 1H, Ar-H), 7.94 (dd, *J* = 7.8, 1.2 Hz, 1H, Ar-H), 7.81 (td, *J* = 7.8, 1.2 Hz, 1H, Ar-H), 7.65 (td, *J* = 7.2, 1.2 Hz, 1H, Ar-H), 7.50 (d, *J* = 8.4 Hz, 1H, Ar-H), 7.26 (t, *J* = 7.8 Hz, 1H, Ar-H), 7.15–7.19 (m, 4H, Ar-H), 7.12 (d, *J* = 8.4 Hz, 1H, Ar-H), 5.18 (s, 2H, NCH_2), 3.81 (s, 3H, OCH_3), 3.80 (s, 3H, OCH_3), 2.02 (s, 6H, 2,6-$(CH_3)_2$); ^{13}C-NMR (DMSO-d_6) δ 158.50, 156.26, 155.50, 151.98, 149.83, 149.51, 145.20, 141.74, 138.71, 134.86, 131.98, 130.50, 129.70, 129.13, 128.47, 127.84, 125.53, 121.19, 121.03, 112.71, 111.99, 97.70, 79.63, 56.04, 55.89, 49.64, 18.32; HRMS (ESI) *m/z* calcd. for $C_{29}H_{28}N_7O_4S$ $[M + H]^+$ 570.1918, found 570.1921.

3-((4-Amino-3-(3-fluoro-4-methoxyphenyl)-1H-pyrazolo[3,4-d]pyrimidin-1-yl)methyl)-2-(2,6-dimethyl-phenyl)-2H-benzo[e][1,2,4]thiadiazine 1,1-dioxide (**15c**)

According to the procedures described for the synthesis of **15a**, compound **15c** were obtained as a white solid (59 mg) in 66% yield, m.p. 226–227 °C; ^{1}H-NMR (DMSO-d_6) δ 8.31 (s, 1H, NH), 8.10 (s, 1H, Ar-H), 7.94 (d, *J* = 7.8 Hz, 1H, Ar-H), 7.81 (t, *J* = 7.8 Hz, 1H, Ar-H), 7.65 (t, *J* = 7.8 Hz, 1H, Ar-H), 7.49 (d, *J* = 8.4 Hz, 1H, Ar-H), 7.43–7.38 (m, 2H, Ar-H), 7.33 (t, *J* = 8.4 Hz, 1H, Ar-H), 7.25 (t, *J* = 7.8 Hz, 1H, Ar-H), 7.15 (d, *J* = 7.8 Hz, 2H, Ar-H), 5.18 (s, 2H, NCH_2), 3.90 (s, 3H, OCH_3), 2.02 (s, 6H, 2,6-$(CH_3)_2$); ^{13}C-NMR (DMSO-d_6) δ 158.50, 156.33, 155.58, 152.84, 152.03 (d, J_{C-F} = 244.6 Hz), 151.85, 148.13 (d, J_{C-F} = 9.1 Hz), 144.02, 141.72, 138.69, 134.86, 131.93, 130.51, 129.71, 128.82 (d, J_{C-F} = 95.1 Hz), 127.82, 125.78 (d, J_{C-F} = 6.0 Hz), 125.21, 121.20, 116.11 (d, J_{C-F} = 19.6 Hz), 114.91, 97.67, 79.65, 56.57, 49.64, 18.32; HRMS (ESI) *m/z* calcd. for $C_{28}H_{25}FN_7O_3S$ $[M + H]^+$ 558.1718, found 558.1733.

3-((4-Amino-3-(6-methoxypyridin-3-yl)-1H-pyrazolo[3,4-d]pyrimidin-1-yl)methyl)-2-(2,6-dimethylphenyl)-2H-benzo[e][1,2,4]thiadiazine 1,1-dioxide (**15d**)

According to the procedures described for the synthesis of **15a**, compound **15d** were obtained as a white solid (41 mg) in 47% yield, m.p. 248–249 °C; ^{1}H-NMR (DMSO-d_6) δ 8.39 (d, *J* = 1.8 Hz, 1H, Ar-H), 8.31 (s, 1H, NH), 8.11 (s, 1H, Ar-H), 7.94 (dd, *J* = 7.8, 1.2 Hz, 1H, Ar-H), 7.92 (dd, *J* = 8.4, 2.4 Hz, 1H, Ar-H), 7.81 (td, *J* = 8.4, 1.2 Hz, 1H, Ar-H), 7.65 (td, *J* =7.8, 1.2 Hz, 1H, Ar-H), 7.49 (d, *J* = 7.8 Hz, 1H, Ar-H), 7.26 (t, *J* = 7.8 Hz, 1H, Ar-H), 7.16 (d, *J* = 7.8 Hz, 2H, Ar-H), 6.98 (d, *J* = 8.4 Hz, 1H, Ar-H), 5.20 (s, 2H, NCH_2), 3.92 (s, 3H, OCH_3), 2.03 (s, 6H, 2,6-$(CH_3)_2$); ^{13}C-NMR (DMSO-d_6) δ 164.14, 158.60, 156.38, 155.61, 151.81, 146.69, 142.36, 141.71, 139.29, 138.69, 134.87, 131.91, 130.51, 129.70, 129.13, 128.50, 127.80, 122.70, 121.19, 111.48, 97.92, 79.64, 53.89, 49.66, 18.33; HRMS (ESI) *m/z* calcd. for $C_{27}H_{25}N_8O_4S$ $[M + H]^+$ 541.1765, found 541.1781.

3-((4-Amino-3-(2,3-dihydrobenzo[b][1,4]dioxin-6-yl)-1H-pyrazolo[3,4-d]pyrimidin-1-yl)methyl)-2-(2,6-dimethylphenyl)-2H-benzo[e][1,2,4]thiadiazine 1,1-dioxide (**15e**)

According to the procedures described for the synthesis of **15a**, compound **15e** were obtained as a white solid (71 mg) in 64% yield, m.p. 225–226 °C; ^{1}H-NMR (DMSO-d_6) δ 8.31 (s, 1H, NH), 8.08 (s, 1H, Ar-H), 7.94 (dd, *J* = 7.8, 1.2 Hz, 1H, Ar-H), 7.82 (td, *J* = 7.8, 1.2 Hz, 1H, Ar-H), 7.65 (td, *J* = 7.8, 1.2 Hz, 1H, Ar-H), 7.51 (d, *J* = 8.4 Hz, 1H, Ar-H), 7.24 (t, *J* = 8.4 Hz, 1H, Ar-H), 7.14 (d, *J* = 7.8 Hz, 2H, Ar-H), 7.11–7.09 (m, 2H, Ar-H), 7.02 (d, *J* = 7.8 Hz, 1H, Ar-H), 5.18 (s, 2H, NCH_2), 4.30 (s, 4H, OCH_2CH_2O), 2.01 (s, 6H, 2,6-$(CH_3)_2$); ^{13}C-NMR (DMSO-d_6) δ 158.45, 156.25, 155.47, 151.92, 144.79, 144.60, 144.23, 141.74, 138.66, 134.86, 131.94, 130.47, 129.68, 129.12, 128.48, 127.83, 126.18, 121.59, 121.19, 118.30, 117.23, 97.63, 79.64, 64.67, 64.59, 49.62, 18.30; HRMS (ESI) *m/z* calcd. for $C_{29}H_{26}N_7O_4S$ $[M + H]^+$ 568.1761, found 568.1775.

3-((4-Amino-3-(benzo[d][1,3]dioxol-5-yl)-1H-pyrazolo[3,4-d]pyrimidin-1-yl)methyl)-2-(2,6-dimethyl-phenyl)-2H-benzo[e][1,2,4]thiadiazine 1,1-dioxide (**15f**)

According to the procedures described for the synthesis of **15a**, compound **15f** were obtained as a white solid (29 mg) in 34% yield, m.p. > 250 °C; ^{1}H-NMR (DMSO-d_6) δ 8.31 (s, 1H, NH), 8.08 (s, 1H, Ar-H), 7.94 (dd, *J* = 7.8, 1.2 Hz, 1H, Ar-H), 7.82 (td, *J* = 7.8, 1.2 Hz, 1H, Ar-H), 7.65 (td, *J* = 7.8, 1.2 Hz, 1H, Ar-H), 7.50 (d, *J* = 7.8 Hz, 1H, Ar-H), 7.25 (t, *J* = 7.8 Hz, 1H, Ar-H), 7.15 (d, *J* = 7.2 Hz, 2H, Ar-H), 7.12–7.09 (m, 2H, Ar-H), 7.07 (d, *J* = 8.4, 1H, Ar-H), 6.10 (s, 2H, OCH_2O), 5.17 (s, 2H, NCH_2), 2.01 (s, 6H, 2,6-$(CH_3)_2$); ^{13}C-NMR (DMSO-d_6) δ 158.44, 156.28, 155.47, 151.89, 148.36, 144.98, 141.73, 138.67, 134.87, 131.93, 130.49, 129.70, 129.14, 128.50, 127.82, 126.85, 122.65, 121.19, 109.44, 108.80, 101.89, 97.65, 79.64, 49.62, 18.30; HRMS (ESI) *m/z* calcd. for $C_{28}H_{24}N_7O_4S$ $[M + H]^+$ 554.1605, found 554.1614.

3-((4-Amino-3-(4-methoxyphenyl)-1H-pyrazolo[3,4-d]pyrimidin-1-yl)methyl)-2-(2,6-dimethylphenyl)-2H-benzo[e][1,2,4]thiadiazine 1,1-dioxide (**15g**)

According to the procedures described for the synthesis of **15a**, compound **15g** were obtained as a white solid (45 mg) in 74% yield, m.p. 248–249 °C; ^{1}H-NMR (DMSO-d_6) δ 8.32 (s, 1H, NH), 8.09 (s, 1H, Ar-H), 7.94 (dd, *J* = 7.8, 1.2 Hz, 1H, Ar-H), 7.82 (td, *J* = 7.8, 1.2 Hz, 1H, Ar-H), 7.65 (td, *J* = 7.8, 1.2 Hz, 1H, Ar-H), 7.57 (d, *J* = 8.4 Hz, 2H, Ar-H), 7.50 (d, *J* = 8.4 Hz, 1H, Ar-H), 7.25 (t, *J* = 7.8 Hz, 1H, Ar-H), 7.15 (d, *J* = 7.8 Hz, 2H, Ar-H), 7.11 (d, *J* = 8.4 Hz, 2H, Ar-H), 5.19 (s, 2H, NCH_2), 3.82 (s, 3H, OCH_3), 2.02 (s, 6H, 2,6-$(CH_3)_2$); ^{13}C-NMR (DMSO-d_6) δ160.18, 158.51, 156.26, 155.51, 151.92, 145.03, 141.75, 138.69, 134.85, 131.93, 130.48, 129.95, 129.69, 129.10, 128.49, 127.82, 125.43, 121.19, 115.12, 97.70, 79.63, 55.72, 49.60, 18.34; HRMS (ESI) *m/z* calcd. for $C_{28}H_{26}N_7O_3S$ $[M + H]^+$ 540.1812, found 540.1829.

3-((4-Amino-3-(3-methoxyphenyl)-1H-pyrazolo[3,4-d]pyrimidin-1-yl)methyl)-2-(2,6-dimethylphenyl)-2H-benzo[e][1,2,4]thiadiazine 1,1-dioxide (**15h**)

According to the procedures described for the synthesis of **15a**, compound **15h** were obtained as a white solid (46 mg) in 59% yield, m.p. 221–222 °C; ^{1}H-NMR (DMSO-d_6) δ 8.31 (s, 1H), 8.10 (s, 1H, Ar-H), 7.94 (dd, *J* = 7.8, 1.2 Hz, 1H, Ar-H), 7.82 (td, *J* = 7.8, 1.2 Hz, 1H, Ar-H), 7.63 (td, *J* = 7.8, 1.2 Hz, 1H, Ar-H), 7.50 (d, *J* = 7.8 Hz, 1H, Ar-H), 7.47 (t, *J* = 7.8 Hz, 1H, Ar-H), 7.26 (t, *J* = 7.8 Hz, 1H, Ar-H), 7.23 (d, *J* = 7.8 Hz, 1H, Ar-H), 7.20–7.11 (m, 3H, Ar-H), 7.06 (dd, *J* = 8.4, 2.4 Hz, 1H, Ar-H), 5.21 (s, 2H, NCH_2), 3.82 (s, 3H, OCH_3), 2.02 (s, 6H, 2,6-$(CH_3)_2$); ^{13}C-NMR (DMSO-d_6) δ 160.11, 158.43, 156.31, 155.56, 151.88, 145.02, 141.72, 138.70, 134.87, 134.36, 131.95, 130.86, 130.51, 129.71, 129.14, 128.48, 127.83, 121.20, 120.76, 115.19, 113.85, 97.74, 79.64, 55.63, 49.68, 18.32; HRMS (ESI) *m/z* calcd. for $C_{28}H_{26}N_7O_3S$ $[M + H]^+$ 540.1812, found 540.1825.

3-((4-Amino-3-(4-(trifluoromethoxy)phenyl)-1H-pyrazolo[3,4-d]pyrimidin-1-yl)methyl)-2-(2,6-dimethyl-phenyl)-2H-benzo[e][1,2,4]thiadiazine 1,1-dioxide (**15i**)

According to the procedures described for the synthesis of **15a**, compound **15i** were obtained as a white solid (61 mg) in 61% yield, m.p. 206–207 °C; ^{1}H-NMR (DMSO-d_6) δ 8.12 (s, 1H, Ar-H), 7.94 (dd, *J*

= 8.4, 1.2 Hz, 1H, Ar-H), 7.81 (dt, J = 8.4, 1.2 Hz, 1H, Ar-H), 7.76 (d, J =8.4 Hz, 2H, Ar-H), 7.65 (dt, J = 8.4, 0.6 Hz, 1H, Ar-H), 7.52 (d, J = 7.8 Hz, 2H, Ar-H), 7.48 (d, J = 7.8 Hz, 1H, Ar-H), 7.26 (t, J = 7.8 Hz, 1H, Ar-H), 7.16 (d, J = 7.8 Hz, 2 H, Ar-H), 5.21 (s, 2H), 2.03 (s, 6H); ^{13}C-NMR (DMSO-d_6) δ 158.52, 156.38, 155.72, 151.77, 149.08, 143.91, 141.70, 138.70, 134.87, 132.28, 131.90, 130.59, 130.53, 129.72, 129.14, 128.50, 127.80, 122.10, 121.21, 120.57 (q, J_{C-F} = 256.70 Hz), 97.73, 49.68, 18.34; HRMS (ESI) *m/z* calcd. for $C_{28}H_{23}F_3N_7O_3S$ [M + H]$^+$ 594.1530, found 594.1547.

3-((4-Amino-3-phenyl-1H-pyrazolo[3,4-d]pyrimidin-1-yl)methyl)-2-(2,6-dimethylphenyl)-2H-benzo[e]-[1,2,4]thiadiazine 1,1-dioxide (**15j**)

According to the procedures described for the synthesis of **15a**, compound **15j** were obtained as a white solid (40 mg) in 73% yield, m.p. 193–194 °C; ^{1}H-NMR (DMSO-d_6) δ 8.30 (s, 1H, NH), 8.09 (s, 1H, Ar-H), 7.92 (dd, J = 7.8, 1.2 Hz, 1H, Ar-H), 7.80 (td, J = 7.8, 1.2 Hz, 1H, Ar-H), 7.66–7.62 (m, 3H, Ar-H), 7.54 (t, J = 7.8 Hz, 2H, Ar-H), 7.52–7.32 (m, 2H, Ar-H), 7.24 (t, J = 7.8 Hz, 2H, Ar-H), 7.14 (d, J = 7.8 Hz, 2H, Ar-H), 5.19 (s, 2H, NCH_2), 2.01 (s, 6H, 2,6-$(CH_3)_2$); ^{13}C-NMR (DMSO-d_6) δ 1158.46, 156.31, 155.60, 151.86, 145.16, 141.72, 138.69, 134.54, 133.53, 132.51, 131.99, 131.92, 130.51, 130.47, 129.71, 129.67, 129.27, 129.20, 128.60, 127.81, 121.20, 97.73, 79.65, 49.65, 18.34; HRMS (ESI) *m/z* calcd. for $C_{27}H_{24}N_7O_2S$ [M + H]$^+$ 510.1707, found 510.1722.

3-((4-Amino-3-(1H-indol-5-yl)-1H-pyrazolo[3,4-d]pyrimidin-1-yl)methyl)-2-(2,6-dimethylphenyl)-7-fluoro-2H-benzo[e][1,2,4]thiadiazine 1,1-dioxide (**16a**)

According to the procedures described for the synthesis of **15a**, compound **16a** were obtained as a white solid (65 mg) in 73% yield, m.p. 132–133 °C; ^{1}H-NMR (DMSO-d_6) δ 8.30 (s, 1H, NH), 8.08 (s, 1H, Ar-H), 7.91 (dd, J = 7.2, 2.4 Hz, 1H, Ar-H), 7.81 (brs, 1H, Ar-H), 7.69 (td, J = 9.6, 3.0 Hz, 1H, Ar-H), 7.61 (dd, J = 9.0, 4.8 Hz, 1H, Ar-H), 7.56 (d, J = 8.4 Hz, 1H, Ar-H), 7.44 (t, J = 3.0 Hz, 1H, Ar-H), 7.36 (dd, J = 8.4, 1.8 Hz, 1H, Ar-H), 7.25 (t, J = 7.28Hz, 1H, Ar-H), 7.16 (t, J = 7.8 Hz, 2H, Ar-H), 6.54 (s, 1H, 3-CH-indolyl), 5.20 (s, 2H, NCH_2), 2.01 (s, 6H, 2,6-$(CH_3)_2$); ^{13}C-NMR (DMSO-d_6) δ 160.08 (d, J_{C-F} = 250.7 Hz), 158.52, 156.23, 155.41, 151.51, 146.84, 138.68, 138.61 (d, J_{C-F} = 3.0 Hz), 136.53, 131.81, 131.44 (d, J_{C-F} = 9.1 Hz), 130.55, 129.74, 128.66 (d, J_{C-F} = 9.1 Hz), 128.46, 127.05, 123.87, 122.67 (d, J_{C-F} = 24.2 Hz), 121.74, 120.52, 112.67, 108.19 (d, J_{C-F} = 27.2 Hz), 102.21, 97.85, 79.65, 49.57, 18.32; HRMS (ESI) *m/z* calcd. for $C_{29}H_{24}FN_8O_2S$ [M + H]$^+$ 567.1721, found 567.1739.

3-((A-amino-3-(3,4-dimethoxyphenyl)-1H-pyrazolo[3,4-d]pyrimidin-1-yl)methyl)-2-(2,6-dimethylphenyl)-7-fluoro-2H-benzo[e][1,2,4]thiadiazine 1,1-dioxide (**16b**)

According to the procedures described for the synthesis of **15a**, compound **16b** were obtained as a white solid (47 mg) in 51% yield, m.p. 229–230 °C; ^{1}H-NMR (DMSO-d_6) δ 8.31 (s, 1H, NH), 8.09 (s, 1H, Ar-H), 7.91 (dd, J = 7.2, 2.4 Hz, 1H, Ar-H), 7.69 (td, J = 9.0, 2.4 Hz, 1H, Ar-H), 7.59 (dd, J = 9.0, 4.8 Hz, 1H, Ar-H), 7.26 (t, J = 7.8 Hz, 1H, Ar-H), 7.21–7.10 (m, 5H, Ar-H), 5.19 (s, 2H, NCH_2), 3.82 (s, 3H, OCH_3), 3.81 (s, 3H, OCH_3), 2.01 (s, 6H, 2,6-$(CH_3)_2$); ^{13}C-NMR (DMSO-d_6) δ 160.78 (d, J_{C-F} = 250.7 Hz), 158.51, 156.27, 155.49, 151.46, 149.84, 149.52, 145.24, 138.70, 138.57 (d, J_{C-F} = 3.0 Hz), 131.84, 131.41 (d, J_{C-F} = 7.6 Hz), 130.57, 129.74, 128.69 (d, J_{C-F} = 7.6 Hz), 125.52, 122.66 (d, J_{C-F} = 24.2 Hz), 121.03, 112.72, 112.02, 108.20 (d, J_{C-F} = 27.2 Hz), 97.71, 79.65, 56.04, 55.89, 49.60, 18.31; HRMS (ESI) *m/z* calcd. for $C_{29}H_{27}FN_7O_4S$ [M + H]$^+$ 588.1824, found 588.1838.

3-((4-Amino-3-(3-fluoro-4-methoxyphenyl)-1H-pyrazolo[3,4-d]pyrimidin-1-yl)methyl)-2-(2,6-dimethyl-phenyl)-7-fluoro-2H-benzo[e][1,2,4]thiadiazine 1,1-dioxide (**16c**)

According to the procedures described for the synthesis of **15a**, compound **16c** were obtained as a white solid (76 mg) in 84% yield, m.p. 201–202 °C; ^{1}H-NMR (DMSO-d_6) δ 8.31 (s, 1H, NH), 8.09 (s, 1H, Ar-H), 7.91 (dd, J = 7.2, 3.0 Hz, 1H, Ar-H), 7.69 (td, J = 7.4, 2.4 Hz, 1H, Ar-H), 7.59 (dd, J = 9.0, 4.2 Hz, 1H, Ar-H), 7.44–7.38 (m, 2H, Ar-H), 7.33 (t, J = 9.0 Hz, 1H, Ar-H), 7.26 (t, J = 7.2 Hz, 1H, Ar-H), 7.15 (d, J = 7.8 Hz, 2H, Ar-H), 5.19 (s, 2H, NCH_2), 3.90 (s, 3H, OCH_3), 2.01 (s, 6H, 2,6-$(CH_3)_2$);

^{13}C-NMR (DMSO-d$_6$) δ 160.89 (d, J_{C-F} = 250.7 Hz), 158.50, 156.34, 155.56, 152.02 (d, J_{C-F} = 246.1 Hz), 151.32, 148.14 (d, J_{C-F} = 10.6 Hz), 144.06, 138.68, 138.62 (d, J_{C-F} = 19.6 Hz), 131.78, 131.44 (d, J_{C-F} = 7.6 Hz), 130.59, 129.74, 128.66 (d, J_{C-F} = 7.6 Hz), 125.76 (d, J_{C-F} = 7.6 Hz), 125.21, 122.68 (d, J_{C-F} = 22.7 Hz), 116.11 (d, J_{C-F} = 19.6 Hz), 114.92, 108.21 (d, J_{C-F} = 25.7 Hz), 97.67, 79.63, 56.59, 49.61, 18.30; HRMS (ESI) *m/z* calcd. for $C_{28}H_{24}F_2N_7O_3S$ [M + H]$^+$ 576.1624, found 576.1637.

3-((4-Amino-3-(6-methoxypyridin-3-yl)-1H-pyrazolo[3,4-d]pyrimidin-1-yl)methyl)-2-(2,6-dimethylphenyl)-7-fluoro-2H-benzo[e][1,2,4]thiadiazine 1,1-dioxide (**16d**)

According to the procedures described for the synthesis of **15a**, compound **16d** were obtained as a white solid (51 mg) in 58% yield, m.p. 225–226 °C; ^{1}H-NMR (DMSO-d$_6$) δ 8.38 (s, 1H, NH), 8.31 (s, 1H, Ar-H), 8.10 (s, 1H, Ar-H), 7.90 (d, *J* = 8.4 Hz, 2H, Ar-H), 7.69 (t, *J* = 7.2 Hz, 1H, Ar-H), 7.59 (dd, *J* = 9.0, 4.2 Hz, 1H, Ar-H), 7.25 (t, *J* = 7.2 Hz, 1H, Ar-H), 7.15 (d, *J* = 8.4 Hz, 2H, Ar-H), 6.97 (d, *J* = 8.4 Hz, 1H, Ar-H), 5.20 (s, 2H, NCH$_2$), 3.92 (s, 3H, OCH$_3$), 2.01 (s, 6H, 2,6-(CH$_3$)$_2$); ^{13}C-NMR (DMSO-d$_6$) δ 164.15, 160.89 (d, J_{C-F} = 250.7 Hz), 158.60, 156.39, 155.59, 151.29, 146.69, 142.41, 139.29, 138.69, 138.54 (d, J_{C-F} = 3.0 Hz), 131.77, 131.45 (d, J_{C-F} = 7.6 Hz), 130.59, 129.74, 128.66 (d, J_{C-F} = 9.1 Hz), 122.75, 122.68, 122.67 (d, J_{C-F} = 22.7 Hz), 111.48, 108.20 (d, J_{C-F} = 27.2 Hz), 97.93, 79.64, 53.89, 49.63, 18.32; HRMS (ESI) *m/z* calcd. for $C_{27}H_{24}FN_8O_3S$ [M + H]$^+$ 559.1671, found 559.1678.

3.2. PI3K Kinase Assay

The ADP-Glo luminescent assay was used for PI3Kδ, PI3Kβ and PI3Kγ isoforms and the kinase-Glo luminescent assay was used for PI3Kα according to the standard protocols of Promega [40]. PI-103 was used as a positive control. The compounds were tested from 1 μM or 10 μM, 3-fold dilution, in duplicate for 10 concentrations. The kinase reaction was done in 384-well plate (Corning, Los Altos, MA, USA). Each well was loaded with test compounds (in 100% DMSO) and reaction buffer containing PI substrate. After the PI3K proteins were then added, the reaction was started by the addition of PIP2 and ATP prepared in the reaction buffer and ran for either 60 (for PI3Kα, PI3Kβ, and PI3Kγ) or 120 min (for PI3Kδ). ADP-Glo reagent was then added to terminate the reavtion. The plates were then read in a Synergy 2 reader (BioTek, Shanghai, China) for luminescence detection.

3.3. Cell Proliferation Assay

Cell proliferation was evaluated by The CellTiter-Glo luminescent cell viability assay (Promega, Shanghai, China) was used to evaluate the inhibitory activity of compounds **15a** and **15b** following the manufacturer's protocol. In brief, SU-DHL-6 (ATCC) cells were seeded in 96-well plates (Corning, Los Altos, MA, USA) at density of 1×10^4 cells per well, and incubated with medium alone or with the tested compounds at the indicated concentrations (50 μM in DMSO, 3-fold dilution, in duplicate for 10 concentrations). 50 μL CellTiter-Glo (Promega, Shanghai, China) reagent was added to each well to induce cell lysis, and the plate was incubated at room temperature for 10 min to stabilize luminescent signal. After 100 μL of the mixture from each well was transferred to a new 96-well black plate, the fluorescence signal was read on EnVision (Shanghai, China) and the data were analysized by XLFit 4 software (IDBS, Berlin, Germany).

3.4. Molecular Docking

X-ray cocrystal structure of PI3Kδ enzyme was downloaded from RCSB Protein Date Bank (PDB ID: 2WXH) [42]. The molecular docking of **15a** and **15b** was carried out following the same procedures as reported for compounds **3** and **4** [33].

4. Conclusions

In a continuous study to find more potent and selective PI3Kδ inhibitors based on the rotation-limiting strategy, we substituted the carbonyl in the quinazolinone core for the sulfonyl group, designed and synthesized a series of novel 2*H*-benzo[*e*][1,2,4]thiadiazine 1,1-dioxide derivatives

15a–J and **16a–d**. In agreement with the quinazolinone derivatives, the introduction of a 5-indolyl or 3,4-dimethoxyphenyl at the affinity pocket generated the most potent analogues **15a** and **15b** with the IC_{50} values of 217 to 266 nM, respectively. In comparison with the quinazolinone lead compounds **3** and **4**, the 2*H*-benzo[*e*][1,2,4]thiadiazine 1,1-dioxide derivatives exhibited much reduced PI3Kδ inhibitory activity, but maintained high selectivity over other PI3K isoforms. Unlike the quinazolinone lead compound **4** that was a dual PI3Kδ/γ inhibitor, the 2*H*-benzo[*e*][1,2,4]thiadiazine 1,1-dioxide **15b** was more than 21-fold selective over PI3Kγ. This may provide a structural base for the further design of more potent and selective PI3Kδ inhibitors. In agreement with their high PI3Kδ inhibitory activity, **15a** and **15b** exhibited high antiproliferative potency against B-cell leukemia SU-DHL-6 cells.

Author Contributions: Conceptualization, Y.-P.G. and Z.-P.L.; methodology, Y.-P.G., L.-Q.T. and T.-S.L.; validation, Y.-P.G., L.-Q.T. and T.-S.L.; formal analysis, L.-Q.T. and Y.-P.G.; investigation, Y.-P.G., L.-Q.T. and T.-S.L.; resources, Z.-P.L.; data curation, L.-Q.T. and Y.-P.G.; writing—original draft preparation, L.-Q.T.; writing—review and editing, Z.-P.L.; visualization, Y.-P.G. and L.-Q.T.; supervision, Z.-P.L.; project administration, Z.-P.L.; funding acquisition, Z.-P.L.

Abbreviations

PI3Ks	Phosphoinositide 3-kinases
PIP2	Phosphatidylinositol 4,5-bisphosphate
NBS	*N*-Bromosuccinimide
ADP	Adenosine diphosphate
ATP	Adenosine triphosphate
DMSO	Dimethyl sulfoxide
APDS	PI3Kδ syndrome
FL	Follicular lymphoma
SLL	Small lymphocytic lymphoma
CLL	Chronic lymphocytic leukemia

References

1. Toker, A.; Cantley, L.C. Signalling through the lipid products of phosphoinositide-3-OH kinase. *Nature* **1997**, *387*, 673–676. [CrossRef] [PubMed]
2. Cantley, L.C. The phosphoinositide 3-kinase pathway. *Science* **2002**, *296*, 1655–1657. [CrossRef] [PubMed]
3. Brachmann, S.M.; Yballe, C.M.; Innocenti, M.; Deane, J.A.; Fruman, D.A.; Thomas, S.M.; Cantley, L.C. Role of phosphoinositide 3-kinase regulatory isoforms in development and actin rearrangement. *Mol. Cell. Biol.* **2005**, *25*, 2593–2606. [CrossRef] [PubMed]
4. Vanhaesebroeck, B.; Guillermet-Guibert, J.; Graupera, M.; Bilanges, B. The emerging mechanisms of isoform specific PI3K signaling. *Nat. Rev. Mol. Cell Biol.* **2010**, *11*, 329–341. [CrossRef]
5. Engelman, J.A.; Luo, J.; Cantley, L.C. The evolution of phosphatidylinositol 3-kinases as regulators of growth and metabolism. *Nat. Rev. Genet.* **2006**, *7*, 606–619. [CrossRef] [PubMed]
6. Jimenez, C.; Hernandez, C.; Pimentel, B.; Carrera, A.C. The p85 regulatory subunit controls sequential activation of phosphoinositide 3-kinase by tyr kinases and ras. *J. Biol. Chem.* **2002**, *277*, 41556–41562. [CrossRef] [PubMed]
7. Brock, C.; Schaefer, M.; Reusch, H.P.; Czupalla, C.; Michalke, M.; Spicher, K.; Schultz, G.; Nurnberg, B. Roles of Gβγ in membrane recruitment and activation of p110γ/p101 phosphoinositide 3-kinase γ. *J. Cell Biol.* **2003**, *160*, 89–99. [CrossRef]
8. Okkenhaug, K.; Vanhaesebroeck, B. PI3K in lymphocyte development, differentiation and activation. *Nat. Rev. Immunol.* **2003**, *3*, 317–330. [CrossRef]

9. Liu, L.; Puri, K.D.; Penninger, J.M.; Kubes, P. Leukocyte PI3Kγ and PI3Kδ have temporally distinct roles for leukocyte recruitment in vivo. *Blood* **2007**, *110*, 1191–1198. [CrossRef]
10. Thomas, M.J.; Smith, A.; Head, D.H.; Milne, L.; Nicholls, A.; Pearce, W.; Vanhaesebroeck, B.; Wymann, M.P.; Hirsch, E.; Trifilieff, A.; et al. Airway inflammation: Chemokine-induced neutrophilia and the class I phosphoinositide 3-kinases. *Eur. J. Immunol.* **2005**, *35*, 1283–1291. [CrossRef]
11. Fruman, D.A.; Rommel, C. PI3K and cancer: Lessons, challenges and opportunities. *Nat. Rev. Drug Discov.* **2014**, *13*, 140–156. [CrossRef] [PubMed]
12. Thorpe, L.M.; Yuzugullu, H.; Zhao, J.J. PI3K in cancer: Divergent roles of isoforms, modes of activation and therapeutic targeting. *Nat. Rev. Cancer* **2015**, *15*, 7–24. [CrossRef] [PubMed]
13. Janku, F. Phosphoinositide 3-kinase (PI3K) pathway inhibitors in solid tumors: From laboratory to patients. *Cancer Treat. Rev.* **2017**, *59*, 93–101. [CrossRef] [PubMed]
14. Fruman, D.A.; Chiu, H.; Hopkins, B.D.; Bagrodia, S.; Cantley, L.C.; Abraham, R.T. The PI3K pathway in human disease. *Cell* **2017**, *170*, 605–635. [CrossRef]
15. Zhao, W.; Qiu, Y.; Kong, D. Class I phosphatidylinositol 3-kinase inhibitors for cancer therapy. *Acta Pharm. Sin. B* **2017**, *7*, 27–37. [CrossRef]
16. Garces, A.E.; Stocks, M.J. Class 1 PI3K clinical candidates and recent inhibitor design strategies: A medicinal chemistry perspective. *J. Med. Chem.* **2019**, *62*, 4815–4850. [CrossRef]
17. Knight, Z.A.; Gonzalez, B.; Feldman, M.E.; Zunder, E.R.; Goldenberg, D.D.; Williams, O.; Loewith, R.; Stokoe, D.; Balla, A.; Toth, B.; et al. A pharmacological map of the PI3-K family defines a role for P110α in insulin signaling. *Cell* **2006**, *125*, 733–747. [CrossRef]
18. Huang, X.; Liu, G.; Guo, J.; Su, Z. The PI3K/AKT Pathway in obesity and type 2 diabetes. *Int. J. Biol. Sci.* **2018**, *14*, 1483–1496. [CrossRef]
19. Jackson, S.P.; Schoenwaelder, S.M.; Goncalves, I.; Nesbitt, W.S.; Yap, C.L.; Wright, C.E.; Kenche, V.; Anderson, K.E.; Dopheide, S.M.; Yuan, Y.; et al. PI 3-Kinase P110β: A new target for antithrombotic therapy. *Nat. Med.* **2005**, *11*, 507–514. [CrossRef]
20. Jackson, S.P.; Schoenwaelder, S.M. Antithrombotic phosphoinositide 3-kinase β inhibitors in humans: A 'shear' delight! *J. Thromb. Haemostasis* **2012**, *10*, 2123–2126. [CrossRef]
21. Cushing, T.D.; Metz, D.P.; Whittington, D.A.; McGee, L.R. PI3Kδ and PI3Kγ as targets for autoimmune and inflammatory diseases. *J. Med. Chem.* **2012**, *55*, 8559–8581. [CrossRef] [PubMed]
22. Rowan, W.C.; Smith, J.L.; Affleck, K.; Amour, A. Targeting phosphoinositide 3-kinase δ for allergic asthma. *Biochem. Soc. Trans.* **2012**, *40*, 240–245. [CrossRef] [PubMed]
23. Yoo, E.J.; Ojiaku, C.A.; Sunder, K.; Panettieri, R.A. Phosphoinositide 3-kinase in asthma: Novel roles and therapeutic approaches. *Am. J. Respir. Cell Mol. Biol.* **2017**, *56*, 700–707. [CrossRef] [PubMed]
24. Perry, M.W.D.; Abdulai, R.; Mogemark, M.; Petersen, J.; Thomas, M.J.; Valastro, B.; Eriksson, A.W. Evolution of PI3Kγ and δ Inhibitors for inflammatory and autoimmune diseases. *J. Med. Chem.* **2019**, *62*, 4783–4814. [CrossRef]
25. Kracker, S.; Curtis, J.; Ibrahim, M.A.A.; Sediva, A.; Salisbury, J.; Campr, V.; Debré, M.; Edgar, J.D.M.; Imai, K.; Picard, C.; et al. Occurrence of B-cell lymphomas in patients with activated phosphoinositide 3-kinase δ syndrome. *J. Allergy Clin. Immunol.* **2014**, *134*, 233–236. [CrossRef]
26. Elkaim, E.; Neven, B.; Bruneau, J.; Mitsui-Sekinaka, K.; Stanislas, A.; Heurtier, L.; Lucas, C.L.; Matthews, H.; Deau, M.-C.; Sharapova, S.; et al. Clinical and immunologic phenotype associated with activated phosphoinositide 3-kinase δ syndrome 2: A cohort study. *J. Allergy Clin. Immunol.* **2016**, *138*, 210–218. [CrossRef]
27. Coulter, T.I.; Chandra, A.; Bacon, C.M.; Babar, J.; Curtis, J.; Screaton, N.; Goodlad, J.R.; Farmer, G.; Steele, C.L.; Leahy, T.R.; et al. Clinical spectrum and features of activated phosphoinositide 3-kinase δ syndrome: A large patient cohort study. *J. Allergy Clin. Immunol.* **2017**, *139*, 597–606. [CrossRef]
28. Conte, E.; Gili, E.; Fruciano, M.; Korfei, M.; Fagone, E.; Iemmolo, M.; Lo Furno, D.; Giuffrida, R.; Crimi, N.; Guenther, A.; et al. PI3K P110γ overexpression in idiopathic pulmonary fibrosis lung tissue and fibroblast cells: In vitro effects of its inhibition. *Lab. Investig.* **2013**, *93*, 566–576. [CrossRef]
29. Furman, R.R.; Sharman, J.P.; Coutre, S.E.; Cheson, B.D.; Pagel, J.M.; Hillmen, P.; Barrientos, J.C.; Zelenetz, A.D.; Kipps, T.J.; Flinn, I.; et al. Idelalisib and rituximab in relapsed chronic lymphocytic leukemia. *N. Engl. J. Med.* **2014**, *370*, 997–1007. [CrossRef]
30. Cheah, C.Y.; Fowler, N.H. Idelalisib in the management of lymphoma. *Blood* **2016**, *128*, 331–336. [CrossRef]

31. Vangapandu, H.V.; Jain, N.; Gandhi, V. Duvelisib: A phosphoinositide-3 kinase δ,γ inhibitor for chronic lymphocytic leukemia. *Expert Opin. Investig. Drugs* **2017**, *26*, 625–636. [CrossRef] [PubMed]
32. Greenwell, I.B.; Flowers, C.R.; Blumb, K.A.; Cohen, J.B. Clinical use of PI3K inhibitors in B-cell lymphoid malignancies: Today and tomorrow. *Expert Rev. Anticancer Ther.* **2017**, *17*, 271–279. [CrossRef] [PubMed]
33. Ma, C.-C.; Zhang, C.-M.; Tang, L.-Q.; Liu, Z.-P. Discovery of novel quinazolinone derivatives as high potent and selective PI3Kδ and PI3Kδ/γ inhibitors. *Eur. J. Med. Chem.* **2018**, *151*, 9–17. [CrossRef] [PubMed]
34. Khan, F.A.; Mushtaq, S.; Naz, S.; Farooq, U.; Zaidi, A.; Bukhari, S.M.; Rauf, A.; Mubarak, M.S. Sulfonamides as potential bioactive scaffolds. *Curr. Org. Chem.* **2018**, *22*, 818–830. [CrossRef]
35. Gulcin, I.; Taslimi, P. Sulfonamide inhibitors: A patent review 2013-present. *Expert Opin. Ther. Pat.* **2018**, *28*, 541–549. [CrossRef]
36. Zhao, C.; Rakesh, K.P.; Ravidar, L.; Fang, W.-Y.; Qin, H.-L. Pharmaceutical and medicinal significance of sulfur (S^{VI})-Containing motifs for drug discovery: A critical review. *Eur. J. Med. Chem.* **2019**, *162*, 679–734. [CrossRef]
37. Rassadin, V.A.; Tomashevskiy, A.A.; Sokolov, V.V.; Ringe, A.; Magull, J.; de Meijere, A. Facile access to bicyclic sultams with methyl-1-sulfonylcyclopropane-1-carboxylate moieties. *Eur. J. Org. Chem.* **2009**, 2635–2641. [CrossRef]
38. Murphy, R.C.; Ojo, K.K.; Larson, E.T.; Castellanos-Gonzalez, A.; Perera, B.G.; Keyloun, K.R.; Kim, J.E.; Bhandari, J.G.; Muller, N.R.; Verlinde, C.L.; et al. Discovery of potent and selective inhibitors of CDPK1 from *C. parvum* and *T. gondii*. *ACS Med. Chem. Lett.* **2010**, *1*, 331–335. [CrossRef]
39. Koresawa, M.; Okabe, T. High-throughput screening with quantitation of ATP consumption: A universal non-radioisotope, homogeneous assay for protein kinase. *Assay Drug Dev. Technol.* **2004**, *2*, 153–160. [CrossRef]
40. Raynaud, F.I.; Eccles, S.A.; Patel, S.; Alix, S.; Box, G.; Chuckowree, I.; Folkes, A.; Gowan, S.; De Haven Brandon, A.; Di Stefano, F.; et al. Biological properties of potent inhibitors of class I phosphatidylinositide 3-kinases: From PI-103 through PI-540, PI-620 to the oral agent GDC-0941. *Mol. Cancer Ther.* **2009**, *8*, 1725–1738. [CrossRef]
41. Freeman, J.H.; Wagner, E.C. 3,4-Dihydro-1,2,4-benzothiadiazine. *J. Org. Chem.* **1951**, *16*, 815–837. [CrossRef]
42. Berndt, A.; Miller, S.; Williams, O.; Le, D.D.; Houseman, B.T.; Pacold, J.I.; Gorrec, F.; Hon, W.C.; Ren, P.; Liu, Y.; et al. The p110δ structure: Mechanisms for selectivity and potency of new PI(3)K inhibitors. *Nat. Chem. Biol.* **2010**, *6*, 117–124. [CrossRef] [PubMed]

4

Organosilicon Compounds, SILA-409 and SILA-421, as Doxorubicin Resistance-Reversing Agents in Human Colon Cancer Cells

Olga Wesołowska [1,*], Krystyna Michalak [1], Maria Błaszczyk [1], Joseph Molnár [2] and Kamila Środa-Pomianek [1]

1 Department of Biophysics and Neuroscience, Wroclaw Medical University, 50-367 Wroclaw, Poland; krystyna.michalak@umed.wroc.pl (K.M.); maria.blaszczyk@student.umed.wroc.pl (M.B.); kamila.sroda-pomianek@umed.wroc.pl (K.Ś.-P.)

2 Institute of Medical Microbiology and Immunobiology, University of Szeged, 6720 Szeged, Hungary; molnar.jozsef@med.u-szeged.hu

* Correspondence: olga.wesolowska@umed.wroc.pl;

Abstract: Multidrug resistance (MDR) that occurs in cancer cells constitutes one of the major reasons for chemotherapy failure. The main molecular mechanism of MDR is overexpression of protein transporters from the ATP-binding cassette (ABC) superfamily, such as ABCB1 (multidrug resistance protein 1 (MDR1), P-glycoprotein). At the expense of ATP hydrolysis, ABCB1 pumps a diverse range of substrates (including anticancer drugs) out of the cell, thereby reducing their intracellular concentration. In the present study, the ability of two patented disiloxanes (SILA-409 and SILA-421) to reverse drug resistance in human colon adenocarcinoma cell lines LoVo and LoVo/Dx was investigated. It was demonstrated that both compounds in concentrations of 0.5–1 μM strongly increased the sensitivity of LoVo/Dx cells to doxorubicin. By means of an accumulation test in which rhodamine 123 was used as an ABCB1 substrate analogue, both organosilicon compounds were also shown to inhibit ABCB1 transport activity. The intracellular accumulation of doxorubicin was also increased, and more drug entered the cellular nuclei of resistant cells in the presence of the studied compounds. In conclusion, both SILA-409 and SILA-421 were demonstrated to be effective MDR reversal agents in resistant human colon cancer cells.

Keywords: organosilicon compounds; SILA-409 (Alis-409); SILA-421 (Alis-421); multidrug resistance (MDR) reversal; ABCB1 (P-glycoprotein); colon cancer

1. Introduction

Since chemotherapy continues to be a method of choice for the treatment of various types of cancer, any factors that undermine its effectiveness constitute a serious therapeutic issue. In the majority of patients, the initial response to chemotherapy is satisfactory; however, the occurrence of multidrug resistance (MDR) during treatment results in a development of progressive disease [1,2]. Cells displaying the MDR phenotype are no longer vulnerable to cytotoxic actions of many functionally and structurally dissimilar anti-cancer drugs.

Among several mechanisms that may lead to the development of MDR, the overexpression of ATP-binding cassette (ABC) transporters such as ABCB1 (P-glycoprotein, MDR1: multidrug resistance protein 1), ABCC1 (MRP1: multidrug resistance-associated protein 1), and ABCG2 (BCRP: breast cancer resistance protein) proteins seems to prevail [3,4]. It was recently reported that non-ABC transporters such as Hedgehog receptor Patched were also engaged in doxorubicin (Dox) efflux and conferred Dox resistance to cancer cells [5,6]. ABCB1 is a transporter that utilizes the energy gained from the hydrolysis of ATP to pump many structurally variable substrates (including xenobiotics and chemotherapeutics) out of the cell [7]. Among the numerous strategies proposed to overcome MDR, the most basic approach is the idea to use the inhibitor of a multidrug transporter (MDR modulator) along with chemotherapy in hopes to increase the intracellular accumulation of an anti-cancer drug and to improve the outcome of the treatment. Although this approach is yet to result in any clinical success [8–10], the search for new substances that could serve as clinically applicable MDR modulators is continuously ongoing.

Silicon is a metalloid, which is a group of chemical elements also called semi-metals [11]. It can form chemical bonds with carbon and oxygen, and silicon-containing compounds are widely used in medicine and engineering. Silicone is a synthetic polymer composed of repeating siloxane units. Due to its high biocompatibility and favorable mechanical properties, silicone is used for the production of various medical implants (e.g., breast or testicle), as well as contact lenses [11]. On the other hand, silica materials are applied as controlled drug delivery systems and three-dimensional scaffolds for tissue engineering [11]. The introduction of a silicon atom to a structure usually yields a molecule of higher lipophilicity than its carbon analogue. The increased anti-cancer activity of silicon–indomethacin derivatives was recorded, and it was claimed that the higher lipophilicity of silicon derivatives resulted in their increased uptake by cancer cells [12]. New sila-organosulfur compounds were recently synthesized that were reported to be effective anti-cancer and antibacterial agents [13].

SILA-409 and SILA-421 are water-soluble disiloxanes that were synthesized and patented as putative MDR modulators [14]. They were previously demonstrated to increase fluorescent dye accumulation in human *ABCB1* gene-transfected mouse lymphoma cells and, to much lesser extent, in colon carcinoma Colo320/MDR1-LRP cells, but not in ABCC1 expressing breast cancer (HTB-26/MRP1) and stomach cancer (257P/MDR) cells, which was attributed to their specific interactions with the ABCB1 transporter [15]. The specificity of disiloxanes toward ABCB1 was corroborated in a study by Kars et al. conducted in a model system of breast cancer cells [16]. Recently, the synergism between disiloxanes and amyloid β-protein in the inhibition of ABCB1 transporter activity was reported [17]. In an in vivo study on mice bearing human pancreatic cancer xenografts, the application of SILA-409 resulted in the reduction of tumor growth that was accompanied by increased apoptosis and a reduced level of ABCB1 protein in cancer cells [18]. SILA-421 was found to cause cell-cycle arrest and apoptosis in several non-MDR cancer cell lines [19]. The analysis of the global gene expression profile of HL-60 leukemia cells treated with this compound revealed multiple cellular pathways affected by SILA-421, including DNA replication and transcription processes. Interference with these processes was also attributed to the antimicrobial activity of SILA-409 and SILA-421 compounds [20–22], as well as their ability to eliminate resistance-bearing plasmids from *Escherichia coli* strains [23]. Additionally, the weak chemopreventive activity of disiloxanes was reported both in vitro and in vivo [24].

In the present work, the ability of SILA-409 and SILA-421 to reverse Dox resistance in human adenocarcinoma cells LoVo/Dx was demonstrated. The disiloxanes inhibited the transport function of ABCB1 protein both in LoVo/Dx cells and in Madin-Darby Canine Kidney (MDCK) cells expressing human ABCB1 (MDCK-MDR1). The amount of Dox accumulated inside LoVo/Dx cells was also elevated in the presence of studied compounds, and its distribution pattern was changed.

2. Results and Discussion

2.1. *Cytotoxicity of Disiloxanes*

A human adenocarcinoma cell line sensitive to Dox (LoVo) and its Dox-resistant counterpart (LoVo/Dx) were employed as a model system. It was previously demonstrated that the increased expression of ABCB1 transporter is mainly responsible for the resistance of LoVo/Dx cells [25]. The cytotoxicity of both SILA-409 and SILA-421 to LoVo and LoVo/Dx cells was comparable (Figure 1). Both compounds were strongly cytotoxic to the cells in concentrations above 10 μM. The half maximal inhibitory concentration (IC_{50}) values of SILA-409 were 15.6 μM and 24.6 μM for LoVo and LoVo/Dx cells, respectively. For SILA-421, IC_{50} values were 8.4 μM in LoVo cells and 9.2 μM in LoVo/Dx cells. SILA-421 was more toxic than SILA-409, which might be the result of the higher lipophilicity of this compound.

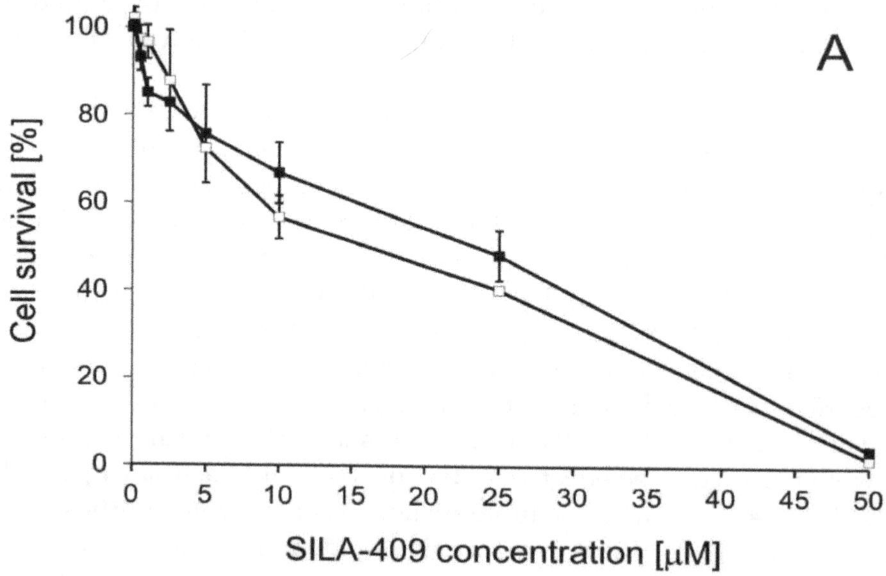

Figure 1. Cytotoxicity of SILA-409 (**A**) and SILA-421 (**B**) to LoVo (open symbols) and LoVo/Dx cells (full symbols). Means of three experiments ± SD are presented.

The cytotoxicity of both disiloxanes to MDCK cells and MDCK transfected with human *ABCB1* gene (MDCK-MDR1) was similar (Figure S1, Supplementary Materials). Both compounds in concentrations below 5 μM slightly stimulated cell growth, whereas, in concentrations of 25 μM and higher, <10% of cells survived. IC_{50} values of SILA-409 in MDCK and MDCK-MDR1 cells were 14.2 μM and 13.9 μM, respectively. For SILA-421, the values of 11.6 μM and 12.1 μM were analogously recorded. Similarly to the findings in colon cancer cells, IC_{50} values for SILA-421 were slightly lower than those for SILA-409.

The cytotoxicity of the studied disiloxanes to various cancer cell lines reported previously [15,19] was similar to the results of the present study. The IC_{50} values of SILA-421 analyzed in several various cancer cell lines, as well as in normal cells HEK-293, lay within the range 5–35 μM [19]. In another study, the cytotoxicity of both SILA-409 and SILA-421 was assessed in a panel of multidrug resistant cancer cell lines of different patterns of expression of MDR-associated transporters [15]. IC_{50} values varied from 8–80 μM depending on cell line. In three out of five cell lines studied, SILA-421 was found to be slightly more cytotoxic than SILA-409.

The analysis of the disiloxanes' chemical structures (Figure S3, Supplementary Materials) and the calculation of their theoretical logP values, performed using the free web tool Molinspiration (https://www.molinspiration.com/cgi-bin/properties), demonstrated that SILA-421 was more lipophilic than SILA-409 (logP values were 5.83 and 9.60 for SILA-409 and SILA-421, respectively). Lipophilicity was observed to positively correlate with the antiproliferative activity of various compounds toward cancer cells [26,27]. However, in other experimental settings, molecular parameters other than lipophilicity were found to affect cytotoxicity to the highest extent [28,29]. Therefore, a larger series of disiloxanes and a characterization of more of their molecular descriptors would be required to determine the effect of lipophilicity on the biological activity of these compounds.

2.2. *Influence of Disiloxanes on Doxorubicin Cytotoxicity*

Next, the influence of the studied modulators on Dox cytotoxicity was investigated (Figure 2). SILA-409 and SILA-421 were applied in concentrations in which they killed <10% of LoVo/Dx cells. The treatment of cells with a combination of either SILA-409 or SILA-421 with Dox significantly reduced the survival rate of resistant colon cancer cells, i.e., the disiloxanes partially reversed Dox resistance. Non-toxic concentrations of SILA-409 and SILA 421 were applied together with doxorubicin. Sensitive LoVo cells were more vulnerable to this anticancer drug (IC_{50} Dox = 4.0 μM) than ABCB1-overexpressing LoVo/Dx cells (IC_{50} Dox = 30.0 μM) [30]. It was demonstrated that both compounds strongly increased the sensitivity of LoVo/Dx cells to doxorubicin without changing the sensitivity of LoVo cells to this drug. The value of IC_{50} for Dox was reduced to 5.7 μM in the presence of SILA-409 at 0.5 μM concentration, and to 6.1 μM in the presence of SILA-421 (1 μM). The isobolographic analysis applied to the obtained results revealed the existence of synergism between Dox and each of the studied disiloxanes (Table 1).

Table 1. Combination of disiloxanes with Dox against LoVo/Dx cell growth.

Concentration (μM)		Ratio	Combination Index
Dox	SILA-409		
8.62	0.5	17.24:1	0.7772
17.24	0.5	34.48:1	0.6136
	SILA-421		
8.62	1	8.62:1	0.6467
17.24	1	17.24:1	0.5632

Dose and effect data were obtained from the sulforhodamine B (SRB) assay (mean values of three experiments) and subjected to CompuSyn analysis. CI (combination index) values were generated by CompuSyn software. CI = 1 indicates additive effect, CI < 1 indicates synergism, and CI > 1 indicates antagonism.

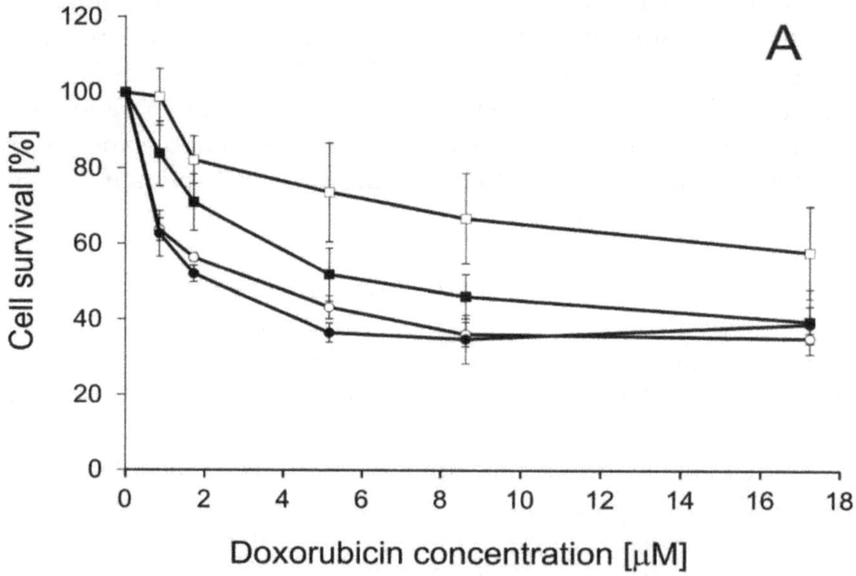

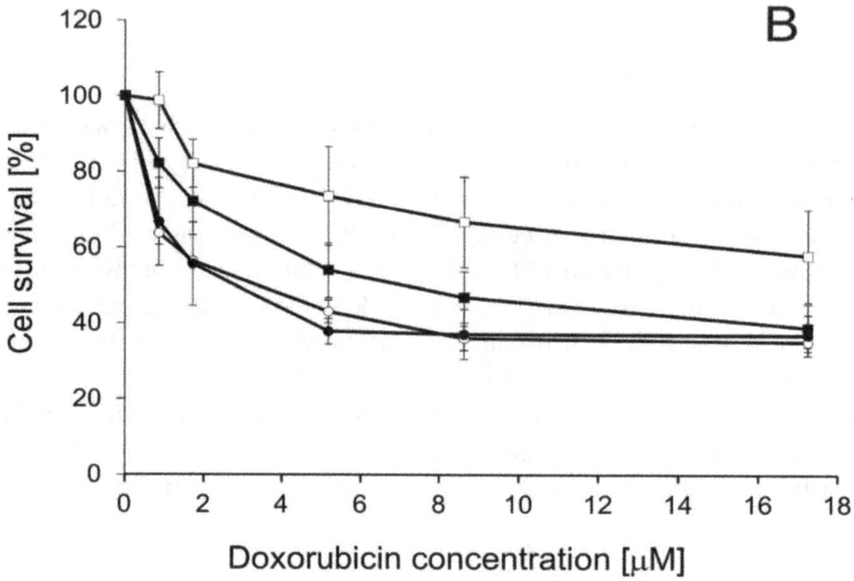

Figure 2. The changes in doxorubicin (Dox) cytotoxicity in LoVo (circles) and LoVo/Dx cells (squares) caused by SILA-409 at 0.5 μM (**A**) and SILA-421 at 1 μM (**B**). Open symbols represent cells treated with Dox only, whereas full symbols represent cells treated with Dox and the modulator. Means of three experiments ± SD are presented.

The reduction of Dox cytotoxicity by SILA-409 and SILA 421 was previously observed in human *ABCB1* gene-transfected mouse lymphoma cells (L5718/MDR) and the resistant colon cancer cell line (Colo320/MDR1-LRP) [15]. Synergism between disiloxanes and Dox was observed in these cell lines but not in breast cancer cell lines MCF-7, T47-D, and HTB-26/MRP1. The authors concluded that the presence of a functional ABCB1 transporter was essential for disiloxanes to be able to revert Dox resistance [15]. This pointed to the specific interactions between SILA-409 and SILA-421 and ABCB1 protein. Similar synergistic interactions with appropriate anticancer drugs were also observed for SILA-409 and SILA-421 in MCF-7 cell lines resistant to paclitaxel and docetaxel, but not in the sublines resistant to Dox and vincristine [16].

Dox cytotoxicity was significantly lower ($p < 0.05$) in LoVo/Dx than in LoVo cells as determined by Student's *t*-test. Significant enhancement ($p < 0.05$) of Dox cytotoxicity was recorded for both SILA-409 and SILA-421in LoVo/Dx cells in the whole concentration range

2.3. Intracellular Accumulation of Rhodamine 123 (R123)

Rhodamine 123 (R123) is popularly used as a fluorescent reporter substrate of the ABCB1 transporter. Both SILA-409 and SILA-421 caused an increase in R123 accumulation in LoVo/Dx and MDCK-MDR1 cells (Figure 3) in a concentration-dependent manner, which suggested that both compounds were inhibitors of ABCB1 transport activity. SILA-421 seemed to exert its inhibitory action in lower concentrations than SILA-409, which significantly elevated fluorescence intensity ratio (FIR) values only in concentrations above 10 μM in Dox-resistant colon cancer cells.

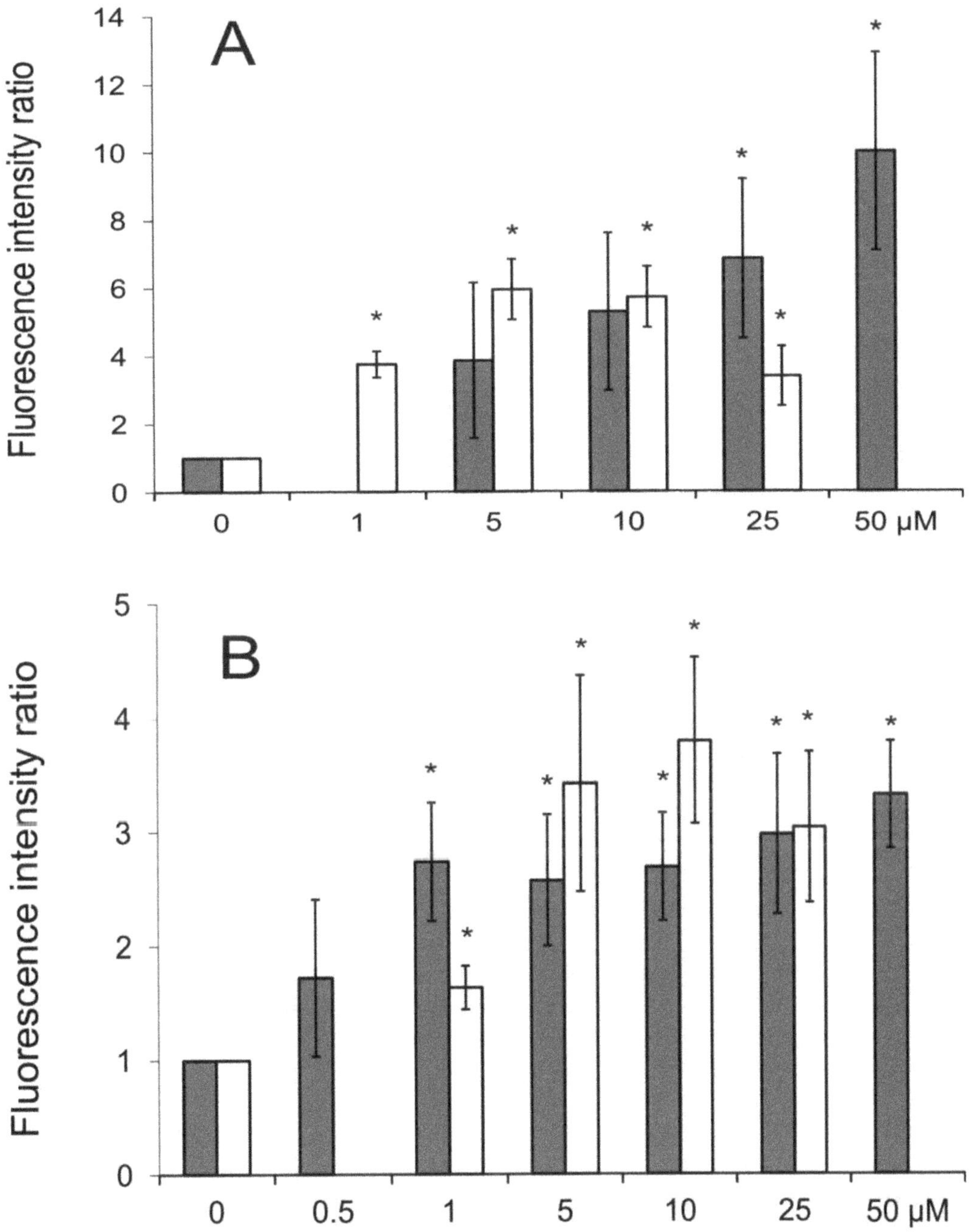

Figure 3. The influence of SILA-409 (gray) and SILA-421 (white) on R123 intracellular accumulation in LoVo/Dx (**A**) and Madin-Darby Canine Kidney-multidrug resistance protein 1 (MDCK-MDR1) cells (**B**). Means ± SD of three experiments are presented. The statistically significant differences from the untreated cells were determined using Student's *t*-test ($^* p < 0.05$).

Molnar et al. [15] also observed increased R123 accumulation in human *ABCB1* gene-transfected mouse lymphoma cells (L5718/MDR) treated with SILA-409 and SILA-421 in concentrations up to 2 μg/mL. Both compounds demonstrated similar activity in this respect. They were, however, unable to affect R123 accumulation in sensitive breast and prostate cancer cells and it was again concluded that the activity of disiloxanes can only be observed in cell lines that express a functional ABCB1 transporter [15]. In the study of Kars et al. [16], both disiloxanes were demonstrated to increase R123 accumulation in a series of breast cancer cell lines resistant to paclitaxel, docetaxel, Dox, and vincristine. In contrast to our findings, SILA-409 was observed to be more active then SILA-421 in this experimental setting.

2.4. Intracellular Accumulation of Doxorubicin

Accumulation of Dox itself by human colon cancer cells was also investigated. As presented in Figure 4, drug-sensitive LoVo cells accumulated more drug than Dox-resistant LoVo/Dx cells. The treatment of cells by disiloxanes at a concentration of 5 μM resulted in a significant increase in Dox accumulation by LoVo/Dx cells with apparently no effect observed in LoVo cells.

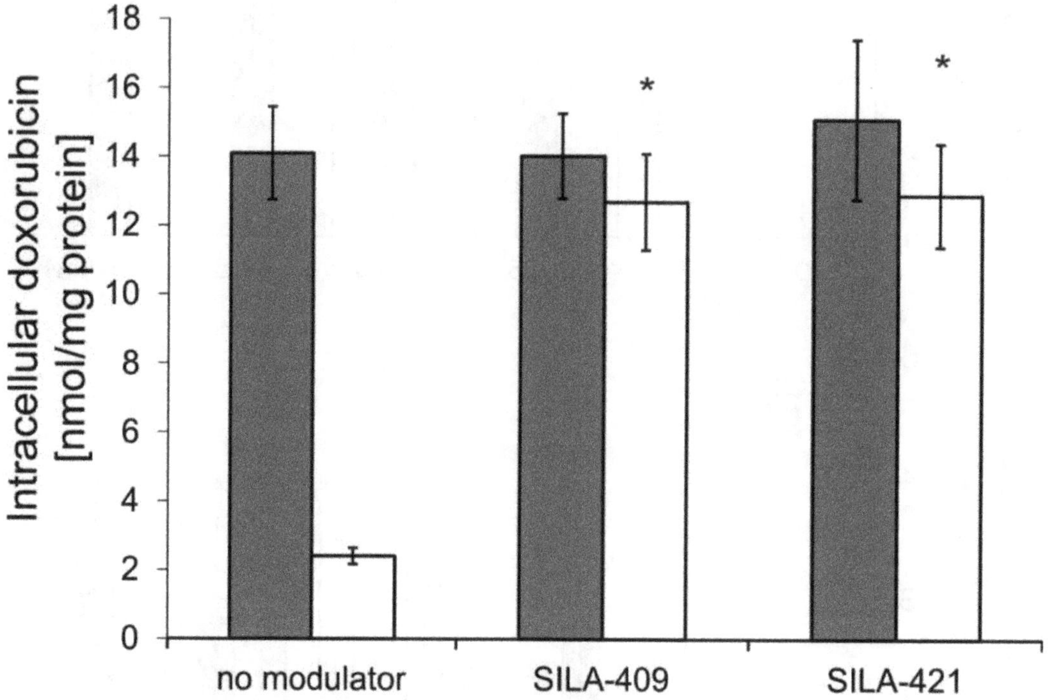

Figure 4. Intracellular doxorubicin (Dox) accumulation in LoVo (gray bars) and LoVo/Dx cells (white bars) treated with SILA-409 and SILA-421 at 5 μM concentration. Means ± SD of three experiments are presented. The statistically significant differences between untreated and disiloxane-treated cells were determined using Student's *t*-test (* $p < 0.05$).

Since Dox is characterized by strong intrinsic fluorescence, its intracellular accumulation may also be examined directly by means of fluorescence microscopy. Again, LoVo cells accumulated more Dox than LoVo/Dx cells (Figure 5 and Figure S2, Supplementary Materials), and the application of disiloxanes at a concentration of 5 μM resulted in an increase in accumulation of the drug in Dox-resistant cells but not in the sensitive ones. SILA-421 was more effective in this respect than SILA-409. The intracellular distribution of Dox was also affected by organosilicon compounds. Dox that was excluded from the nuclei of untreated resistant cells was demonstrated to localize within these organelles in modulator-treated LoVo/Dx cells.

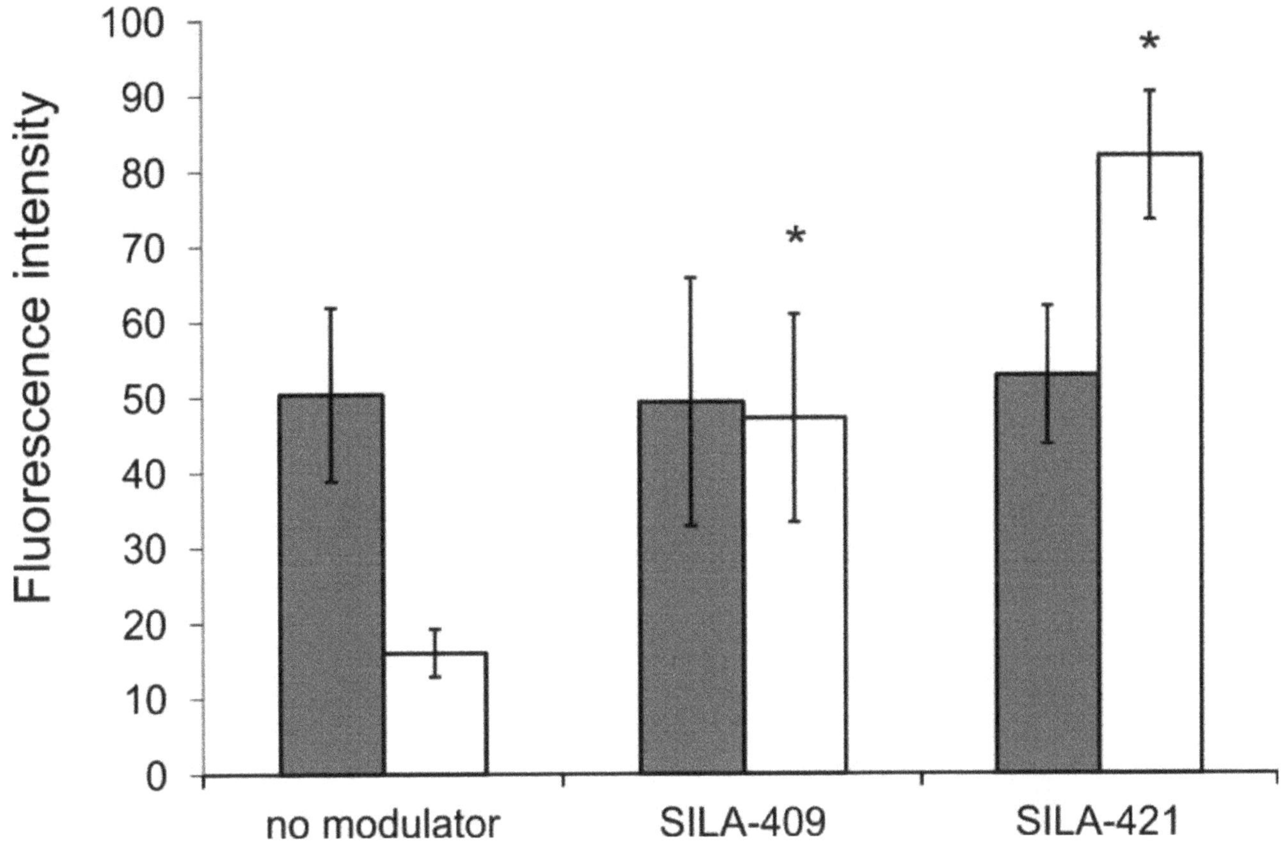

Figure 5. Intensity of intracellular fluorescence of Dox, measured by ImageJ software, in LoVo (gray bars) and LoVo/Dx cells (white bars) treated with 5 μM of SILA-409 and SILA-421 is presented as the mean fluorescence values ± SD measured in 20 representative cells. The statistically significant differences from the untreated cells were determined using Student's *t*-test (* $p < 0.05$).

According to our best knowledge, the influence of SILA-409 and SILA-421 on Dox accumulation and cellular localization was not previously studied. The pattern of changes in Dox accumulation caused by disiloxanes was similar to the changes caused by verapamil (a well-known inhibitor of ABCB1 protein) observed previously in the same colon cancer cell lines as those used in the present work [25].

2.5. Expression of ABCB1 Transporter

Additionally, the influence of disiloxanes on ABCB1 transporter expression was analyzed by Western blotting (Figure 6). Both SILA-409 and SILA-421 significantly decreased ABCB1 protein level in LoVo/Dx cells during 48 h of treatment. SILA-421 turned out to be more active in this respect in comparison with SILA-409. No effect of organosilicon compounds on ABCB1 protein level was noted during 60 min of treatment with modulators (data not shown).

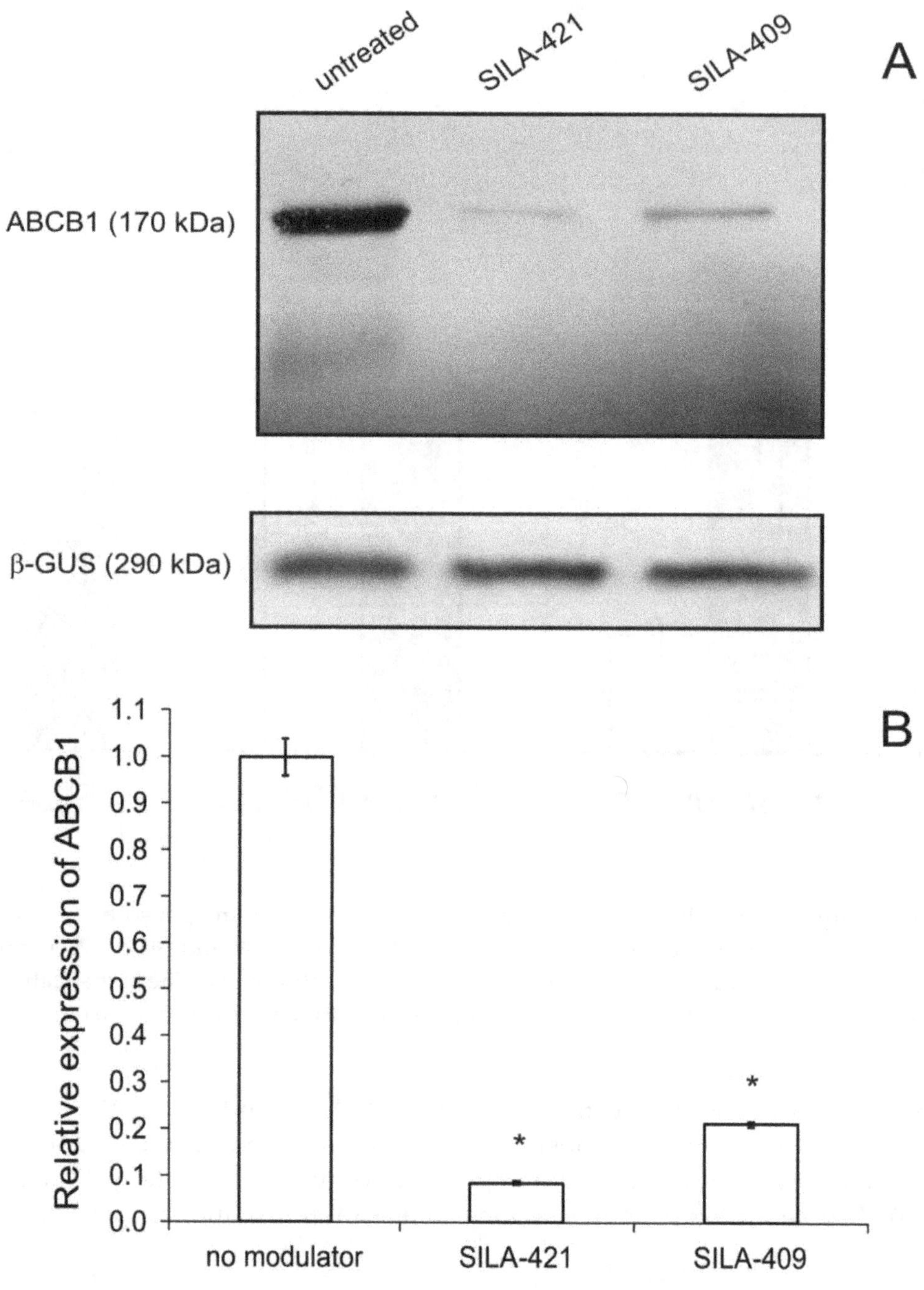

Figure 6. Western blot analysis of ATP-binding cassette B1 (ABCB1) protein level (**A**) in LoVo/Dx cells cultured with 0.5 μM SILA-409 and SILA-421 for 48 h. The molecular masses of the proteins are indicated on the left side of the gel. β-Glucuronidase (β-GUS) was used as a reference protein. The relative level of ABCB1 expression (**B**) was normalized to the control derived from non-treated LoVo/Dx cells. The results of three experiments ± SD are presented. The statistically significant differences from the untreated controls were determined using Student's *t*-test (* $p < 0.05$).

The downregulation of ABCB1 expression was previously demonstrated using immunohistochemical methods in pancreatic tumor samples isolated from mice treated with SILA-409 [18]. On the other hand, no influence of disiloxanes (tested in concentrations of 380–500 μg/mL) on *ABCB1* expression level was detected in mouse T-lymphoma cells transfected with human *ABCB1* [15].

3. Materials and Methods

3.1. Chemicals

Orgasnosilicon compounds 1,3-dimethyl-1,3-bis(4-fluorophenyl)-1,3-bis(3-morpholino-propyl)disiloxan dihydrochloride (SILA-409) and 1,3-dimethyl-1,3-bis(4-fluorophenyl)-1,3-bis{3-[1(4-butylpiperazinyl)]-propyl}-disiloxan tetrahydrochloride (SILA-421) were synthesized and patented [14]. Their chemical structures are presented in Figure S3 (Supplementary Materials). Stock solutions of organosilicon compounds were prepared in dimethyl sulfoxide (DMSO). Sulforhodamine B (SRB), rhodamine 123 (R123), and doxorubicin (Dox) were obtained from Sigma-Aldrich (Poznan, Poland) and dissolved in water.

3.2. Cell Culture

Human colorectal adenocarcinoma cell line, LoVo, and its resistant subline, LoVo/Dx, obtained by prolonged exposure to Dox [31], were obtained from the Institute of Immunology and Experimental Therapy of Polish Academy of Science (Wroclaw, Poland). Cultivation conditions were Ham's F12 medium (with the addition of 10% fetal bovine serum, L-glutamine, antibiotics, and, in the case of LoVo/Dx cells, Dox at 100 ng/mL), at 37 °C and 5% CO_2.

Madin-Darby Canine Kidney cells (MDCK) and MDCK cells expressing human ABCB1 (MDCK-MDR1) [32] were purchased from the Netherlands Cancer Institute (NKI-AVL, Amsterdam, the Netherlands). The cells were cultured in DMEM medium supplemented with 10% fetal bovine serum, L-glutamine, and antibiotics at 37 °C and 5% CO_2.

3.3. Cell Viability Assay

The SRB assay [33] with minor modifications was used for the estimation of the effect of the studied compounds on cell growth. Cells were seeded in 96-well flat-bottom microtiter plates in 75 µL of medium and allowed to attach (60 min, 37 °C). Then, 75 µL of medium containing an amount of the studied compounds (such that a desired compound concentration was obtained in a final sample volume) was added to each well, with the exception of the control wells, which contained medium only. The culture plates were then incubated for 48 h at 37 °C. The further procedure was carried out as previously described [34]. Cytotoxicity of DMSO to LoVo and LoVo/Dx cells was negligible.

3.4. Isobolographic Analysis

Combination index (CI) values were calculated using the CompuSyn software (www.combosyn.com, ComboSyn, Inc., Paramus, USA) according to the classic median-effect equation as described by Chou and Martin [35].

$$CI = \frac{(D)_1}{(Dx)_1} + \frac{(D)_2}{(Dx)_2}, \tag{1}$$

where $(Dx)_1$ is the dose of drug 1 alone that inhibits a system by x%, $(Dx)_2$ is the dose of drug 2 alone that inhibits a system by x%, and $(D)_1 + (D)_2$ are doses of drugs 1 and 2 in combination that also inhibit a system by x%.

3.5. Accumulation of Rhodamine 123 in Cancer Cells

In order to determine R123 accumulation, the cells were harvested and incubated (300,000 cells/mL) with the appropriate concentration of the studied compound (15 min; 25 °C). Next, R123 (10 µM) was added, and the cells were incubated for 60 min at 37 °C. After centrifugation, the samples were washed twice with ice-cold phosphate-buffered saline (PBS) and dissolved in lysis buffer (20 mM Tris-HCl, 0.2% SDS, pH = 7.7). Intracellular fluorescence (λ_{ex} = 485 nm, λ_{em} = 538 nm) was collected with the use of an Infinite M200Pro plate reader (Tecan Instruments, Maennedorf, Switzerland). Based on measured the fluorescence intensity (FL) of the treated and control samples (without modulator), the fluorescence intensity ratio (FIR) was calculated according to the following equation:

$$FIR = \frac{(FL_{LoVoDx\ or\ MDCK-MDR1\ treated})/(FL_{LoVoDx\ or\ MDCK-MDR1\ control})}{(FL_{LoVo\ or\ MDCK\ treated})/(FL_{LoVo\ or\ MDCK\ control})}. \quad (2)$$

3.6. Intracellular Accumulation of Doxorubicin

Intracellular Dox accumulation was detected with a fluorimetry based assay as described previously [36]. Briefly, cells were seeded (800,000/well) onto a six-well plate and incubated for 24 h at 37 °C. Then, the cells were incubated in PBS containing Dox (4 μM) and treated with the modulators. After 48 h of incubation, cells were washed twice in ice-cold PBS and detached. Next, cells were centrifuged and lysed. The cellular protein content was determined using the standard method of Bradford reaction [37]. Dox content was measured using an LS-5 spectrofluorimeter (Perkin-Elmer, Beaconsfield, UK). Excitation and emission wavelengths were 475 and 553 nm, respectively. Fluorescence was expressed in ng of Dox per mg of cellular protein with the use of the calibration curve prepared previously.

For fluorescence microscopic experiments, LoVo and LoVo/Dx cells were cultivated on eight-well μ-Slide microscopy chambers (Ibidi, Munich, Germany) for 48 h. For the experiment, a fresh portion of F12 medium was added containing 50 μM Dox (plus 5 μM of the studied compounds in treated samples), and cells were incubated for 60 min at 37 °C. After incubation, the chambers were washed with PBS and with serum- and phenol red-free F12 medium. The images were collected with a Nikon Eclipse TE2000-E microscope. Fluorescence was excited in the range 528–553 nm and collected in the range 578–633 nm.

3.7. Expression of ABCB1 Protein

Cell lysates were prepared in ice-cold lysis buffer (1% Triton X-100, 50 mM Hepes, 150 mM NaCl, 1.5 mM $MgCl_2$, 1 mM ethylene glycol-bis(β-aminoethyl ether)-*N,N,N′,N′*-tetraacetic acid (EGTA), 1 mM phenylmethylsulfonyl fluoride (PMSF), 100 mM NaF, 10 mM sodium pyrophosphate, 10 μg/mL aprotinin, and 10% glycerol, pH 7.4). After centrifugation of whole-cell lysates (13,000× *g*, 10 min, 4 °C), the supernatants were taken for analysis. The standard method of Bradford reaction was used to measure protein content (Bradford, 1976). The proteins were subjected to SDS-PAGE, transferred to polyvinylidene difluoride (PVDF) membranes, and detected using primary antibodies in tris-buffered saline with Tween (TBS-T) buffer (0.1% Triton X-100, 50 mM Tris-HCl, 150 mM NaCl, 1, pH 7.4) with 5% bovine serum albumin (BSA). The anti-ABCB1 mouse monoclonal primary antibodies (C494) (Alexis) were used at dilution 1:1000. The level of β-glucuronidase (β-GUS) was also determined as a reference protein (anti-glucuronidase mouse monoclonal antibody, diluted 1:1000, Thermo Scientific). After incubation (overnight at 4 °C), the membranes were washed in TBS-T and incubated with rabbit anti-mouse immunoglobulin G (IgG) secondary antibody conjugated to horseradish peroxidase (HRP) (dilution 1:1000, Thermo Scientific) for 30 min at 4 °C. The membranes were then washed with TBS-T, and the proteins were visualized. The relative amount of protein normalized to the control (non-treated cells) was determined. The optical density of the bands on the electrophoregram was detected with the Image J softwar version 1.43m.

3.8. Statistical Analysis

Data represent the means ± standard deviation (SD) of at least three replications. Student's *t*-test was applied, and *p*-values less than 0.05 were considered to be statistically significant.

4. Conclusions

Organosilicon compounds, SILA-409 and SILA-421, were demonstrated to reverse doxorubicin resistance in a human colon cancer cell line. Both compounds were inhibitors of the transport function of ABCB1 protein judging from the increased accumulation of R123 by modulator-treated cells. Intracellular accumulation of Dox was also increased, and more drug entered cellular nuclei in the presence of the studied compounds. SILA-421 demonstrated slightly higher activity than SILA-409. Additionally, the decreased expression of ABCB1 protein after treatment with disiloxanes was recorded. Therefore, the studied compounds acted as resistance-reversing agents via two mechanisms. They were effective inhibitors of the ABCB1 transport function, and its reduction was easily observed after 60 min of disiloxane treatment (e.g., in fluorescence microscopy and R123 accumulation experiments). Moreover, after prolonged treatment with SILA-409 and SILA-421, the reduction of ABCB1 protein level that occurred certainly increased the MDR-reversing potency of these compounds. In conclusion, both SILA-409 and SILA-421 were demonstrated to be effective anti-MDR agents in resistant human colon cancer cells.

Author Contributions: Conceptualization, O.W. and K.M.; Validation, O.W.; Formal analysis, O.W. and K.Ś.-P.; Investigation, O.W., K.Ś.-P., and M.B.; Resources, J.M.; Writing—Original draft preparation, O.W.; Writing—Review and editing, O.W., K.Ś.-P., J.M. and K.M.; Visualization, O.W.; Supervision, K.M.; Funding acquisition, K.M. All authors have read and approved the final version of the manuscript.

References

1. Gottesman, M.M. Mechanisms of cancer drug resistance. *Ann. Rev. Med.* **2002**, *53*, 615–627. [CrossRef] [PubMed]
2. Li, W.; Zhang, H.; Assaraf, Y.G.; Zhao, K.; Xu, X.; Xie, J.; Yang, D.H.; Chen, Z.S. Overcoming ABC transporter-mediated multidrug resistance: Molecular mechanisms and novel therapeutic drug strategies. *Drug Resist. Updat.* **2016**, *27*, 14–29. [CrossRef] [PubMed]
3. Szakacs, G.; Paterson, J.K.; Ludwig, J.A.; Booth-Genthe, C.; Gottesman, M.M. Targeting multidrug resistance in cancer. *Nat. Rev. Drug Discov.* **2006**, *5*, 219–234. [CrossRef] [PubMed]
4. Choi, Y.H.; Yu, A.M. ABC transporters in multidrug resistance and pharmacokinetics, and strategies for drug development. *Curr. Pharm. Des.* **2014**, *20*, 793–807. [CrossRef] [PubMed]
5. Bidet, M.; Tomico, A.; Martin, P.; Guizouarn, H.; Mollat, P.; Mus-Veteau, I. The Hedgehog receptor patched functions in multidrug transport and chemotherapy resistance. *Mol. Cancer Res.* **2012**, *10*, 1496–1508. [CrossRef]
6. Hasanovic, A.; Ruggiero, C.; Jung, S.; Rapa, I.; Signetti, L.; Ben Hadj, M.; Terzolo, M.; Beuschlein, F.; Volante, M.; Hantel, C.; et al. Targeting the multidrug transporter Patched potentiates chemotherapy efficiency on adrenocortical carcinoma in vitro and in vivo. *Int. J. Cancer* **2018**, *143*, 199–211. [CrossRef]
7. Sharom, F.J. ABC multidrug transporters: Structure, function and role in chemoresistance. *Pharmacogenomics* **2008**, *9*, 105–127. [CrossRef]
8. Shukla, S.; Wu, C.P.; Ambudkar, S.V. Development of inhibitors of ATP-binding cassette drug transporters: Present status and challenges. *Expert Opin. Drug Metab. Toxicol.* **2008**, *4*, 205–223. [CrossRef]
9. Kelly, R.J.; Draper, D.; Chen, C.C.; Robey, R.W.; Figg, W.D.; Piekarz, R.L.; Chen, X.; Gardner, E.R.; Balis, F.M.; Venkatesan, A.M.; et al. A pharmacodynamic study of docetaxel in combination with the P-glycoprotein antagonist tariquidar (XR9576) in patients with lung, ovarian, and cervical cancer. *Clin. Cancer Res.* **2011**, *17*, 569–580. [CrossRef]
10. Cripe, L.D.; Uno, H.; Paietta, E.M.; Litzow, M.R.; Ketterling, R.P.; Bennett, J.M.; Rowe, J.M.; Lazarus, H.M.; Luger, S.; Tallman, M.S. Zosuquidar, a novel modulator of P-glycoprotein, does not improve the outcome of older patients with newly diagnosed acute myeloid leukemia: A randomized, placebo-controlled trial of the Eastern Cooperative Oncology Group 3999. *Blood* **2010**, *116*, 4077–4085. [CrossRef]
11. Sekhon, B.S. Metalloid compounds as drugs. *Res. Pharm. Sci.* **2013**, *8*, 145–158. [PubMed]
12. Gately, S.; West, R. Novel therapeutics with enhanced biological activity generated by the strategic introduction of silicon isosteres into known drug scaffolds. *Drug Develop. Res.* **2007**, *68*, 156–163. [CrossRef]
13. Mousazadeh, H.; Milani, M.; Zarghami, N.; Alizadeh, E.; Safa, K.D. Study of the cytotoxic and bactericidal effects of sila-substituted thioalkyne and mercapto-thione compounds based on 1,2,3-triazole scaffold. *Basic Clin. Pharmacol Toxicol.* **2017**, *121*, 390–393. [CrossRef] [PubMed]

14. Varga, A.; Hegyes, P.; Molnar, J.; Mucsi, I.; Hever, A.; Szabo, D.; Kiesig, S.; Lage, H.; Gaal, D.; Nacsa, J. Substituted Disiloxanes, Method for the Production Thereof and the Use Thereof for Reversal of Multidrug Resistance (MDR). EP Patent 1 432 717 B1, 19 May 1999.
15. Molnar, J.; Mucsi, I.; Nacsa, J.; Hever, A.; Gyemánt, N.; Ugocsai, K.; Hegye, P.; Kiessig, S.T.; Gaal, D.; Lage, H.; et al. New silicon compounds as resistance modifiers against multidrug-resistant cancer cells. *Anticancer Res.* **2004**, *24*, 865–872. [PubMed]
16. Kars, M.D.; Iseri, O.D.; Gunduz, U.; Ural, A.U.; Arpaci, F.; Molnar, J. Development of rational in vitro models for drug resistance in breast cancer and modulation of MDR by selected compounds. *Anticancer Res.* **2006**, *26*, 4559–4568.
17. Molnar, J.; Ocsovszki, I.; Pusztai, R. Amyloid-beta interactions with ABC transporters and resistance modifiers. *Anticancer Res.* **2018**, *38*, 3407–3410. [CrossRef]
18. Zalatnai, A.; Molnar, J. Effect of SILA-409, a new organosilicon multidrug- resistance modifier, on human pancreatic cancer xenografts. *In Vivo* **2006**, *20*, 137–140.
19. Olszewski, U.; Zeillinger, R.; Kars, M.D.; Zalatnai, A.; Molnar, J.; Hamilton, G. Anticancer effects of the organosilicon multidrug-resistance modulator SILA 421. *Anticancer Agents Med. Chem.* **2012**, *12*, 663–671. [CrossRef]
20. Martins, M.; Viveiros, M.; Ramos, J.; Couto, I.; Molnar, J.; Boeree, M.; Amaral, L. SILA-421, an inhibitor of efflux pumps of cancer cells, enhances the killing of intracellular extensively drug-resistant tuberculosis (XDR-TB). *Int. J. Antimicrob. Ag.* **2009**, *33*, 479–482. [CrossRef]
21. Simons, S.O.; Kristiansen, J.E.; Hajos, G.; van der Laan, T.; Molnár, J.; Boeree, M.J.; van Ingen, J.; Christensen, J.B.; Viveiros, M.; Riedl, Z.; et al. Activity of the efflux pump inhibitor SILA 421 against drug-resistant tuberculosis. *Int. J. Antimicrob. Ag.* **2013**, *41*, 488–489. [CrossRef]
22. De Knegt, G.J.; Bakker-Woudenberg, I.A.; van Soolingen, D.; Aarnoutse, R.; Boeree, M.J.; de Steenwinkel, J.E. SILA-421 activity in vitro against rifampicin-susceptible and rifampicin-resistant Mycobacterium tuberculosis, and in vivo in a murine tuberculosis model. *Int. J. Antimicrob. Ag.* **2015**, *46*, 66–72. [CrossRef] [PubMed]
23. Schelz, Z.; Martins, M.; Martins, A.; Viveiros, M.; Molnar, J.; Amaral, L. Elimination of plasmids by SILA compounds that inhibit efflux pumps of bacteria and cancer cells. *In Vivo* **2007**, *21*, 635–639.
24. Tokuda, H.; Maoka, T.; Suzuiki, N.; Hohmann, J.; Vasas, A.; Engi, H.; Mucsi, I.; Olszewski, U.; Hamilton, G.; Amaral, L.; et al. Effects of two disiloxanes ALIS-409 and ALIS-421 on chemoprevention in model experiments. *Anticancer Res.* **2013**, *33*, 2021–2027. [PubMed]
25. Wesołowska, O.; Wiśniewski, J.; Środa, K.; Krawczenko, A.; Bielawska-Pohl, A.; Paprocka, M.; Duś, D.; Michalak, K. 8-Prenylnaringenin is an inhibitor of multidrug resistance associated transporters, P-glycoprotein and MRP1. *Eur. J. Pharmacol.* **2010**, *644*, 32–40. [CrossRef] [PubMed]
26. Dobhal, M.P.; Li, G.; Gryshuk, A.; Graham, A.; Bhatanager, A.K.; Khaja, S.D.; Joshi, Y.C.; Sharma, M.C.; Oseroff, A.; Pandey, R.K. Structural modifications of plumieride isolated from *Plumeria bicolor* and the effect of these modifications on in vitro anticancer activity. *J. Org. Chem.* **2004**, *69*, 6165–6172. [CrossRef] [PubMed]
27. Carella, A.; Roviello, V.; Iannitti, R.; Palumbo, R.; La Manna, S.; Marasco, D.; Trifuoggi, M.; Diana, R.; Roviello, G.N. Evaluating the biological properties of synthetic 4-nitrophenyl functionalized benzofuran derivatives with telomeric DNA binding and antiproliferative activities. *Int. J. Biol. Macromol.* **2019**, *121*, 77–88. [CrossRef]
28. Środa-Pomianek, K.; Michalak, K.; Świątek, P.; Poła, A.; Palko-Łabuz, A.; Wesołowska, O. Increased lipid peroxidation, apoptosis and selective cytotoxicity in colon cancer cell line LoVo and its doxorubicin-resistant subline LoVo/Dx in the presence of newly synthesized phenothiazine derivatives. *Biomed. Pharmacother.* **2018**, *106*, 624–636. [CrossRef]
29. Deo, K.M.; Sakoff, J.; Gilbert, J.; Zhang, Y.; Aldrich Wright, J.R. Synthesis, characterisation and influence of lipophilicity on cellular accumulation and cytotoxicity of unconventional platinum(iv) prodrugs as potent anticancer agents. *Dalton Trans.* **2019**, *48*, 17228–17240. [CrossRef]
30. Środa-Pomianek, K.; Michalak, K.; Palko-Łabuz, A.; Poła, A.; Dzięgiel, P.; Puła, B.; Świątek, P.; Wesołowska, O. Cytotoxic and multidrug resistance reversal activity of phenothiazine derivative is strongly enhanced by theobromine, a phytochemical from cocoa. *Eur. J. Pharmacol.* **2019** *849*, 124–134. [CrossRef]
31. Grandi, M.; Geroni, C.; Giuliani, F.C. Isolation and characterization of a human colon adenocarcinoma cell line resistant to doxorubicin. *Br. J. Cancer* **1986**, *54*, 515–518. [CrossRef]

32. Pastan, I.; Gottesman, M.M.; Ueda, K.; Lovelace, E.; Rutherford, A.V.; Willingham, M.C. A retrovirus carrying an MDR1 cDNA confers multidrug resistance and polarized expression of P-glycoprotein in MDCK cells. *Proc. Natl. Acad. Sci. USA* **1988**, *85*, 4486–4490. [CrossRef] [PubMed]
33. Skehan, P.; Storeng, R.; Scudiero, D.; Monks, A.; McMahon, J.; Vistica, D.; Warren, J.T.; Bokesch, H.; Kenney, S.; Boyd, M.R. New colorimetric cytotoxicity assay for anticancer-drug screening. *J. Natl. Cancer Inst.* **1990**, *82*, 1107–1112. [CrossRef] [PubMed]
34. Palko-Łabuz, A.; Środa-Pomianek, K.; Uryga, A.; Kostrzewa-Susłow, E.; Michalak, K. Anticancer activity of baicalein and luteolin studied in colorectal adenocarcinoma LoVo cells and in drug-resistant LoVo/Dx cells. *Biomed. Pharmacother.* **2017**, *88*, 232–241. [CrossRef]
35. Chou, T.C.; Martin, N. *CompuSyn for Drug Combinations: PC Software and User's Guide: A Computer Program for Quantitation of Synergism and Antagonism in Drug Combinations, and the Determination of IC50 and ED50 and LD50 Values*; ComboSyn Inc.: Paramus, NJ, USA, 2005.
36. Riganti, C.; Miraglia, E.; Viarisio, D.; Costamagna, C.; Pescarmona, G. Nitric oxide reverts the resistance to doxorubicin in human colon cancer cells by inhibiting the drug efflux. *Cancer Res.* **2005**, *65*, 516–525.
37. Bradford, M.M. A rapid and sensitive method for the quantitation of microgram quantities of protein utilizing the principle of protein-dye binding. *Anal. Biochem.* **1976**, *72*, 248–254. [CrossRef]

5

Bioactive Compounds and Metabolites from Grapes and Red Wine in Breast Cancer Chemoprevention and Therapy

Danielly C. Ferraz da Costa [1], Luciana Pereira Rangel [2], Julia Quarti [3], Ronimara A. Santos [1], Jerson L. Silva [4,*] and Eliane Fialho [3,*]

1 Departamento de Nutrição Básica e Experimental, Instituto de Nutrição, Universidade do Estado do Rio de Janeiro, Rio de Janeiro 20550-013, Brazil; daniellyferraz@ymail.com (D.C.F.d.C.); ronimaras@gmail.com (R.A.S.)

2 Faculdade de Farmácia, Universidade Federal do Rio de Janeiro, Rio de Janeiro 21941-902, Brazil; lprangel@pharma.ufrj.br

3 Departamento de Nutrição Básica e Experimental, Instituto de Nutrição Josué de Castro, Universidade Federal do Rio de Janeiro, Rio de Janeiro 21941-902, Brazil; julia_quarti@hotmail.com

4 Programa de Biologia Estrutural, Instituto de Bioquímica Médica Leopoldo de Meis, Instituto Nacional de Ciência e Tecnologia de Biologia Estrutural e Bioimagem, Universidade Federal do Rio de Janeiro, Rio de Janeiro 21941-902, Brazil

* Correspondences: jerson@bioqmed.ufrj.br (J.L.S.); fialho@nutricao.ufrj.br (E.F.);

Academic Editors: José Antonio Lupiáñez, Amalia Pérez-Jiménez, Eva E. Rufino-Palomares and Luca Rolle

Abstract: Phytochemicals and their metabolites are not considered essential nutrients in humans, although an increasing number of well-conducted studies are linking their higher intake with a lower incidence of non-communicable diseases, including cancer. This review summarizes the current findings concerning the molecular mechanisms of bioactive compounds from grapes and red wine and their metabolites on breast cancer—the most commonly occurring cancer in women—chemoprevention and treatment. Flavonoid compounds like flavonols, monomeric catechins, proanthocyanidins, anthocyanins, anthocyanidins and non-flavonoid phenolic compounds, such as resveratrol, as well as their metabolites, are discussed with respect to structure and metabolism/bioavailability. In addition, a broad discussion regarding in vitro, in vivo and clinical trials about the chemoprevention and therapy using these molecules is presented.

Keywords: bioactive compounds; metabolites; wine; grapes; breast cancer; chemoprevention; chemotherapy

---

1. Introduction

Breast cancer was ranked as the fifth leading cause of death (627,000 deaths, 6.6%) worldwide in 2018 [1]. During the last decade, new strategies based on the use of dietary chemopreventive agents for breast cancer management have been developed. Several in vitro and in vivo studies have reported the beneficial effects promoted by bioactive compounds from grapes and its derivative products [2]. The positive impact on health has been attributed to its phenolic compounds, such as flavonoids, stilbenes, anthocyanins and other molecules. This review aims to summarize the current findings regarding the role of bioactive compounds from grapes and red wine and their metabolites on breast cancer chemoprevention and treatment by exploring its molecular targets and mechanisms of action [3].

In cancer research, a wide variety of established breast cancer cell lines are used as experimental models. Most of them resemble the different subtypes of breast cancer seen in the clinic. These cell lines offer an infinite supply of a relatively homogeneous cell population that is capable of self-replication in standard cell culture medium and are available through commercial cell banks. The most commonly used breast cancer cell line in the world, MCF-7, was established in 1973 at the Michigan Cancer Foundation. With different molecular characteristics, MDA-MB-231, MDA-MB-453, MDA-MB-468, TD47D, among others, are frequently used in studies, as will be described below [4].

2. Anticancer Effects Produced by Grapes and Seed Extracts

Grapes and their derivative products are a rich source of bioactive molecules, including flavonoid compounds (flavonols, monomeric catechins, proanthocyanidins, anthocyanins, anthocyanidins) and non-flavonoid phenolic compounds (resveratrol), as well as their metabolites. Several molecular pathways involved in breast cancer cell signaling and differentiation, cell cycle arrest, apoptosis, and metastasis can be modulated by these compounds, as described below (Figure 1).

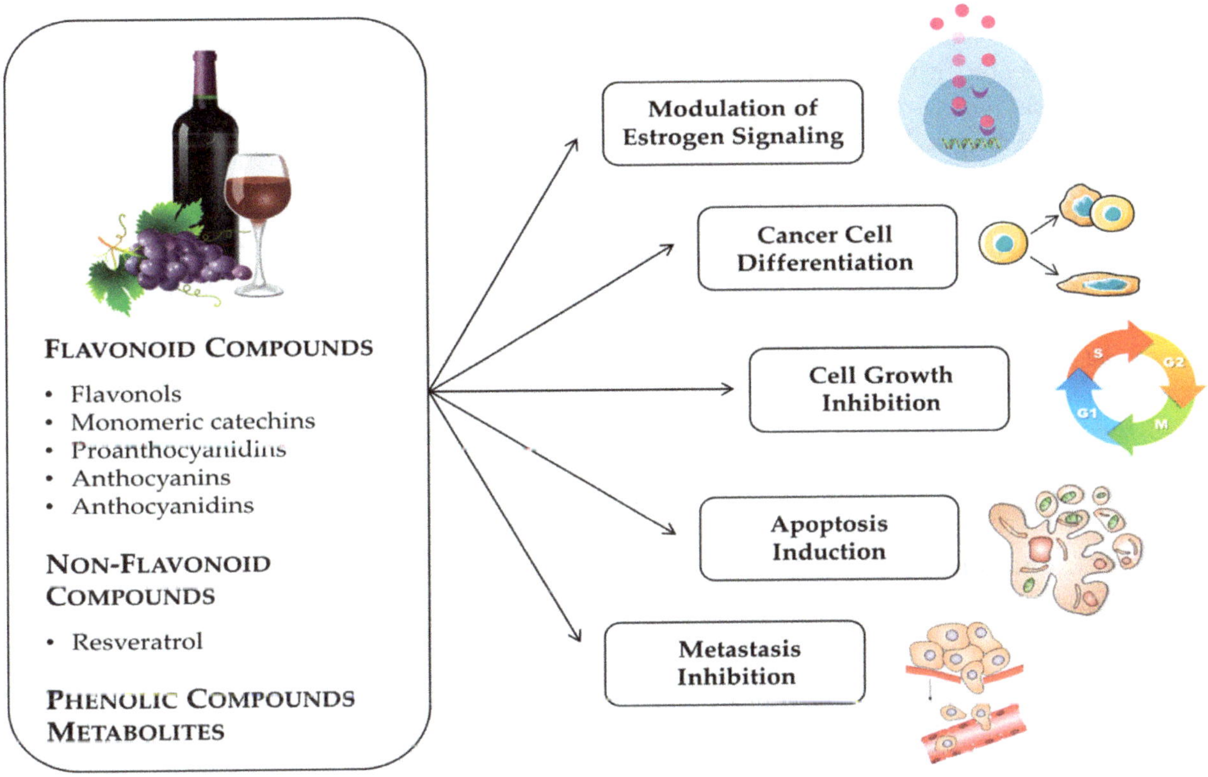

Figure 1. Anticancer activities promoted by phenolic compounds from grapes and red wine and their metabolites.

A polyphenolic fraction isolated from grape seeds (GSP) containing 50% of procyanidins, 5% of catechin and 6% of epicatechin that has been described to cause irreversible inhibition growth of MDA-MB-468, a metastatic breast cancer cell line, by a mechanism involving activation of MAPK/ERK1/2 and MAPK/p38, the two MAPK pathways associated with cell growth and differentiation. GSP also promoted the induction of CDKI Cip1/p21 and a decrease in CDK4, resulting in G1 arrest [5]. Polyphenols obtained by hydroalcoholic extraction from grape seeds promoted a selective inhibition of cell viability and induction of apoptotic cell death on MCF-7 cells. The authors hypothesize that this effect is mediated by gap-junction-mediated cell-cell communications improvement via re-localization of Cx43 proteins and up-regulation of CX43 gene, since gap junctions have been associated with the apoptotic process [6].

Extracellular matrix remodeling, which is influenced by urokinase-type plasminogen activator (uPA) and matrix metalloproteinases (MMPs), is a critical event in the metastasizing process. Dinicola et al. [7] have studied the effect of grape seed extract (GSE) containing 6.2 mg/g of catechins and 5,6 mg/g of procyanidins on metastatic human breast carcinoma cell line focusing on migration and invasion processes. Low GSE concentrations (25 μg/mL) were reported to strongly inhibit MDA-MB-231 cell migration and invasion by decreasing uPA, MMP-2 and MMP-9 activity, as well as down-regulating β-catenin, fascin and NF-κB expression. On the other hand, high GSE concentration (50 and 100 μg/mL) triggered proliferation arrest and apoptosis.

Another target in the treatment of several cancers is the inhibition of angiogenesis, which is supported by vascular endothelial growth factor (VEGF). A study by Lu et al. [8] showed that GSE (85% procyanidins) reduced VEGF expression in both U251 human glioma cells and MDA-MB-231 human breast cancer cells, supporting the hypothesis that GSE may be a natural anti-angiogenesis source of compounds.

Previous studies described many phytochemicals found in grapes and wine as aromatase inhibitors [9]. Polyphenols were demonstrated to modulate estrogen signaling and to compete for steroid-binding sites. Kijima et al. [10] reported that GSP (74–78% proanthocyanidins and <6% catechin, epicatechin, and their gallic acid esters) suppressed aromatase expression and activity on MCF-7aro (aromatase transfected MCF-7 cells) and SK-BR-3 cells. Aromatase catalyzes critical reactions of estrogen synthesis, converting androgen to estrogen, which is known to stimulate breast cancer cell growth by binding to the estrogen receptor (ER). Another approach includes the combination of therapeutic compounds, like doxorubicin (Dox), and phytochemicals for cancer management. GSE (95% procyanidins) increases the efficacy of Dox in human breast cancer MCF-7, MDA-MB468, and MDA-MB231 cells suggesting a strong possibility of a synergistic effect of GSE and Dox combination, independent of the estrogen receptor status of cells [11].

Grape seed proanthocyanidin extract (GSPE) showed also a promising therapeutic role against adverse effects of the chemotherapeutic agents carboplatin and thalidomide. Administration of these agents in rats led to an enhancement in the TNF-α and IL-6 cytokine levels, which could be partially reversed by administration of GSPE. In addition, GSPE reduced free radicals like thiobarbituric acid-reactive substances and nitric oxide and increased glutathione and antioxidant enzymes in liver and heart [12].

3. Flavonoid Compounds

3.1. Flavonols

Flavonols are a subgroup of the flavonoids group, structurally resembling flavones, with the presence of an additional hydroxyl in position 3 of the A ring of the flavones general backbone (3-hidroxyflavone) (Figure 2). The most abundant flavonols present in wine are quercetin, a majoritary compound in this beverage, kaempferol, myricetin, isorhamnetin (quercetin 3′-methylether), and rutin, a glucoside derivative of quercetin [13].

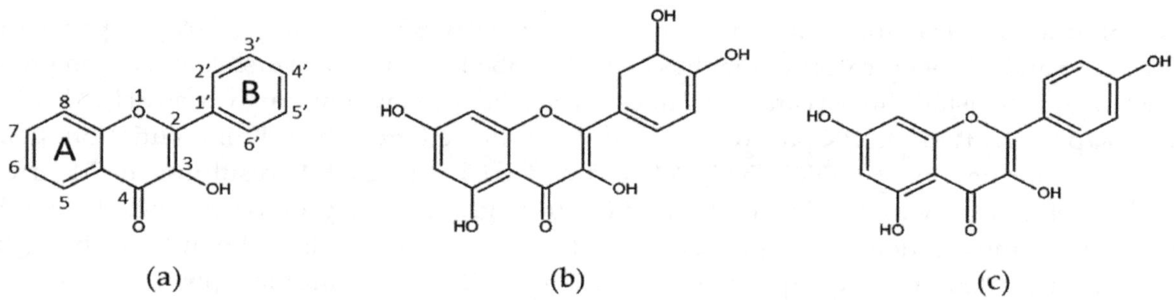

Figure 2. (**a**) Basic structure of flavonols. (**b**) Kaempferol. (**c**) Quercetin.

In red wine, flavonol (aglycones and glycosides) concentration ranges from around 3 to 50 mg/L [14,15], while quercetin varies from around 1 to 10 mg/L in different wines from different regions of the world [16,17]. Flavonol concentration appears to be related to the degree of sun exposure of the grapes while cultivated and the degradation is both related to UV exposure and temperature [13,18]. Moreover, flavonol content is dramatically altered during the processing of grapes, wine production, and storage [13,19,20].

Flavonol bioavailability may vary according to the substitutions found in the molecule, e.g., sugars (mostly glycosides). A relevant example is rutin, a glycosidic disaccharide conjugate of quercetin [13]. The glycosylated forms are the most frequently found in wine and these compounds appear to be more resistant to degradation than their correspondent aglycones [21].

We discuss below the particular effects of quercetin and kaempferol, the most abundant flavonols in wine, on breast cancer. Their effects encompass both chemoprevention and therapy. Although their aglycone forms share a high structural resemblance, the targets, mechanisms of action and bioavailability of these compounds may vary according to the metabolites produced and substitutions found [22,23].

The anticancer effects of kaempferol and quercetin have been described in several different cancer types, such as bladder, breast, prostate, ovarian, liver, and colon. A special feature is given to breast cancer due to a superior number of published works. The few epidemiological studies available using flavonoids such as quercetin or kaempferol on breast cancer involve the observation of their dietary contribution. However, their findings vary from null to positive effects in cancer prevention [24–26]. It is important to mention that, in spite of the larger number of basic research papers published so far, there is a small number of pre-clinical and clinical studies using kaempferol or quercetin as anticancer agents [27,28]. This is due to their low bioavailability, which is around 2% for kaempferol [29,30] and 20% for quercetin, while only 1% was found in the free form in serum [31,32]. This has inspired several works describing drug delivery systems including quercetin and other drugs, such as doxorubicin [33–35]. Likewise, the blending of kaempferol and other flavonoids, either in a complex mixture [36] or simply in combination with quercetin, has been described to increase their anticancer properties [37].

In a general way, the anticancer activities of these two flavonols in breast cancer can be organized in three groups: apoptosis induction, growth inhibition (cell cycle arrest), and inhibition of the metastatic behavior: invasion, migration and epithelial-mesenchymal transition (EMT). Several different papers describe the effects of kaempferol and quercetin in the induction of apoptosis in breast cancer cells, such as MCF-7, MDA-MB-453, SK-BR-3, and MDA-MB-231 [38–40]. Kaempferol and quercetin decrease the growth of MCF-7 and MDA-MB-231 cells with micromolar concentrations. However, the MCF-7 cell line appeared to be more sensitive to quercetin than MDA-MB-231 [41–44]. The same was observed for kaempferol in an MCF-7 3-D model, with ERK signaling being responsible for the apoptotic death [45] and cell cycle arrest at the sub-G1 phase [40].

Kaempferol was found to inhibit the RhoA and RacA signaling pathways, leading to cell migration and invasion inhibition in MDA-MB-231 and MDA-MB-453, triple negative breast cancer (TNBC) cells [41]. This compound was also found to promote PARP cleavage for apoptosis induction through the downregulation of Bcl-2 and BAX induction [38]. On the other hand, kaempferol demonstrated a strong antioxidant activity that was able to attenuate ROS-induced hemolysis and to promote an antiproliferative effect on different tumor cell lines, including MCF-7 cells [46].

Quercetin has been widely reported for its activity against breast cancer cell lines such as MCF-7 and MDA-MB-231 [47–49]. The mechanisms of action involved apoptosis induction through different pathways, such as caspase activation through the mitochondrial pathway [50,51], inhibition of the Akt signaling pathways [52,53], and cell cycle arrest in the G2/M phase [39,44,50,54]. These effects have been shown in vitro, but also in vivo [22]. Quercetin induces necroptosis, with an increase in BAX expression and Bcl-2 inhibition [55]. In combination with chloramphenicol, isorhamnetin, the main metabolite of quercetin in mammals, was shown to induce mitochondrial fission through CaMKII/Drp1, leading to apoptosis [56]. Also, quercetin-3-*O*-d-galactopyranoside induced apoptosis via ROS through the inhibition of NFκβ signaling pathway and activation of the BAX-caspase 3 axis [57]. Dietary quercetin has demonstrated an inverted "U"-shaped dose-dependent curve on the C3(1)/SV40 Tag breast cancer mouse model [58].

The antimetastatic potential of these compounds involves their ability to inhibit the expression of metalloproteinases such as MMP-3 and MMP-9 [53,59,60]. EMT and angiogenesis in breast cancer cells are also inhibited by quercetin [61,62].

Fatty acid synthase inhibition by flavonoids has been reported and associated with modulation of cell growth and promotion of apoptosis [63]. Quercetin led MDA-MB-231 and MCF-7 cells to EGFR reduction and this signaling promoted fatty acid alterations, including fatty acid isomerization and free radicals production [64].

The structure similarity of estradiol and flavones confers on them a potential to interfere in tumor growth and development through the interaction with ERs [65–68] and aromatase [69,70]. Preliminary reports show an anti-estrogenic activity for quercetin [71,72], but kaempferol stood out in a panel of phytoestrogens as the one with the most affinity with ERα, which enhances estrogen-dependent cell proliferation [68], displaying estrogenic affinity at 5 μM in a luciferase model in MCF-7 cells. Also, in this cell line, kaempferol revealed a dual effect, according to the concentration used: at the 10 μM range, it was described as an ER competitor with estrogen, since the increase in estrogen concentration was able to impair its functions. On the other hand, at a higher concentration of kaempferol, 100 μM, increments in estrogen concentration were unable to block the kaempferol effect, suggesting different pathways for activation by this compound [73].

In this sense, kaempferol is able to overcome the effects produced by triclosan and bisphenol A, exogenous xenoestrogenic compounds considered endocrine-disrupting chemicals (EDCs) with anti-apoptosis effects [74]. Kaempferol was shown to reverse these effects, increasing BAX levels and reducing Bcl-2 levels, leading VM7Luc4E2 cells to apoptosis [75]. Kaempferol was also able to suppress the EMT and metastatic-related behaviors of MCF-7 cells induced by triclosan [76] and to reverse triclosan-induced phosphorylation of IRS-1, AKT, MEK1/2 and ERK. In a 17β-estradiol (E2) or triclosan tumor growth-induced in vivo xenograft mouse model, co-treatment with kaempferol inhibited tumor growth [74].

Quercetin has been described as a multidrug resistance (MDR) inhibitor in several different works. It is defined as an inhibitor of p-glycoprotein by direct binding to this efflux pump, but also through the downregulation of p-gp expression [77–79]. Furthermore, quercetin was shown to potentiate the doxorubicin effect and to reduce its toxicity and side effects, both in vitro and in vivo [33,80]. Similar effects were seen with other drugs such as docetaxel [81], tamoxifen [82], paclitaxel and vincristine [79] using different drug delivery systems. Kaempferol is able to reverse drug resistance promoted by ABCG2 [83,84] and to inhibit quercetin efflux by this transporter [85].

Multidrug transporters are also acknowledged in the metabolization/elimination of quercetin and kaempferol. ABCG2 and ABCC2 participate in kaempferol-3-glucuronide (the major metabolite of kaempferol) elimination in vivo [86]. Finally, the cooperation between ABC transporters and UDP-glucuronosyltransferases appears to regulate kaempferol glucuronidation, thus regulating its accumulation in cells (in comparison to the glucuronide forms) with effects on the pharmacological properties of this compound [87].

3.2. Monomeric Catechins and Proanthocyanidins

Catechins, epicatechins, and proanthocyanidins are naturally occurring flavan-3-ols, typically found in tea, cocoa, grape, and wine [88]. Proanthocyanidins are the major phenolic compounds in grape seed and skin [89] and catechins are present in large amounts in green and black teas [90] and in red wine [91]. Proantocyanidins, also known as condensed tannins, are phenolic compounds that take the form of dimers, trimers, and highly polymerized oligomers of flavan-3-ol units [92,93]. Therefore, proanthocyanidins are metabolized to catechins and catechin derivatives [94].

Previous studies indicated that (+)-catechin and (−)-epicatechin (Figure 3) are rapidly absorbed from the upper portion of the small intestine in both human and animal organisms [95]. Catechin bioavailability is inversely proportional to its molecular masses. For example, although the (−)-epigallocatechin-3-gallate (EGCG) content in tea is much higher than other catechins, the peak plasma levels for EGCG (458 Da), (−)-epigallocatechin (306 Da), and (−)-epicatechin (290 Da) are 0.26, 0.48, and 0.19 μM, respectively. Plasma (+)-catechin concentrations increased in response to the ingestion of a single serving of reconstituted red wine. A maximum level of (+)-catechin at 76.7 nmol/L was detected in humans at 1.4 h after intake of both dealcoholized and reconstituted wine [91]. The bioavailability of procyanidins closely resembles that of flavan-3-ol monomers. Different studies, following the ingestion of GSE and GSPE, have shown that during digestion, the oligomers are fragmented into monomeric units of (+)-catechin and (−)-epicatechin and free forms of dimers and trimers have been detected in rat plasma [96,97]. Procyanidin B1 was also detected in human serum 2 h after intake of GSE [98]. Biotransformation of catechins directly undergoes phase II of metabolism, where they can be methylated by catechol-*O*-methyltransferase (COMT), glucuronidated by UDP-glucuronosyltransferase (UGT) or sulfated by sulfotransferase (SULT) [99]. Catechins can also be degraded in the intestinal tract by microorganisms to ring fission metabolites M4, M6, and M6′ [100].

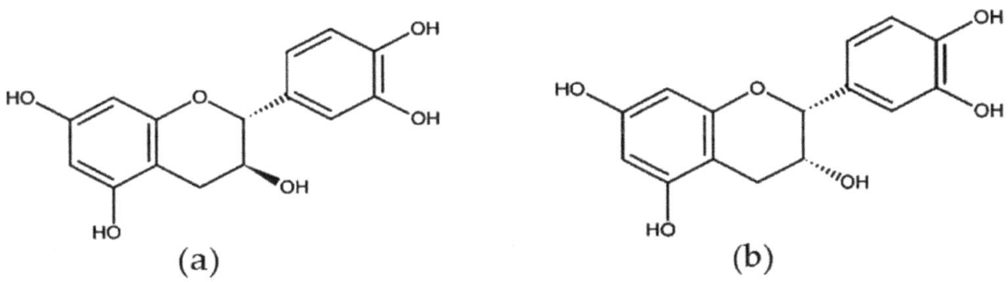

Figure 3. Structures of (**a**) (+)-catechin and (**b**) (−)-epicatechin.

The biological activities of these polyphenols that exert an effect on breast cancer were obtained from a variety of studies, including in vitro and in vivo data. Isolated catechin decreased cell viability and proliferation of MCF-7 human breast cancer cells at 30 and 60 μg/mL [101]. Alshatwi et al. [102] demonstrated that catechin hydrate (150 μg/mL and 300 μg/mL) effectively induced apoptosis in MCF-7 cells through increased expression levels of caspases -3, -8, -9 and p53.

Interestingly, inhibition of cell proliferation by purified (+)-catechin and (−)-epicatechin was more effective in hormone-sensitive breast cancer cells (MCF-7 and T47D), also demonstrating a possible implication of steroid hormone receptors in the action of polyphenols, and in fact, a competition of epicatechin for ER was reported [103].

The anti-carcinogenic activity of wine polyphenols is related to the protection of DNA damages by chemically reactive molecules, such as ROS (reactive oxygen species). The antioxidant effect of purified polyphenols was investigated in three types of breast cancer cells. The treatment with catechin and epicatechin decreased about 80% of ROS production on T47D cells, while no effect was noticed on MDA-MB-231 and MCF-7 cells. The authors attributed the results to different constitutive ROS production between cell lines, hormone receptor spectrum (considering interaction of ROS and these molecules) and limitations of the method [103].

The chemopreventive activity of GSP was demonstrated in an established carcinogen-induced animal model of breast cancer. Adult rats that received 5% GSE (86% proanthocyanidins) showed 44% reduction in the number of DMBA (7,12-dimethylbenz(a)anthracene)-induced mammary tumors [94]. The same effect was observed on a xenograft model using BALB/c nu/nu, athymic, ovariectomized mice carrying MCF-7aro tumors. Mice gavaged with GSE (74–78% proanthocyanidins and <6% catechin, epicatechin and their gallic acid esters) had a 70% reduction in tumor growth, indicating that GSE could suppress aromatase-positive tumors in vivo [10]. On the other hand, diets supplemented with 0.1%, 0.5% and 1.0% of grape seed proanthocyanidins (3.8% of catechin and epicatechin, 96.2% of oligomers and polymers) were not effective in reducing DMBA-induced rat mammary carcinogenesis. The authors attributed the results to the poor absorption of the components and, thus, insufficient amounts being available in the mammary gland to modulate tumorigenesis [104].

In humans, a pilot study with daily doses of grape GSPE failed to decrease plasma estrogens in postmenopausal women [105], despite the same extract exhibit inhibition in cell growth on MCF-7 cells in culture [106]. A double-blind placebo-controlled randomized phase II trial investigated the efficacy of IH636 GSPE in patients with tissue induration, considered a late adverse effect of curative radiotherapy for early breast cancer. In this study, 44 volunteers were given 100 mg of GSPE three times a day orally for six months. The authors considered that the study failed to demonstrate the efficacy of orally-administered GSPE, since there was no significant difference between the groups in terms of external assessments (tissue hardness, breast appearance) or patient self-assessments (breast hardness, pain or tenderness), 12 months post-randomization [107], although the same extract exhibited inhibition in cell growth of MCF-7 cells in culture at 25 mg/L [106].

Additionally, other health effects attributed to GSE and GSPE demonstrated potential to improve antioxidant cell defenses and modulate proinflammatory cytokines, which possibly complement the antitumoral functions of these matrices [108].

3.3. *Anthocyanins and Anthocyanidins*

Anthocyanins are the most abundant flavonoid pigments in young red wines, being responsible for their intense red color [109]. To date, the number of reported types of anthocyanins exceeds 600 [110], but the most common anthocyanidins, aglycone forms of anthocyanins, are cyanidin, pelargonidin, delphinidin, peonidin, petunidin, and malvidin [111] (Figure 4). Anthocyanidins could be immediately metabolized after ingestion of anthocyanins since the β-glucosidase found in intestinal bacteria can easily hydrolyze respective anthocyanins (glycosides) to anthocyanidins (aglycones) [112]. Anthocyanins are known for their apparent poor bioavailability (less to 1–2%). However, presystemic metabolism of these compounds may underestimate their bioavailability if only parent compounds and/or phenolic acid breakdown products are targeted in bioassays. Taking into account the original parent compounds, generated metabolites (from phase I and phase II metabolism and from microbiota-generated) and conjugated products, total bioavailability is much higher than previously credited, after all, anthocyanins are very influential to health [113].

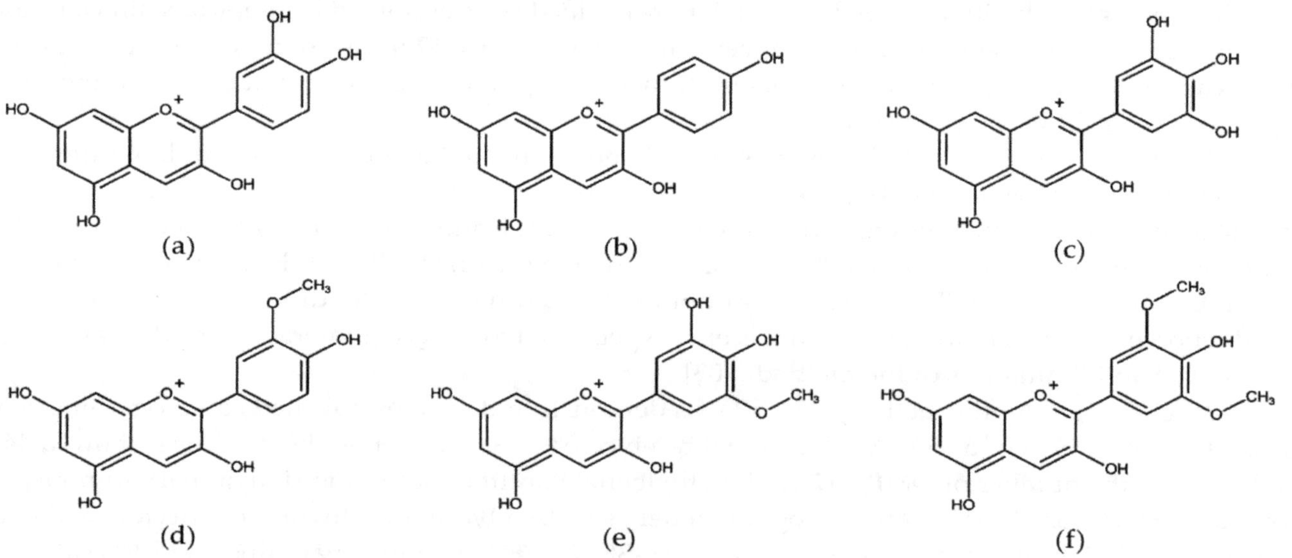

Figure 4. The most frequent anthocyanidins. (**a**) cyanidin, (**b**) pelargonidin, (**c**) delphinidin, (**d**) peonidin, (**e**) petunidin, (**f**) malvidin.

Anthocyanins show a range of antitumor activity in vitro and in vivo, from chemoprevention to chemotherapy. Their potential antitumor effects include antioxidant activities, anti-inflammatory effects, anti-mutagenesis, induction of differentiation and cell cycle arrest, stimulation of apoptosis, autophagy modulation, anti-metastasis, reversion of drug resistance and increasing the sensitivity of cancer cells to chemotherapy [114].

The effects of anthocyanins on breast cancer are some of the most studied, both concerning prevention and treatment of this disease. One of the proposed mechanisms of carcinogenesis is the formation of carcinogen-DNA adducts in target tissues, which is essential to the initiation of chemically induced breast cancer [115]. Singletary et al. [116] evaluated an anthocyanin-rich extract from Concord grapes and the major anthocyanins detected in this extract, delphinidin aglycone and its glucoside, for their capacity to inhibit DNA adduct formation due to the environmental carcinogen benzo[a]pyrene (BP) in a noncancerous, immortalized human breast epithelial cell line (MCF-10F). These authors observed that both grape extract (10 and 20 μg/mL) and isolated compounds (0.6 μM) inhibited BP–DNA adduct formation, through enhancing phase II metabolizing enzymes (GST and NQO1) activities, and suppressed reactive metabolites such as ROS.

Syed et al. [117] also showed that delphinidin, the most common anthocyanidin monomer, could prevent tumor development and malignant progression through inhibition of breast oncogenesis. These authors also assessed experiments with the MCF-10A cell line, a non-tumorigenic mammary epithelial cell line for studying normal breast cell function and transformation, and demonstrated that delphinidin (5 to 40 μM) inhibited HGF-induced early biochemical effects, blocking proliferation and migration of this cell line.

Hepatocyte growth factor (HGF) is produced mainly by mesenchymal cells and acts primarily through its only receptor, c-Met [118]. A variety of cellular responses are activated by c-Met/HGF signaling and mediate critical physiological processes for tumor growth and metastasis in human cancers, including angiogenesis [119], cellular invasion [120–122], and morphogenic differentiation [123]. In addition to observing effects on non-tumor breast cells, Syed et al. [117] showed that delphinidin treatment caused growth inhibition of breast cancer cells that express HGF, suggesting that this compound could prevent HGF-mediated activation of signaling pathways implicated in breast cancer.

The chemopreventive effects of delphinidin-3-glucoside were also evaluated on breast carcinogenesis [124]. Yang et al. [124] described that this phytochemical effectively suppressed carcinogenic transformation of MCF-10A cells induced by carcinogen treatment (NNK and BP). After that, these authors investigated the molecular mechanism related to lncRNA HOX transcript antisense RNA (HOTAIR) modulation. Long non-coding RNAs (lncRNA) are usually related to a group of RNAs with more than 200 nucleotides and are not involved in protein generation, despite being involved in different regulatory processes, such as modulation of gene expression [125]. HOTAIR, which is over-expressed in different types of cancers, is a lncRNA that plays a role in carcinogenesis and cancer progression by promoting cancer cell viability, growth, and metastasis [126]. In its turn, HOTAIR is regulated by the interferon regulatory factor-1 (IRF1) protein, which decreases HOTAIR expression. On the other hand, Akt activation decreases IRF1 expression and, consequently, elevates HOTAIR levels [127,128]. Yang et al. [124] observed that delphinidin-3-glucoside treatment (40 μM) inhibited HOTAIR expression in breast carcinogenesis and breast cancer cells. Besides that, these researchers also found the same results in xenografted breast tumors in athymic mice. Mechanistically, in this study delphinidin-3-glucoside down-regulates HOTAIR by inhibiting Akt activation and promoting IRF1.

The first report of tumor cell proliferation inhibitory activity of anthocyanidins from grape skin was published by Zhang et al. [129]. These authors tested the cell proliferation inhibitory activity of five anthocyanidins (cyanidin, delphinidin, pelargonidin, petunidin, and malvidin) and four anthocyanins (cyanidin-3-glucoside, cyanidin-3-galactoside, delphinidin-3-galactoside, and pelargonidin-3-galactoside) against diverse human cancer cell lines. Although anthocyanins did not inhibit proliferation of any cell line tested, even at the highest concentration (200 μg/mL), anthocyanidins inhibited cancer cell proliferation, with malvidin and pelargonidin being the most promising compounds, since they affected many different cancer cells at the same time.

Afaq et al. [130] evaluated the effect of delphinidin (5–40 μM) on epidermal growth factor receptor (EGFR)-positive breast cancer AU-565 cells and non-tumorigenic MCF-10A cells. EGFR is overexpressed in about 20% of invasive breast carcinoma [131] and has been implicated in tumor progression since it promotes a loss of balance between proliferation and apoptosis. The authors showed that this compound is an inhibitor of EGFR and its downstream signaling, the PI3K/AKT and MAPK pathways, both of which play a significant role in the mitogenic and cell survival responses mediated by EGFR. This same study also demonstrated that delphinidin treatment caused more dramatic inhibition of growth of AU-565 cells than MCF-10A cells and had minimal effect on normal mammary epithelial 184A1 cells, which express very low levels of EGFR, suggesting an important contribution of EGFR in delphinidin action. Moreover, delphinidin treatment of AU-565 cells resulted in induction of caspase 3-dependent apoptosis.

Delphinidin has also been shown to induce apoptosis and autophagy in MDA-MB-453 (concentrations of 20, 40 and 80 μM) and BT474 (concentrations of 60, 100 and 140 μM) cell lines [132]. In this study, the autophagy inhibitors, 3-methyladenine (3-MA) or bafilomycin A1 (BA1), enhanced the delphinidin-induced apoptosis in both breast cancer cell lines, suggesting that autophagy might exert a protective effect in this experimental model. In addition, these authors showed that delphinidin induced autophagy via the mTOR and AMPK signaling pathways.

The effect of cyanidin-3-glucoside, the main anthocyanin studied in breast cancer cells, was evaluated on breast cancer-induced angiogenesis [133]. This anthocyanin attenuated breast cancer-induced angiogenesis via inhibiting the expression and secretion of VEGF, the most important angiogenic cytokine, in a dose-dependent manner (concentrations up to 20 μM). The mechanism proposed by these authors involves the downregulation of STAT3, at both mRNA and protein level, via inducing miR-124, resulting in VEGF inhibition. Thus, the inhibitory effect of cyanidin-3-glucoside on the endogenous STAT3 may occur in a non-canonical way, via miRNAs, which could downregulate target gene expression with mRNA degradation.

Recently, Liang et al. [134] reported that cyanidin-3-glucoside (20 μM) decreased the migratory and invasive nature of triple-negative breast cancer cell lines through reversion of the EMT, which is highly associated with cancer metastasis. Cyanidin-3-glucoside increased epithelial markers (E-cadherin and zonula occludens-1), decreased mesenchymal markers (vimentin and N-cadherin) and EMT-associated transcription factors (Snail1, Snail2). Mechanistically, this phytochemical also attenuated the pivotal factor for EMT, NF-κB, and induced the inhibitor Sirt1 in triple-negative breast cancer cell lines.

There is currently available evidence that endogenous estrogens play a critical role in the development of breast cancer [135]. Despite the fact that triple-negative breast cancer is characterized by a lack of ERα expression [136], data suggest that estrogen still plays a critical role in the etiology of this type of cancer since a 36-kDa variant of ERα, known as ER alpha 36 (ERα36), is highly expressed in triple-negative breast cancer [137] and is involved in rapid estrogen signaling [138]. Studies also emphasize the causal link between ERα36 and EGFR, since this receptor is one of the most critical downstream targets of activated ERα36 signaling [138].

Wang et al. [139] found that cyanidin-3-glucoside (150 μM) preferentially promotes cell death, by the extrinsic apoptosis pathway of triple-negative breast cancer cells (MDA-MB-231) that co-express ERα36 and EGFR. Cyanidin-3-glucoside directly binds to the ERα36 receptor, which in turn inhibits its downstream signaling, the EGFR/AKT pathway leading to EGFR degradation through the proteasome system. A xenograft mouse model also confirmed these properties of cyanidin-3-glucoside.

Fernandes et al. [140] evaluated the effect of cyanidin-3-glucoside, delphinidin-3-glucoside, and vinylpyranoanthocyanin-catechins (portisins) on MCF-7 cells. Overall, the studied compounds inhibited, in a dose-dependent manner (12.5–100 μM), the growth of MCF-7 cells, however, delphinidin-3-glucoside and its respective portisin presented the highest cytotoxic effect. This same study also highlighted a structural requirement for a more potent cytotoxicity effect on MCF-7 cells, characterized by an ortho- trihydroxylated substituent attached to the phenolic ring. Nevertheless, this study was unable to elucidate whether anthocyanins antiproliferative effect could be dependent or independent of ERs or other molecular pathways involved.

Although the monoclonal antibody trastuzumab improves survival of patients with HER2-positive breast cancers [141], the majority of patients who initially respond to this therapy demonstrate disease progression within 12–24 months [142]. Thereby, identifying alternative strategies to overcome trastuzumab resistance targeting HER2 may improve treatment response in breast cancer. Li et al. [143] investigated the antitumor properties of anthocyanins, peonidin-3-glucoside, and cyanidin-3-glucoside, on parental HER2-positive cells and their trastuzumab-resistant cell lines. Treatment with cyanidin-3-glucoside and peonidin-3-glucoside significantly inhibited cell growth in the parental and trastuzumab-resistant cells in a dose-dependent manner. The authors also observed that the mechanisms of action of cyanidin-3-glucoside (5 μg/mL) and peonidin-3-glucoside (5 μg/mL) involve the inhibition of HER2 phosphorylation, the induction of apoptosis in both sensitive and trastuzumab-resistant cell lines, and in a higher anthocyanins concentration (1 mg/mL), an inhibition of trastuzumab-resistant cells migration and invasion was also observed. Besides that, treatment with both anthocyanins (6 mg/Kg/twice weekly, intraperitoneal) reduced trastuzumab-resistant cell-mediated tumor growth in vivo.

As described above, cyanidin-3-glucoside can act alone against breast cancer. However, it has also been shown to be effective in combination with trastuzumab in three representative HER2-positive breast cancer cell lines [144]. These researchers demonstrated that HER2 inactivation seems to represent a central role in the synergistic effect between cyanidin-3-glucoside and trastuzumab in all HER2-positive breast cancer cells tested. Moreover, cyanidin-3-glucoside (5 μg/mL) alone and in combination with trastuzumab (5 μg/mL) induced cell apoptosis in HER2-positive cell lines. These authors also evaluated, in an in vivo xenograft model in mice, the effect of 6 mg/mL cyanidin-3-glucoside in association with 6 mg/mL trastuzumab intraperitoneally twice a week for 25 days. These results demonstrated that anthocyanins were able to significantly enhance trastuzumab-induced tumor growth inhibition.

4. Non-Flavonoid Phenolic Compounds

Resveratrol

Natural stilbenes are an important group of non-flavonoid polyphenols characterized by the presence of a 1,2-diphenylethylene nucleus in their structure [145]. Among them, resveratrol (3,4′,5-trihydroxy-*trans*-stilbene) is a phenolic compound derived from grapes, berries, peanuts, and other plant sources. The molecule consists of two aromatic rings that are connected through a methylenic bridge and exists as *cis*- and *trans*-resveratrol isomers (Figure 5), and their glucosides, *cis*- and *trans*-piceid [146]. Resveratrol was originally identified as a phytoalexin by Langcake and Pryce [147] and is produced by a wide range of plant species under stressful environmental conditions, such as pathogen infection and ultraviolet radiation. Grapes and their derivative products, particularly red wine, are the most important natural sources of resveratrol. The resveratrol composition of wines depends on the grape varieties used, as well as the growing conditions and the wine-making methods, which may vary. In fresh grape skin, the concentration of this compound is in the range of 50–100 μg per gram, and red wine contains about 1.9 ± 1.7 mg/L of *trans*-resveratrol [148–152].

In humans, resveratrol is extensively metabolized and rapidly eliminated. When consumed orally, the molecule is absorbed via passive diffusion or by membrane transporters in the intestine, and then conjugated into glucuronides and sulfates. Although oral absorption is around 75%, only a small fraction of resveratrol ingested from dietary sources reaches the bloodstream and body tissues. It was previously described that metabolism in the liver and intestine results in oral bioavailability of about 1–2% of *trans*-resveratrol [153–155]. Rapid conjugation and low bioavailability are some of the major limitations and challenges of the in vivo use of this compound. Different methodological approaches, such as encapsulation in liposomes, emulsions, micelles, insertion into polymeric nanoparticles, solid dispersions, and nanocrystals, have been developed to improve the low aqueous solubility and the poor bioavailability of resveratrol [156]. Furthermore, the use of naturally occurring or synthetic resveratrol derivatives, with a better pharmacokinetic profile, low toxicity, less side effects, and improved biological activities, are promising strategies for clinical applications of stilbene compounds [157].

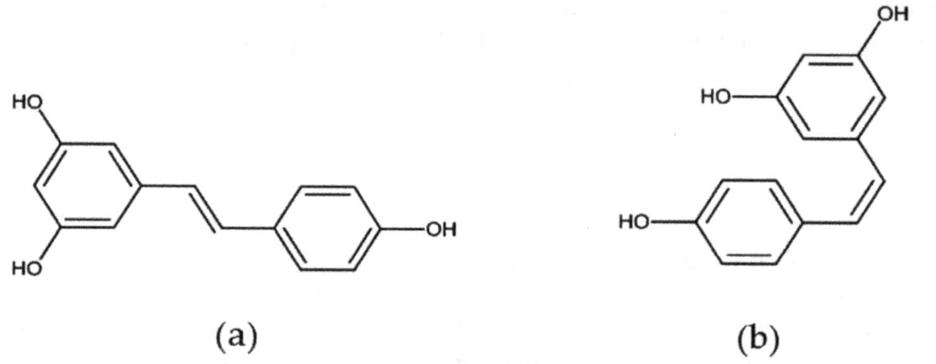

(a) (b)

Figure 5. Structures of stilbenes. (**a**) Trans- resveratrol and (**b**) cis-resveratrol.

Resveratrol exhibits multiple bioactivities, including anti-oxidative, anti-inflammatory, cardioprotective, neuroprotective, anti-aging and anticancer properties. Accumulated experimental and clinical evidence clearly shows the chemopreventive and chemotherapeutic potential of resveratrol, as reviewed in our recent publication [158]. Scientific interest in this molecule has grown considerably during the last 23 years, since Jang and colleagues first demonstrated the ability of resveratrol to inhibit in vivo carcinogenesis in a mouse skin cancer model [159,160]. Resveratrol is reported to act as a multi-target suppressor of all three carcinogenesis stages (initiation, promotion, and progression), by regulating signal transduction pathways that control cell division and growth, apoptosis, inflammation, angiogenesis, and metastasis. Furthermore, resveratrol increases the efficacy of traditional chemotherapy and radiotherapy by reducing drug resistance and sensitizing tumor cells to a chemotherapeutic agent [160–163].

A plethora of studies, including in vitro and in vivo investigations, have suggested that resveratrol triggers chemopreventive and therapeutic responses against several tumor types, such as skin, breast, prostate, lung, colon, and liver cancer [163,164]. As indicated by a recent search on PubMed (accessed in April 2020), most of these studies (570 of 3524 hits) have been reported in breast cancer models. In 2005, it was shown for the first time that resveratrol from grape consumption is inversely related to breast cancer risk, as reported in a case-control study conducted between 1993 and 2003 in the Swiss Canton of Vaud on 369 cases and 602 controls [165]. Among its wide range of biological properties, resveratrol has attracted considerable attention in breast carcinogenesis because of its role as a phytoestrogen. This compound can compete with natural estrogens for binding to ERs, thus modulating its biological responses [146,155,166,167].

Hormone-dependent tumors may be prevented by regular exposition to selective estrogen receptor modulators (SERMs). These compounds exhibit different levels of estrogen agonism or antagonism, depending on the cell type and gene expression targeted by ERs [168]. Gehm and colleagues were the first to investigate whether resveratrol would have estrogenic activity due to its structural similarity to the synthetic estrogen diethylstilbestrol (DES; 4,4′-dihydroxy-*trans*-α, β-diethylstilbene). Based on its ability to compete with E2 for binding to and modulating the activity of ERα, resveratrol was characterized as a phytoestrogen [169]. It binds to ER at a low micromolar range (3–10 μM) and with lower affinity than estradiol. Despite this, resveratrol may act as a superagonist in activating hormone receptor-mediated gene transcription in MCF-7 cells [169,170]. In contrast, the antiestrogenic activity of resveratrol in breast cancer was also reported, being related to pathways that inhibit estrogen-induced cellular outcomes, such as proliferation, tumoral transformation, and progression [146]. Lu and Serrero reported ER antagonism of resveratrol (5 μM) in the presence of E2 and partial agonism in its absence [171]. It was also demonstrated that resveratrol exerted a mixed agonist/antagonist action in cells transiently transfected with ER, and mediated higher transcriptional activity when bound to ERβ than to ERα. Moreover, resveratrol showed antagonist activity with ERα, but not with ERβ [172]. Based on these reports, resveratrol may be categorized as a natural SERM, since it behaves as both agonist and antagonist of ERs. These opposite responses vary according to cell type, resveratrol concentration, hormone competition and ERs expression [155,173]. Resveratrol also modulates the expression of the progesterone receptor (PR). It was previously reported that resveratrol produces greater transcriptional activation of PR than estradiol. In MCF-7 cells, resveratrol was as effective as a maximal dose of estradiol in activating PR gene expression [169].

In tumors, expression of aromatase is upregulated compared to that of surrounding noncancerous tissue. The suppression of in situ estrogen formation by using aromatase inhibitors is a promising route for chemoprevention against breast cancer. In SK-BR-3 cells, resveratrol significantly reduced aromatase mRNA and protein expression in a dose-dependent manner [174]. Resveratrol also inhibits the expression and enzyme activity of aromatase, thus reducing localized estrogen production in breast cancer cells [175]. When tested in a co-culture system of T47D breast cancer cells with human breast adipose fibroblasts (BAFs), resveratrol (20 μM) promoted an aromatase inhibitory effect as potent as 20 nM of letrozole, which is a clinically used anti-aromatase drug in breast cancer treatment [176].

As reviewed by different authors, several experimental approaches have been used to describe the molecular mechanisms of resveratrol in breast carcinogenesis [155,158,162,177]. In addition to the phytoestrogenic action, resveratrol modulates xenobiotic metabolism by altering ABCG2 and CYP1A1 activities [178]; decreases the production of prostaglandins by inhibiting COX-2 expression and activity at multiple levels [177]; suppresses the growth of different breast cancer cell lines and induces a number of biological pathways, thus leading to cell growth arrest and apoptosis [155,165,177,179,180]; modulates the p53 tumor suppressor protein by inducing post-translational modifications [158,180]; prevents mutant p53 aggregation in breast cancer cells and in breast tumor xenografts [181]; regulates extracellular growth factors and receptor tyrosine kinases [162]; induces epigenetic mechanisms by modulation of histone acetylation/methylation [182]; inhibits angiogenesis, EMT, and metastasis [155]; acts as an MDR reversion molecule [183] and sensitizes breast cancer cells toward chemotherapy [161]. In animal studies, resveratrol inhibits chemically-induced breast carcinogenesis; it reduces tumor growth, decreases angiogenesis and increases the apoptotic index in xenograft breast cancer models; delays the tumor development, reduces the mean number and size of tumors and diminished the number of lung metastases in spontaneous breast tumor models [155]. In recent years, accumulating evidence also suggests that resveratrol may be effective in breast cancer management when given in combination with other naturally occurring and chemotherapeutic agents, thus suggesting that resveratrol can enhance the efficacy of other compounds [184].

Although the antitumor activity of resveratrol in in vitro and animal breast cancer models is well established, the clinical evidence regarding its therapeutic effect against breast cancer is still limited. Considering that preclinical and clinical studies suggested that resveratrol may modulate several hormone-related factors involved in breast cancer risk, a pilot phase I clinical study was conducted in a group of forty postmenopausal women with high body mass index, to determine the clinical effect of resveratrol on systemic sex steroid hormones. The resveratrol intervention (1 g daily, for 12 weeks) did not result in significant changes in serum concentrations of estradiol, estrone, or testosterone, but had favorable effects on estrogen metabolism and steroid hormone-binding globulin (SHBG) [185]. Further clinical trials are required to ascertain and validate the efficacy of resveratrol on breast cancer.

5. Grape and Wine Metabolites and Breast Cancer (In Vitro and In Vivo Studies)

The health-promoting effect of wine can be focused on consumption, bioavailability, metabolism and microbiota influence on bioactive compounds. There is now strong evidence that the molecules responsible for those effects are probably not the ingested ones but rather their metabolites that occur after the action of microbiota and absorption process. The identification and quantification of these metabolites has not been an easy task, but improvement of analytical methods and sensitivity has allowed some advances in metabolomics area [186].

The WinMet database contains 2030 putative compounds present in oenological matrices covering 10 different families, such as phenols, organic acids, biogenic amines, sugars, polyols, fatty acids, higher alcohols, aldehydes, lignans, and ketones [187]. These molecules can be divided into primary metabolites (e.g., sugars, amino acids, and short chain organic acids) and secondary metabolites (flavonoids and phenol compounds) and are well documented in the literature about wines [188].

Wine is a complex mixture of many different molecules and several factors interfere in its composition, such as grape type, fermentation process, aging, among others. For example, catechin and epicatechin decrease during aging in all wines, while gallic acid increases in almost all red wines [189]. Thus, the purpose of this section will be to discuss in vitro and in vivo studies related to the metabolites of the flavonoid and non-flavonoid compounds present in red wine described previously in this review, and the relationship between these molecules and breast cancer.

The majority of phenolic compounds from grapes and wine are metabolized in the gastrointestinal tract, where they are broken down by gut microbiota and typically involve deglycosylation, followed by breakdown of ring structures to produce phenolic acids and aldehydes. These metabolites can be detected in bloodstream, urine, and fecal samples by using sophisticated instrumentation methods for quantitation and identification at low concentrations [190].

An intervention study with red wine offered to eight healthy adults for 20 days revealed significant changes in eight metabolites: 3,5-dihydroxybenzoic acid, 3-*O*-methylgallic acid, p-coumaric acid, phenylpropionic acid, protocatechuic acid, vanillic acid, syringic acid and 4-hydroxy-5-(phenyl)valeric acid without any influence of ethanol on the microbial action [191]. The same research group characterized the metabolome of human feces after moderate consumption of red wine by healthy subjects during four weeks and showed 37 metabolites related to wine intake, from which 20 could be tentatively or completely identified, including the following: wine compounds, microbial-derived metabolites of wine polyphenols and endogenous metabolites and/or others derived from different nutrient pathways. After wine consumption, fecal metabolome is usually enriched in flavan-3-ols metabolites [192].

To determine which compounds in grapes and wine are the most bioactive, their effects in disease models must be known, including absorption and metabolism. Rats that consume a red wine extract have elevated levels of the microbial phenolic acid metabolites 3-hydroxyphenylpropionic, 3-hydroxybenzoic, 3-hydroxyhippuric, hippuric, p-coumaric, vanillic, 4-hydroxybenzoic, and 3-hydroxyphenylacetic acids in urine. These urine metabolites account for roughly 10% of the administered red wine polyphenols [193]. Most grape and wine flavonoids and others are rapidly metabolized in the human body, making it difficult to determine whether these compounds are effective against disease.

Based on these metabolites, the combination of hippuric acid (HA) nanocomposite (intercalation of hippuric acid into a zinc-layered hydroxide) with doxorubicin and oxaliplatin induced cytotoxicity in MDA-MB-231 and MCF-7 cell lines [194]. 4-Hydroxybenzoic acid (4-HBA) and a histone deacetylase 6 (HDAC6) inhibitor could successfully reverse adryamicin (ADM) resistance in human breast cancer cells. 4-HBA significantly promoted the anticancer effect of ADM on apoptosis induction, as evidenced by the increased expressions of caspase-3 and PARP cleavage, which were associated with the promotion of p53 and homeodomain interacting protein kinase-2 (HIPK2) expressions in ADM-resistant breast cancer cells. Therefore, 4-HBA could be applied as an effective HDAC6 inhibitor to reverse human breast cancer resistance. Herein, the 4-HBA and ADM combination might represent a useful therapeutic strategy to prevent human breast cancer [195].

Apoptotic effects of protocatechuic acid (PCA), another metabolite of wine, were examined on MCF-7 cells. Results showed that PCA concentration-dependently decreased cell viability, increased lactate dehydrogenase leakage, enhanced DNA fragmentation, reduced mitochondrial membrane potential and lowered Na^+-K^+-ATPase activity. PCA also concentration-dependently elevated caspases-3 and -8 activities and significantly inhibited cell adhesion. These findings suggest that PCA is a potent anticancer agent to cause apoptosis or retard invasion and metastasis in breast cancer and other cells [196].

The metabolites gallic acid, 4-*O*-methylgallic acid and 3-*O*-methylgallic acid are detected in the plasma of humans who consume 300 mL of red wine [197]. In fact, the metabolites gallic acid and 4-*O*-methylgallic acid are well correlated with wine consumption and may be used as urinary biomarkers for wine intake in health-related studies [198]. Phenolic acid metabolites are mainly formed from gut microbiota metabolism and could be responsible for much of the disease reduction associated with consuming wine and grape phenolics.

Gallic acid (GA) possesses potential for antitumoral activity on different types of malignancies. GA treatment significantly decreased the cell viability of MDA-MB-231 and HS578T cells in a dose-dependent manner. In addition, GA exerted relatively lower cytotoxicity on non-cancer breast fibroblast MCF-10F. The changes in cell cycle distribution in response to GA treatment led to an increase of G0/G1 and sub-G1 phase ratio in MDA-MB-231 cells. GA also downregulated cyclin D1/CDK4 and cyclin E/CDK2, upregulated p21Cip1 and p27Kip1 and induced activation of caspase-9 and caspase-3. In addition, it modulated p38 mitogen-activated protein kinase that was involved in the GA-mediated cell-cycle arrest and apoptosis. GA inhibited the cell viability of TNBC cells, which may be related to the G1 phase arrest and cellular apoptosis via p38 mitogen-activated protein kinase/p21/p27 axis. Thus, GA could be beneficial for TNBC treatment [199]. GA also promoted inhibition of proliferation and induction of apoptosis in MCF-7 cells. The results revealed that GA induced apoptosis by triggering the extrinsic or Fas/FasL pathway as well as the intrinsic or mitochondrial pathway. Furthermore, the apoptotic signaling induced by GA was amplified by a cross-link between the two pathways. Taken together, these findings may be useful for understanding the mechanism of action of GA on breast cancer cells and provide new insights into the possible application of such a compound and its derivatives in breast cancer therapy [200].

5.1. *Resveratrol Metabolites*

Resveratrol is a minor component of red wines and, following its ingestion, it is converted to glucuronide and sulfate metabolites, which are present in the circulatory system in nanomolar concentrations [201]. Nevertheless, the by far most commonly studied form of resveratrol is the aglycone, often at concentrations largely exceeding those attainable in vivo. By contrast, very little is known about the biological activity of the resveratrol metabolites formed upon intestinal absorption, which represent the major circulating forms of resveratrol; in particular, the glucuronic acid and the sulfate conjugates of trans-resveratrol, which are produced at the enterocyte and hepatocyte level [202]. Besides dihydroresveratrol, Bode et al. [203] found, in vivo and in vitro, bacterial trans-resveratrol metabolites: 3′,4-dihydroxy-trans-stilbene and 3′,4′-dihydroxybibenzyl (lunularin). In estrogen-sensitive cancer cells, like MCF-7, 3′,4-dihydroxy-trans-stilbene showed agonist properties [204].

Resveratrol-3-*O*-sulfate (R3S), but no other resveratrol derivative, exerted a pronounced antiestrogenic activity on both receptors (α and β), with a marked preference for ER. R3S, the main resveratrol metabolite accumulating in human plasma after ingestion of dietary amounts of resveratrol, is an effective ER-preferential anti-estrogen in both yeast and mammalian cells [205]. A significant increase in MCF-7 cancer cells growth rates was shown in the presence of picomolar concentrations of dihydroresveratrol (DH-RSV) because this polyphenol has a profound proliferative effect on hormone-sensitive tumor cell lines such as MCF-7.

The proliferative effect of DH-RSV was not observed in cell lines that do not express hormone receptors (MDA-MB-231, BT-474 and K-562) [206]. Human MCF-7 (wild-type p53), MDA-MB-231 (mutant p53) and nontumorigenic MCF-10A cells are treated with resveratrol and physiological-derived metabolites (RSV-3-*O*-glucuronide, RSV-3-*O*-sulfate, RSV-4′-*O*-sulfate, DH-RSV and DH-RSV-3-*O*-glucuronide). Cellular senescence is measured by SA-β-gal activity and senescence-associated markers (p53, p21Cip1/Waf1, p16INK4a and phosphorylation status of retinoblastoma (pRb/tRb). While no effect is observed in MDA-MB-231 and normal cells, resveratrol metabolites induce cellular senescence in MCF-7 cells by reducing their clonogenic capacity and arresting cell cycle at the G2M/S phase, but do not induce apoptosis. Senescence is induced through the p53/p21Cip1/Waf1 and p16INK4a/Rb pathways, depending on the resveratrol metabolite, and requires ABC transporters, but not ERs. Recent evidence demonstrates that resveratrol metabolites, but not free resveratrol, reach malignant tumors (MT) in breast cancer (BC) patients. Since these metabolites, as detected in MT, do not exert short-term antiproliferative or estrogenic/antiestrogenic activities, long-term tumor senescent chemoprevention has been hypothesized. These data suggest that resveratrol metabolites, as found in MT from BC patients, are not deconjugated to release free resveratrol, but enter the cells and may exert long-term tumor-senescent chemoprevention [207].

5.2. Catechins Metabolites

Catechin appears to be metabolized only if absorbed from the small intestinal lumen. Both 3′-*O*-methylcatechin-glucuronide and catechin-glucuronide are produced in intestinal cells and methylation and sulfation of catechin metabolites occur in the liver [208]. Catechin glucuronide and 3′-*O*-methylcatechin glucuronide are mainly found in plasma of rats after ingestion of catechins [208,209]. Large amounts of the 3′-*O*-methyl metabolite are also found to be glucuronidated and sulfated on the same compound, presumably produced in the liver, and are only detected in the bile [208]. In humans, between 3.0 and 10.3% of ingested catechins from red wine are accounted for in urine, mostly as catechin and its 39-*O*-methyl-glucuronide and sulfate metabolites [210].

Aside from metabolism that occurs in intestinal cells and liver, catechins can also be metabolized by gut microbiota to produce phenolic acid metabolites. In rats, these metabolites can be found in urine, being 3-hydroxyphenylpropionic acid, 3-hydroxybenzoic acid and 3-hydroxyhippuric acid present in the highest concentrations [193]. When catechin is incubated with human gut microbiota, it is metabolized to 4-hydroxybenzoic acid, 2,4,6-trihydroxybenzaldehyde, phloroglucinol and 4-methoxysalicylic acid [211], again emphasizing the effects of individual microbiota profiles on gut metabolism. We have not found much research showing the association of catechin metabolites with breast cancer, only with the use of phloroglucinol, as can be seen above.

Metastasis is a challenging clinical problem and the primary cause of death in breast cancer patients. Treatment with phloroglucinol (PG) effectively inhibited mesenchymal phenotypes of basal type breast cancer cells through downregulation of SLUG without causing a cytotoxic effect. Importantly, PG decreased SLUG through inhibition of PI3K/AKT and RAS/RAF-1/ERK signaling. Treatment with PG sensitized breast cancer cells to anticancer drugs such as cisplatin, etoposide, and taxol, as well as to ionizing radiation. Taken together, these data indicate PG to be a good candidate to target breast cancer stem-like cells (BCSCs) and to prevent disease relapse [212,213].

5.3. Anthocyanins Metabolites

In humans, nanomolar plasma concentrations of anthocyanins are found after they are consumed. Anthocyanins such as cyanidin-3-glucoside and pelargonidin-3-glucoside could be absorbed in their intact form into the gastrointestinal wall, undergo extensive first-pass metabolism, and enter the systemic circulation as metabolites. Phenolic acid metabolites were found in the bloodstream in much higher concentrations than their parent compounds. These metabolites could be responsible for the health benefits associated with anthocyanins [214].

After rats ate cyanidin-3-glucoside, the aglycone was only found in the small intestine, cyanidin-3-glucoside was found in the plasma, and methylated cyanidin-3-glucoside was found in the liver and kidney [215]. Cyanidin-3-glucoside attenuates the angiogenesis of breast cancer via inhibiting STAT3/VEGF pathway [133].

In humans and Caco-2 cells, cyanidin-3-*O*-glucoside's major metabolites are protocatechuic acid (PCA) and phloroglucinaldehyde which are also subjected to entero-hepatic recycling, although caffeic acid and peonidin-3-glucoside seem to be strictly produced in the large bowel and renal tissues [216].

Previous studies evaluated the bioavailability of anthocyanins using red wine and dealcoholized red wine [217,218]. One of the first studies is the work of Bub and co-workers who only detected the main native anthocyanin in plasma and urine with no effect of ethanol on the amount quantified [217]. Ethanol enhances cyanidin-3-*O*-glucoside's metabolism potentiating its conversion into methylated and glucuronidated derivatives, showing an increase in the two main anthocyanin conjugates, methyl-cyanidin-glucuronide and 3′-methyl-cyanidin-3-*O*-glucoside, of 59% and 57%, respectively. But in this case, the food matrix used was blackberry puree with or without ethanol, and not wine or grapes [219].

The accumulation of multiple phenolic metabolites might ultimately be responsible for reported anthocyanin bioactivity, with the gut microbiota apparently playing an important role in the biotransformation process. Nevertheless, phase II conjugates of cyanidin-3-*O*-glucoside and cyanidin (cyanidin-glucuronide, methyl cyanidin and methyl-cyanidin-glucuronide) were also detected in plasma and urine [186]. The most important metabolites corresponded to products of anthocyanin degradation (i.e., benzoic, phenylacetic and phenylpropenoic acids, phenolic aldehydes and hippuric acid) and their phase II conjugates, which were found at 60- and 45-fold higher concentrations than their parent compounds in urine and plasma, respectively [220].

Delphinidin-3-glucoside, cyanidin-3-glucoside and petunidin-3-glucoside methylated metabolites were obtained by enzymatic hemi-synthesis and decreased or did not alter the antiproliferative effect of the original anthocyanin in MCF-7 cells [221]. The methylation reaction alters the number of hydroxyl and methoxyl groups in ring B, so these metabolites are likely to have different antioxidant activities in comparison with the original anthocyanins. Generally, the health effects of anthocyanins are associated with an increase in the endogenous antioxidant defenses. In a paper by Fernandes et al. [221] the synthetized methylated metabolites still displayed some antiproliferative activities for the three cell lines although not as intense as parental anthocyanin. The biological studies conducted with the metabolites in comparison with the native compounds allow understanding of the real contribution of methylation towards the antioxidant and antiproliferative effects of anthocyanins. However, this subject is new and needs more publications for a good discussion, especially from methylated anthocyanin-derived metabolites.

5.4. Quercetin Metabolites

Quercetin or its metabolites may have cytotoxic activities [222]. Studies on the metabolism of quercetin suggest degradation by intestinal microbiota and relatively low absorption [223], limiting its use as a biomarker. Metabolism of quercetin includes 3,4-dihydroxyphenylacetic acid (DHPAA) as homoprotocatechuic acid, m-hydroxyphenylacetic acid (mHPAA), and 3-methoxy-4-hydroxyphenylacetic acid as homovanillic acid (HVA) [224]. These three metabolites are excreted in the urine of rats, rabbits, and humans [224,225].

Recently, Yamazaki et al. [226,227] investigated the effects of quercetin and its main circulating metabolite quercetin-3-*O*-glucuronide on MCF-10A and MDA-MB-231 cells and suggested that these flavonoids may suppress invasion of these cells by controlling β_2-adrenergic signaling, and may be a dietary chemopreventive factor for stress-related breast cancer.

5.5. Metabolites and Breast Cancer Patients

In relation to breast cancer patients, previous reports have shown that glycolysis, lipogenesis and the production of volatile organic metabolites were increased in the serum of these patients compared to healthy women [228]. The serum levels of choline, tyrosine, valine, lactate, isoleucine are up-regulated, and glutamate levels are downregulated in patients with early-stage breast cancer [229]. These studies reveal that metabolic alterations are important indications for breast cancer. There is evidence that metabolic changes are correlated with metastasis and metabolism of tumors [230–232]. Metabolism changes are often associated with resistance to chemotherapy and therapeutic sensitivity in clinical chemotherapy. Breast cancer cells not only show significant differences in metabolism compared with healthy breast cells, but also show differences in drug resistance [233,234]. Cancer and metabolism are deeply interconnected, studies indicate that cancer evolution is associated with abnormal glucose metabolism that is related to high proliferation, metastasis and clinical characteristics and is allied to the action of a particular drug. In this context, chemoresistance enables cancer cells to survive drug action and proliferate uncontrollably, which may lead to strong metastatic potential and cancer progression [230–234].

A recent clinical trial has reported resveratrol accumulation, mainly as sulfates and glucuronides, in normal and malignant human breast tissues. Although phase-II conjugation might hamper a direct anticancer activity, long-term tumor-senescent chemoprevention cannot be discarded [235]. Metabolites of wine bioactive compounds have been positively related to in vitro and in vivo breast anticancer properties and this evidence was associated with the ingestion of several flavonoids present in large amounts in red wine. However, the concentration required to trigger a biological event is dependent not only on the amount ingested, but also on critical variables that include bioaccessibility, bioavailability, stability under in vivo conditions, and so on. Many studies are still required to clarify the role of many of these metabolites with regard to the health-promoting properties of wine.

Table 1 summarizes the data collected from the literature about the metabolite dosage used or found in the different in vitro and in vivo models mentioned in this review.

Table 1. Summary of metabolites found or used in different in vitro and in vivo models.

Dietary Factor/Isolated Compound	Model (Human/Animal/Cancer Cell Lines)	Sample Type	Discriminating Metabolites	Average of Metabolites (Found or Used)	Primary Reference
Red wine	Human (healthy subjects)	Plasma	catechin gallic acid 4-*O*-methylgallic acid 3-*O*-methylgallic acid caffeic acid	0.13–1.5 µmol/L	[197]
Red wine resveratrol in capsules	Human (healthy subjects)	Plasma	*trans*-resveratrol *trans*-resveratrol-4′-*O*-glucuronide *trans*-resveratrol-3′-*O*-glucuronide resveratrol resveratrol-*O*-glucuronide resveratrol-*O*-sulfate	0–0.03 µM 0–3.9 µM 0–2.7 µM 0.04–0.23 µM 0.56–2.90 µM 0.75–4.78 µM	[201]
Red wine and red grape juice	Human (male healthy subjects)	Plasma Urine	cyanidin 3-glucoside, delphinidin 3-glucoside, malvidin 3-glucoside, peonidin 3-glucoside, petunidin 3-glucoside	0.42–48.8 ng/mL (maximum) 0.66–86.7 µg/h	[218]
Red wine, dealcoholized red wine and grape juice	Human (male healthy subjects)	Plasma Urine	malvidin-3-glucoside	1.38 nM (maximum) 13.3–27.0 µg	[217]
Habitual diets	Human (healthy subjects)	Urine	3,4-dihydroxyphenylacetic acid *m*-hydroxyphenylacetic acid homovanillic acid	0.7 µg/mL 4.8 µg/mL 2.8 µg/mL	[225]
Red wine and dealcoholized red wine	Human (healthy subjects)	Urine	catechin (unmethylated conjugates) catechin (methylated conjugates)	5.32 µmol 1.27 µmol	[210]
Wine	Human (healthy subjects)	Urine	gallic acid 4-*O*-methylgallic acid	1.6–6.1 µmol/d	[198]
Red wine and dealcoholized red wine	Human (healthy adults)	Human feces	3,5-dihydroxybenzoic acid, protocatechuic acid, 3-*O*-methylgallic acid, vanillic acid, syringic acid, p-coumaric acid, phenylpropionic acid, 4-hydroxy-5-(phenyl)valeric acid, 2-hydroxyglutaric acid, 2-methylbutyric acid, 2,3-pentanedione, diethylmalonate, 2-phenethyl butyrate, 2-phenylethyl hexanoate, 5-(3′,4′-dihydroxyphenyl)gamma-valerolactone, 3-(3′-hydroxyphenyl)propionic acid, 4-hydroxy-5-(3′-hydroxyphenyl)valeric acid, benzoic acid, 4-hydroxy-5-(phenyl)valeric acid	0.2–50 µg/g	[191]
Catechin	Human (healthy subjects)	Feces	4-hydroxybenzoic acid 2,4,6-trihydroxybenzoic acid phloroglucinol 4-methoxysalicylic acid	Not determined	[211]
Trans-resveratrol	Human (healthy subjects)	Feces	dihydroresveratrol 3,4′-dihydroxy-*trans*-stilbene 3,4′-dihydroxybibenzyl (lunularin)	0–86.9 µmol/L 0–11.1 µmol/L 0–79.8 µmol/L	[203]

Table 1. *Cont.*

Dietary Factor/Isolated Compound	Model (Human/Animal/Cancer Cell Lines)	Sample Type	Discriminating Metabolites	Average of Metabolites (Found or Used)	Primary Reference
Fried onions, quercetin rutinoside, quercetin aglycone	Human (healthy ileostomy subjects)	Ileostomy effluent urine	quercetin	37–72 mg 73–275 μg	[223]
Isotopically labeled cyanidin-3-glucoside (6,8,10,3′,5′-13C_5-C3G)	Human (male healthy subjects)	Serum Urine	24 labeled metabolites were identified (cyanidin-glucuronide, methyl cyanidin-glucuronide, methyl C3G-glucuronide, protocatechuic acid (PCA), phloroglucinaldehyde, phloroglucinaldehyde, PCA-3-glucuronide, PCA-4-glucuronide, PCA-3-sulfate, PCA-4-sulfate, vanillic acid, isovanillic acid, vanillic acid-glucuronide, isovanillic acid-glucuronide, vanillic acid-sulfate, isovanillic acid-sulfate, methyl 3,4-dihydroxybenzoate, 2-hydroxy-4-methoxybenzoic acid, methyl vanillate, 3,4-dihydroxyphenylacetic acid, 4-hydroxyphenylacetic acid, caffeic acid, ferulic acid, hippuric acid)	6.11 μmol/L (maximum) 15.69 μmol/L (maximum)	[220]
Red wine powder	Animal (male Wistar rats)	Urine Plasma	aromatic acids catechins hippuric acid hippuric acid	4.7–2790 μg/d 0–8 mg/d 0.6–3 mg/d 60–110 μmol/L	[193]
(+)-Catechin	Animal (male Wistar rats)	Plasma	catechin glucuronide catechin glucuronide + sulfate 3′-*O*-methyl catechin-glucuronide 3′-*O*-methyl catechin-glucuronide + sulfate	0.2–2.8 μmol/L 0.1–0.8 μmol/L 0.3–19.3 μmol/L 16.8–38.3 μmol/L	[208]
(+)-Catechin (−)-Epicatechin (+)-Catechin + (−)-Epicatechin	Animal (male Sprague-Dawley rats)	Plasma Urine	catechin epicatechin 3′-*O*-methyl-catechin 3′-*O*-methyl-epicatechin catechin epicatechin 3′-*O*-methyl-catechin 3′-*O*-methyl-epicatechin	0.15–44.2 μmol.h.L^{-1} 0–41.9 μmol.h.L^{-1} 0–23.0 μmol.h.L^{-1} 0.82–78.3 μmol.h.L^{-1} 0.01–8.85 μmol.h.L^{-1} 0.03–16.6 μmol.h.L^{-1} 0–3.60 μmol.h.L^{-1} 0–9.45 μmol.h.L^{-1}	[209]
Cyanidin 3-*O*-β-D-glucoside	Animal (male Wistar rats)	Plasma Kidney Liver	cyanidin 3-*O*-β-D-glucoside protocatechuic acid cyanidin 3-*O*-β-D-glucoside methylated cyanidin 3-*O*-β-D-glucoside cyanidin 3-*O*-β-D-glucoside methylated cyanidin 3-*O*-β-D-glucoside	0–0.31 μmol/L 0–2.56 μmol/L 0–3.20 μmol/L 0–1.32 μmol/L 0 μmol/L 0–0.64 μmol/L	[215]
Rutin Quercetin	Animal (rabbits)	Urine	3,4-dihydroxyphenylacetic acid *m*-hydroxyphenylacetic acid *p*-hydroxyphenylacetic acid homovanillic acid	Not determined	[224]
Phloroglucinol	Animal (athymic Balb/c female nude mice)	Mice	phloroglucinol	25 mg of phloroglucinol/kg of body	[213]
Hippuric acid associated with doxorubicin or oxaliplatin	Cancer cell lines (MDA-MB-231, MCF-7, Caco-2)	Cells	Hippuric acid associated with doxorubicin or oxaliplatin	0.13–20 μg/mL (IC_{50})	[194]
4-hydroxybenzoic acid	Cancer cell lines (MCF-7, adriamycin-resistant cells MCF-7/ADM, MDA-MB-231, MDA-MB-468, 4T1) Animal (BALB/c mice)	Cells Tumor	4-hydroxybenzoic acid	0–20 μM 2 mg/Kg	[195]

Table 1. *Cont.*

Dietary Factor/Isolated Compound	Model (Human/Animal/Cancer Cell Lines)	Sample Type	Discriminating Metabolites	Average of Metabolites (Found or Used)	Primary Reference
Protocatechuic acid	Cancer cell lines (MCF-7, A549, HepG2, HeLa, LNCap)	Cells	protocatechuic acid	1–8 μmol/L	[196]
Gallic acid	Cancer cell lines (MDA-MB-231, HS578T, MCF-7)	Cells	gallic acid	5–400 μM	[199]
Resveratrol Hydrosystilbenes Dihydroresveratrol	Cancer cell lines (MCF-7, MDA-MB-231, 3T-474, K-562)	Cells	resveratrol hydrosystilbenes dihydroresveratrol	1 nM–10 μM	[206]
Resveratrol-3-*O*-sulfate	Cancer cell line (MCF-7)	Cells	resveratrol-3-*O*-sulfate	500 nM–100 μM	[205]
Resveratrol Resveratrol-3′-*O*-glucuronide Resveratrol 3′-*O*-sulfate Resveratrol 4′-*O*-sulfate Dihydroresveratrol Dihydroresveratrol-3′-*O*-glucuronide	Cancer cell lines (MCF-7, MDA-MB-231)	Cells	resveratrol resveratrol-3′-*O*-glucuronide resveratrol 3′-*O*-sulfate resveratrol 4′-*O*-sulfate dihydroresveratrol dihydroresveratrol-3′-*O*-glucuronide	0.4–10 μmol/L	[207]
Phloroglucinol	Cancer cell lines (BT549, MDA-MB-231, MCF-7, SK-BR3, BT549)	Cells	phloroglucinol	0–100 μM	[212]
Delphinidin-3-glucuronide Cyanidin-3-glucuronide Petunidin-3-glucuronide	Cancer cell lines (MKN-28, Caco-2, MCF-7)	Cells	delphinidin-3-glucuronide cyanidin-3-glucuronide petunidin-3-glucuronide	6.3–100 μM	[221]
Quercetin-3-*O*-glucuronide	Non-tumorigenic cell line (MCF-10A) and cancer cell line (MDA-MB-231)	Cells	quercetin-3-*O*-glucuronide	0.01–μM	[226]

6. Conclusions

As can be seen in this compilation, grapes and wines are rich and complex sources of bioactive molecules with multiple targets and effects. The natural polyphenols from these dietary products belong to different classes of compounds, both flavonoid and non-flavonoid, and have been studied in different models of breast cancer, both in vivo and in vitro. The major anticancer activities promoted by these compounds are summarized in Figure 1 and include modulation of estrogen cell signaling, cancer cell differentiation, cell growth inhibition, apoptosis induction and suppression of the metastatic behavior.

Based on dietary source, bioactive compounds or their metabolites used in different in vitro and in vivo studies for breast cancer, we conclude that there is a great variation of doses utilized or found. When the studies utilize wine or grape as a bioactive compound source, it is possible to observe a great variation on metabolite quality and quantity. On the other hand, when the isolated metabolite or its precursor were used, mainly in cancer cell lines, variations from 1 nM until 100 μM were used, and some authors justify the use of these concentrations to approximate the physiological concentrations. It is also important to point out that the effects produced by the glycosidic forms and the aglycones might lead to different routes of absorption and/or metabolization, leading to important variations in bioavailability and global effects produced.

The bioavailability of these compounds is another important issue that must be circumvented to improve local biological effects. In this way, grape and wine have long been used as sources of lead compounds in the search for breast cancer chemotherapy candidates and should be further explored in clinical studies, along with the biotechnological improvements necessary for their application.

Author Contributions: Writing—original draft preparation—D.C.F.d.C., L.P.R., J.Q., R.A.S., E.F.; writing and editing—D.C.F.d.C., L.P.R., J.L.S., E.F.; All authors have read and agreed to the published version of the manuscript.

References

1. The International Agency for Research on Cancer (IARC) Report, World Health Organization (WHO). *Latest Global Cancer Data: Cancer Burden Rises to 18.1 Million New Cases and 9.6 Million Cancer Deaths in 2018*; IARC: Lyon, France, 2018.
2. Teixeira, A.; Baenas, N.; Dominguez-Perles, R.; Barros, A.; Rosa, E.; Moreno, D.A.; Garcia-Viguera, C. Natural bioactive compounds from winery by-products as health promoters: A review. *Int. J. Mol. Sci.* **2014**, *15*, 15638–15678. [CrossRef]
3. Amor, S.; Châlons, P.; Aires, V.; Delmas, D. Polyphenol Extracts from Red Wine and Grapevine: Potential Effects on Cancers. *Diseases* **2018**, *6*, 106. [CrossRef] [PubMed]
4. Holliday, D.L.; Speirs, V. Choosing the right cell line for breast cancer research. *Breast Cancer Res.* **2011**, *13*, 1–7. [CrossRef] [PubMed]
5. Agarwal, C.; Sharma, Y.; Zhao, J.; Agarwal, R. A polyphenolic fraction from grape seeds causes irreversible growth inhibition of breast carcinoma MDA-MB468 cells by inhibiting mitogen- activated protein kinases activation and inducing G1 arrest and differentiation. *Clin. Cancer Res.* **2000**, *6*, 2921–2930. [PubMed]
6. Leone, A.; Longo, C.; Gerardi, C.; Trosko, J.E. Pro-apoptotic effect of grape seed extract on MCF-7 involves transient increase of gap junction intercellular communication and Cx43 up-regulation: A mechanism of chemoprevention. *Int. J. Mol. Sci.* **2019**, *20*, 3244. [CrossRef]
7. Dinicola, S.; Pasqualato, A.; Cucina, A.; Coluccia, P. Grape seed extract suppresses MDA-MB231 breast cancer cell migration and invasion. *Eur. J. Nutr.* **2014**, *53*, 421–431. [CrossRef]
8. Lu, J.; Zhang, K.; Chen, S.; Wen, W. Grape seed extract inhibits VEGF expression via reducing HIF-1α protein expression. *Carcinogenesis* **2009**, *30*, 636–644. [CrossRef]

9. Eng, E.T.; Williams, D.; Mandava, U.; Kirma, N.; Tekmal, R.R.; Chen, S. Anti-Aromatase Chemicals in Red Wine. *Ann. N. Y. Acad. Sci.* **2006**, *963*, 239–246. [CrossRef]
10. Kijima, I.; Phung, S.; Hur, G.; Kwok, S.L.; Chen, S. Grape seed extract is an aromatase inhibitor and a suppressor of aromatase expression. *Cancer Res.* **2006**, *66*, 5960–5967. [CrossRef]
11. Sharma, G.; Tyagi, A.K.; Singh, R.P.; Chan, D.C.F.; Agarwal, R. Synergistic anti-cancer effects of grape seed extract and conventional cytotoxic agent doxorubicin against human breast carcinoma cells. *Breast Cancer Res. Treat.* **2004**, *85*, 1–12. [CrossRef]
12. Yousef, M.I.; Mahdy, M.A.; Abdou, H.M. The potential protective role of grape seed proanthocyanidin extract against the mixture of carboplatin and thalidomide induced hepatotoxicity and cardiotoxicity in male rats. *Prev. Med. Commun. Health* **2020**, *2*, 1–7. [CrossRef]
13. Makris, D.P.; Kallithraka, S.; Kefalas, P. Flavonols in grapes, grape products and wines: Burden, profile and influential parameters. *J. Food Compos. Anal.* **2006**, *19*, 396–404. [CrossRef]
14. Simonetti, P.; Pietta, P.; Testolin, G. Polyphenol content and total antioxidant potential of selected Italian wines. *J. Agric. Food Chem.* **1997**, *45*, 1152–1155. [CrossRef]
15. Gardner, P.T.; McPhail, D.B.; Crozier, A.; Duthie, G.G. Electron spin resonance (ESR) spectroscopic assessment of the contribution of quercetin and other flavonols to the antioxidant capacity of red wines. *J. Sci. Food Agric.* **1999**, *79*, 1011–1014. [CrossRef]
16. McDonald, M.S.; Hughes, M.; Burns, J.; Lean, M.E.J.; Matthews, D.; Crozier, A. Survey of the Free and Conjugated Myricetin and Quercetin Content of Red Wines of Different Geographical Origins. *J. Agric. Food Chem.* **1998**, *46*, 368–375. [CrossRef]
17. Dabeek, W.M.; Marra, M.V. Dietary quercetin and kaempferol: Bioavailability and potential cardiovascular-related bioactivity in humans. *Nutrients* **2019**, *11*, 2288. [CrossRef]
18. Kennedy, J.A. Grape and wine phenolics: Observations and recent findings. *Ciencia e Investigación Agraria* **2008**, *35*, 107–120. [CrossRef]
19. Fernández de Simón, B.; Hernández, T.; Cadahía, E.; Dueñas, M.; Estrella, I. Phenolic compounds in a Spanish red wine aged in barrels made of Spanish, French and American oak wood. *Eur. Food Res. Technol.* **2003**, *216*, 150–156. [CrossRef]
20. Castellari, M.; Piermattei, B.; Arfelli, G.; Amati, A. Influence of aging conditions on the quality of red Sangiovese wine. *J. Agric. Food Chem.* **2001**, *49*, 3672–3676. [CrossRef]
21. Makris, D.P.; Rossiter, J.T. Heat-induced, metal-catalyzed oxidative degradation of quercetin and rutin (quercetin 3-*O*-rhamnosylglucoside) in aqueous model systems. *J. Agric. Food Chem.* **2000**, *48*, 3830–3838. [CrossRef]
22. Hashemzaei, M.; Far, A.D.; Yari, A.; Heravi, R.E.; Tabrizian, K.; Taghdisi, S.M.; Sadegh, S.E.; Tsarouhas, K.; Kouretas, D.; Tzanakakis, G.; et al. Anticancer and apoptosis-inducing effects of quercetin in vitro and in vivo. *Oncol. Rep.* **2017**, *38*, 819–828. [CrossRef] [PubMed]
23. Imran, M.; Salehi, B.; Sharifi-Rad, J.; Gondal, T.A.; Saeed, F.; Imran, A.; Shahbaz, M.; Fokou, P.V.T.; Arshad, M.U.; Khan, H.; et al. Kaempferol: A key emphasis to its anticancer potential. *Molecules* **2019**, *24*, 2277. [CrossRef] [PubMed]
24. Franke, A.A.; Custer, L.J.; Wilkens, L.R.; Le Marchand, L.; Nomura, A.M.Y.; Goodman, M.T.; Kolonel, L.N. Liquid chromatographic-photodiode array mass spectrometric analysis of dietary phytoestrogens from human urine and blood. *J. Chromatogr. B Anal. Technol. Biomed. Life Sci.* **2002**, *777*, 45–59. [CrossRef]
25. Wang, L.; Lee, I.M.; Zhang, S.M.; Blumberg, J.B.; Buring, J.E.; Sesso, H.D. Dietary intake of selected flavonols, flavones, and flavonoid-rich foods and risk of cancer in middle-aged and older women. *Am. J. Clin. Nutr.* **2009**, *89*, 905–912. [CrossRef] [PubMed]
26. Mokbel, K.; Mokbel, K. Chemoprevention of Breast Cancer with Vitamins and Micronutrients: A Concise Review. *In Vivo* **2019**, *33*, 983–997. [CrossRef]
27. Wang, X.; Yang, Y.; An, Y.; Fang, G. The mechanism of anticancer action and potential clinical use of kaempferol in the treatment of breast cancer. *Biomed. Pharmacother.* **2019**, *117*, 109086. [CrossRef]
28. Tang, S.M.; Deng, X.T.; Zhou, J.; Li, Q.P.; Ge, X.X.; Miao, L. Pharmacological basis and new insights of quercetin action in respect to its anti-cancer effects. *Biomed. Pharmacother.* **2020**, *121*, 109604. [CrossRef]
29. Barve, A.; Chen, C.; Hebbar, V.; Desiderioa, J.; Constance Lay-Lay Saw, A.-N.K. Metabolism, oral bioavailability and pharmacokinetics of chemopreventive kaempferol in rats. *Biopharm. Drug Dispos.* **2009**, *30*, 356–365. [CrossRef]

30. Zabela, V.; Sampath, C.; Oufir, M.; Moradi-Afrapoli, F.; Butterweck, V.; Hamburger, M. Pharmacokinetics of dietary kaempferol and its metabolite 4-hydroxyphenylacetic acid in rats. *Fitoterapia* **2016**, *115*, 189–197. [CrossRef]
31. Lamson, D.W.; Brignall, M.S. Antioxidants and cancer III: Quercetin. *Altern. Med. Rev.* **2000**, *5*, 196–208.
32. Cai, X.; Fang, Z.; Dou, J.; Yu, A.; Zhai, G. Bioavailability of Quercetin: Problems and Promises. *Curr. Med. Chem.* **2013**, *20*, 2572–2582. [CrossRef] [PubMed]
33. Liu, S.; Li, R.; Qian, J.; Sun, J.; Li, G.; Shen, J.; Xie, Y. The combination therapy of doxorubicin and quercetin on multidrug resistant breast cancer and their sequential delivery by reduction-sensitive hyaluronic acid-based conjugate/D-α-tocopheryl polyethylene glycol 1000 succinate mixed micelles. *Mol. Pharm.* **2020**, *17*, 1415–1427. [CrossRef] [PubMed]
34. Liu, Z.; Balasubramanian, V.; Bhat, C.; Vahermo, M.; Mäkilä, E.; Kemell, M.; Fontana, F.; Janoniene, A.; Petrikaite, V.; Salonen, J.; et al. Quercetin-Based Modified Porous Silicon Nanoparticles for Enhanced Inhibition of Doxorubicin-Resistant Cancer Cells. *Adv. Healthc. Mater.* **2017**, *6*, 1–11. [CrossRef] [PubMed]
35. Lv, L.; Liu, C.; Chen, C.; Yu, X.; Chen, G.; Shi, Y.; Qin, F.; Ou, J.; Qiu, K.; Li, G. Quercetin and doxorubicin co-encapsulated biotin receptortargeting nanoparticles for minimizing drug resistance in breast cancer. *Oncotarget* **2016**, *7*, 32184–32199. [CrossRef]
36. Kubatka, P.; Kapinová, A.; Kello, M.; Kruzliak, P.; Kajo, K.; Výbohová, D.; Mahmood, S.; Murin, R.; Viera, T.; Mojžiš, J.; et al. Fruit peel polyphenols demonstrate substantial anti-tumour effects in the model of breast cancer. *Eur. J. Nutr.* **2015**, *55*, 955–965. [CrossRef]
37. Leigh Ackland, M.; Van De Waarsenburg, S.; Jones, R. Synergistic antiproliferation action of the flavonols quercetin and kaempferol in cultured human cancer cell lines. *In Vivo* **2005**, *19*, 69–76.
38. Yi, X.; Zuo, J.; Tan, C.; Xian, S.; Luo, C.; Chen, S.; Yu, L.; Luo, Y. Kaempferol, a flavonoid compound from gynura medica induced apoptosis and growth inhibition in MCF-7 breast cancer cell. *Afr. J. Tradit. Complement. Altern. Med.* **2016**, *13*, 210–215. [CrossRef]
39. Choi, E.J.; Ahn, W.S. Kaempferol induced the apoptosis via cell cycle arrest in human breast cancer MDA-MB-453 cells. *Nutr. Res. Pract.* **2008**, *2*, 322–325. [CrossRef]
40. Kang, G.Y.; Lee, E.R.; Kim, J.H.; Jung, J.W.; Lim, J.; Kim, S.K.; Cho, S.G.; Kim, K.P. Downregulation of PLK-1 expression in kaempferol-induced apoptosis of MCF-7 cells. *Eur. J. Pharmacol.* **2009**, *611*, 17–21. [CrossRef]
41. Li, S.; Yan, T.; Deng, R.; Jiang, X.; Xiong, H.; Wang, Y.; Yu, Q.; Wang, X.; Chen, C.; Zhu, Y. Low dose of kaempferol suppresses the migration and invasion of triple-negative breast cancer cells by downregulating the activities of RhoA and Rac1. *OncoTargets Ther.* **2017**, *10*, 4809–4819. [CrossRef]
42. Zhu, L.; Xue, L. Kaempferol suppresses proliferation and induces cell cycle arrest, apoptosis, and DNA damage in breast cancer cells. *Oncol. Res.* **2019**, *27*, 629–634. [CrossRef] [PubMed]
43. Ranganathan, S.; Halagowder, D.; Sivasithambaram, N.D. Quercetin suppresses twist to induce apoptosis in MCF-7 breast cancer cells. *PLoS ONE* **2015**, *10*, 1–21. [CrossRef] [PubMed]
44. Kabała-Dzik, A.; Rzepecka-Stojko, A.; Kubina, R.; Iriti, M.; Wojtyczka, R.D.; Buszman, E.; Stojko, J. Flavonoids, bioactive components of propolis, exhibit cytotoxic activity and induce cell cycle arrest and apoptosis in human breast cancer cells MDA-MB-231 and MCF-7—A comparative study. *Cell. Mol. Biol.* **2018**, *64*, 1–10. [CrossRef] [PubMed]
45. Kim, B.W.; Lee, E.R.; Min, H.; Jeong, H.S.; Ahn, J.Y.; Kim, J.H.; Choi, H.Y.; Choi, H.; Eun, Y.K.; Se, P.P.; et al. Sustained ERK activation is involved in the kaempferol-induced apoptosis of breast cancer cells and is more evident under 3-D culture condition. *Cancer Biol. Ther.* **2008**, *7*, 1080–1089. [CrossRef]
46. Liao, W.; Chen, L.; Ma, X.; Jiao, R.; Li, X.; Wang, Y. Protective effects of kaempferol against reactive oxygen species-induced hemolysis and its antiproliferative activity on human cancer cells. *Eur. J. Med. Chem.* **2016**, *114*, 24–32. [CrossRef]
47. Zhang, H.; Zhang, M.; Yu, L.; Zhao, Y.; He, N.; Yang, X. Antitumor activities of quercetin and quercetin-5′,8-disulfonate in human colon and breast cancer cell lines. *Food Chem. Toxicol.* **2012**, *50*, 1589–1599. [CrossRef]
48. Wu, Q.; Needs, P.W.; Lu, Y.; Kroon, P.A.; Ren, D.; Yang, X. Different antitumor effects of quercetin, quercetin-3′-sulfate and quercetin-3-glucuronide in human breast cancer MCF-7 cells. *Food Funct.* **2018**, *9*, 1736–1746. [CrossRef]
49. Niazvand, F.; Orazizadeh, M.; Khorsandi, L.; Abbaspour, M.; Mansouri, E.; Khodadadi, A. Effects of Quercetin-Loaded Nanoparticles on MCF-7 Human Breast Cancer Cells. *Medicina* **2019**, *55*, 114. [CrossRef]

50. Chou, C.C.; Yang, J.S.; Lu, H.F.; Ip, S.W.; Lo, C.; Wu, C.C.; Lin, J.P.; Tang, N.Y.; Chung, J.G.; Chou, M.J.; et al. Quercetin-mediated cell cycle arrest and apoptosis involving activation of a caspase cascade through the mitochondrial pathway in human breast cancer MCF-7 cells. *Arch. Pharm. Res.* **2010**, *33*, 1181–1191. [CrossRef]
51. Chien, S.Y.; Wu, Y.C.; Chung, J.G.; Yang, J.S.; Lu, H.F.; Tsou, M.F.; Wood, W.; Kuo, S.J.; Chen, D.R. Quercetin-induced apoptosis acts through mitochondrial- and caspase-3-dependent pathways in human breast cancer MDA-MB-231 cells. *Hum. Exp. Toxicol.* **2009**, *28*, 493–503. [CrossRef]
52. Balakrishnan, S.; Mukherjee, S.; Das, S.; Bhat, F.A.; Raja Singh, P.; Patra, C.R.; Arunakaran, J. Gold nanoparticles–conjugated quercetin induces apoptosis via inhibition of EGFR/PI3K/Akt–mediated pathway in breast cancer cell lines (MCF-7 and MDA-MB-231). *Cell Biochem. Funct.* **2017**, *35*, 217–231. [CrossRef] [PubMed]
53. Lin, C.W.; Hou, W.C.; Shen, S.C.; Juan, S.H.; Ko, C.H.; Wang, L.M.; Chen, Y.C. Quercetin inhibition of tumor invasion via suppressing PKCδ/ERK/AP-1-dependent matrix metalloproteinase-9 activation in breast carcinoma cells. *Carcinogenesis* **2008**, *29*, 1807–1815. [CrossRef] [PubMed]
54. Li, J.; Zhu, F.; Lubet, R.A.; De Luca, A.; Grubbs, C.; Ericson, M.E.; D'Alessio, A.; Normanno, N.; Dong, Z.; Bode, A.M. Quercetin-3-methyl ether inhibits lapatinib-sensitive and -resistant breast cancer cell growth by inducing G2/M arrest and apoptosis. *Mol. Carcinog.* **2013**, *52*, 134–143. [CrossRef] [PubMed]
55. Khorsandi, L.; Orazizadeh, M.; Niazvand, F.; Abbaspour, M.R.; Mansouri, E.; Khodadadi, A. Quercetin induces apoptosis and necroptosis in MCF-7 breast cancer cells. *Bratislava Med. J.* **2017**, *118*, 123–128. [CrossRef]
56. Hu, J.; Zhang, Y.; Jiang, X.; Zhang, H.; Gao, Z.; Li, Y.; Fu, R.; Li, L.; Li, J.; Cui, H.; et al. ROS-mediated activation and mitochondrial translocation of CaMKII contributes to Drp1-dependent mitochondrial fission and apoptosis in triple-negative breast cancer cells by isorhamnetin and chloroquine. *J. Exp. Clin. Cancer Res.* **2019**, *38*, 1–16. [CrossRef]
57. Qiu, J.; Zhang, T.; Zhu, X.; Yang, C.; Wang, Y.; Zhou, N.; Ju, B.; Zhou, T.; Deng, G.; Qiu, C. Hyperoside induces breast cancer cells apoptosis via ROS-mediated NF-κB signaling pathway. *Int. J. Mol. Sci.* **2020**, *21*, 131. [CrossRef]
58. Steiner, J.L.; Davis, J.M.; McClellan, J.L.; Enos, R.T.; Carson, J.A.; Fayad, R.; Nagarkatti, M.; Nagarkatti, P.S.; Altomare, D.; Creek, K.E.; et al. Dose-dependent benefits of quercetin on tumorigenesis in the C3(1)/SV40Tag transgenic mouse model of breast cancer. *Cancer Biol. Ther.* **2014**, *15*, 1456–1467. [CrossRef]
59. Phromnoi, K.; Yodkeeree, S.; Anuchapreeda, S.; Limtrakul, P. Inhibition of MMP-3 activity and invasion of the MDA-MB-231 human invasive breast carcinoma cell line by bioflavonoids. *Acta Pharmacol. Sin.* **2009**, *30*, 1169–1176. [CrossRef]
60. Li, C.; Yang, D.; Zhao, Y.; Qiu, Y.; Cao, X.; Yu, Y.; Guo, H.; Gu, X.; Yin, X. Inhibitory Effects of Isorhamnetin on the Invasion of Human Breast Carcinoma Cells by Downregulating the Expression and Activity of Matrix Metalloproteinase-2/9. *Nutr. Cancer* **2015**, *67*, 1191–1200. [CrossRef]
61. Balakrishnan, S.; Bhat, F.A.; Raja Singh, P.; Mukherjee, S.; Elumalai, P.; Das, S.; Patra, C.R.; Arunakaran, J. Gold nanoparticle–conjugated quercetin inhibits epithelial–mesenchymal transition, angiogenesis and invasiveness via EGFR/VEGFR-2-mediated pathway in breast cancer. *Cell Prolif.* **2016**, *49*, 678–697. [CrossRef]
62. Oh, S.J.; Kim, O.; Lee, J.S.; Kim, J.A.; Kim, M.R.; Choi, H.S.; Shim, J.H.; Kang, K.W.; Kim, Y.C. Inhibition of angiogenesis by quercetin in tamoxifen-resistant breast cancer cells. *Food Chem. Toxicol.* **2010**, *48*, 3227–3234. [CrossRef] [PubMed]
63. Brusselmans, K.; Vrolix, R.; Verhoeven, G.; Swinnen, J.V. Induction of cancer cell apoptosis by flavonoids is associated with their ability to inhibit fatty acid synthase activity. *J. Biol. Chem.* **2005**, *280*, 5636–5645. [CrossRef] [PubMed]
64. Hanikoglu, A.; Kucuksayan, E.; Hanikoglu, F.; Ozben, T.; Menounou, G.; Sansone, A.; Chatgilialoglu, C.; Di Bella, G.; Ferreri, C. Effects of somatostatin, curcumin, and quercetin on the fatty acid profile of breast cancer cell membranes. *Can. J. Physiol. Pharmacol.* **2020**, *98*, 131–138. [CrossRef] [PubMed]
65. Kuiper, G.G.J.M.; Lemmen, J.G.; Carlsson, B.; Corton, J.C.; Safe, S.H.; Van Der Saag, P.T.; Van Der Burg, B.; Gustafsson, J.Å. Interaction of estrogenic chemicals and phytoestrogens with estrogen receptor β. *Endocrinology* **1998**, *139*, 4252–4263. [CrossRef] [PubMed]
66. Hung, H. Inhibition of Estrogen Receptor Alpha Expression and Function in MCF-7 Cells by Kaempferol. *J. Cell. Physiol.* **2004**, *198*, 197–208. [CrossRef] [PubMed]

67. Yiğitaslan, S.; Erol, K.; Özatik, F.Y.; Özatik, O.; Şahin, S.; Çengelli, Ç. Estrogen-like activity of quercetin in female rats. *Erciyes Tip Derg.* **2016**, *38*, 53–58. [CrossRef]
68. Puranik, N.V.; Srivastava, P.; Bhatt, G.; John Mary, D.J.S.; Limaye, A.M.; Sivaraman, J. Determination and analysis of agonist and antagonist potential of naturally occurring flavonoids for estrogen receptor (ERα) by various parameters and molecular modelling approach. *Sci. Rep.* **2019**, *9*, 1–11. [CrossRef] [PubMed]
69. Park, Y.J.; Choo, W.H.; Kim, H.R.; Chung, K.H.; Oh, S.M. Inhibitory aromatase effects of flavonoids from ginkgo biloba extracts on estrogen biosynthesis. *Asian Pac. J. Cancer Prev.* **2015**, *16*, 6317–6325. [CrossRef]
70. Kao, Y.C.; Zhou, C.; Sherman, M.; Laughton, C.A.; Chen, S. Molecular basis of the inhibition of human aromatase (estrogen synthetase) by flavone and isoflavone phytoestrogens: A site-directed mutagenesis study. *Environ. Health Perspect.* **1998**, *106*, 85–92. [CrossRef]
71. van Meeuwen, J.A.; ter Burg, W.; Piersma, A.H.; van den Berg, M.; Sanderson, J.T. Mixture effects of estrogenic compounds on proliferation and pS2 expression of MCF-7 human breast cancer cells. *Food Chem. Toxicol.* **2007**, *45*, 2319–2330. [CrossRef]
72. Resende, F.A.; de Oliveira, A.P.S.; de Camargo, M.S.; Vilegas, W.; Varanda, E.A. Evaluation of Estrogenic Potential of Flavonoids Using a Recombinant Yeast Strain and MCF7/BUS Cell Proliferation Assay. *PLoS ONE* **2013**, *8*, 1–7. [CrossRef] [PubMed]
73. Seung, M.O.; Yeon, P.K.; Kyu, H.C. Biphasic effects of kaempferol on the estrogenicity in human breast cancer cells. *Arch. Pharm. Res.* **2006**, *29*, 354–362.
74. Kim, S.H.; Hwang, K.A.; Choi, K.C. Treatment with kaempferol suppresses breast cancer cell growth caused by estrogen and triclosan in cellular and xenograft breast cancer models. *J. Nutr. Biochem.* **2016**, *28*, 70–82. [CrossRef] [PubMed]
75. Lee, G.A.; Choi, K.C.; Hwang, K.A. Treatment with phytoestrogens reversed triclosan and bisphenol A-induced anti-apoptosis in breast cancer cells. *Biomol. Ther.* **2018**, *26*, 503–511. [CrossRef] [PubMed]
76. Lee, G.A.; Choi, K.C.; Hwang, K.A. Kaempferol, a phytoestrogen, suppressed triclosan-induced epithelial-mesenchymal transition and metastatic-related behaviors of MCF-7 breast cancer cells. *Environ. Toxicol. Pharmacol.* **2017**, *49*, 48–57. [CrossRef] [PubMed]
77. Mei, Y.Q.; Kai, L.; Qun, S.; Qingyue, L.; Jinghui, H.; Fangxuan, H.; Ren-Wang, J. Reversal of multidrug resistance in cancer by multi-functional flavonoids. *Front. Oncol.* **2019**, *9*, 487.
78. Soo, Y.C.; Min, K.S.; Na, H.K.; Jung, O.J.; Eun, J.G.; Hwa, J.L. Inhibition of P-glycoprotein by natural products in human breast cancer cells. *Arch. Pharm. Res.* **2005**, *28*, 823–828.
79. Li, S.; Yuan, S.; Zhao, Q.; Wang, B.; Wang, X.; Li, K. Quercetin enhances chemotherapeutic effect of doxorubicin against human breast cancer cells while reducing toxic side effects of it. *Biomed. Pharmacother.* **2018**, *100*, 441–447. [CrossRef]
80. Li, S.; Zhao, Q.; Wang, B.; Yuan, S.; Wang, X.; Li, K. Quercetin reversed MDR in breast cancer cells through down-regulating P-gp expression and eliminating cancer stem cells mediated by YB-1 nuclear translocation. *Phyther. Res.* **2018**, *32*, 1530–1536. [CrossRef]
81. Desale, J.P.; Swami, R.; Kushwah, V.; Katiyar, S.S.; Jain, S. Chemosensitizer and docetaxel-loaded albumin nanoparticle: Overcoming drug resistance and improving therapeutic efficacy. *Nanomedicine* **2018**, *13*, 2759–2776. [CrossRef]
82. Kumar, M.; Sharma, G.; Misra, C.; Kumar, R.; Singh, B.; Katare, O.P.; Raza, K. N-desmethyl tamoxifen and quercetin-loaded multiwalled CNTs: A synergistic approach to overcome MDR in cancer cells. *Mater. Sci. Eng. C* **2018**, *89*, 274–282. [CrossRef] [PubMed]
83. Imai, Y.; Tsukahara, S.; Asada, S.; Sugimoto, Y. Phytoestrogens/flavonoids reverse breast cancer resistance protein/ABCG2-mediated multidrug resistance. *Cancer Res.* **2004**, *64*, 4346–4352. [CrossRef] [PubMed]
84. Fan, X.; Bai, J.; Zhao, S.; Hu, M.; Sun, Y.; Wang, B.; Ji, M.; Jin, J.; Wang, X.; Hu, J.; et al. Evaluation of inhibitory effects of flavonoids on breast cancer resistance protein (BCRP): From library screening to biological evaluation to structure-activity relationship. *Toxicol. Vitr.* **2019**, *61*, 104642. [CrossRef] [PubMed]
85. An, G.; Gallegos, J.; Morris, M.E. The bioflavonoid kaempferol is an Abcg2 substrate and inhibits Abcg2-mediated quercetin efflux. *Drug Metab. Dispos.* **2011**, *39*, 426–432. [CrossRef]
86. Zheng, L.; Zhu, L.; Zhao, M.; Shi, J.; Li, Y.; Yu, J.; Jiang, H.; Wu, J.; Tong, Y.; Liu, Y.; et al. In Vivo Exposure of Kaempferol Is Driven by Phase II Metabolic Enzymes and Efflux Transporters. *AAPS J.* **2016**, *18*, 1289–1299. [CrossRef]

87. Li, Y.; Lu, L.; Wang, L.; Qu, W.; Liu, W.; Xie, Y.; Zheng, H.; Wang, Y.; Qi, X.; Hu, M.; et al. Interplay of Efflux Transporters with Glucuronidation and Its Impact on Subcellular Aglycone and Glucuronide Disposition: A Case Study with Kaempferol. *Mol. Pharm.* **2018**, *15*, 5602–5614. [CrossRef]
88. Yao, L.H.; Jiang, Y.M.; Shi, J.; Tomás-Barberán, F.A.; Datta, N.; Singanusong, R.; Chen, S.S. Flavonoids in food and their health benefits. *Plant Foods Hum. Nutr.* **2004**, *59*, 113–122. [CrossRef]
89. Pastrana-Bonilla, E.; Akoh, C.C.; Sellappan, S.; Krewer, G. Phenolic Content and Antioxidant Capacity of Muscadine Grapes. *J. Agric. Food Chem.* **2003**, *51*, 5497–5503. [CrossRef]
90. Graham, H.N. Green tea composition, consumption, and polyphenol chemistry. *Prev. Med.* **1992**, *21*, 334–350. [CrossRef]
91. Bell, J.R.C.; Donovan, J.L.; Wong, R.; Waterhouse, A.L.; German, J.B.; Walzem, R.L. (+)-Catechin in human plasma after ingestion of a single serving of reconstituted red wine. *Am. J. Clin. Nutr.* **2000**, *71*, 103–108. [CrossRef]
92. Silva, J.M.R.; Rigaud, J.; Cheynier, V.; Cheminat, A.; Moutounet, M. Procyanidin dimers and trimers from grape seeds. *Phytochemistry* **1991**, *30*, 1259–1264. [CrossRef]
93. Prieur, C.; Rigaud, J.; Cheynier, V.; Moutounet, M. Oligomeric and polymeric procyanidins from grape seeds. *Phytochemistry* **1994**, *36*, 781–784. [CrossRef]
94. Kim, H.; Hall, P.; Smith, M.; Kirk, M.; Prasain, J.K.; Barnes, S.; Grubbs, C. Chemoprevention by Grape Seed Extract and Genistein in Carcinogen- induced Mammary Cancer in Rats Is Diet Dependent 1, 2. *Int. Res. Conf. Food Nutr. Cancer* **2004**, 3445–3452. [CrossRef] [PubMed]
95. Ou, K.; Gu, L. Absorption and metabolism of proanthocyanidins. *J. Funct. Foods* **2014**, *7*, 43–53. [CrossRef]
96. Tsang, C.; Auger, C.; Mullen, W.; Bornet, A.; Rouanet, J.-M.; Crozier, A.; Teissedre, P.-L. The absorption, metabolism and excretion of flavan-3-ols and procyanidins following the ingestion of a grape seed extract by rats. *Br. J. Nutr.* **2005**, *94*, 170–181. [CrossRef]
97. Serra, A.; MacI, A.; Romero, M.P.; Valls, J.; Bladé, C.; Arola, L.; Motilva, M.J. Bioavailability of procyanidin dimers and trimers and matrix food effects in in vitro and in vivo models. *Br. J. Nutr.* **2010**, *103*, 944–952. [CrossRef]
98. Sano, A.; Yamakoshi, J.; Tokutake, S.; Tobe, K.; Kubota, Y.; Kikuchi, M. Procyanidin B1 is detected in human serum after intake of proanthocyanidin-rich grape seed extract. *Biosci. Biotechnol. Biochem.* **2003**, *67*, 1140–1143. [CrossRef]
99. Yang, C.S.; Sang, S.; Lambert, J.D.; Lee, M.J. Bioavailability issues in studying the health effects of plant polyphenolic compounds. *Mol. Nutr. Food Res.* **2008**, *52*, 139–151. [CrossRef]
100. Meng, X.; Sang, S.; Zhu, N.; Lu, H.; Sheng, S.; Lee, M.J.; Ho, C.T.; Yang, C.S. Identification and characterization of methylated and ring-fission metabolites of tea catechins formed in humans, mice, and rats. *Chem. Res. Toxicol.* **2002**, *15*, 1042–1050. [CrossRef]
101. Faria, A.; Calhau, C.; De Freitas, V.; Mateus, N. Procyanidins as antioxidants and tumor cell growth modulators. *J. Agric. Food Chem.* **2006**, *54*, 2392–2397. [CrossRef]
102. Alshatwi, A.A. Catechin hydrate suppresses MCF-7 proliferation through TP53/Caspase-mediated apoptosis. *J. Exp. Clin. Cancer Res.* **2010**, *29*, 1–9. [CrossRef] [PubMed]
103. Damianaki, A.; Bakogeorgou, E.; Kampa, M.; Notas, G.; Hatzoglou, A.; Panagiotou, S.; Gemetzi, C.; Kouroumalis, E.; Martin, P.M.; Castanas, E. Potent inhibitory action of red wine polyphenols on human breast cancer cells. *J. Cell. Biochem.* **2000**, *78*, 429–441. [CrossRef]
104. Singletary, K.W.; Meline, B. Effect of Grape Seed Proanthocyanidins on Colon Aberrant Crypts and Breast Tumors in a Rat Dual-Organ Tumor Model. *Nutr. Cancer* **2001**, *39*, 252–258. [CrossRef] [PubMed]
105. Wahner-roedler, D.L.; Bauer, B.A.; Loehrer, L.L.; Cha, S.S.; Vera, J.; Hoskin, T.L.; Olson, J.E. The Effect of Grape Seed Extract on Estrogen Levels of Postmenopausal Women—A Pilot Study. *J. Diet. Suppl.* **2016**, *11*, 184–197. [CrossRef]
106. Ye, X.; Krohn, R.L.; Liu, W.; Joshi, S.S.; Kuszynski, C.A.; McGinn, T.R.; Bagchi, M.; Preuss, H.G.; Stohs, S.J.; Bagchi, D. The cytotoxic effects of a novel IH636 grape seed proanthocyanidin extract on cultured human cancer cells. *Stress Adapt. Prophyl. Treat.* **1999**, *196*, 99–108.
107. Brooker, S.; Martin, S.; Pearson, A.; Bagchi, D.; Earl, J.; Gothard, L.; Hall, E.; Porter, L.; Yarnold, J. Double-blind, placebo-controlled, randomised phase II trial of IH636 grape seed proanthocyanidin extract (GSPE) in patients with radiation-induced breast induration. *Radiother. Oncol.* **2006**, *79*, 45–51. [CrossRef]

108. Ma, Z.F.; Zhang, H. Phytochemical constituents, health benefits, and industrial applications of grape seeds: A mini-review. *Antioxidants* **2017**, *6*, 71. [CrossRef]
109. Tang, K.; Liu, T.; Han, Y.; Xu, Y.; Li, J.M. The Importance of Monomeric Anthocyanins in the Definition of Wine Colour Properties. *S. Afr. J. Enol. Vitic.* **2017**, *38*, 1–10. [CrossRef]
110. Zhang, Y.; Butelli, E.; Martin, C. Engineering anthocyanin biosynthesis in plants. *Curr. Opin. Plant Biol.* **2014**, *19*, 81–90. [CrossRef]
111. Khoo, H.E.; Azlan, A.; Tang, S.T.; Lim, S.M. Anthocyanidins and anthocyanins: Colored pigments as food, pharmaceutical ingredients, and the potential health benefits. *Food Nutr. Res.* **2017**, *61*, 1361779. [CrossRef]
112. Tsuda, T.; Watanabe, M.; Ohshima, K.; Norinobu, S.; Choi, S.W.; Kawakishi, S.; Osawa, T. Antioxidative Activity of the Anthocyanin Pigments Cyanidin 3-*O*-β-d-Glucoside and Cyanidin. *J. Agric. Food Chem.* **1994**, *42*, 2407–2410. [CrossRef]
113. Lila, M.A.; Burton-Freeman, B.; Grace, M.; Kalt, W. Unraveling Anthocyanin Bioavailability for Human Health. *Annu. Rev. Food Sci. Technol.* **2016**, *7*, 375–393. [CrossRef] [PubMed]
114. Lin, B.W.; Gong, C.C.; Song, H.F.; Cui, Y.Y. Effects of anthocyanins on the prevention and treatment of cancer. *Br. J. Pharmacol.* **2017**, *174*, 1226–1243. [CrossRef] [PubMed]
115. Hemmlnki, K. DNA adducts, mutations and cancer. *Carcinogenesis* **1993**, *14*, 2007–2012. [CrossRef]
116. Singletary, K.W.; Jung, K.J.; Giusti, M. Anthocyanin-rich grape extract blocks breast cell DNA damage. *J. Med. Food* **2007**, *10*, 244–251. [CrossRef]
117. Syed, D.N.; Afaq, F.; Sarfaraz, S.; Khan, N.; Kedlaya, R.; SAetaluri, V.; Mukhtar, H. Delphinidin inhibits cell proliferation and invasion via modulation of Met receptor phosphorylation. *Toxicol. Appl. Pharmacol.* **2008**, *231*, 52–60. [CrossRef]
118. Jeffers, M.; Schmidt, L.; Nakaigawa, N.; Webb, C.P.; Weirich, G.; Kishida, T.; Zbar, B.; Vande Woude, G.F. Activating mutations for the Met tyrosine kinase receptor in human cancer. *Proc. Natl. Acad. Sci. USA* **1997**, *94*, 11445–11450. [CrossRef]
119. Ding, S.; Merkulova-Rainon, T.; Han, Z.C.; Tobelem, G. HGF receptor up-regulation contributes to the angiogenic phenotype of human endothelial cells and promotes angiogenesis in vitro. *Blood* **2003**, *101*, 4816–4822. [CrossRef]
120. Bae-Jump, V.; Segreti, E.M.; Vandermolen, D.; Kauma, S. Hepatocyte growth factor (HGF) induces invasion of endometrial carcinoma cell lines in vitro. *Gynecol. Oncol.* **1999**, *73*, 265–272. [CrossRef]
121. Jeffers, M.; Rong, S.; Woude, G.F. Enhanced tumorigenicity and invasion-metastasis by hepatocyte growth factor/scatter factor-met signalling in human cells concomitant with induction of the urokinase proteolysis network. *Mol. Cell. Biol.* **1996**, *16*, 1115–1125. [CrossRef]
122. Murray, D.W.; Didier, S.; Chan, A.; Paulino, V.; Van Aelst, L.; Ruggieri, R.; Tran, N.L.; Byrne, A.T.; Symons, M. Guanine nucleotide exchange factor Dock7 mediates HGF-induced glioblastoma cell invasion via Rac activation. *Br. J. Cancer* **2014**, *110*, 1307–1315. [CrossRef]
123. Yang, Y.; Spitzer, E.; Meyer, D.; Sachs, M.; Niemann, C.; Hartmann, G.; Weidner, K.M.; Birchmeier, C.; Birchmeier, W. Sequential requirement of hepatocyte growth factor and neuregulin in the morphogenesis and differentiation of the mammary gland. *J. Cell Biol.* **1995**, *131*, 215–226. [CrossRef] [PubMed]
124. Yang, X.; Luo, E.; Liu, X.; Han, B.; Yu, X.; Peng, X. Delphinidin-3-glucoside suppresses breast carcinogenesis by inactivating the Akt/HOTAIR signaling pathway. *BMC Cancer* **2016**, *16*, 423. [CrossRef] [PubMed]
125. Khorkova, O.; Hsiao; Wahlestedt, C. Basic Biology and Therapeutic Implications of lncRNA. *Physiol. Behav.* **2015**, *87*, 15–24. [CrossRef] [PubMed]
126. Hajjari, M.; Salavaty, A. HOTAIR: An oncogenic long non-coding RNA in different cancers. *Cancer Biol. Med.* **2015**, *12*, 1–9. [PubMed]
127. Yang, G.; Zhang, S.; Gao, F.; Liu, Z.; Lu, M.; Peng, S.; Zhang, T.; Zhang, F. Osteopontin enhances the expression of HOTAIR in cancer cells via IRF1. *Biochim. Biophys. Acta Gene Regul. Mech.* **2014**, *1839*, 837–848. [CrossRef]
128. Chen, J.; Lin, C.; Yong, W.; Ye, Y.; Huang, Z. Calycosin and genistein induce apoptosis by inactivation of HOTAIR/p-akt signaling pathway in human breast cancer MCF-7 cells. *Cell. Physiol. Biochem.* **2015**, *35*, 722–728. [CrossRef]
129. Zhang, Y.; Vareed, S.K.; Nair, M.G. Human tumor cell growth inhibition by nontoxic anthocyanidins, the pigments in fruits and vegetables. *Life Sci.* **2005**, *76*, 1465–1472. [CrossRef]

130. Afaq, F.; Zaman, N.; Khan, N.; Syed, D.N.; Sarfaraz, S.; Zaid, M.A.; Mukhtar, H. Inhibition of epidermal growth factor receptor signaling pathway by delphinidin, an anthocyanidin in pigmented fruits and vegetables. *Int. J. Cancer* **2008**, *123*, 1508–1515. [CrossRef]
131. Abd El-Rehim, D.M.; Pinder, S.E.; Paish, C.E.; Bell, J.A.; Rampaul, R.S.; Blamey, R.W.; Robertson, J.F.R.; Nicholson, R.I.; Ellis, I.O. Expression and co-expression of the members of the epidermal growth factor receptor (EGFR) family in invasive breast carcinoma. *Br. J. Cancer* **2004**, *91*, 1532–1542. [CrossRef]
132. Chen, J.; Zhu, Y.; Zhang, W.; Peng, X.; Zhou, J.; Li, F.; Han, B.; Liu, X.; Ou, Y.; Yu, X. Delphinidin induced protective autophagy via mTOR pathway suppression and AMPK pathway activation in HER-2 positive breast cancer cells. *BMC Cancer* **2018**, *18*, 342. [CrossRef] [PubMed]
133. Ma, X.; Ning, S. Cyanidin-3-glucoside attenuates the angiogenesis of breast cancer via inhibiting STAT3/VEGF pathway. *Phyther. Res.* **2019**, *33*, 81–89. [CrossRef] [PubMed]
134. Liang, L.; Liu, X.; He, J.; Shao, Y.; Liu, J.; Wang, Z.; Xia, L.; Han, T.; Wu, P. Cyanidin-3-glucoside induces mesenchymal to epithelial transition via activating Sirt1 expression in triple negative breast cancer cells. *Biochimie* **2019**, *162*, 107–115. [CrossRef] [PubMed]
135. Samavat, H.; Kurzer, M.S. Estrogen Metabolism and Breast Cancer. *Cancer Lett.* **2015**, *356*, 231–243. [CrossRef]
136. Reis-Filho, J.S.; Tutt, A.N.J. Triple negative tumours: A critical review. *Histopathology* **2008**, *52*, 108–118. [CrossRef]
137. Zhang, X.T.; Kang, L.G.; Ding, L.; Vranic, S.; Gatalica, Z.; Wang, Z.Y. A positive feedback loop of ER-α36/EGFR promotes malignant growth of ER-negative breast cancer cells. *Oncogene* **2011**, *30*, 770. [CrossRef]
138. Wang, Z.Y.; Zhang, X.T.; Shen, P.; Loggie, B.W.; Chang, Y.C.; Deuel, T.F. A variant of estrogen receptor-α, hER-α36: Transduction of estrogen- and antiestrogen-dependent membrane-initiated mitogenic signaling. *Proc. Natl. Acad. Sci. USA* **2006**, *103*, 9063–9068. [CrossRef]
139. Wang, L.; Li, H.; Yang, S.; Ma, W.; Liu, M.; Guo, S.; Zhan, J.; Zhang, H.; Tsang, S.Y.; Zhang, Z.; et al. Cyanidin-3-o-glucoside directly binds to ERa36 and inhibits EGFR-positive triple-negative breast cancer. *Oncotarget* **2016**, *7*, 68864. [CrossRef]
140. Fernandes, I.; Faria, A.; Azevedo, J.; Soares, S.; Calhau, C.; De Freitas, V.; Mateus, N. Influence of anthocyanins, derivative pigments and other catechol and pyrogallol-type phenolics on breast cancer cell proliferation. *J. Agric. Food Chem.* **2010**, *58*, 3785–3792. [CrossRef]
141. Swain, S.M.; Baselga, J.; Kim, S.B.; Ro, J.; Semiglazov, V.; Campone, M.; Ciruelos, E.; Ferrero, J.; Schneeweiss, A.; Heeson, S.; et al. Pertuzumab, trastuzumab, and docetaxel in HER2-positive metastatic breast cancer. *N. Engl. J. Med.* **2015**, *372*, 724–734. [CrossRef]
142. Witzel, I.; Müller, V.; Abenhardt, W.; Kaufmann, M.; Schoenegg, W.; Schneeweis, A.; Jänicke, F. Long-term tumor remission under trastuzumab treatment for HER2 positive metastatic breast cancer—Results from the HER-OS patient registry. *BMC Cancer* **2014**, *14*, 806. [CrossRef] [PubMed]
143. Li, X.; Xu, J.; Tang, X.; Liu, Y.; Yu, X.; Wang, Z.; Liu, W. Anthocyanins inhibit trastuzumab-resistant breast cancer in vitro and in vivo. *Mol. Med. Rep.* **2016**, *13*, 4007–4013. [CrossRef] [PubMed]
144. Liu, W.; Xu, J.; Liu, Y.; Yu, X.; Tang, X.; Wang, Z.; Li, X. Anthocyanins potentiate the activity of trastuzumab in human epidermal growth factor receptor 2-positive breast cancer cells in vitro and in vivo. *Mol. Med. Rep.* **2014**, *10*, 1921–1926. [CrossRef] [PubMed]
145. Shen, T.; Wang, X.N.; Lou, H.X. Natural stilbenes: An overview. *Nat. Prod. Rep.* **2009**, *26*, 916–935. [CrossRef]
146. Signorelli, P.; Ghidoni, R. Resveratrol as an anticancer nutrient: Molecular basis, open questions and promises. *J. Nutr. Biochem.* **2005**, *16*, 449–466. [CrossRef]
147. Langcake, P.; Pryce, R.J. The production of resveratrol by Vitis vinifera and other members of the Vitaceae as a response to infection or injury. *Physiol. Plant Pathol.* **1976**, *9*, 77–86. [CrossRef]
148. Jeandet, P.; Bessis, R.; Gautheron, B. The production of resveratrol (3, 5, 4′-trihydroxystilbene) by grape berries in different developmental stages. *Am. J. Enol. Vitic.* **1991**, *42*, 41–46.
149. Goldberg, D.M.; Yan, J.; Ng, E.; Diamandis, E.P.; Karumanchiri, A.; Soleas, G.; Waterhouse, A.L. A global survey of trans-resveratrol concentrations in commercial wines. *Am. J. Enol. Vitic.* **1995**, *46*, 159–165.
150. Romero-Pérez, A.I.; Lamuela-Raventós, R.M.; Waterhouse, A.L.; De La Torre-Boronat, M.C. Levels of cis- and trans-Resveratrol and Their Glucosides in White and Rosé Vitis vinifera Wines from Spain. *J. Agric. Food Chem.* **1996**, *44*, 2124–2128. [CrossRef]

151. Pace-Asciak, C.; Rounova, O.; Hahn, S.E.; Diamandis, E.P.; Goldberg, D.M. Wines and grape juices as modulators of platelet aggregation in healthy human subjects. *Clin. Chim. Acta* **1996**, *246*, 163–182. [CrossRef]
152. Weiskirchen, S.; Weiskirchen, R. Resveratrol: How Much Wine Do You Have to Drink to Stay Healthy? *Adv. Nutr. An Int. Rev. J.* **2016**, *7*, 706–718. [CrossRef] [PubMed]
153. Goldberg, D.M.; Yan, J.; Soleas, G.J. Absorption of three wine-related polyphenols in three different matrices by healthy subjects. *Clin. Biochem.* **2003**, *36*, 79–87. [CrossRef]
154. Walle, T. Bioavailability of resveratrol. *Ann. N. Y. Acad. Sci.* **2011**, *1215*, 9–15. [CrossRef] [PubMed]
155. Sinha, D.; Sarkar, N.; Biswas, J.; Bishayee, A. Resveratrol for breast cancer prevention and therapy: Preclinical evidence and molecular mechanisms. *Semin. Cancer Biol.* **2016**, *40*, 209–232. [CrossRef] [PubMed]
156. Chimento, A.; De Amicis, F.; Sirianni, R.; Sinicropi, M.S.; Puoci, F.; Casaburi, I.; Saturnino, C.; Pezzi, V. Progress to improve oral bioavailability and beneficial effects of resveratrol. *Int. J. Mol. Sci.* **2019**, *20*, 1381. [CrossRef] [PubMed]
157. Nawaz, W.; Zhou, Z.; Deng, S.; Ma, X.; Ma, X.; Li, C.; Shu, X. Therapeutic versatility of resveratrol derivatives. *Nutrients* **2017**, *9*, 1188. [CrossRef] [PubMed]
158. da Costa, D.C.F.; Fialho, E.; Silva, J.L. Cancer chemoprevention by resveratrol: The P53 tumor suppressor protein as a promising molecular target. *Molecules* **2017**, *22*, 1014. [CrossRef]
159. Jang, M.; Cai, L.; Udeani, G.O.; Slowing, K.V.; Thomas, C.F.; Beecher, C.W.W.; Fong, H.H.S.; Farnsworth, N.R.; Kinghorn, A.D.; Mehta, R.G.; et al. Cancer chemopreventive activity of resveratrol, a natural product derived from grapes. *Science* **1997**, *275*, 218–220. [CrossRef]
160. Pezzuto, J.M. Resveratrol: Twenty years of growth, development and controversy. *Biomol. Ther.* **2019**, *27*, 1. [CrossRef]
161. Casanova, F.; Quarti, J.; Da Costa, D.C.F.; Ramos, C.A.; Da Silva, J.L.; Fialho, E. Resveratrol chemosensitizes breast cancer cells to melphalan by cell cycle arrest. *J. Cell. Biochem.* **2012**, *113*, 2586–2596. [CrossRef]
162. Varoni, E.M.; Lo Faro, A.F.; Sharifi-Rad, J.; Iriti, M. Anticancer Molecular Mechanisms of Resveratrol. *Front. Nutr.* **2016**, *3*, 8. [CrossRef] [PubMed]
163. Ko, J.H.; Sethi, G.; Um, J.Y.; Shanmugam, M.K.; Arfuso, F.; Kumar, A.P.; Bishayee, A.; Ahn, K.S. The role of resveratrol in cancer therapy. *Int. J. Mol. Sci.* **2017**, *18*, 2589. [CrossRef] [PubMed]
164. Ndiaye, M.; Kumar, R.; Ahmad, N. Resveratrol in cancer management: Where are we and where we go from here? *Ann. N. Y. Acad. Sci.* **2011**, *1215*, 144–149. [CrossRef] [PubMed]
165. Levi, F.; Pasche, C.; Lucchini, F.; Ghidoni, R.; Ferraroni, M.; La Vecchia, C. Resveratrol and breast cancer risk. *Eur. J. Cancer Prev.* **2005**, *14*, 139–142. [CrossRef] [PubMed]
166. Chakraborty, S.; Levenson, A.S.; Biswas, P.K. Structural insights into Resveratrol's antagonist and partial agonist actions on estrogen receptor alpha. *BMC Struct. Biol.* **2013**, *13*, 27. [CrossRef]
167. Poschner, S.; Maier-Salamon, A.; Thalhammer, T.; Jäger, W. Resveratrol and other dietary polyphenols are inhibitors of estrogen metabolism in human breast cancer cells. *J. Steroid Biochem. Mol. Biol.* **2019**, *190*, 11–18. [CrossRef]
168. Jordan, V.C. Antiestrogens and Selective Estrogen Receptor Modulators as Multifunctional Medicines. 2. Clinical Considerations and New Agents. *J. Med. Chem.* **2003**, *46*, 1081–1111. [CrossRef]
169. Gehm, B.D.; McAndrews, J.M.; Chien, P.Y.; Jameson, J.L. Resveratrol, a polyphenolic compound found in grapes and wine, is an agonist for the estrogen receptor. *Proc. Natl. Acad. Sci. USA* **1997**, *94*, 14138–14143. [CrossRef]
170. Levenson, A.S.; Gehm, B.D.; Pearce, S.T.; Horiguchi, J.; Simons, L.A.; Ward, J.E.; Jameson, J.L.; Jordan, V.C. Resveratrol acts as an estrogen receptor (ER) agonist in breast cancer cells stably transfected with ERα. *Int. J. Cancer* **2003**, *104*, 587–596. [CrossRef]
171. Lu, R.; Serrero, G. Resveratrol, a natural product derived from grape, exhibits antiestrogenic activity and inhibits the growth of human breast cancer cells. *J. Cell. Physiol.* **1999**, *179*, 297–304. [CrossRef]
172. Bowers, J.L.; Tyulmenkov, V.V.; Jernigan, S.C.; Klinge, C.M. Resveratrol acts as a mixed agonist/antagonist for estrogen receptors α and β. *Endocrinology* **2000**, *141*, 3657–3667. [CrossRef] [PubMed]
173. Gehm, B.D.; Levenson, A.S.; Liu, H.; Lee, E.J.; Amundsen, B.M.; Cushman, M.; Jordan, V.C.; Jameson, J.L. Estrogenic effects of resveratrol in breast cancer cells expressing mutant and wild-type estrogen receptors: Role of AF-1 and AF-2. *J. Steroid Biochem. Mol. Biol.* **2004**, *88*, 223–234. [CrossRef] [PubMed]

174. Simpson, E.R.; Michael, M.D.; Agarwal, V.R.; Hinshelwood, M.M.; Bulun, S.E.; Zhao, Y. Cytochromes P450 11: Expression of the CYP19 (aromatase) gene: An unusual case of alternative promoter usage. *FASEB J.* **1997**, *11*, 29–36. [CrossRef]
175. Wang, Y.; Lee, K.W.; Chan, F.L.; Chen, S.; Leung, L.K. The red wine polyphenol resveratrol displays bilevel inhibition on aromatase in breast cancer cells. *Toxicol. Sci.* **2006**, *92*, 71–77. [CrossRef]
176. Chottanapund, S.; Van Duursen, M.B.M.; Navasumrit, P.; Hunsonti, P.; Timtavorn, S.; Ruchirawat, M.; Van den Berg, M. Anti-aromatase effect of resveratrol and melatonin on hormonal positive breast cancer cells co-cultured with breast adipose fibroblasts. *Toxicol. In Vitro* **2014**, *28*, 1215–1221. [CrossRef]
177. Le Corre, L.; Chalabi, N.; Delort, L.; Bignon, Y.J.; Bernard-Gallon, D.J. Resveratrol and breast cancer chemoprevention: Molecular mechanisms. *Mol. Nutr. Food Res.* **2005**, *49*, 462–471. [CrossRef] [PubMed]
178. Sinha, R.; Caporaso, N. Diet, Genetic Susceptibility and Human Cancer Etiology. *J. Nutr.* **1999**, *129*, 556S–559S. [CrossRef]
179. Pozo-Guisado, E.; Alvarez-Barrientos, A.; Mulero-Navarro, S.; Santiago-Josefat, B.; Fernandez-Salguero, P.M. The antiproliferative activity of resveratrol results in apoptosis in MCF-7 but not in MDA-MB-231 human breast cancer cells: Cell-specific alteration of the cell cycle. *Biochem. Pharmacol.* **2002**, *64*, 1375–1386. [CrossRef]
180. Da Costa, D.C.F.; Casanova, F.A.; Quarti, J.; Malheiros, M.S.; Sanches, D.; dos Santos, P.S.; Fialho, E.; Silva, J.L. Transient Transfection of a Wild-Type p53 Gene Triggers Resveratrol-Induced Apoptosis in Cancer Cells. *PLoS ONE* **2012**, *7*, 1–12.
181. Da Costa, D.C.F.; Campos, N.P.C.; Santos, R.A.; Guedes-da-Silva, F.H.; Martins-Dinis, M.M.D.C.; Zanphorlin, L.; Ramos, C.; Rangel, L.P.; Silva, J.L. Resveratrol prevents p53 aggregation in vitro and in breast cancer cells. *Oncotarget* **2018**, *9*, 29112–29122. [CrossRef]
182. Chang, L.C.; Yu, Y.L. Dietary components as epigenetic-regulating agents against cancer. *Biomedicine* **2016**, *6*, 1–8. [CrossRef]
183. Alamolhodaei, N.S.; Tsatsakis, A.M.; Ramezani, M.; Hayes, A.W.; Karimi, G. Resveratrol as MDR reversion molecule in breast cancer: An overview. *Food Chem. Toxicol.* **2017**, *103*, 223–232. [CrossRef]
184. Singh, C.K.; George, J.; Ahmad, N. Resveratrol-based combinatorial strategies for cancer management. *Ann. N. Y. Acad. Sci.* **2014**, *1290*, 113–121. [CrossRef] [PubMed]
185. Chow, H.H.S.; Garland, L.L.; Heckman-Stoddard, B.M.; Hsu, C.H.; Butler, V.D.; Cordova, C.A.; Chew, W.M.; Cornelison, T.L. A pilot clinical study of resveratrol in postmenopausal women with high body mass index: Effects on systemic sex steroid hormones. *J. Transl. Med.* **2014**, *12*, 1–7. [CrossRef]
186. Fernandes, I.; Pérez-Gregorio, R.; Soares, S.; Mateus, N.; De Freitas, V.; Santos-Buelga, C.; Feliciano, A.S. Wine flavonoids in health and disease prevention. *Molecules* **2017**, *22*, 292. [CrossRef] [PubMed]
187. Arbulu, M.; Sampedro, M.C.; Gómez-Caballero, A.; Goicolea, M.A.; Barrio, R.J. Untargeted metabolomic analysis using liquid chromatography quadrupole time-of-flight mass spectrometry for non-volatile profiling of wines. *Anal. Chim. Acta* **2015**, *858*, 32–41. [CrossRef] [PubMed]
188. Alves Filho, E.G.; Silva, L.M.A.; Ribeiro, P.R.V.; de Brito, E.S.; Zocolo, G.J.; Souza-Leão, P.C.; Marques, A.T.B.; Quintela, A.L.; Larsen, F.H.; Canuto, K.M. 1 H NMR and LC-MS-based metabolomic approach for evaluation of the seasonality and viticultural practices in wines from São Francisco River Valley, a Brazilian semi-arid region. *Food Chem.* **2019**, *289*, 558–567. [CrossRef] [PubMed]
189. Cassino, C.; Tsolakis, C.; Bonello, F.; Gianotti, V.; Osella, D. Wine evolution during bottle aging, studied by 1H NMR spectroscopy and multivariate statistical analysis. *Food Res. Int.* **2019**, *116*, 566–577. [CrossRef]
190. Forester, S.C.; Waterhouse, A.L. Metabolites Are Key to Understanding Health Effects of Wine Polyphenolics. *J. Nutr.* **2009**, *139*, 1824S–1831S. [CrossRef]
191. Jiménez-Girón, A.; Queipo-Ortuño, M.; Boto-Ordóñez, M.; Muñoz-Gonzáles, I.; Sánches-Patán, F.; Monagas, M.; Martín-Álvarez, P.; Murri, M.; Tinahones, J.F.; Abdrés-Lacueva, C.; et al. Comparative Study of Microbial-Derived Phenolic Metabolites in Human Feces after Intake of Gin, Red Wine, and Dealcoholized Red Wine. *J. Agric. Food Chem.* **2013**, *61*, 3909–3915. [CrossRef]
192. Jiménez-Girón, A.; Ibáñez, C.; Cifuentes, A.; Simó, C.; Muñoz-González, I.; Martín-Álvarez, P.J.; Bartolomé, B.; Moreno-Arribas, M.V. Faecal metabolomic fingerprint after moderate consumption of red wine by healthy subjects. *J. Proteome Res.* **2015**, *14*, 897–905. [CrossRef] [PubMed]

193. Gonthier, M.-P.; Cheynier, V.; Donovan, J.L.; Manach, C.; Morand, C.; Mila, I.; Lapierre, C.; Rémésy, C.; Scalbert, A. Microbial Aromatic Acid Metabolites Formed in the Gut Account for a Major Fraction of the Polyphenols Excreted in Urine of Rats Fed Red Wine Polyphenols. *J. Nutr.* **2003**, *133*, 461–467. [CrossRef] [PubMed]
194. Al Ali, S.H.H.; Al-Qubaisi, M.; Hussein, M.Z.; Ismail, M.; Bullo, S. Hippuric acid nanocomposite enhances doxorubicin and oxaliplatin-induced cytotoxicity in MDA-MB231, MCF-7 and Caco2 cell lines. *Drug Des. Devel. Ther.* **2013**, *7*, 25. [CrossRef]
195. Wang, X.N.; Wang, K.Y.; Zhang, X.S.; Yang, C.; Li, X.Y. 4-Hydroxybenzoic acid (4-HBA) enhances the sensitivity of human breast cancer cells to adriamycin as a specific HDAC6 inhibitor by promoting HIPK2/p53 pathway. *Biochem. Biophys. Res. Commun.* **2018**, *504*, 812–819. [CrossRef] [PubMed]
196. Yin, M.C.; Lin, C.C.; Wu, H.C.; Tsao, S.M.; Hsu, C.K. Apoptotic effects of protocatechuic acid in human breast, lung, liver, cervix, and prostate cancer cells: Potential mechanisms of action. *J. Agric. Food Chem.* **2009**, *57*, 6468–6473. [CrossRef]
197. Cartron, E.; Fouret, G.; Carbonneau, M.A.; Lauret, C.; Michel, F.; Monnier, L.; Descomps, B.; Léger, C.L. Red-wine beneficial long-term effect on lipids but not on antioxidant characteristics in plasma in a study comparing three types of wine—Description of two O-methylated derivatives of gallic acid in humans. *Free Radic. Res.* **2003**, *37*, 1021–1035. [CrossRef]
198. Mennen, L.I.; Sapinho, D.; Ito, H.; Bertrais, S.; Galan, P.; Hercberg, S.; Scalbert, A. Urinary flavonoids and phenolic acids as biomarkers of intake for polyphenol-rich foods. *Br. J. Nutr.* **2006**, *96*, 191–198. [CrossRef]
199. Lee, H.L.; Lin, C.S.; Kao, S.H.; Chou, M.C. Gallic acid induces G1 phase arrest and apoptosis of triple-negative breast cancer cell MDA-MB-231 via p38 mitogen-activated protein kinase/p21/p27 axis. *Anticancer Drugs* **2017**, *28*, 1150–1156. [CrossRef]
200. Wang, K.; Zhu, X.; Zhang, K.; Zhu, L.; Zhou, F. Investigation of Gallic Acid Induced Anticancer Effect in Human Breast Carcinoma MCF-7 Cells. *J. Biochem. Mol. Toxicol.* **2014**, *28*, 387–393. [CrossRef]
201. Vitaglione, P.; Sforza, S.; Del Rio, D. Occurrence, Bioavailability, and Metabolism of Resveratrol. In *Flavonoids and Related Compounds: Bioavailability and Function*, 1st ed.; Spencer, J.P.E., Crozier, A., Eds.; CRC Press: Boca Raton, FL, USA, 2012; pp. 167–182.
202. Henry-Vitrac, C.; Desmoulière, A.; Girard, D.; Mérillon, J.M.; Krisa, S. Transport, deglycosylation, and metabolism of trans-piceid by small intestinal epithelial cells. *Eur. J. Nutr.* **2006**, *45*, 376–382. [CrossRef]
203. Bode, L.M.; Bunzel, D.; Huch, M.; Cho, G.S.; Ruhland, D.; Bunzel, M.; Bub, A.; Franz, C.M.A.P.; Kulling, S.E. In vivo and in vitro metabolism of trans-resveratrol by human gut microbiota. *Am. J. Clin. Nutr.* **2013**, *97*, 295–309. [CrossRef] [PubMed]
204. Lappano, R.; Rosano, C.; Madeo, A.; Albanito, L.; Plastina, P.; Gabriele, B.; Forti, L.; Stivala, L.A.; Iacopetta, D.; Dolce, V.; et al. Structure-activity relationships of resveratrol and derivatives in breast cancer cells. *Mol. Nutr. Food Res.* **2009**, *53*, 845–858. [CrossRef] [PubMed]
205. Ruotolo, R.; Calani, L.; Fietta, E.; Brighenti, F.; Crozier, A.; Meda, C.; Maggi, A.; Ottonello, S.; Del Rio, D. Anti-estrogenic activity of a human resveratrol metabolite. *Nutr. Metab. Cardiovasc. Dis.* **2013**, *23*, 1086–1092. [CrossRef] [PubMed]
206. Gakh, A.A.; Anisimova, N.Y.; Kiselevsky, M.V.; Sadovnikov, S.V.; Stankov, I.N.; Yudin, M.V.; Rufanov, K.A.; Krasavin, M.Y.; Sosnov, A.V. Dihydro-resveratrol—A potent dietary polyphenol. *Bioorganic Med. Chem. Lett.* **2010**, *20*, 6149–6151. [CrossRef]
207. Giménez-Bastida, J.A.; Ávila-Gálvez, M.Á.; Espín, J.C.; González-Sarrías, A. Conjugated Physiological Resveratrol Metabolites Induce Senescence in Breast Cancer Cells: Role of p53/p21 and p16/Rb Pathways, and ABC Transporters. *Mol. Nutr. Food Res.* **2019**, *63*, 1900629. [CrossRef]
208. Donovan, J.L.; Crespy, V.; Manach, C.; Morand, C.; Besson, C.; Scalbert, A.; Rémésy, C. Catechin Is Metabolized by Both the Small Intestine and Liver of Rats. *J. Nutr.* **2001**, *131*, 1753–1757. [CrossRef]
209. Baba, S.; Osakabe, N.; Natsume, M.; Muto, Y.; Takizawa, T.; Terao, J. In Vivo Comparison of the Bioavailability of (+)-Catechin, (−)-Epicatechin and Their Mixture in Orally Administered Rats. *J. Nutr.* **2001**, *131*, 2885–2891. [CrossRef]
210. Donovan, J.L.; Kasim-Karakas, S.; German, J.B.; Waterhouse, A.L. Urinary excretion of catechin metabolites by human subjects after red wine consumption. *Br. J. Nutr.* **2002**, *87*, 31–37. [CrossRef]

211. Kim, D.H.; Jung, E.A.; Sohng, I.S.; Han, J.A.; Kim, T.H.; Han, M.J. Intestinal bacterial metabolism of flavonoids and its relation to some biological activities. *Arch. Pharm. Res.* **1998**, *21*, 17–23. [CrossRef]
212. Kim, R.K.; Suh, Y.; Yoo, K.C.; Cui, Y.H.; Hwang, E.; Kim, H.J.; Kang, J.S.; Kim, M.J.; Lee, Y.Y.; Lee, S.J. Phloroglucinol suppresses metastatic ability of breast cancer cells by inhibition of epithelial-mesenchymal cell transition. *Cancer Sci.* **2015**, *106*, 94–101. [CrossRef]
213. Kim, R.K.; Uddin, N.; Hyun, J.W.; Kim, C.; Suh, Y.; Lee, S.J. Novel anticancer activity of phloroglucinol against breast cancer stem-like cells. *Toxicol. Appl. Pharmacol.* **2015**, *286*, 143–150. [CrossRef] [PubMed]
214. Fang, J. Bioavailability of anthocyanins. *Drug Metab. Rev.* **2014**, *46*, 508–520. [CrossRef] [PubMed]
215. Tsuda, T.; Horio, F.; Osawa, T. Absorption and metabolism of cyanidin 3-*O*-β-D-glucoside in rats. *FEBS Lett.* **1999**, *449*, 179–182. [CrossRef]
216. Olivas-Aguirre, F.J.; Rodrigo-García, J.; Martínez-Ruiz, N.D.R.; Cárdenas-Robles, A.I.; Mendoza-Díaz, S.O.; Álvarez-Parrilla, E.; González-Aguilar, G.A.; De La Rosa, L.A.; Ramos-Jiménez, A.; Wall-Medrano, A. Cyanidin-3-*O*-glucoside: Physical-chemistry, foodomics and health effects. *Molecules* **2016**, *21*, 1264. [CrossRef] [PubMed]
217. Bub, A.; Watzl, B.; Heeb, D.; Rechkemmer, G.; Briviba, K. Malvidin-3-glucoside bioavailability in humans after ingestion of red wine, dealcoholized red wine and red grape juice. *Eur. J. Nutr.* **2001**, *40*, 113–120. [CrossRef]
218. Bitsch, R.; Netzel, M.; Frank, T.; Strass, G.; Bitsch, I. Bioavailability and biokinetics of anthocyanins from red grape juice and red wine. *J. Biomed. Biotechnol.* **2004**, *2004*, 293–298. [CrossRef]
219. Marques, C.; Fernandes, I.; Norberto, S.; Sá, C.; Teixeira, D.; de Freitas, V.; Mateus, N.; Calhau, C.; Faria, A. Pharmacokinetics of blackberry anthocyanins consumed with or without ethanol: A randomized and crossover trial. *Mol. Nutr. Food Res.* **2016**, *60*, 2319–2330. [CrossRef]
220. Czank, C.; Cassidy, A.; Zhang, Q.; Morrison, D.J.; Preston, T.; Kroon, P.A.; Botting, N.P.; Kay, C.D. Human metabolism and elimination of the anthocyanin, cyanidin-3-glucoside: A ^{13}C-tracer study. *Am. Clin. Nutr.* **2013**, *97*, 995–1003. [CrossRef]
221. Fernandes, I.; Marques, F.; De Freitas, V.; Mateus, N. Antioxidant and antiproliferative properties of methylated metabolites of anthocyanins. *Food Chem.* **2013**, *141*, 2923–2933. [CrossRef]
222. Geahlen, R.L.; Koonchanok, N.M.; McLaughlin, J.L.; Pratt, D.E. Inhibition of protein-tyrosine kinase activity by flavanoids and related compounds. *J. Nat. Prod.* **1989**, *52*, 982–986. [CrossRef]
223. Hollman, P.C.; de Vries, J.H.; van Leeuwen, S.D.; Mengelers, M.J.; Katan, Martijn, K.B. Absorption of dietary quercetin glycosides and quercetin healthy ileostomy volunteers. *Am. J. Clin. Nutr.* **1995**, *62*, 1276–1282. [CrossRef] [PubMed]
224. Booth, A.N.; Murray, C.W.; Jones, F.T.; Deeds, F. The Metabolic Fate of Rutin and Quercetin in the Animal Body. *J. Biol. Chem.* **1956**, *233*, 251–257.
225. Gross, M.; Pfeiffer, M.; Martini, M.; Campbell, D.; Slavin, J.; Potter, J. The quantitation of metabolites of quercetin flavonols in human urine. *Cancer Epidemiol. Biomarkers Prev.* **1996**, *5*, 711–720. [PubMed]
226. Yamazaki, S.; Sakakibara, H.; Takemura, H.; Yasuda, M.; Shimoi, K. Quercetin-3-*O*-glucronide inhibits noradrenaline binding to α2-adrenergic receptor, thus suppressing DNA damage induced by treatment with 4-hydroxyestradiol and noradrenaline in MCF-10A cells. *J. Steroid Biochem. Mol. Biol.* **2014**, *143*, 122–129. [CrossRef] [PubMed]
227. Yamazaki, S.; Miyoshi, N.; Kawabata, K.; Yasuda, M.; Shimoi, K. Quercetin-3-*O*-glucuronide inhibits noradrenaline-promoted invasion of MDA-MB-231 human breast cancer cells by blocking β2-adrenergic signaling. *Arch. Biochem. Biophys.* **2014**, *557*, 18–27. [CrossRef] [PubMed]
228. Hadi, N.I.; Jamal, Q.; Iqbal, A.; Shaikh, F.; Somroo, S.; Musharraf, S.G. Serum Metabolomic Profiles for Breast Cancer Diagnosis, Grading and Staging by Gas Chromatography-Mass Spectrometry. *Sci. Rep.* **2017**, *7*, 1–11. [CrossRef]
229. Jové, M.; Collado, R.; Quiles, J.L.; Ramírez-Tortosa, M.C.; Sol, J.; Ruiz-Sanjuan, M.; Fernandez, M.; Cabrera, C.d.l.T.; Ramírez-Tortosa, C.; Granados-Principal, S.; et al. A plasma metabolomic signature discloses human breast cancer. *Oncotarget* **2017**, *8*, 19522. [CrossRef]
230. Liu, H.; Liu, Y.; Zhang, J.T. A new mechanism of drug resistance in breast cancer cells: Fatty acid synthase overexpression-mediated palmitate overproduction. *Mol. Cancer Ther.* **2008**, *7*, 263–270. [CrossRef]

231. Wang, J.B.; Erickson, J.W.; Fuji, R.; Ramachandran, S.; Gao, P.; Dinavahi, R.; Wilson, K.F.; Ambrosio, A.L.B.; Dias, S.M.G.; Dang, C.V.; et al. Targeting mitochondrial glutaminase activity inhibits oncogenic transformation. *Cancer Cell* **2010**, *18*, 207–219. [CrossRef]
232. Wang, G.; Li, Y.; Yang, Z.; Xu, W.; Yang, Y.; Tan, X. ROS mediated EGFR/MEK/ERK/HIF-1α Loop Regulates Glucose metabolism in pancreatic cancer. *Biochem. Biophys. Res. Commun.* **2018**, *500*, 873–878. [CrossRef]
233. Cardoso, M.R.; Santos, J.C.; Ribeiro, M.L.; Talarico, M.C.R.; Viana, L.R.; Derchain, S.F.M. A metabolomic approach to predict breast cancer behavior and chemotherapy response. *Int. J. Mol. Sci.* **2018**, *19*, 617. [CrossRef] [PubMed]
234. Gomes, L.; Viana, L.; Silva, J.L.; Mermelstein, C.; Atella, G.; Fialho, E. Resveratrol Modifies Lipid Composition of Two Cancer Cell Lines. *Biomed Res. Int.* **2020**, *2020*, 1–10. [CrossRef] [PubMed]
235. Ávila-Gálvez, M.Á.; García-Villalba, R.; Martínez-Díaz, F.; Ocaña-Castillo, B.; Monedero-Saiz, T.; Torrecillas-Sánchez, A.; Abellán, B.; González-Sarrías, A.; Espín, J.C. Metabolic Profiling of Dietary Polyphenols and Methylxanthines in Normal and Malignant Mammary Tissues from Breast Cancer Patients. *Mol. Nutr. Food Res.* **2019**, *63*, 1801239. [CrossRef] [PubMed]

6

Synthesis, Docking Studies and Biological Activity of New Benzimidazole-Triazolothiadiazine Derivatives as Aromatase Inhibitor

Ulviye Acar Çevik [1,2], Betül Kaya Çavuşoğlu [3], Begüm Nurpelin Sağlık [1,2], Derya Osmaniye [1,2], Serkan Levent [1,2], Sinem Ilgın [4], Yusuf Özkay [1,2,*] and Zafer Asım Kaplancıklı [1]

1 Department of Pharmaceutical Chemistry, Faculty of Pharmacy, Anadolu University, Eskisehir 26470, Turkey; uacar@anadolu.edu.tr (U.A.Ç.); bnsaglik@anadolu.edu.tr (B.N.S.); dosmaniye@anadolu.edu.tr (D.O.); serkanlevent@anadolu.edu.tr (S.L.); zakaplan@anadolu.edu.tr (Z.A.K.)
2 Doping and Narcotic Compounds Analysis Laboratory, Faculty of Pharmacy, Anadolu University, Eskisehir 26470, Turkey
3 Department of Pharmaceutical Chemistry, Faculty of Pharmacy, Bülent Ecevit University, Zonguldak 67100, Turkey; betulkaya@anadolu.edu.tr
4 Department of Pharmaceutical Toxicology, Faculty of Pharmacy, Anadolu University, Eskisehir 26470, Turkey; silgin@anadolu.edu.tr
* Correspondence: yozkay@anadolu.edu.tr;

Academic Editor: Filippo Minutolo

Abstract: In the last step of estrogen biosynthesis, aromatase enzyme catalyzes the conversion of androgens to estrogens. Aromatase inhibition is an important way to control estrogen-related diseases and estrogen levels. In this study, sixteen of benzimidazole-triazolothiadiazine derivatives have been synthesized and studied as potent aromatase inhibitors. First, these compounds were tested for their anti-cancer properties against human breast cancer cell line (MCF-7). The most active compounds **5c**, **5e**, **5k**, and **5m** on MCF-7 cell line were subject to further in vitro aromatase enzyme inhibition assays to determine the possible mechanisms of action underlying their activity. Compound **5e** showed slight less potent aromatase inhibitory activity than that of letrozole with $IC_{50} = 0.032 \pm 0.042$ µM, compared to $IC_{50} = 0.024 \pm 0.001$ µM for letrozole. Furthermore, compound **5e** and reference drug letrozole were docked into human placental aromatase enzyme to predict their possible binding modes with the enzyme. Finally, ADME parameters (absorption, distribution, metabolism, and excretion) of synthesized compounds (**5a–5p**) were calculated by QikProp 4.8 software.

Keywords: aromatase; MCF-7; NIH3T3; benzimidazole; triazolothiadiazine; docking; ADME

---

1. Introduction

Aromatase is a member of the cytochrome P450 enzyme that catalyzes the biosynthesis of estrogens from androgens [1,2]. Estrogen levels have been shown to be higher in breast cancer cells. Inhibition of aromatase is one of the effective current therapeutic strategies for controlling estrogen-dependent breast cancer. Therefore, one of the commonly used classes of drugs for the management of estrogen-dependent cancer is aromatase inhibitors (AIs) [1,3,4].

Aromatase inhibitors that have been used clinically can be categorized as first-, second-, and third generations based on their evolution time or steroidal or steroidal or non-steroidal aromatase inhibitors (NSAIs) based on their structural similarity with steroids [5,6].

Aminoglutethimide is the prototype nonsteroidal inhibitor of aromatase. Problems with the side effects and selectivity of aminoglutethimide led to the development of the second-generation of nonsteroidal aromatase inhibitor (Fadrazole bearing imidazole structure) [7]. However, this

compound still has some nonselective inhibitory activity with respect to progesterone, corticosterone, and aldosterone biosynthesis. Competitive nonsteroidal inhibitors can also be constructed with a triazole ring, which is found in the third generation of aromatase inhibitors [8–10]. Most of the nonsteroidal aromatase inhibitors of therapeutic importance act covalently bind to the substrate-binding site of aromatase by coordinate the heme iron [11–13]. Especially, the heterocyclic nitrogen atom of triazole and imidazole plays an important role by coordinating with the heme iron of the aromatase enzyme [12,13]. Some studies have shown that imidazole and triazole derivatives have promising aromatase inhibition [14–17].

Recent clinical studies have shown that aromatase inhibitors, especially the third-generation, are more effective than fulvestrant and tamoxifen because of their lower side effects and higher clinical efficacy. Nevertheless, the development of acquired resistance after prolonged AIs therapy, undesirable side effects (bone loss, cardiac events, increased rash, insomnia, headaches, and arthralgia) limits their use in clinical practice. Thus, the search for new potent molecules that impair cancer growth, strongly inhibit aromatase enzyme, and present fewer side effects is of major importance [18–21].

In the previous study, 3-[4-(5-methyl-1*H*-benzo[*d*]imidazol-2-yl)phenyl]-6- (substituted phenyl) -7H-[1,2,4] triazolo [3,4-b] [1,3,4]thiadiazines derivatives have been synthesized and promising compounds have been obtained that need further development as a new class of aromatase inhibitors [22]. In this study, new benzimidazole-triazolothiadiazine derivatives were synthesized and structure of these compounds was characterized by spectroscopic data. Their antiproliferative activities against MCF-7 were evaluated. To identify the possible modes of action, aromatase inhibition experiments were performed for the most active compounds against the MCF-7 cell line. Finally, in silico prediction of pharmacokinetic profiles (ADME) were calculated for physicochemical properties of these drug candidates.

2. Results and Discussion

2.1. Chemistry

Synthesis of the target compounds was accomplished according to the steps illustrated in Scheme 1. Substituents of the synthesized compounds (**5a–5p**) were shown in Table 1. The starting intermediated compound (**1a,1b**) was prepared by the reaction of 1,2-phenylenediamine and sodium metabisulfite with 4-formylbenzoic acid methyl ester as described in a previous study [23]. The ester derivative (**1a,1b**) reacted with hydrazine hydrate producing compounds **2a, 2b** in a microwave synthesis reactor. Then, the compounds-(5-substitüe-1*H*-benzimidazol-2-yl)benzoic acid hydrazide derivatives (**2a,2b**) were treated with carbon disulfide in NaOH solution affording, after acidic treatment, compounds **3a, 3b**. The reaction of compound **3a, 3b** with hydrazine hydrate in the presence of ethanol produced compounds **4a, 4b**. Then cyclization of compounds **4a, 4b** with appropriate phenacyl bromide in the presence of anhydrous ethanol provided the desired final products (**5a–5p**). The characterization of these new derivatives was done by their spectroscopic (^{1}H NMR, ^{13}C NMR and Mass) data. ^{1}H NMR and ^{13}C NMR spectra of the synthesized compounds were observed at the expected region. Mass spectra (HRMS) of all the synthesized compounds showed that the molecular ion $[M + H]^+$ peak is in agreement with their molecular formula (see Supplementary Materials).

6

Synthesis, Docking Studies and Biological Activity of New Benzimidazole-Triazolothiadiazine Derivatives as Aromatase Inhibitor

Ulviye Acar Çevik [1,2], Betül Kaya Çavuşoğlu [3], Begüm Nurpelin Sağlık [1,2], Derya Osmaniye [1,2], Serkan Levent [1,2], Sinem Ilgın [4], Yusuf Özkay [1,2,*] and Zafer Asım Kaplancıklı [1]

1 Department of Pharmaceutical Chemistry, Faculty of Pharmacy, Anadolu University, Eskisehir 26470, Turkey; uacar@anadolu.edu.tr (U.A.Ç.); bnsaglik@anadolu.edu.tr (B.N.S.); dosmaniye@anadolu.edu.tr (D.O.); serkanlevent@anadolu.edu.tr (S.L.); zakaplan@anadolu.edu.tr (Z.A.K.)

2 Doping and Narcotic Compounds Analysis Laboratory, Faculty of Pharmacy, Anadolu University, Eskisehir 26470, Turkey

3 Department of Pharmaceutical Chemistry, Faculty of Pharmacy, Bülent Ecevit University, Zonguldak 67100, Turkey; betulkaya@anadolu.edu.tr

4 Department of Pharmaceutical Toxicology, Faculty of Pharmacy, Anadolu University, Eskisehir 26470, Turkey; silgin@anadolu.edu.tr

* Correspondence: yozkay@anadolu.edu.tr;

Academic Editor: Filippo Minutolo

Abstract: In the last step of estrogen biosynthesis, aromatase enzyme catalyzes the conversion of androgens to estrogens. Aromatase inhibition is an important way to control estrogen-related diseases and estrogen levels. In this study, sixteen of benzimidazole-triazolothiadiazine derivatives have been synthesized and studied as potent aromatase inhibitors. First, these compounds were tested for their anti-cancer properties against human breast cancer cell line (MCF-7). The most active compounds **5c**, **5e**, **5k**, and **5m** on MCF-7 cell line were subject to further in vitro aromatase enzyme inhibition assays to determine the possible mechanisms of action underlying their activity. Compound **5e** showed slight less potent aromatase inhibitory activity than that of letrozole with $IC_{50} = 0.032 \pm 0.042$ μM, compared to $IC_{50} = 0.024 \pm 0.001$ μM for letrozole. Furthermore, compound **5e** and reference drug letrozole were docked into human placental aromatase enzyme to predict their possible binding modes with the enzyme. Finally, ADME parameters (absorption, distribution, metabolism, and excretion) of synthesized compounds (**5a–5p**) were calculated by QikProp 4.8 software.

Keywords: aromatase; MCF-7; NIH3T3; benzimidazole; triazolothiadiazine; docking; ADME

---

1. Introduction

Aromatase is a member of the cytochrome P450 enzyme that catalyzes the biosynthesis of estrogens from androgens [1,2]. Estrogen levels have been shown to be higher in breast cancer cells. Inhibition of aromatase is one of the effective current therapeutic strategies for controlling estrogen-dependent breast cancer. Therefore, one of the commonly used classes of drugs for the management of estrogen-dependent cancer is aromatase inhibitors (AIs) [1,3,4].

Aromatase inhibitors that have been used clinically can be categorized as first-, second-, and third generations based on their evolution time or steroidal or steroidal or non-steroidal aromatase inhibitors (NSAIs) based on their structural similarity with steroids [5,6].

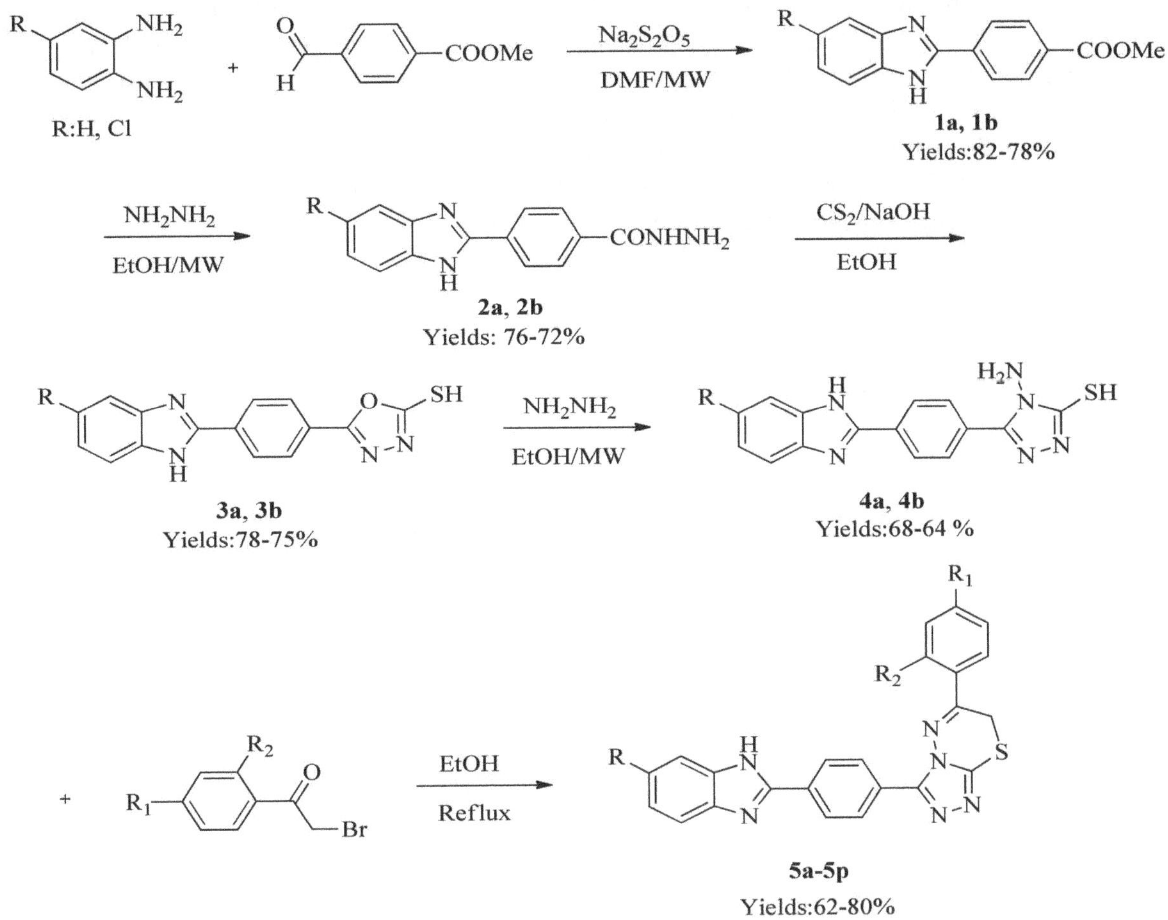

Scheme 1. The reaction sequence for the synthesis of the compounds (**5a–5p**).

Table 1. The synthesized compounds (**5a–5p**).

Comp.	R	R[1]	R[2]
5a	-H	-H	-H
5b	-H	-Cl	-H
5c	-H	-F	-H
5d	-H	$-CH_3$	-H
5e	-H	-CN	-H
5f	-H	-Br	-H
5g	-H	-F	-F
5h	-H	-Cl	-Cl
5i	-Cl	-H	-H
5j	-Cl	-Cl	-H
5k	-Cl	-F	-H
5l	-Cl	$-CH_3$	-H
5m	-Cl	-CN	-H
5n	-Cl	-Br	-H
5o	-Cl	-F	-F
5p	-Cl	-Cl	-Cl

2.2. *Cytotoxicity Assay*

The newly synthesized compounds were evaluated for their in vitro anticancer potential against MCF-7 breast cancer cell lines by MTT assay [24] using cisplatin as a reference standard. The 50% inhibitory concentration (IC_{50}) values were determined for these compounds. In addition, the cytotoxic activities of compounds **5c**, **5e**, **5k**, and **5m** were assessed against healthy NIH3T3 [25] cells, in order to express the selectivity toward carcinogenic cells. The IC_{50} values of test compounds were determined as the mean IC_{50} of 4 independent experiments. Results are presented in Table 2, as IC_{50} values are in μM and revealed that some of the tested compounds were remarkably more cytotoxic than the cisplatin against MCF-7 cell lines. Concerning MCF-7 cell line, the most potent compounds were the 4-cyano derivatives **5e** and **5m** with IC_{50} = 0.016 ± 0.001 and 0.018 ± 0.001 μM, respectively compared to IC_{50} = 0.020 ± 0.009 μM for the reference drug cisplatin. Furthermore, the most promising activity was observed for the compounds **5c** and **5k** bearing 4-fluorophenyl derivatives with IC_{50}= 0.119 ± 0.005 and 0.110 ± 0.005 μM, respectively compared to IC_{50} = 0.020 ± 0.009 μM for the reference drug cisplatin.

Table 2. IC_{50} (μM) values of compounds (**5a–5p**) (n = 4).

Comp.	MCF-7	NIH3T3
5a	0.142 ± 0.007	-
5b	0.0414 ± 0.001	-
5c	**0.119 ± 0.005**	**81.8 ± 2.4**
5d	0.194 ± 0.006	-
5e	**0.016 ± 0.001**	**≥1000**
5f	0.318 ± 0.019	-
5g	0.245 ± 0.004	-
5h	0.342 ± 0.017	-
5ı	0.205 ± 0.005	-
5j	0.258 ± 0.011	-
5k	**0.110 ± 0.005**	**77.6 ± 2.1**
5l	0.352 ± 0.019	-
5m	**0.018 ± 0.001**	**≥1000**
5n	0.264 ± 0.011	-
5o	0.373 ± 0.011	-
5p	0.147 ± 0.001	-
Cisplatin	**0.020 ± 0.009**	**≥1000**

Benzimidazole-triazolothiadiazine derivatives led to a promising increase in the anti-proliferative activity. The synthesized compounds can be divided into two groups as nonsubstituted benzimidazole and 5-chlorobenzimidazole. Test compounds showed variable activities against MCF-7. In particular, compounds **5e** and **5m** displayed the highest cytotoxic activity against MCF-7 cell line. The most active compounds **5e** and **5m** carried a 4-cyanophenyl substituent. The chlorine substituent in the fifth position (**5m**) of the benzimidazole ring did not significantly affect the activity. Compounds **5c** and **5k** carrying fluorine substituents in the fourth position of the phenyl ring showed lower activity than compounds **5e** and **5m** bearing cyano group in the fourth position of the phenyl ring.

2.3. Aromatase Inhibition Assay

The in vitro anti-aromatase activity of the most active compounds **5c**, **5e**, **5k,** and **5m** was valued using commercial fluorometric assay kit (Aromatase-CYP19A Inhibitor Screening kit, Bio Vision) with letrozole as the reference drug. Results are presented in Table 3. The IC_{50} values of compounds were in the sub-micromolar range (2.276 ± 0.106–0.03 2 ± 0.001 μM). The best value was shown by compound **5e** with IC_{50} value (0.032 ± 0.001 μM).

Table 3. IC_{50} (μM) values of compounds **5c**, **5e**, **5k**, **5m,** and letrozole.

Comp.	Aromatase Inhibition
5c	1.716 ± 0.042
5e	**0.032 ± 0.001**
5k	2.276 ± 0.106
5m	1.562 ± 0.064
Letrozole	**0.024 ± 0.001**

2.4. Molecular Docking

After the most active derivative was selected as compound **5e** according to in vitro aromatase enzyme inhibition assay and letrozole, molecular docking studies were performed to explain its binding modes with human aromatase enzyme active site. For this purpose, the crystal structure of human aromatase enzyme (PDB ID: 3EQM) [26] was retrieved from the Protein Data Bank server (www.pdb.org). The 2D and 3D docking poses of compound 5e are presented in Figures 1 and 2. The docking poses of letrozole are presented in Figures 3 and 4.

According to docking poses, it is understood that compound 5e displays compatible settlement with the enzyme active region. The benzimidazole ring in the structure forms two π–π interactions with Arg115 and Phe134. Also, it can be seen from 2D docking pose, this compound is in interaction with Hem molecules and Cys437 via its nitrogen atoms of triazolothiadiazine ring by salt bridge. There is another π–π interaction between 4-cyanophenyl ring and HEM molecule. The nitrogen atom of cyano group at C-4 position of phenyl ring interacts with hydroxyl of Ser314 doing hydrogen bonding. It is thought that this interaction is important for compound **5e** in terms of explaining its inhibitory activity. It is seen that the presence of an electron withdrawing group such as cyano at this position is a positive contribution to the activity.

As seen in the docking poses, letrozole is settled down in the enzyme active site properly. For letrozole, it is seen that benzonitrile ring creates π–π interaction with HEM molecule. Another π–π interaction is observed between 1,2,4-triazole ring and Arg115. Also, this 1,2,4-triazole ring forms two hydrogen bonds via its second and fourth nitrogen atoms with amino groups of Ala438 and Arg115, respectively.

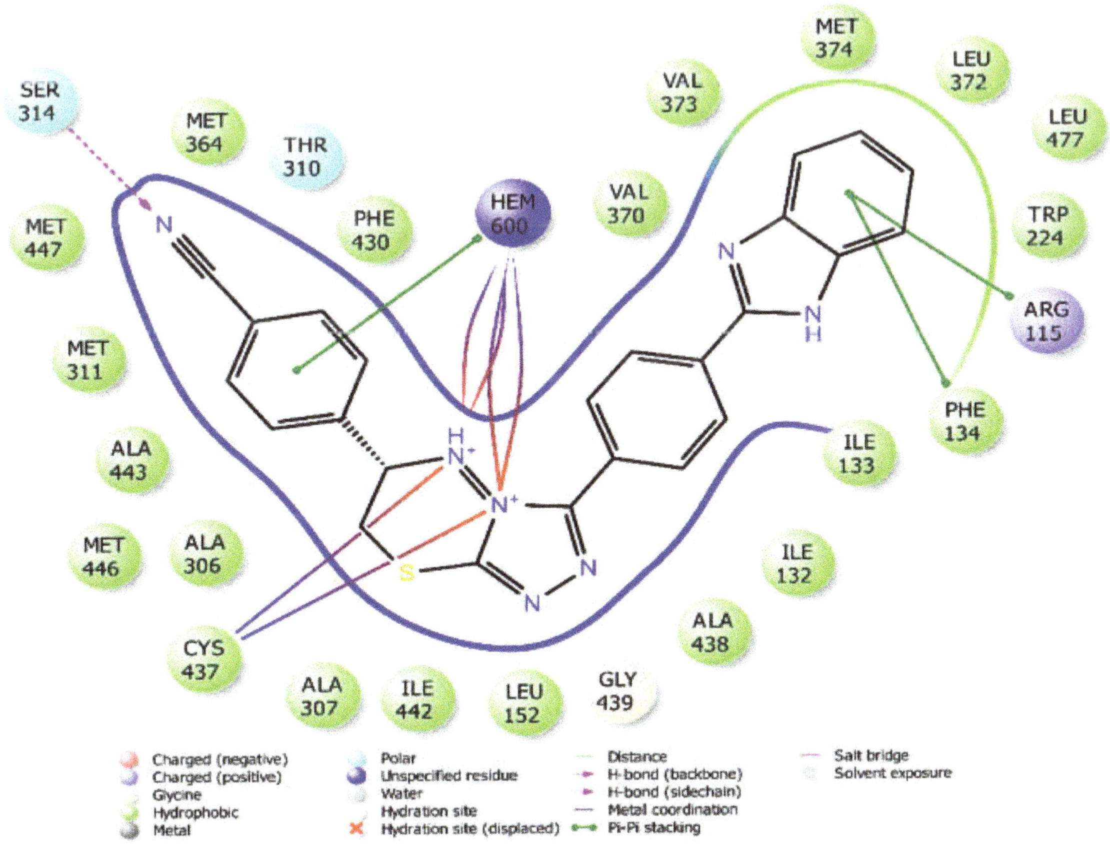

Figure 1. Two-dimensional interaction mode of compound **5e** in the enzyme active site (Human aromatase PDB Code: 3EQM).

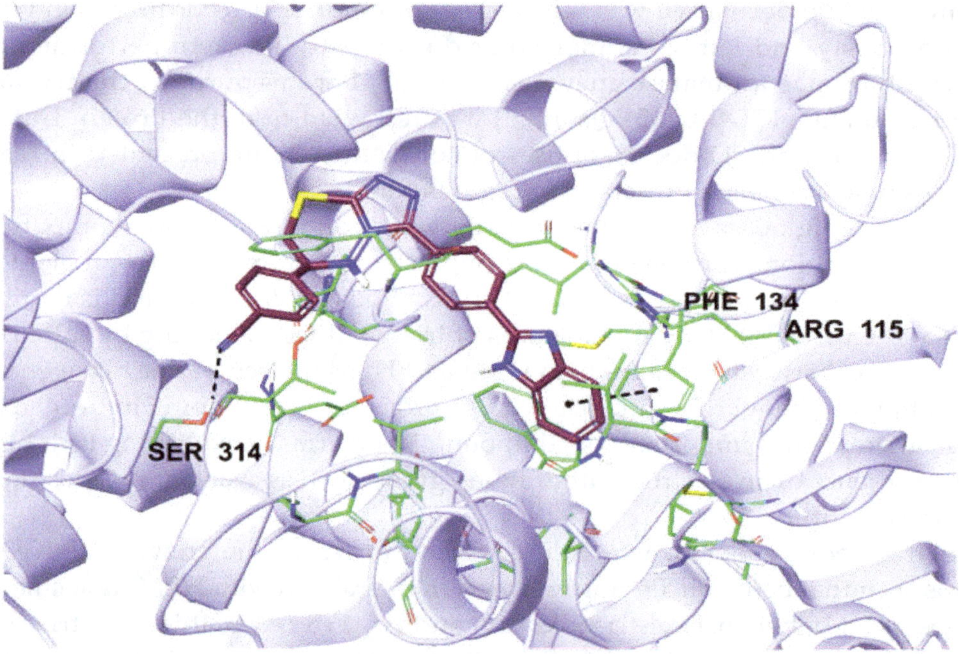

Figure 2. The interacting mode of compound **5e** in the active region of human aromatase. The inhibitor, colored with maroon, and the important residues, colored with purple, in the active site of the enzyme are presented by tube model.

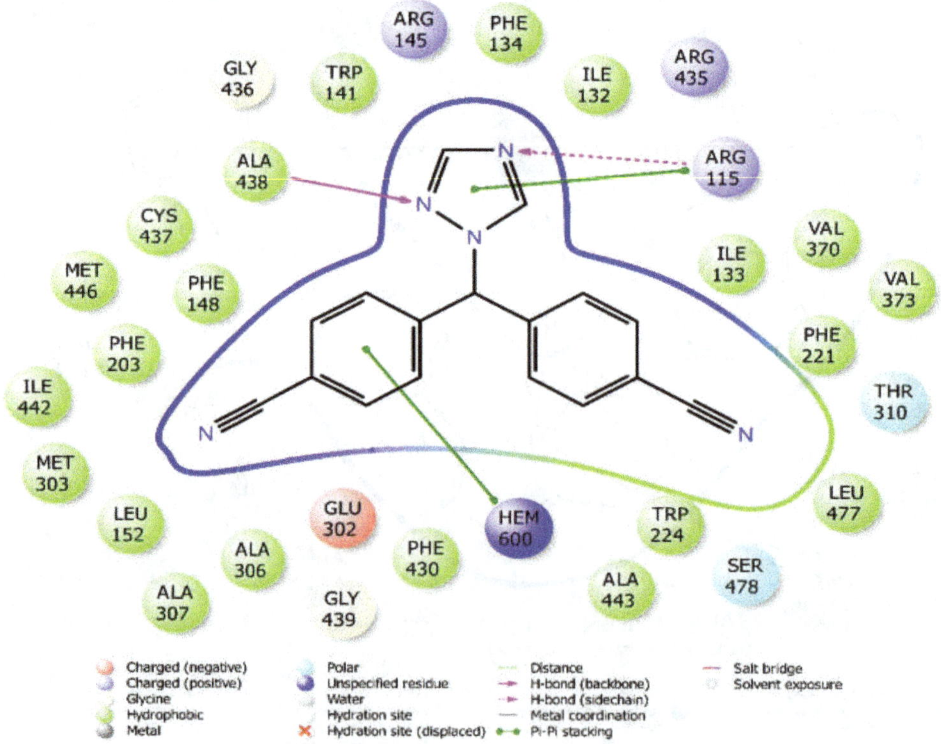

Figure 3. Two-dimensional interaction mode of letrozole in the enzyme active site (Human aromatase PDB Code: 3EQM).

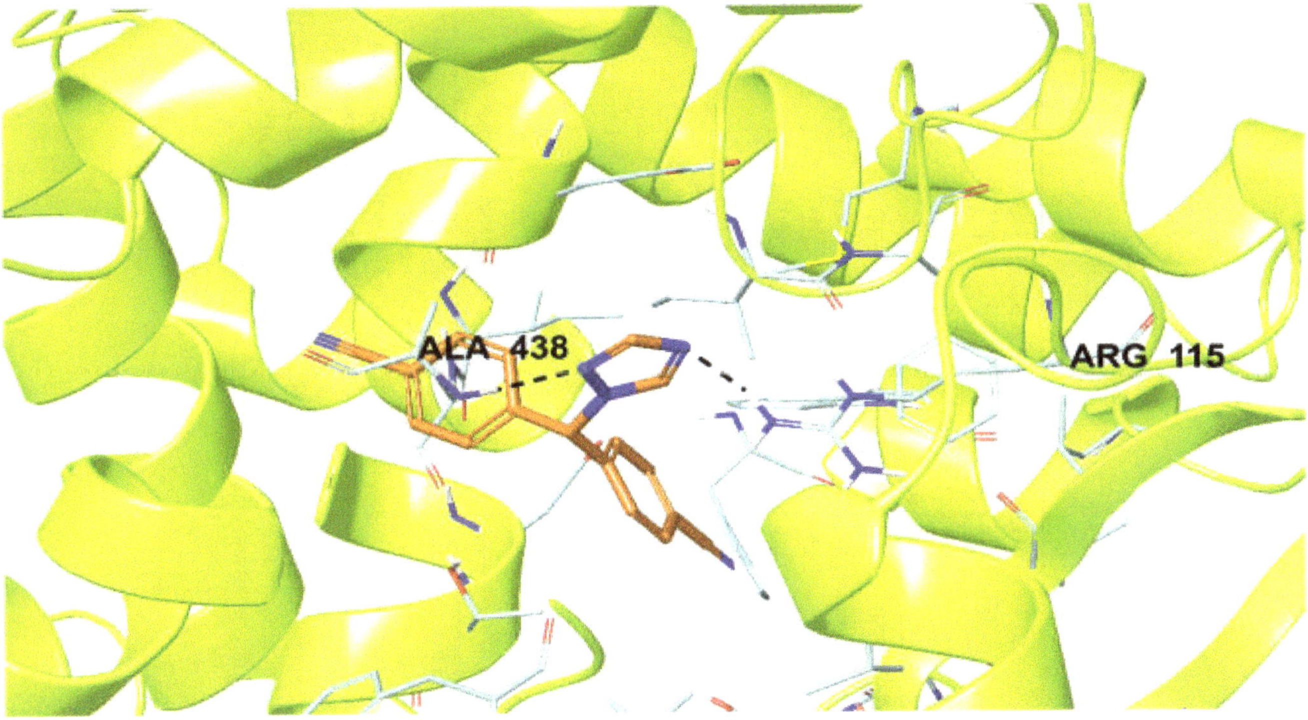

Figure 4. The interacting mode of letrozole in the active region of human aromatase. The inhibitor, colored with orange, and the important residues, colored with turquoise, in the active site of the enzyme are presented by tube model.

2.5. Theoretical Determination of ADME Properties

QikProp allows to provide acceptable ranges for comparing the predicted properties of compounds with those of 95% of known drugs and estimate drug-likeness properties. The drug-likeness of a compound was assessed according to Jorgensen's rule of three [27], which regards PCaco (>22 nm/s), logS (>−5.7), primary metabolites (PM) (<7), and Lipinski's rule of five [28], which considers number of hydrogen bond acceptors (≤10) and donors (≤5), molecular weight (<500 Da), and octanol/water partition coefficient (≤5).

Table 4. presents the predicted ADME properties of all compounds. According to Lipinski's rule of five and Jorgensen's rule of three, all compounds (**5a–5p**) are in accordance with the rule by causing no more than one violation. Consequently, according to predictions of ADME properties, it can be suggested that the active compounds may have a good pharmacokinetic profile.

Table 4. Calculated ADME parameters.

Comp.	MW	RB	DM	MV	DHB	AHB	PSA	logP	logS	PCaco	logBB	PMDCK	PM	CNS	%HOA	VRF	VRT
5a	408.48	0	13.539	1230.58	1	4.5	66.81	5.226	−7.577	1145.907	−0.361	1066.282	2	0	100	1	1
5b	442.925	0	11.536	1274.691	1	4.5	66.813	5.722	−8.323	1145.871	−0.207	2630.568	2	0	100	1	1
5c	426.47	0	11.294	1246.689	1	4.5	66.815	5.463	−7.944	1145.883	−0.255	1928.038	2	0	100	1	1
5d	422.506	0	14.175	1289.517	1	4.5	66.81	5.533	−8.145	1145.907	−0.388	1066.282	3	0	100	1	1
5e	433.489	1	7.968	1297.278	1	6	92.606	4.468	−8.534	236.976	−1.255	194.119	2	−2	95.607	0	1
5f	487.376	0	11.913	1283.596	1	4.5	66.813	5.799	−8.439	1145.858	−0.198	2828.358	2	0	100	1	1
5g	444.461	0	12.598	1251.337	1	4.5	65.595	5.544	−8.02	1167.271	−0.2	2431.401	2	0	100	1	1
5h	477.37	0	12.709	1287.743	1	4.5	64.6	5.897	−8.422	1199.257	−0.099	3927.141	2	0	100	1	1
5i	442.925	0	12.609	1274.528	1	4.5	66.806	5.721	−8.321	1145.207	−0.208	2625.13	2	0	100	1	1
5j	477.37	0	10.697	1318.639	1	4.5	66.809	6.217	−9.068	1145.171	−0.054	6476.318	2	0	100	1	1
5k	460.915	0	10.455	1290.637	1	4.5	66.811	5.957	−8.688	1145.183	−0.101	4746.726	2	0	100	1	1
5l	456.951	0	13.229	1333.465	1	4.5	66.806	6.028	−8.891	1145.207	−0.235	2625.13	3	0	100	1	1
5m	467.934	1	7.409	1341.226	1	6	92.602	4.96	−9.274	236.832	−1.117	477.911	2	−2	100	0	1
5n	521.821	0	11.046	1327.544	1	4.5	66.809	6.294	−9.184	1145.158	−0.044	6963.267	2	0	92.631	2	1
5o	478.906	0	11.99	1295.266	1	4.5	65.591	6.038	−8.764	1166.535	−0.046	5985.589	2	0	100	1	1
5p	511.815	0	12.056	1331.676	1	4.5	64.597	6.391	−9.166	1198.487	0.055	9667.877	2	1	93.553	2	1

MW: Molecular weight **RB:** Number of rotatable bonds (recommended value: 0-15) **DM:** Computed dipole moment (recommended value: 1-12.5) **MV:** Total solvent-accessible volume (recommended value: 500-2000) **DHB:** Estimated number of hydrogen bond donors (recommended value: 0-6) **AHB:** Estimated number of hydrogen bond acceptors (recommended value: 2-20) **PSA:** Van der Waals surface area of polar nitrogen and oxygen atoms and carbonyl carbon atoms (recommended value: 7-200) **logP:** Predicted octanol/water partition coefficient (recommended value: -2-6.5) **logS:** Predicted aqueous solubility (recommended value: -6.5-0.5) **PCaco:** Predicted apparent Caco-2 cell permeability (recommended value: <25 poor, >500 great) **logBB:** Predicted brain/blood partition coefficient (recommended value: -3-1.2) **PMDCK:** Predicted apparent MDCK cell permeability (recommended value: <25 poor, >500 great) **PM:** Number of likely metabolic reactions (recommended value: 1-8) **CNS:** Predicted central nervous system activity (recommended value: −2 (inactive), +2 (active)) **%HOA:** Predicted human oral absorption percent (recommended value: >80% is high, <25% is poor) **VRF:** Number of violations of Lipinski's rule of five. The rules are: MW < 500, logP < 5, DHB ≤ 5, AHB≤ 10, Positive PSA value. **VRT:** Number of violations of Jorgensen's rule of three. The three rules are: logS > -5.7, PCaco > 22 nm/s, PM < 7.

3. Materials and Methods

3.1. Chemistry

Whole chemicals employed in the synthetic procedure were purchased from Sigma-Aldrich Chemicals (Sigma-Aldrich Corp., St. Louis, MO, USA) or Merck Chemicals (Merck KGaA, Darmstadt, Germany). Melting points of the obtained compounds were determined by MP90 digital melting point apparatus (Mettler Toledo, OH, USA) and were uncorrected. Microwave syntheses were realized by using a Monowave 300 high-performance microwave reactor (Anton-Paar, Austria). ^{1}H NMR and ^{13}C NMR spectra of the synthesized compounds were registered by a Bruker 300 MHz and 75 MHz digital FT-NMR spectrometer (Bruker Bioscience, Billerica, MA, USA) in DMSO-d_6, respectively. Splitting patterns were designated as follows: s: singlet; d: doublet; t: triplet; m: multiplet in the NMR spectra. Coupling constants (*J*) were reported as Hertz. M+1 peaks were determined by Shimadzu LC/MS ITTOF system (Shimadzu, Tokyo, Japan). All reactions were monitored by thin-layer chromatography (TLC) using Silica Gel 60 F254 TLC plates (Merck KGaA, Darmstadt, Germany).

3.1.1. Synthesis of 4-(5-substitüe-1H-benz[d]imidazol-2-yl)benzoic Acid Methyl Ester (**1a,1b**)

Yields: 82–78%. 4-(5-substitüe-1*H*-benz[*d*]imidazol-2-yl)benzoic acid hydrazide derivatives (**2a,2b**) (yields: 76–72%) and 5-[4-(5(6)-substituted-1*H*-benz[*d*]imidazol-2-yl)phenyl]-1,3,4-oxadiazole-2-thiol derivatives (**3a,3b**) (yields: 78–7 %) were prepared following the reported procedures [23].

3.1.2. 4-Amino-5-(4-(5-substitüe-1H-benzo[d]imidazol-2-yl)phenyl)-4H-1,2,4-triazole-3-thiol (**4a,4b**)

Compound **3a** or **3b** (0.02 mol) was dissolved in ethanol. Hydrazine hydrate (5 mL) was added to the mixture. The reaction mixture was heated at 240 °C and 10 bar for 10 min under microwave synthesis reactor (Anton-Paar Monowave 300). After the reaction ended, the product was washed with water, dried, and crystallized using ethanol (96%) [22]. Yields: 68–64%.

3.1.3. 3-(4-(5-substitüe-1H-benzo[d]imidazol-2-yl)phenyl)-6-(substitüephenyl)-7H-[1,2,4]triazole [3,4-b][1,3,4]thiadiazine (**5a–5p**)

Compound **4a** or **4b** (0.003 mol) and appropriate phenacyl bromide (0.003 mol) in ethanol was heated under reflux for 8 h. After the reaction ended, the product was filtered and dried [22].

3-(4-(1H-benzo[d]imidazol-2-yl)phenyl)-6-phenyl-7H-[1,2,4]triazole[3,4-b][1,3,4] thiadiazine (5a): Yields: 77%. Mp 230.7–232.9 °C. ^{1}H-NMR (300 MHz, DMSO-d_6): δ = 4.52 (2H, s, -CH_2-), 7.52-7.55 (2H, m, aromatic CH), 7.59–7.67 (3H, m, Aromatic CH), 7.83–7.86 (2H, m, aromatic CH), 8.06–8.09 (2H, m, aromatic CH), 8.34 (2H, d, *J*=8.67 Hz, 1,4-disubstitutedbenzene), 8.43 (2H, d, *J*=8.64 Hz, 1,4-disubstitutedbenzene). ^{13}C-NMR (75 MHz, DMSO-d6): δ = 23.31, 114.89, 125.84, 126.55, 128.13, 128.50, 129.13, 129.65, 132.64, 133.78, 134.17, 143.96, 149.21, 151.22, 156.82, 163.07. HRMS (*m*/*z*): $[M + H]^+$ calcd for $C_{23}H_{16}N_6S$: 409.1224; found: 409.1230.

3-(4-(1H-benzo[d]imidazol-2-yl)phenyl)-6-(4-chlorophenyl)-7H-[1,2,4]triazole[3,4-b][1,3,4] thiadiazine (**5b**): Yields: 72%. Mp 190.9–192.6 °C. ^{1}H-NMR (300 MHz, DMSO-d_6): δ = 4.50 (2H, s, -CH_2-), 7.56–7.59 (2H, m, aromatic CH), 7.65–7.70 (3H, m, aromatic CH), 7.86–7.89 (2H, m, aromatic CH), 8.06–8.09 (2H, m, aromatic CH), 8.31 (2H, d, *J*=8.61 Hz, 1,4-disubstitutedbenzene), 8.57 (2H, d, *J*=8.61 Hz, 1,4-Disubstitutedbenzene). ^{13}C-NMR (75 MHz, DMSO-d_6): δ=23.27, 114.67, 125.49, 126.35, 128.87, 129.11, 129.32, 129.45, 129.73, 129.92, 130.11, 130.71, 132.62, 133.01, 137.50, 144.01, 148.52, 151.17, 156.87. HRMS (*m*/*z*): $[M + H]^+$ calcd for $C_{23}H_{15}N_6SCl$: 443.0843; found: 443.0840.

3-(4-(1*H*-benzo[*d*]imidazol-2-yl)phenyl)-6-(4-fluorophenyl)-7H-[1,2,4]triazole[3,4-b][1,3,4] thiadiazine (**5c**): Yields: 69%. Mp 274.2–277.1 °C. ^{1}H-NMR (300 MHz, DMSO-d_6): δ = 4.50 (2H, s, -CH_2-), 7.12 (1H, s, aromatic CH), 7.29 (1H, s, aromatic CH), 7.46–7.52 (4H, m, aromatic CH), 7.81–7.84 (2H, m, aromatic CH), 8.33 (2H, d, *J* = 8.64 Hz, 1,4-disubstitutedbenzene), 8.51 (2H, d, J=8.76 Hz, 1,4-disubstitutedbenzene).

^{13}C-NMR (75 MHz, DMSO-d_6): δ = 23.27, 114.32, 114.90, 116.76 (d, J = 21.98 Hz), 126.40, 127.68, 127.96, 128.43, 128.56, 128.69, 128.87, 128.95, 130.32 (d, J = 2.77 Hz), 130.78 (d, J = 8.43 Hz), 134.60, 143.66, 151.30, 155.71, 166.36 (d, J = 249.53 Hz). HRMS (m/z): $[M + H]^+$ calcd for $C_{23}H_{15}N_6FS$: 427.1137; found: 427.1136.

3-(4-(1H-benzo[d]imidazol-2-yl)phenyl)-6-(4-methylphenyl)-7H-[1,2,4]triazole[3,4-b][1,3,4] thiadiazine (**5d**): Yields: 70%. Mp 207.5–209.1 °C. ^{1}H-NMR (300 MHz, DMSO-d_6): δ = 2.41 (3H, s, CH_3), 4.49 (2H, s, -CH_2-), 7.41 (2H, d, J = 8.13 Hz, 1,4-disubstitutedbenzene), 7.52–7.55 (2H, m, benzimidazole CH), 7.83–7.86 (2H, m, benzimidazole CH), 7.97 (2H, d, J = 8.25 Hz, 1,4-disubstitutedbenzene), 8.33 (2H, d, J = 8.58 Hz, 1,4-disubstitutedbenzene), 8.43 (2H, d, J = 8.61 Hz, 1,4-disubstitutedbenzene). ^{13}C-NMR (75 MHz, DMSO-d_6): δ=21.55, 23.18, 114.86, 125.84, 126.42, 128.08, 128.24, 128.47, 129.02, 129.22, 129.71, 130.20, 130.90, 134.11, 142.96, 144.00, 147.35, 149.13, 151.07, 156.69. HRMS (m/z): $[M + H]^+$ calcd for $C_{24}H_{18}N_6S$: 423.1381; found: 423.1386.

3-(4-(1H-benzo[d]imidazol-2-yl)phenyl)-6-(4-cyanophenyl)-7H-[1,2,4]triazole[3,4-b][1,3,4] thiadiazine (**5e**): Yields: 68%. Mp 259.3–263.1 °C. ^{1}H-NMR (300 MHz, DMSO-d_6): δ = 4.53 (2H, s, -CH_2-), 7.56–7.58 (2H, m, benzimidazole CH), 7.85–7.88 (2H, m, benzimidazole CH), 8.06 (2H, d, J = 8.37 Hz, 1,4-disubstitutedbenzene), 8.21 (2H, d, J = 8.46 Hz, 1,4-disubstitutedbenzene), 8.30 (2H, d, J = 8.49 Hz, 1,4-disubstitutedbenzene), 8.42 (2H, d, J = 8.49 Hz, 1,4-disubstitutedbenzene). ^{13}C-NMR (75 MHz, DMSO-d_6): δ = 23.35, 114.58, 114.71, 118.68, 125.51, 126.39, 127.20, 128.48, 128.74, 128.87, 129.19, 129.43, 129.84, 133.03, 133.44, 137.97, 143.97, 148.72, 151.25, 155.45. HRMS (m/z): $[M + H]^+$ calcd for $C_{24}H_{15}N_7S$: 434.1186; found: 434.1182.

3-(4-(1H-benzo[d]imidazol-2-yl)phenyl)-6-(4-bromophenyl)-7H-[1,2,4]triazole[3,4-b][1,3,4] thiadiazine (**5f**): Yields: 74%. Mp 284.8–286.2 °C. ^{1}H-NMR (300 MHz, DMSO-d_6): δ = 4.50 (2H, s, -CH_2-), 7.53–7.56 (3H, m, aromatic CH), 7.81–7.85 (3H, m, aromatic CH), 7.99–8.02 (2H, m, aromatic CH), 8.32 (2H, d, J = 8.64 Hz, 1,4-disubstitutedbenzene), 8.42 (2H, d, J = 8.70 Hz, 1,4-disubstitutedbenzene). ^{13}C-NMR (75 MHz, DMSO-d_6): δ = 23.20, 114.91, 125.04, 125.96, 126.50, 127.03, 128.56, 129.19, 130.09, 130.90, 132.37, 132.67, 133.00, 142.94, 143.96, 147.34, 149.17, 151.22, 155.95. HRMS (m/z): $[M + H]^+$ calcd for $C_{23}H_{15}N_6SBr$: 487.0311; found: 487.0335.

3-(4-(1H-benzo[d]imidazol-2-yl)phenyl)-6-(2,4-difluorohenyl)-7H-[1,2,4]triazole [3,4-b][1,3,4] thiadiazine (**5g**): Yields: 72%. Mp 208.5–210.7 °C. ^{1}H-NMR (300 MHz, DMSO-d_6): δ = 4.42 (2H, s, -CH_2-), 7.46–7.49 (4H, m, aromatic CH), 7.79–7.82 (3H, m, aromatic CH), 7.29–7.35 (2H, m, aromatic CH), 8.45–8.51 (2H, m, aromatic CH). ^{13}C-NMR (75 MHz, DMSO-d_6): δ = 25.37, 113.01 (dd, J_1 = 3.08 Hz, J_2 = 21.45 Hz), 106.08 (d, J = 26.01 Hz), 114.05, 114.45, 119.72 (dd, J_1 = 3.02 Hz, J_2 = 11.51 Hz), 126.56, 127.17, 128.25, 128.75, 129.15, 132.37, 132.67 (dd, J_1 = 3.12 Hz, J_2 = 10.36 Hz), 134.23, 135.55, 143.74, 148.22, 151.06, 153.70, 164.66 (d, J = 251.18 Hz), 164.83 (d, J = 250.91 Hz). HRMS (m/z): $[M + H]^+$ calcd for $C_{23}H_{14}N_6SF_2$: 445.1053; found: 445.1041.

3-(4-(1H-benzo[d]imidazol-2-yl)phenyl)-6-(2,4-dichlorophenyl)-7H-[1,2,4]triazole[3,4-b] [1,3,4] thiadiazine (**5h**): Yields: 77%. Mp 190.7–193.4 °C. ^{1}H-NMR (300 MHz, DMSO-d_6): δ = 4.36 (2H, s, -CH_2-), 7.34–7.37 (3H, m, aromatic CH), 7.65 (1H, dd, J_1 = 2.04 Hz, J_2 = 8.34 Hz, aromatic CH), 7.70–7.73 (2H, m, aromatic CH), 7.78–7.81 (1H, m, aromatic CH), 8.20 (2H, d, J = 8.64 Hz, 1,4-disubstitutedbenzene), 8.40 (2H, d, J = 8.61 Hz, 1,4-disubstitutedbenzene). ^{13}C-NMR (75 MHz, DMSO-d_6): δ = 26.23, 115.05, 115.32, 124.22, 124.72, 126.99, 127.78, 128.08, 128.29, 128.57, 128.96, 129.59, 130.38, 132.93, 133.05, 133.74, 136.86, 143.65, 149.92, 151.62, 156.53. HRMS (m/z): $[M + H]^+$ calcd for $C_{23}H_{14}N_6SCl_2$: 477.0457; found: 477.0450.

3-(4-(5-chloro-1H-benzo[d]imidazol-2-yl)phenyl)-6-phenyl-7H-[1,2,4]triazole[3,4-b][1,3,4] thiadiazine (**5i**): Yields: 80%. Mp: 247.3–249.6 °C. ^{1}H-NMR (300 MHz, DMSO-d_6): δ = 4.50 (2H, s, -CH_2-), 7.49 (1H, dd, J_1 = 1.89 Hz, J_2=8.67 Hz, aromatic CH), 7.59–7.62 (3H, m, aromatic CH), 7.78–7.84 (2H, m, aromatic

CH), 8.03–8.06 (2H, m, aromatic CH), 8.27 (2H, d, J = 8.64 Hz, 1,4-disubstitutedbenzene), 8.37 (2H, d, J = 8.64 Hz, 1,4-disubstitutedbenzene). ^{13}C-NMR (75 MHz, DMSO-d_6): δ = 23.32, 114.60, 116.29, 125.95, 126.40, 128.11, 128.47, 128.97, 129.20, 129.63, 129.94, 132.62, 133.27, 133.71, 135.39, 143.97, 150.42, 151.04, 156.76. HRMS (*m/z*): [M + H]$^+$ calcd for $C_{23}H_{15}N_6SCl$: 443.0826; found: 443.0840.

3-(4-(5-chloro-1*H*-benzo[*d*]imidazol-2-yl)phenyl)-6-(4-chlorophenyl)-7H-[1,2,4]triazole [3,4-b][1,3,4] thiadiazine (**5j**): Yields: 70%. Mp: 226.0–228.9 °C. ^{1}H-NMR (300 MHz, DMSO-d_6): δ = 4.46 (2H, s, -CH_2-), 7.33–7.37 (1H, m, benzimidazole CH), 7.63 (2H, d, J = 8.61 Hz, 1,4-disubstitutedbenzene), 7.68–7.73 (2H, m, benzimidazole CH), 8.04 (2H, d, J = 8.61 Hz, 1,4-disubstitutedbenzene), 8.19 (2H, d, J = 8.46 Hz, 1,4-disubstitutedbenzene), 8.39 (2H, d, J = 8.43 Hz, 1,4-disubstitutedbenzene). ^{13}C-NMR (75 MHz, DMSO-d_6): δ = 23.13, 115.14, 116.51, 124.18, 127.79, 128.20, 128.33, 128.83, 128.98, 129.19, 129.68, 129.87, 130.51, 131.57, 132.60, 137.42, 143.58, 151.40, 155.59. HRMS (*m/z*): [M + H]$^+$ calcd for $C_{23}H_{14}N_6SCl_2$: 477.0427; found: 477.0450.

3-(4-(5-chloro-1*H*-benzo[*d*]imidazol-2-yl)phenyl)-6-(4-fluorophenyl)-7H-[1,2,4]triazole [3,4-b][1,3,4] thiadiazine (**5k**): Yields: 71%. Mp: 249.1–250.9 °C. ^{1}H-NMR (300 MHz, DMSO-d_6): δ = 4.48 (2H, s, -CH_2-), 7.38 (1H, dd, J_1 = 1.98 Hz, J_2 = 8.58 Hz, aromatic CH), 7.46–7.48 (2H, m, aromatic CH), 7.71–7.74 (1H, m, aromatic CH), 7.77 (1H, s, aromatic CH), 8.12–8.14 (2H, m, aromatic CH), 8.25 (2H, d, J = 8.64 Hz, 1,4-disubstitutedbenzene), 8.40 (2H, d, J = 8.61 Hz, 1,4-disubstitutedbenzene). ^{13}C-NMR (75 MHz, DMSO-d_6): δ = 23.45, 114.95, 116.45, 116.77 (d, J = 22.09 Hz), 124.83, 128.07, 128.21, 128.39, 128.84, 128.89, 130.30 (d, J = 2.99 Hz), 130.85 (d, J = 8.93 Hz), 135.26, 137.58, 143.69, 150.99, 151.27, 155.73, 164.82 (d, J = 249.42 Hz). HRMS (*m/z*): [M + H]$^+$ calcd for $C_{23}H_{14}N_6FSCl$: 461.0741; found: 461.0746.

3-(4-(5-chloro-1*H*-benzo[*d*]imidazol-2-yl)phenyl)-6-(4-methylphenyl)-7H-[1,2,4]triazole [3,4-b][1,3,4] thiadiazine (**5l**): Yields: 65%. Mp: 250.7–252.3 °C. ^{1}H-NMR (300 MHz, DMSO-d_6): δ = 4.46 (2H, s, -CH2-), 7.40 (2H, d, J = 8.07 Hz, 1,4-disubstitutedbenzene), 7.45 (1H, dd, J_1 = 1.95 Hz, J_2 = 8.67 Hz, benzimidazole CH), 7.76–7.79 (1H, m, benzimidazole CH), 7.82–7.83 (1H, m, benzimidazole CH), 7.95 (2H, d, J = 8.31 Hz, 1,4-disubstitutedbenzene), 8.28 (2H, d, J = 8.67 Hz, 1,4-disubstitutedbenzene), 8.37 (2H, d, J = 8.67 Hz, 1,4-disubstitutedbenzene). ^{13}C-NMR (75 MHz, DMSO-d_6): δ = 21.54, 23.15, 114.88, 116.44, 125.26, 127.74, 128.08, 128.21, 128.95, 129.24, 129.72, 130.21, 130.90, 134.62, 136.89, 142.95, 143.90, 150.99, 151.15, 156.66. HRMS (*m/z*): [M + H]$^+$ calcd for $C_{24}H_{17}N_6SCl$: 457.0994; found: 457.0997.

3-(4-(5-chloro-1*H*-benzo[*d*]imidazol-2-yl)phenyl)-6-(4-cyanophenyl)-7H-[1,2,4]triazole [3,4-b][1,3,4] thiadiazine (**5m**): Yields: 62%. Mp: 254.0–255.7 °C. ^{1}H-NMR (300 MHz, DMSO-d_6): δ = 4.53 (2H, s, -CH_2-), 7.50 (1H, dd, J_1 = 1.95 Hz, J_2 = 8.70 Hz, benzimidazole CH), 7.85–7.86 (1H, m, aromatic CH), 8.06–8.08 (3H, m, aromatic CH), 8.21 (2H, d, J = 8.61 Hz, 1,4-disubstitutedbenzene), 8.26 (2H, d, J = 8.64 Hz, 1,4-disubstitutedbenzene), 8.38 (2H, d, J = 8.64 Hz, 1,4-disubstitutedbenzene). ^{13}C-NMR (75 MHz, DMSO-d_6): δ = 23.30, 114.57, 114.71, 118.70, 125.83, 126.85, 128.48, 128.86, 129.11, 129.37, 129.81, 133.46, 133.58, 135.73, 137.98, 143.88, 150.56, 151.33, 155.41. HRMS (*m/z*): [M + H]$^+$ calcd for $C_{24}H_{14}N_7SCl$: 468.0782; found: 468.0793.

3-(4-(5-chloro-1*H*-benzo[*d*]imidazol-2-yl)phenyl)-6-(4-bromophenyl)-7H-[1,2,4]triazole [3,4-b][1,3,4] thiadiazine (**5n**): Yields: 76%. Mp: 243.4–247.3 °C. ^{1}H-NMR (300 MHz, DMSO-d_6): δ = 4.48 (2H, s, -CH_2-), 7.43 (1H, dd, J_1 = 1.98 Hz, J_2 = 8.67 Hz, benzimidazole CH), 7.75 (1H, s, aromatic CH), 7.80–7.82 (3H, m, aromatic CH), 7.99 (2H, d, J = 8.70 Hz, 1,4-disubstitutedbenzene), 8.26 (2H, d, J = 8.58 Hz, 1,4-disubstitutedbenzene), 8.37 (2H, d, J = 8.64 Hz, 1,4-disubstitutedbenzene). ^{13}C-NMR (75 MHz, DMSO-d_6): δ=23.14, 115.01, 116.52, 124.92, 126.45, 128.10, 129.05, 130.07, 131.76, 132.00, 132.15, 132.67, 133.00, 141.45, 143.77, 148.89, 149.69, 151.39, 155.91. HRMS (*m/z*): [M + H]$^+$ calcd for $C_{23}H_{14}N_6SClBr$: 520.9930; found: 520.9945.

3-(4-(5-chloro-1*H*-benzo[*d*]imidazol-2-yl)phenyl)-6-(2,4-difluorohenyl)-7H-[1,2,4]triazole [3,4-b][1,3,4] thiadiazine (**5o**): Yields: 66%. Mp: 182.2–185.0 °C. ^{1}H-NMR (300 MHz, DMSO-d_6): δ = 4.39 (2H, s,

-CH_2-), 7.28–7.34 (1H, m, aromatic CH), 7.42–7.48 (1H, m, aromatic CH), 7.48–7.52 (2H, m, aromatic CH), 7.77–7.83 (2H, m, aromatic CH), 7.93–8.01 (1H, m, aromatic CH), 8.25 (2H, d, J = 8.64 Hz, 1,4-disubstitutedbenzene), 8.44 (2H, d, J = 8.58 Hz, 1,4-disubstitutedbenzene). ^{13}C-NMR (75 MHz, DMSO-d_6): δ = 25.31, 105.76 (d, J = 26.01 Hz), 106.28, 113.19 (dd, J_1 = 2.63 Hz, J_2 = 20.86 Hz), 114.74, 116.39, 119.76 (dd, J_1 = 3.73 Hz, J_2 = 7.83 Hz), 125.45, 127.49, 128.32, 128.94, 129.14, 129.40, 132.71 (dd, J_1 = 3.21 Hz, J_2 = 9.80 Hz), 134.22, 143.80, 151.60, 151.26, 153.78, 161.28 (d, J = 252.62 Hz), 164.46 (d, J = 256.22 Hz). HRMS (m/z): $[M + H]^+$ calcd for $C_{23}H_{13}N_6F_2SCl$: 479.0632; found: 479.0652.

3-(4-(5-chloro-1*H*-benzo[*d*]imidazol-2-yl)phenyl)-6-(2,4-dichlorophenyl)-7H-[1,2,4]triazole [3,4-b][1,3,4] thiadiazine (**5p**): Yields: 68%. Mp: 114.4–116.5 °C. ^{1}H-NMR (300 MHz, DMSO-d_6): δ = 4.35 (2H, s, -CH_2-), 7.25 (1H, dd, J_1 = 1.74 Hz, J_2 = 8.52 Hz, aromatic CH), 7.65 (2H, dd, J_1 = 2.07 Hz, J_2 = 8.34 Hz, aromatic CH), 7.88 (2H, d, J = 8.34 Hz, aromatic CH), 7.90 (1H, m, aromatic CH), 8.16 (2H, d, J = 8.61 Hz, 1,4-disubstitutedbenzene), 8.32 (2H, d, J = 8.58 Hz, 1,4-disubstitutedbenzene). ^{13}C-NMR (75 MHz, DMSO-d_6): δ = 26.33, 106.76, 125.55, 127.29, 127.35, 128.58, 128.90, 129.64, 130.37, 131.63, 132.35, 132.96, 133.06, 133.44, 133.77, 136.56, 136.84, 143.51, 149.25, 151.77, 156.48. HRMS (m/z): $[M + H]^+$ calcd for $C_{23}H_{13}N_6SCl_3$: 511.0037; found: 511.0061.

3.2. Cytotoxicity Assay

The anticancer activity of compounds **5a–5p** were screened according to the MTT assays. The MTT assays were performed as previously described [24,25]. Cisplatin was used as the reference drug for the MCF7 cell line in the MTT assays.

3.3. Aromatase Inhibition Assay

This method was carried out according to the kit procedure (Bio Vision, Aromatase (CYP19A) Inhibitor Screening Kit (Fluorometric)). The compounds were dissolved in dimethyl sulfoxide (DMSO) and added to the assay in at least seven concentrations ranging from 10^{-3}–10^{-9} M. The recombinant human aromatase stock was prepared by reconstituting with 1 mL of aromatase assay buffer. The contents were mixed thoroughly by vortexing to obtain a homogeneous solution and the solution was transferred to a 15-mL conical tube. The volume was brought to 2450 μL with the aromatase assay buffer and 50 μl of NADPH production system (100X) was added for a final total volume of 2.5 mL. Letrozole was used as a positive inhibition control. For solvent control, a small aliquot of aromatase assay buffer containing the organic solvent was used to dissolve the test compounds that were prepared. Reaction wells containing test compounds and the corresponding no inhibitor controls (which may also serve as a solvent control), as well as a background control (containing no fluorogenic Aromatase Substrate) were prepared. The plate was incubated for at least 10 min at 37 °C to allow test ligands to interact with the aromatase. After incubation, 30 μl of the aromatase substrate/NADP+ mixture was added to each well. Immediately (within 1 min), the fluorescence at Ex/Em = 488/527 nm was measured.

3.4. Molecular Docking

A structure-based in silico procedure was applied to discover the binding modes of compound 5e to human aromatase enzyme active site. The crystal structures of human aromatase (PDB ID: 3EQM) [26] was retrieved from the Protein Data Bank server (www.pdb.org).

The structures of ligands were built using the Schrödinger Maestro [29] interface and then were submitted to the Protein Preparation Wizard protocol of the Schrödinger Suite 2016 Update 2 [30]. The ligands were prepared by the LigPrep 3.8 [31] to assign the protonation states at pH 7.4 ± 1.0 and the atom types, correctly. Bond orders were assigned, and hydrogen atoms were added to the structures. The grid generation was formed using Glide 7.1 [32]. Flexible docking runs were performed with single precision docking mode (SP).

3.5. Theoretical Determination of ADME Properties

Physicochemical parameters of obtained compounds (**5a–5p**) were evaluated by using QikProp 4.8 [33].

4. Conclusions

Inhibition of aromatase has proved to be an effective approach for the treatment of hormone-dependent breast cancer in the postmenopausal women. Imidazole and triazole groups are important rings for the development new potent aromatase inhibitors with high affinity for the enzyme. A series of benzimidazole-triazolothiadiazine derivatives have been synthesized with different substituents at benzimidazole and phenyl rings. The newly synthesized compounds were tested for their anti-cancer properties against human breast cancer cell line (MCF-7). The synthesized compounds were then tested in in vitro aromatase assay and two compounds (**5e** and **5m**) exhibited activity similar to letrozole.

Author Contributions: Z.A.K., Y.Ö., conceived and designed the experiments; D.O., U.A.Ç. performed the synthesis; S.L. performed analysis studies; B.N.S., U.A.Ç., and S.I. performed activity tests; D.O., U.A.Ç., B.N.S., B.K.Ç. wrote the paper. All authors have read and agreed to the published version of the manuscript.

Acknowledgments: This study was financially supported by Anadolu University Scientific Projects Fund, Project No: 1905S032.

References

1. Chamduang, C.; Pingaew, R.; Prachayasittikul, V.; Prachayasittikul, S.; Ruchirawat, S.; Prachayasittikul, V. Novel triazole-tetrahydroisoquinoline hybrids as human aromatase inhibitors. *Bioorg. Chem.* **2019**, *93*, 103327. [CrossRef] [PubMed]
2. Doiron, J.; Richard, R.; Touré, M.M.; Picot, N.; Richard, R.; Čuperlović-Culf, M.; Robichaud, G.A.; Touaibia, M. Synthesis and structure–activity relationship of 1-and 2-substituted-1, 2, 3-triazole letrozole-based analogues as aromatase inhibitors. *Eur. J. Med. Chem.* **2011**, *46*, 4010–4024. [CrossRef] [PubMed]
3. Henneberta, O.; Montes, M.; Favre-Reguillon, A.; Chermetted, H.; Ferroudc, C.; Mortin, R. Epimerase activity of the human 11β-hydroxysteroid dehydrogenase type 1 on 7-hydroxylated C19-steroids. *J. Steroid Biochem. Mol. Biol.* **2009**, *114*, 57–63. [CrossRef] [PubMed]
4. Leechaisit, R.; Pingaew, R.; Prachayasittikul, V.; Worachartcheewan, A.; Prachayasittikul, S.; Ruchirawat, S.; Prachayasittikul, V. Synthesis, molecular docking, and QSAR study of bis-sulfonamide derivatives as potential aromatase inhibitors. *Bioorg. Med. Chem.* **2019**, *27*, 115040. [CrossRef]
5. Brueggemeier, R.W.; Hackett, J.C.; Diaz-Cruz, E.S. Aromatase inhibitors in the treatment of breast cancer. *Endocr. Rev.* **2005**, *26*, 331–345. [CrossRef]
6. Cepa, M.M.; da Silva, E.J.T.; Correia-da-Silva, G.; Roleira, F.M.; Teixeira, N.A. Synthesis and biochemical studies of 17-substituted androst-3-enes and 3,4-epoxyandrostanes as aromatase inhibitors. *Steroids* **2008**, *73*, 1409–1415. [CrossRef]
7. Bonfield, K.; Amato, E.; Bankemper, T.; Agard, H.; Steller, J.; Keeler, J.M.; Roy, D.; McCallum, A.; Paula, S.; Ma, L. Development of a new class of aromatase inhibitors: Design, synthesis and inhibitory activity of 3-phenylchroman-4-one (isoflavanone) derivatives. *Bioorg. Med. Chem.* **2012**, *20*, 2603–2613. [CrossRef]
8. Rampogu, S.; Baek, A.; Bavi, R.S.; Son, M.; Cao, G.P.; Kumar, R.; Park, C.; Zeb, A.; Rana, R.M.; Park, S.J.; et al. Identification of Novel Scaffolds with Dual Role as Antiepileptic and Anti-Breast Cancer. *IEEE/ACM Trans. Comput. Biol. Bioinform.* **2018**, *16*, 1663–1674. [CrossRef]
9. Trunet, P.F.; Vreeland, F.; Royce, C.; Chaudri, H.A.; Cooper, J.; Bhatnagar, A.S. Clinical use of aromatase inhibitors in the treatment of advanced breast cancer. *J. Steroid. Biochem. Mol. Biol.* **1997**, *61*, 241–245. [CrossRef]

10. Steele, R.E.; Mellor, L.B.; Sawyer, W.K.; Wasvary, J.M.; Browne, L.J. In vitro and in vivo studies demonstrating potent and selective estrogen inhibition with the nonsteroidal aromatase inhibitor CGS 16949A. *Steroids* **1987**, *50*, 147161. [CrossRef]
11. Kato, S.; Endoh, H.; Masuhiro, Y.; Kitamoto, T.; Uchiyama, S.; Sasaki, H.; Masushige, S.; Gotoh, Y.; Nishida, E.; Kawashima, H.; et al. Activation of the estrogen receptor through phosphorylation by mitogen-activated protein kinase. *Science* **1995**, *270*, 1491–1494. [CrossRef] [PubMed]
12. Sable, P.M.; Potey, L.C. Synthesis and antiproliferative activity of imidazole and triazole derivatives of flavonoids. *Pharm. Chem. J.* **2018**, *52*, 438–443. [CrossRef]
13. Gilardi, G.; Di Nardo, G. Heme iron centers in cytochrome P450: Structure and catalytic activity. *Rend. Lincei* **2017**, *28*, 159–167. [CrossRef]
14. Asadi, P.; Khodarahmi, G.; Farrokhpour, H.; Hassanzadeh, F.; Saghaei, L. Quantum mechanical/molecular mechanical and docking study of the novel analogues based on hybridization of common pharmacophores as potential anti-breast cancer agents. *Res. Pharm. Sci.* **2017**, *12*, 233.
15. Mojaddami, A.; Sakhteman, A.; Fereidoonnezhad, M.; Faghih, Z.; Najdian, A.; Khabnadideh, S.; Rezaei, Z. Binding mode of triazole derivatives as aromatase inhibitors based on docking, protein ligand interaction fingerprinting, and molecular dynamics simulation studies. *Res. Pharm. Sci.* **2017**, *12*, 21. [CrossRef]
16. Song, Z.; Liu, Y.; Dai, Z.; Liu, W.; Zhao, K.; Zhang, T.; Dai, Y. Synthesis and aromatase inhibitory evaluation of 4-N-nitrophenyl substituted amino-4H-1,2,4-triazole derivatives. *Bioorg. Med. Chem.* **2016**, *24*, 4723–4730. [CrossRef]
17. Adhikari, N.; Amin, S.A.; Jha, T.; Gayen, S. Integrating regression and classification-based QSARs with molecular docking analyses to explore the structure-antiaromatase activity relationships of letrozole-based analogs. *Can. J. Chem.* **2017**, *95*, 1285–1295. [CrossRef]
18. Prachayasittikul, V.; Pingaew, R.; Worachartcheewan, A.; Sitthimonchai, S.; Nantasenamat, C.; Prachayasittikul, S.; Ruchirawat, S.; Prachayasittikul, V. Aromatase inhibitory activity of 1, 4-naphthoquinone derivatives and QSAR study. *EXCLI J.* **2017**, *16*, 714.
19. Augusto, T.V.; Amaral, C.; Varela, C.L.; Bernardo, F.; da Silva, E.T.; Roleira, F.F.; Costa, S.; Teixeria, N.; Correia-da-Silva, G. Effects of new C6-substituted steroidal aromatase inhibitors in hormone-sensitive breast cancer cells: Cell death mechanisms and modulation of estrogen and androgen receptors. *J. Steroid. Biochem. Mol. Biol.* **2019**, *195*, 105486. [CrossRef]
20. Shoombuatong, W.; Schaduangrat, N.; Nantasenamat, C. Towards understanding aromatase inhibitory activity via QSAR modeling. *EXCLI J.* **2018**, *17*, 688.
21. Prior, A.M.; Yu, X.; Park, E.J.; Kondratyuk, T.P.; Lin, Y.; Pezzuto, J.M.; Sun, D. Structure-activity relationships and docking studies of synthetic 2-arylindole derivatives determined with aromatase and quinone reductase 1. *Bioorg. Med. Chem. Lett.* **2017**, *27*, 5393–5399. [CrossRef] [PubMed]
22. Acar Çevik, U.; Sağlık, B.N.; Osmaniye, D.; Levent, S.; Kaya Çavuşoğlu, B.; Karaduman, A.B.; Ozkay, Y.; Kaplancıklı, Z.A. Synthesis and docking study of benzimidazole–triazolothiadiazine hybrids as aromatase inhibitors. *Arch. Pharm.* **2020**, e2000008. [CrossRef] [PubMed]
23. Çevik, U.A.; Osmaniye, D.; Çavuşoğlu, B.K.; Sağlik, B.N.; Levent, S.; Ilgin, S.; Ozkay, Y.; Kaplancikli, Z.A. Synthesis of novel benzimidazole–oxadiazole derivatives as potent anticancer activity. *Med. Chem. Res.* **2019**, *28*, 2252–2261. [CrossRef]
24. Evren, A.E.; Yurttaş, L.; Eksellı, B.; Akalın-Cıftcı, G. Novel tri-substituted thiazoles bearing piperazine ring: Synthesis and evaluation of their anticancer activity. *Lett. Drug Des. Discov.* **2019**, *16*, 547–555. [CrossRef]
25. Çevik, U.A.; Sağlık, B.N.; Ardıç, C.M.; Özkay, Y.; Atlı, Ö. Synthesis and evaluation of new benzimidazole derivatives with hydrazone moiety as anticancer agents. *Turk. J. Biochem.* **2018**, *43*, 151–158. [CrossRef]
26. Ghosh, D.; Griswold, J.; Erman, M.; Pangborn, W. Structural basis for androgen specificity and oestrogen synthesis in human aromatase. *Nature* **2009**, *457*, 219. [CrossRef]
27. Jorgensen, W.L.; Duffy, E.M. Prediction of drug solubility from structure. *Adv. Drug Deliv. Rev.* **2002**, *54*, 355–366. [CrossRef]
28. Lipinski, C.A.; Lombardo, F.; Dominy, B.W.; Feeney, P.J. Experimental and computational approaches to estimate solubility and permeability in drug discovery and development settings. *Adv. Drug Deliv. Rev.* **1997**, *23*, 3–25. [CrossRef]
29. *Maestro*, version 10.6; Schrödinger, LLC: New York, NY, USA, 2016.
30. *The Schrödinger Suite 2016 Update 2*; Schrödinger, LLC: New York, NY, USA, 2016.

7

Characterization of an Isogenic Model of Cisplatin Resistance in Oesophageal Adenocarcinoma Cells

Amy M. Buckley [1], Becky AS. Bibby [2], Margaret R. Dunne [1], Susan A. Kennedy [1], Maria B. Davern [1], Breandán N. Kennedy [3], Stephen G. Maher [1,†] and Jacintha O'Sullivan [1,*,†]

1 Department of Surgery, Trinity Translational Medicine Institute, St. James's Hospital, Trinity College Dublin, Dublin 8, Ireland; bucklea6@tcd.ie (A.M.B.); margaret.a.dunne@gmail.com (M.R.D.); KENNES21@tcd.ie (S.A.K.); DAVERNMA@tcd.ie (M.B.D.); MAHERST@tcd.ie (S.G.M.)

2 Translational Radiobiology Group, Division of Cancer Sciences, University of Manchester, Manchester Academic Health Science Centre, Christie Hospital, Manchester M20 4BX, UK; becky.bibby@manchester.ac.uk

3 UCD Conway Institute & UCD School of Biomolecular and Biomedical Science, University College Dublin, Dublin 4, Ireland; brendan.kennedy@ucd.ie

* Correspondence: osullij4@tcd.ie

† These authors contributed equally to this work.

Abstract: Cisplatin (cis-diamminedichloroplatinum) is widely used for the treatment of solid malignancies; however, the development of chemoresistance hinders the success of this chemotherapeutic in the clinic. This study provides novel insights into the molecular and phenotypic changes in an isogenic oesophageal adenocarcinoma (OAC) model of acquired cisplatin resistance. Key differences that could be targeted to overcome cisplatin resistance are highlighted. We characterise the differences in treatment sensitivity, gene expression, inflammatory protein secretions, and metabolic rate in an isogenic cell culture model of acquired cisplatin resistance in OAC. Cisplatin-resistant cells (OE33 Cis R) were significantly more sensitive to other cytotoxic modalities, such as 2 Gy radiation ($p = 0.0055$) and 5-fluorouracil (5-FU) ($p = 0.0032$) treatment than parental cisplatin-sensitive cells (OE33 Cis P). Gene expression profiling identified differences at the gene level between cisplatin-sensitive and cisplatin-resistant cells, uncovering 692 genes that were significantly altered between OE33 Cis R cells and OE33 Cis P cells. OAC is an inflammatory-driven cancer, and inflammatory secretome profiling identified 18 proteins secreted at significantly altered levels in OE33 Cis R cells compared to OE33 Cis P cells. IL-7 was the only cytokine to be secreted at a significantly higher levels from OE33 Cis R cells compared to OE33 Cis P cells. Additionally, we profiled the metabolic phenotype of OE33 Cis P and OE33 Cis R cells under normoxic and hypoxic conditions. The oxygen consumption rate, as a measure of oxidative phosphorylation, is significantly higher in OE33 Cis R cells under normoxic conditions. In contrast, under hypoxic conditions of 0.5% O_2, the oxygen consumption rate is significantly lower in OE33 Cis R cells than OE33 Cis P cells. This study provides novel insights into the molecular and phenotypic changes in an isogenic OAC model of acquired cisplatin resistance, and highlights therapeutic targets to overcome cisplatin resistance in OAC.

Keywords: oesophageal cancer; treatment resistance; cisplatin; metabolism; inflammation; radiation

---

1. Introduction

Oesophageal cancer is the sixth most common cause of cancer-related mortality globally, and unfortunately, the five-year survival rates remain low at <20% [1,2]. Oesophageal cancer consists of two different histological subtypes: oesophageal squamous cell carcinoma (OSCC) and oesophageal adenocarcinoma (OAC) [1]. In recent years, the epidemiology of oesophageal cancer dramatically shifted, wherein OAC is now the most prevalent subtype in the Western world [3]. The increasing OAC incidence in Western countries has paralleled the increasing rates of obesity, which is a known risk factor for OAC [4].

The current standard treatment of care for oesophageal cancer focusses on neoadjuvant treatment with chemotherapy alone (neoCT) or in combination with radiation, and neoadjuvant chemoradiation (neoCRT) for locally advanced tumours prior to surgery [5]. Despite the improvements demonstrated with neoadjuvant treatment versus surgery alone, only ~30% of patients achieve a complete pathological response to neoadjuvant treatment, which is a proxy for improved overall survival [6]. Surgery offers the best chance of locoregional control, and neoadjuvant treatment aims to reduce tumour burden prior to surgery to improve post-operative outcome. Thus, it is critical to improve response rates to neoadjuvant therapy to increase patient survival [5,7,8]. Treatment resistance is a major cause of treatment failure, and it is crucial to understand the molecular mechanisms and markers governing the treatment resistance phenotype.

Cisplatin is a platinum-based chemotherapy that is used to treat a wide number of solid cancers [9]. Cisplatin is administered as part of a neoadjuvant chemotherapy regimen, and is referred to as MAGIC for the treatment of OAC [10]. The MAGIC chemotherapy protocol consists of the administration of epirubicin, cisplatin, and 5-fluorouracil pre-operatively and post-operatively [11,12]. One mechanism by which cisplatin exerts its anti-cancer effect is through the generation of DNA lesions, resulting in the activation of the DNA damage response and the subsequent induction of mitochondrial-mediated apoptosis [9]. Initial responses to cisplatin are often quite promising; however, chemoresistance to cisplatin frequently develops, leading to treatment failure, and a poor response to neoadjuvant treatment is associated with poor outcome. Thus, it is critical to understand the molecular mechanisms governing resistance to cisplatin in OAC. Our first findings investigate cross-resistance and sensitivity to other cytotoxic treatments, including radiation and 5-fluorouracil (5-FU).

OAC is an inflammatory-driven upper gastrointestinal malignancy, and previous studies have reported on the role of inflammation as a negative regulator of response to radiation treatment in OAC [4,13]. Inflammation is linked with cisplatin resistance, and Cui et al. demonstrated that interleukin-7 (IL-7) upregulation was associated with cisplatin resistance in glioma cells [14]. Targeting IL-7 improved cisplatin sensitivity [14]. In the present study, we identify changes in the inflammatory secretome in an isogenic OAC model of cisplatin resistance to increase our understanding of inflammation in cisplatin resistance. Inflammation is also tightly linked to metabolism, as inflammatory cells rely on metabolites generated from the metabolic cycle to maintain their function [15]. Tumours rely on metabolism to fuel their growth, and altered energy metabolism is an emerging hallmark of cancer [16]. Metabolic alterations correlate with treatment resistance in OAC, wherein increased oxygen consumption is linked with a radioresistant phenotype in an isogenic model of OAC radioresistance [17,18]. Furthermore, in a lung cancer model, cisplatin-resistant cells have significantly elevated oxygen consumption rates compared to parental cisplatin-sensitive cells [19]. This paradigm has not yet been explored in a cisplatin-resistant model of OAC.

In this study, we examined the key differences in chemosensitivity, radiosensitivity, gene expression, inflammatory secretions, and metabolism between matched OAC cisplatin-sensitive (OE33 Cis P) cells and OAC cisplatin-resistant (OE33 Cis R) cells. Cisplatin-resistant cells are more sensitive to radiation and 5-FU treatment than cisplatin-sensitive cells. Cisplatin resistance was associated with a number of significant changes in gene expression, where KEGG pathway analysis identified four pathways upregulated in chemoresistant OE33 Cis R cells, including pathways in cancer, tumour growth factor (TGF)-beta signalling, Wnt signalling, and steroid biosynthesis. Eighteen proteins were secreted at significantly altered levels in OE33 Cis R cells compared to OE33 Cis P, with IL-7 secretion at a significantly higher level from chemoresistant OE33 Cis R cells compared with OE33 Cis P cells. Metabolic profiling revealed that the oxygen consumption rate, as a measure of oxidative phosphorylation, was significantly higher in OE33 Cis R cells under normoxic conditions ($p = 0.0040$). In contrast, under hypoxic conditions, the oxygen consumption rate was significantly lower in OE33 Cis R cells than in OE33 Cis P cells ($p = 0.0078$). This study highlights molecular and phenotypical changes in an isogenic OAC model of acquired cisplatin resistance, and highlights key differences that could be therapeutically targeted to overcome cisplatin resistance in OAC.

2. Results

2.1. OE33 Cis R Cells Are More Sensitive to Radiation and 5-Fluorouracil (5-FU) Treatment

The relative cisplatin sensitivity of the parental cell line, OE33 Cis P, and the age and passage-matched cisplatin resistant subclone, OE33 Cis R, was evaluated by clonogenic assay. The treatment of cisplatin-sensitive OAC cells with the IC_{50} of cisplatin was previously determined in CCK8 assay (Figure 1); 1.3 μM of cisplatin significantly reduced the surviving fraction of OE33 Cis P cells to 0.303 compared to untreated OE33 Cis P cells, $p = 0.0108$ (Figure 2A). However, 1.3 μM of cisplatin did not significantly alter the surviving fraction of OE33 Cis R cells (0.944 $\pm$ 0.042 compared to untreated OE33 Cis R cells), which in itself was significantly higher than the surviving fraction of the OE33 Cis P cells treated with 1.3 μM of cisplatin, $p = 0.0011$ (Figure 2A). A ~two-fold higher concentration, 2.8 μM of cisplatin, significantly reduced the surviving fraction of OE33 Cis R cells to 0.604 $\pm$ 0.045, which was a reduction of ~39%, $p = 0.0043$ (Figure 2A). Notably, OE33 Cis P cells were not clonogenically viable with 2.8 μM of cisplatin. To investigate whether OE33 cells with acquired cisplatin resistance had altered sensitivity to other treatments, we investigated the response to both clinically relevant doses of radiation and 5-FU. The basal cell survival and radiosensitivity of cisplatin-sensitive OE33 Cis P cells and cisplatin-resistant OE33 Cis R OAC cells were assessed by clonogenic assay. Basal cell survival was assessed in OE33 Cis P and OE33 Cis R to determine if in the absence of any irradiation, there was a difference in surviving fraction. No significant difference was observed between the two cell lines under basal conditions, indicating that there is no longer-term proliferation differences between these cell lines, which might correlate with the altered radiosensitivity phenotypes (Figure 2B). To assess whether acquired cisplatin resistance conferred altered radiosensitivity, OE33 Cis P and OE33 Cis R cells were either mock-irradiated or treated with a single dose of 2 Gy X-ray radiation. Interestingly, OE33 Cis R cells were significantly more radiosensitive than OE33 Cis P cells, $p = 0.0055$ (Figure 2C). Similarly, OE33 Cis R cells were significantly more sensitive to 5-FU compared to the OE33 Cis P cells following 72 h of 5-FU treatment, $p = 0.0032$ (Figure 2D). In summary, OE33 Cis R cells were more radiosensitive and 5-FU chemosensitive when compared to the parental OE33 Cis P cells.

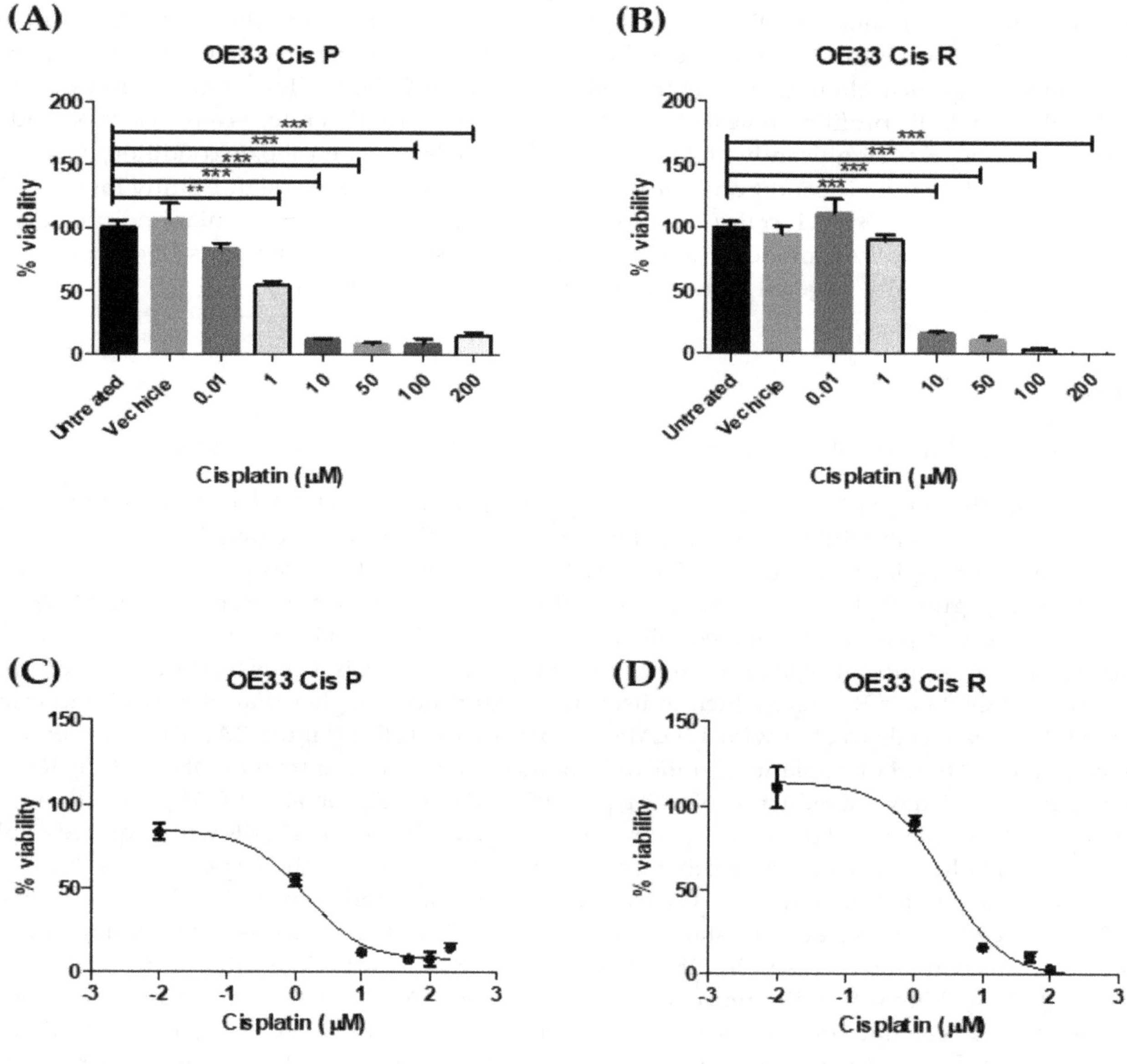

Figure 1. Oesophageal adenocarcinoma (OAC) cisplatin-sensitive (OE33 Cis P) cells were significantly more sensitive to cisplatin-induced cell death than OAC cisplatin-resistant (OE33 Cis R) cells. The toxicity to a range of increasing concentrations of cisplatin in (**A**) OE33 Cis P and (**B**) OE33 Cis R cells following 48 h of treatment was determined using a CCK-8 assay. The 48-h IC_{50} for (**C**) OE33 Cis P cells and (D) OE33 Cis R cells was 1.3 μM and 2.8 μM, respectively (n = 3). ** $p < 0.01$, *** $p < 0.001$ by an unpaired two-tailed *t*-test.

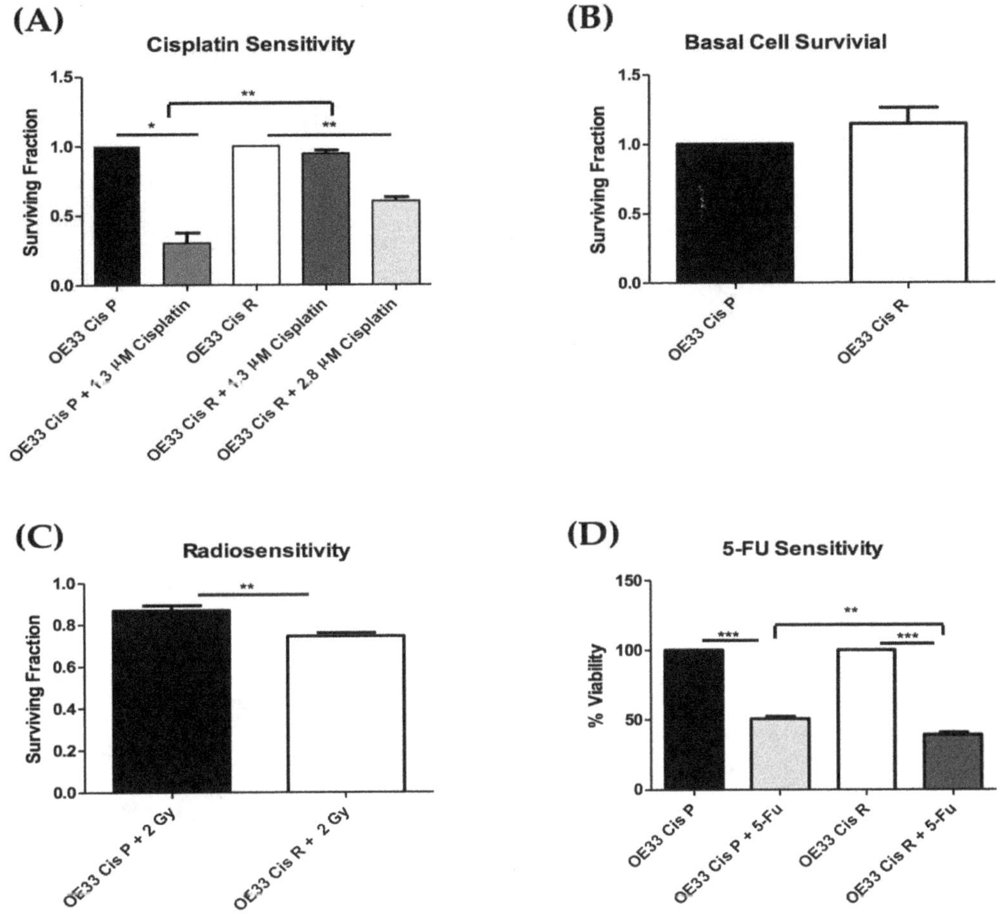

Figure 2. Cisplatin-resistant (OE33 Cis R) oesophageal adenocarcinoma cells are more radiosensitive than cisplatin-sensitive (OE33 Cis P) oesophageal adenocarcinoma (OAC) cells. (**A**) The sensitivity of cisplatin-sensitive (OE33 Cis P) and cisplatin-resistant (OE33 Cis R) OAC cells to cisplatin was assessed by clonogenic assay (n = 3). (**B**) There is no difference in the basal cell surviving fraction of cisplatin-sensitive and cisplatin-resistant OAC cells cultured in RPMI media, (n = 3). (**C**) Surviving fraction of Cis P and Cis R OAC cells following treatment of one 2 Gy fraction of irradiation, (n = 3). (**D**) The viability of the OE33 Cis R cells was significantly decreased compared to the OE33 Cis P when treated with 12 µM of 5-fluorouracil (5-FU) (n = 4). An unpaired t-test was used to compare between different cell lines, and a paired t-test was used to compare between the same cell line. Data presented as ±SEM * $p < 0.05$, ** $p < 0.01$, *** $p < 0.0001$.

2.2. Gene Expression Is Significantly Altered in OE33 Cis R Cells

OE33 Cis R cells have increased ALDH1 activity, which is a marker of stemness, compared to OE33 Cis P cells [20]. Thus, we investigated whether acquired cisplatin resistance was associated with significant changes in gene expression by whole genome digital gene expression analysis. Of the ~25,000 genes detected, 692 genes were significantly altered, 278 were upregulated, and 414 were downregulated between OE33 Cis P and OE33 Cis R cell lines. Applying a threshold of ±twofold change expression, 42 genes were upregulated (Figure 3A), and 104 genes were downregulated (Figure 3B) in the OE33 Cis R cell line compared to the OE33 Cis P cell line. Kyoto Encyclopedia of Genes and Genomes (KEGG) pathway analysis identified four pathways that were significantly upregulated in OE33 Cis R cells based on the gene expression findings, including: pathways in cancer, TGF-beta signalling, Wnt signalling, and steroid biosynthesis (Table 1A). Furthermore, eight KEGG pathways were downregulated in OE33 Cis R cells, including the MAPK signalling pathway, complement and coagulation cascades, RIG-I-like receptor signalling, sulfur metabolism, NOD-like receptor signalling, cell adhesion molecules, B cell receptor signalling, and Notch signalling (Table 1B).

In summary, OE33 Cis R cells with acquired cisplatin resistance have a significantly altered gene expression profile compared to matched cisplatin sensitive OE33 Cis P cells.

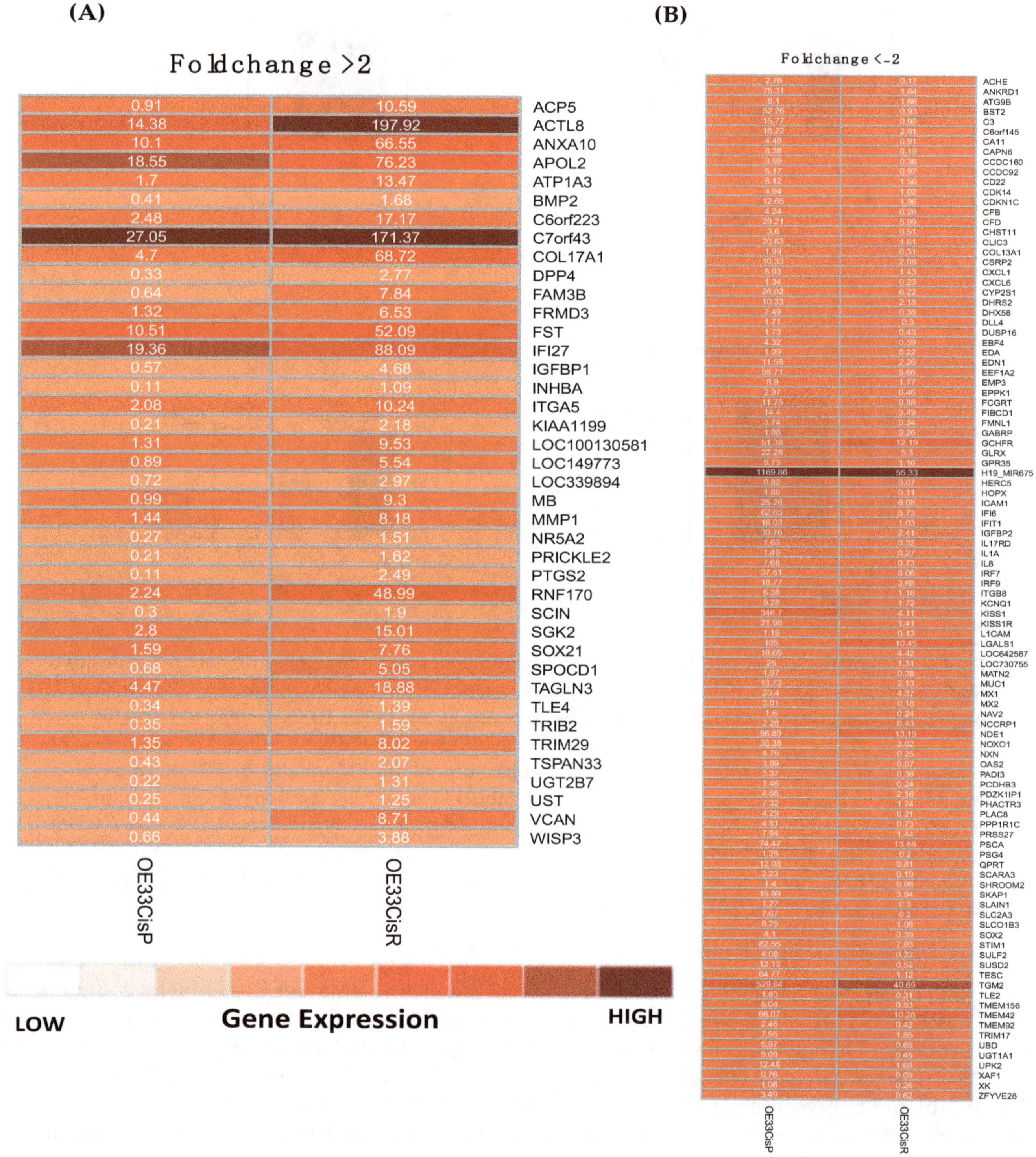

Figure 3. OE33 Cis R cells have a significantly altered gene expression profile compared to OE33 Cis P cells. Heatmaps were generated from gene expression data after applying a fold change filter ±two. (**A**) Heatmap showing 42 genes that were significantly upregulated in OE33 Cis R cells with a fold change of greater than two. (**B**) Heatmap showing 104 genes which were significantly downregulated in OE33 Cis R cells with a fold change of less than minus two. Gene expression values shown as Fragments Per Kilobase of transcript per Million mapped reads (FKPM).

Table 1. Kyoto Encyclopaedia of Genes and Genomes (KEGG) pathway analysis identifies significant pathway differences in OE33 Cis P versus OE33 Cis R cells. (**A**) KEGG pathway analysis of gene expression data identified four pathways that were significantly upregulated in OE33 Cis R cells compared to OE33 Cis P cells. (**B**) KEGG pathway analysis of gene expression data identified eight pathways that were significantly downregulated in OE33 Cis R cells compared to OE33 Cis P cells.

(**A**)

KEGG Pathway Term	Number of Identified Genes Involved	p Value	Gene Names
hsa05200:Pathways in cancer	13	5.29×10^{-3}	BMP4, PPARD, BMP2, BCR, PTGS2, EPAS1, PIK3CB, FOXO1, KITLG, MLH1, MMP1, RAC2, WNT9A
hsa04350:TGF-beta signalling pathway	6	1.21×10^{-2}	BMP4, INHBA, BMP2, ID2, ID1, FST
hsa00100:Steroid biosynthesis	3	2.92×10^{-2}	CYP27B1, LIPA, DHCR24
hsa04310:Wnt signalling pathway	6	9.19×10^{-2}	SENP2, PPARD, RAC2, PRICKLE2, FRAT2, WNT9A

(**B**)

KEGG Pathway Term	Number of Identified Genes Involved	p Value	Gene Names
hsa04010:MAPK signaling pathway	17	2.61×10^{-4}	FGFR3, PDGFA, RELB, CACNG6, CACNG4, NR4A1, STK3, JMJD7-PLA2G4B, RASGRP3, DUSP14, JMJD7, DUSP16, RRAS, HSPB1, TRAF6, GADD45B, PLA2G4B, IL1A, DUSP6
hsa04610:Complement and coagulation cascades	7	4.23×10^{-3}	PLAT, C3, CFB, SERPINA1, CFD, F2R, PLAUR
hsa04622:RIG-I-like receptor signaling pathway	6	2.09×10^{-2}	IFIH1, ISG15, IL8, IRF7, TRAF6, DHX58
hsa00920:Sulfur metabolism	3	2.84×10^{-2}	CHST11, CHST13, SULT2B1
hsa04621:NOD-like receptor signaling pathway	5	4.95×10^{-2}	CXCL1, IL8, IL18, TRAF6, BIRC3
hsa04514:Cell adhesion molecules (CAMs)	7	7.50×10^{-2}	ICAM1, CLDN9, CLDN3, ITGB8, PVRL2, CD22, L1CAM
hsa04662:B cell receptor signaling pathway	5	8.68×10^{-2}	RASGRP3, CD22, PIK3AP1, MALT1, VAV1
hsa04330:Notch signaling pathway	4	8.75×10^{-2}	HES5, DTX2, DLL4, RBPJ

2.3. Acquisition of Cisplatin Resistance Results in an Alerted Inflammatory Secretome

OAC is an inflammatory-driven upper gastrointestinal cancer, and previous studies have reported inflammation as a negative regulator of response to radiation treatment in OAC [13,21]. However, a link between inflammation and cisplatin resistance in OAC has not yet been investigated. To determine if cisplatin-resistant OE33 Cis R cells have an altered inflammatory secretome to cisplatin-sensitive OE33 Cis P OAC cells, a 47-analyte multiplex enzyme linked immunosorbent assay (ELISA) was conducted. Twenty-three proteins of 47 analytes were detected in either one or both cell lines. IL-7 was secreted at significantly higher levels from OE33 Cis R cells, $p = 0.0191$ (Figure 4A). Seventeen proteins were secreted at significantly lower levels from OE33 Cis R cells compared OE33 Cis P cells, including C-reactive protein (CRP), IL-12p70, IL-10, TNFα, macrophage-derived chemokine (MDC), intracellular adhesion molecule 1 (ICAM-1), IL-6, IL-1β, IL-13, serum amyloid A (SAA), TARC, IL-4, IL-8, IL-1RA, IL-1α, IL-2, and IP-10, as shown in Figure 4 ($p < 0.05$). There was no significant difference in the secreted levels of five of the 23 proteins detected; MCP-1, VEGF-A, VCAM, GM-CSF, and IL-15 between the cell lines (Supplemental Figure S1). OE33 Cis R cells have an altered inflammatory secretome compared to cisplatin-sensitive OE33 Cis P cells, where OE33 Cis R cells have reduced levels of a number of inflammatory chemokines and cytokines and vascular injury proteins except for IL-7, which is secreted at significantly higher levels from OE33 Cis R OAC cells.

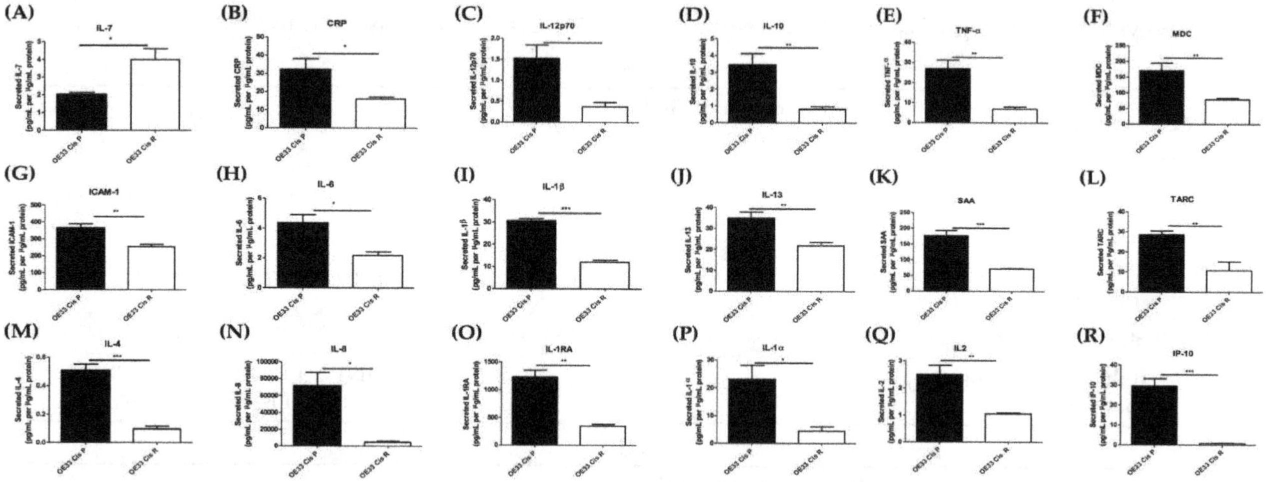

Figure 4. Inflammatory protein secretions are significantly different in cisplatin-sensitive (OE33 Cis P) versus cisplatin-resistant (OE33 Cis R) OAC cells. The secreted levels of 47 proteins in Cis P and Cis R cells was evaluated by multiplex ELISA; 23 proteins were detected in supernatant of Cis P and Cis R cells; 18 proteins were significantly different between the two cell lines, and interleukin-7 was significantly higher in Cis R cells compared to Cis P cells. Secreted levels of (**A**) Interleukin-7 (IL-7) (**B**) C-reactive protein (CRP) (**C**) Interleukin 12p70 (IL-12p70) (**D**) Interleukin 10 (IL-10) (**E**) Tumour necrosis factor α (TNF-α) (**F**) Macrophage-derived chemokine (MDC) (**G**) Intracellular adhesion molecule 1 (ICAM-1) (**H**) Interleukin 6 (IL-6) (**I**) Interleukin 1β (IL-1β) (**J**) Interleukin 13 (IL-13) (**K**) Serum amyloid A (SAA) (**L**) Thymus and activation regulated chemokine (TARC) (**M**) Interleukin 4 (IL-4) (**N**) Interleukin 8 (IL-8) (**O**) Interleukin 1 receptor antagonist (IL-1RA) (**P**) Interleukin 1α (IL-1α) (**Q**) Interleukin 2 (IL-2) (**R**) Interferon gamma-induced protein 10 (IP-10) in OE33 Cis P and OE33 Cis R cells, all secretions normalised to protein content. (n = 4). Unpaired *t*-test. * $p < 0.05$, ** $p < 0.01$, *** $p < 0.001$. Date expressed as ±SEM.

We also compared our findings from our gene expression study (Figure 3) to our inflammatory secretome data described in this section to determine if there was any overlap between the two datasets. In both our gene expression data (Figure 3B) and inflammatory secretome dataset (Figure 4G, 4N, 4P) ICAM-1, IL-8, and IL-1α were both expressed and secreted at significantly lower levels from OE33 Cis R cells compared to OE33 Cis P cells (Table 2).

Table 2. Differences in gene expression and protein secretion values of ICAM-1, IL-8, and IL-1α in OE33 Cis P and OE33 Cis R cells. This table shows the mean values of data that were used to calculate the significant differences in gene expression and protein secretions previously illustrated in Figures 3B and 4G, 4N, 4P. Fragments Per Kilobase of transcript per Million mapped reads (FKPM).

Protein	OE33 Cis P Mean Gene Expression (FPKM)	OE33 Cis R Mean Gene Expression (FPKM)	OE33 Cis P Mean Protein Secretion (pg/mL per µg/mL Protein)	OE33 Cis R Mean Protein Secretion (pg/mL per µg/mL Protein)
ICAM-1	25.26	6.08	365.64	254.39
IL-8	7.68	0.73	71822.10	4611.60
IL-1$^{\alpha}$	1.49	0.27	23.10	4.56

2.4. OE33 Cis R Cells Have an Altered Metabolic Phenotype Compared to the Parental OE33 Cis P Cells

Altered mitochondrial function is linked with treatment resistance in OAC; thus, we wanted to investigate the association between cisplatin resistance and metabolism in our model of OAC-acquired cisplatin resistance [17]. To investigate whether cisplatin-resistant OE33 Cis R cells have altered energy metabolism, we measured the two major energy pathway—oxidative phosphorylation and glycolysis—using the Seahorse XFe24 analyser under normoxic and hypoxic conditions. OE33 Cis R cells have a significantly higher ($p = 0.0040$) oxygen consumption rate (OCR), which is a measure of oxidative phosphorylation compared to OE33 Cis P cells, under normoxia. However, the oxygen consumption rate of OE33 Cis R cells was significantly lower than OE33 Cis P cells under low oxygen conditions (0.5% O_2), $p = 0.0078$, (Figure 5A). There was no significant difference in the extracellular acidification rate (ECAR), which is a measure of glycolysis, between the two cell lines under normoxic or hypoxic conditions (Figure 5B). To further investigate changes in cellular energetics both OE33 Cis P and OE33 Cis R cells were treated with oligomycin (a mitochondrial complex V inhibitor and antimycin A (a mitochondrial complex III inhibitor), which inhibit specific processes in the electron transport chain. Oligomycin and antimycin produced a similar level of OCR inhibition in both OE33 Cis P and OE33 Cis R cells, and there was no significant difference in the rate of ATP production or proton leak between cisplatin-sensitive and cisplatin-resistant cells under normoxic or hypoxic conditions (Figure 5C,D). Furthermore, treatment of OE33 Cis P and OE33 Cis R cells with the uncoupling agent carbonyl cyanide-*p*-trifluoromethoxyphenylhydrazone (FCCP) showed no significant difference in maximal respiration rate between the cell lines (Figure 5E). In addition, the rate of non-mitochondrial respiration was not significantly altered between the two cell lines (Figure 5F). In summary, OE33 Cis R cells have an alerted metabolic phenotype whereby they have a significantly elevated OCR compared to parental OE33 Cis P cells under normoxic conditions, and OE33 Cis R cells have significantly lower OCR under hypoxic conditions.

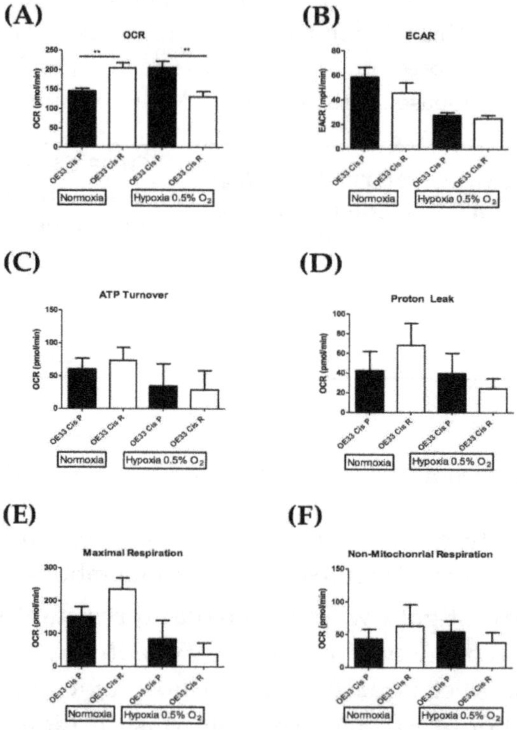

Figure 5. Cisplatin-resistant (OE33 Cis R) oesophageal adenocarcinoma cells have an altered metabolic phenotype compared to cisplatin-sensitive (OE33 Cis P) cells under normoxic and hypoxic conditions (0.5% O_2). (**A**) The oxygen consumption rate (OCR), which is a measure of oxidative phosphorylation, was evaluated in OE33 Cis P and OE33 Cis R OAC cells using the Seahorse Biosciences XFe24 extracellular flux analyser cultured under normoxic and hypoxic conditions (0.5% O_2). OE33 Cis R cells have a significantly higher OCR when compared to OE33 Cis P; cisplatin-sensitive cells, under normoxic conditions (n = 5), unpaired *t*-test, ** $p < 0.01$. (**B**) The extracellular acidification rate (ECAR), which is a measure glycolysis, was evaluated in OE33 Cis P and OE33 Cis R cells using the Seahorse Biosciences XFe24 extracellular flux analyser cultured under normoxic and hypoxic conditions (0.5% O_2), (n = 5), unpaired *t*-test. (**C**) Difference in the rate of ATP production in OE33 Cis P and OE33 Cis R cells cultured under normoxic and hypoxic conditions (0.5% O_2), (n = 5), unpaired *t*-test. (**D**) Difference in the rate of proton leak in OE33 Cis P and OE33 Cis R cells cultured under normoxic and hypoxic conditions (0.5% O_2), (n = 5), unpaired *t*-test. (**E**) Difference in maximal respiration rate in OE33 Cis P and OE33 Cis R cells cultured under normoxic and hypoxic conditions (0.5% O_2), (n = 5), unpaired *t*-test. (**F**) Difference in non-mitochondrial respiration in OE33 Cis P and OE33 Cis R cells cultured under normoxic and hypoxic conditions (0.5% O_2), (n = 5), unpaired *t*-test. Data presented as $\pm$SEM.

3. Discussion

Cisplatin is a widely use chemotherapeutic drug for the treatment of solid cancers, including OAC; however, the development of chemoresistance to cisplatin hinders the success of this agent [9]. Previous studies in cisplatin-resistant cancer cell lines of various tissue origin report multiple mechanisms responsible for enhanced resistance, and that the cisplatin-resistant phenotype is the result of multiple microRNA, gene, and protein expression changes [22–24]. Molecular mechanisms commonly associated with cisplatin resistance include alterations in DNA repair, drug influx/efflux, drug detoxification, cell cycle dysregulation, and evasion of apoptosis [25]. In this study, we sought to characterise the key differences linked to resistance in an isogenic model of OAC cisplatin resistance, including relative chemosensitivity and radiosensitivity, whole gene expression, inflammatory protein secretions, and metabolic phenotype.

Chemoresistant OE33 Cis R cells have a significant acquired resistance to cisplatin compared to cisplatin-sensitive OE33 Cis P cells. Interestingly, cisplatin-resistant OE33 Cis R cells are more radiosensitive than matched OE33 Cis P cells. Cisplatin is often administered in combination with radiation for the treatment of numerous solid cancers, including oesophageal, head, neck, and cervical cancer [26–29]. Cisplatin has been widely shown to enhance radiosensitivity, which is potentially through the non-homologous end joining (NHEJ) DNA repair pathway [30,31]. As cisplatin is often given in combination with radiation to improve response, it was surprising that OE33 Cis R cells are more radiosensitive than OE33 Cis P cells. OE33 Cis R cells can overcome cytotoxic insult from cisplatin to a greater degree than OE33 Cis P cells, but cannot overcome radiation-induced DNA damage as efficiently as they could before the acquisition of cisplatin resistance. Whilst it was unexpected that OE33 Cis R cells are more radiosensitive, as DNA is the common target of both cisplatin and radiation, the mechanisms of action in yielding lethal events, delivery methods, and repair systems as a result of both treatments are very different. Cisplatin has to cross the plasma membrane and traffic to the nucleus; this is a process during which it can be affected in several ways, such as influx via CTR1, efflux via ABC transporters, detoxification by glutathione, trapping in lysosomes, altered trafficking between the plasma membrane and the nucleus, as well as DNA repair proficiency [32,33]. Radiation, on the other hand, largely influences DNA damage through water radiolysis (70%), and has direct effects on DNA bases (30%), but is also subject to energy transfer, glutathione scavenging, oxygen fixation, and DNA repair proficiency [34]. Radiation is responsible for the induction of double-strand breaks in DNA, whereas cisplatin treatment results in the formation of DNA adducts as a result of covalent bonds [31]. Additionally, cisplatin largely employs homologous recombination and nucleotide excision repair as its major pathways of repair, while radiation employs non-homologous end joining, base excision repair, single-strand break repair and, to a much lesser extent, homologous recombination. Thus, the DNA repair mechanics that were employed by cancer cells following either radiation or cisplatin treatment are quite different, and the significance of DNA repair in potentially driving this phenotype requires further mechanistic investigation in the future. Furthermore, OE33 Cis R cells were found to be more sensitive to 5-FU treatment compared to OE33 Cis P cells. A previous study established cisplatin-resistant and 5-FU-resistant OAC OE19 cell lines [35]. Interestingly, miRNA expression profiling in the OE19 cisplatin-resistant cell line and the OE19 5-FU-resistant cell line identified a large number of miRNA that were significantly differentially expressed in comparison to the relatively chemosensitive controls [23,31]. In the OE19 cisplatin-resistant cells 18 miRNAs were significantly dysregulated compared to controls (13 downregulated, five upregulated), of which 11 were validated including: miR-455-3p, miR-200b-3p, let-7e-5p, miR-181b-5p, miR-125a-5p, miR-181a-5p, miR-200b-5p, miR-31-5p, miR-200a-3p, miR-638, and miR-191-5p. Interestingly, the miRNA expression profile of the cisplatin-resistant cell line differed from the miRNA expression profile of the 5-FU-resistant cell line [23,31]. The differential miRNA expression profiles may be associated with the different mechanisms by which cisplatin and 5-FU induce cytotoxic damage.

The gene expression data that were presented in this study provide indications as to the potential mechanisms associated with enhanced resistance to cisplatin in the OE33 Cis R cells compared to the OE33 Cis P cells. Cell membrane transporter genes *ATP1A3*, *ABCA12*, *TMEM199*, and *TMEM22* were upregulated in the OE33 Cis R, and *TMEM156* and *TMEM42* were downregulated. The existing literature is limited with regards to these genes; however, they are members of cell membrane transporter families, some of which are associated with transport and the cellular accumulation of cisplatin, such as ATP7A/B and TMEM205 [25]. Upregulated Wnt signalling and the EMT pathway are also associated with cisplatin resistance [36,37]. The upregulation of the *PRICKLE2* gene may contribute to an increase in Wnt signalling in the OE33 Cis R cell line [38]. The *CDKN1C* gene produces the cyclin-dependent kinase inhibitor p57, which functions as a tumour suppressor in multiple cancer types [39]. Furthermore, the overexpression of p57 has been shown to enhance cisplatin sensitivity in-vitro via intrinsic mitochondrial apoptosis [40]. The downregulation of the *CDKN1C* gene in the OE33 Cis R cell line may contribute to the evasion of apoptosis and cellular resistance to cisplatin. Interestingly, TGF-β signalling, which was identified by KEGG pathway analysis to be upregulated in OE33 Cis R cells, has previously been linked to cisplatin resistance in nasopharyngeal and head and neck cancer; it would be of interest in the future to further understand the role Of TGF-β signalling in cisplatin resistance in OAC [41,42].

KEGG pathway analysis also revealed that the complement pathway was downregulated in cisplatin-resistant cells; this was an interesting finding, as levels of complement C3a and C4a of the classically activated pathway have previously been shown to be predictive of response to neoadjuvant chemoradiation therapy in OAC [13]. Considering this, we sought to investigate the larger inflammatory secretome of OAC cisplatin-resistant OE33 Cis R cells compared to that of cisplatin-sensitive OE33 Cis P cells. OAC is an inflammatory-driven cancer; thus, it is vital to understand the potential contributions of inflammatory secretions to cisplatin resistance. OE33 Cis R cells have a significantly altered inflammatory profile; only one protein, IL-7, was secreted at higher levels from OE33 Cis R cells. Whereas, 17 proteins (CRP, IL-12p70, IL-10, TNFα, MDC, ICAM-1, IL-6, IL-1β, IL-13, SAA, TARC, IL-4, IL-8, IL-1RA, IL-1α, IL-2, and IP-10) were secreted at significantly lower levels from in OE33 Cis R cells compared OE33 Cis P cells. Three of the proteins detected—ICAM-1, IL-1α and IL-8—were also found to be altered at the gene level, where they were both expressed and secreted at significantly lower levels from OE33 Cis R cells compared with OE33 Cis P cells. In a human glioma cancer model, the expression of IL-7 was positively correlated with the IC_{50} of cisplatin in both cell lines and glioma patient samples, and the overexpression of IL-7 further increased cisplatin resistance in glioma cancer cells [14]. This study supports our findings and further highlights IL-7 as a potential mediator of cisplatin resistance in OAC. IL-7 may be a useful therapeutic target for enhancing cisplatin sensitivity in OAC, and this warrants further investigation in the future.

Interleukin-1 alpha (IL-1α) is a potent inflammatory cytokine that plays a pivotal role in the inflammatory response [43]. IL-1α was both expressed and secreted at significantly lower levels from OE33 Cis R cells when compared to OE33 Cis P cells. Interestingly, IL-1α has previously been shown to play a key role in cisplatin sensitivity in human ovarian cancer cells, whereby IL-1α was shown to enhance sensitivity to cisplatin [44]. IL-1α given in combination with cisplatin was shown to enhance the anti-proliferative effect of cisplatin, increase cisplatin uptake, and increase DNA-platination in human ovarian OVCAR-3 cells [44]. Given that we have shown IL-1α to be expressed and secreted at a lower level in cisplatin resistant cells, it would be of interest to evaluate the potential chemosensitising effect of combining IL-1α with cisplatin in OE33 Cis R cells.

Similarly, intracellular adhesion molecule-1 (ICAM-1) was found to be both expressed and secreted at significantly lower levels from OE33 Cis R cells compared to cisplatin-sensitive OE33 Cis P cells. The role of ICAM-1 in carcinogenesis and drug resistance is often dependent on the cancer and cell type. ICAM-1 has previously been shown to have anti-cancer activity in numerous studies through its recruitment of immune cells to the tumour [45–47]. Furthermore, cisplatin treatment has been shown to induce ICAM-1 expression in cancer cells; thus, it is not surprising that ICAM-1 is found at lower levels in the cisplatin-resistant cells compared to the OAC cisplatin-sensitive cells [48]. On the other hand, in an oesophageal SCC cancer study, ICAM-1 was reported to enhance cisplatin resistance and tumourigenicity in-vivo. However, it is important to note that this study was carried out in immunodeficient mice [49]. Thus, the potential of targeting ICAM-1 to alter cisplatin sensitivity in OAC needs further exploration, as it has direct effects on numerous cell types, including both cancer and endothelial cells, and is reliant on interactions with the tumour microenvironment.

Inflammation and metabolism are tightly interlinked biological processes whereby inflammatory cells rely on metabolites generated from the metabolic cycle to maintain their function. Given the significant differences in inflammatory protein secretions from OE33 Cis R cells compared to OE33 Cis P cells, we sought to investigate the metabolic profile of our model of acquired cisplatin resistance. Cisplatin-resistant OE33 Cis R cells have an altered metabolic phenotype compared to matched OE33 Cis P cisplatin-sensitive cells. OE33 Cis R cells have an ~40% higher rate of oxygen consumption rate than OAC cisplatin-sensitive cells. Interestingly, a previous study by Lynam-Lennon et al. demonstrated that increased oxygen consumption rate was linked with a radioresistant phenotype in OAC [17]. However, to date, the role of oxidative phosphorylation in cisplatin resistance in OAC has been underexplored. In a human ovarian cancer model of cisplatin resistance, SKOV3/DPP cisplatin-resistant cells had a significantly higher oxygen consumption rate when compared to SKOV3 cisplatin-sensitive cells [50]. The treatment of ovarian cisplatin-resistant cells with a Bcl-2 inhibitor was found to reduce the oxygen consumption rate and enhance cisplatin sensitivity [50]. Additionally, a study by Catanzaro et al. demonstrated that the inhibition of glucose-6-phosphate dehydrogenase could sensitise cisplatin-resistant ovarian cancer cells to cytotoxic death, further highlighting the role of the oxidative phosphorylation pathway in cisplatin resistance [51]. An elevated oxygen consumption rate has also been linked to chemoresistance with other chemotherapies, such as 5-FU. A study by Denise et al. demonstrated that 5-FU-resistant colorectal cancer cells have a significantly higher oxygen consumption rate compared to parental 5-FU sensitive cells. Furthermore, an increased oxygen consumption rate has also been linked to chemoresistance in docetaxel-resistant prostate cancer cells, where treatment with metformin to inhibit oxygen consumption was found to increase chemosensitivity [52]. Thus, it would be of interest to target oxidative phosphorylation in OAC OE33 Cis R cells as a potential mechanism to enhance cisplatin sensitivity. Metabolism is also tightly influenced by environmental conditions, whereby low oxygen conditions can result in the upregulation of hypoxia-inducible glucose transporters [53]. Thus, we investigated the metabolic rate of OE33 Cis P and Cis R cells under hypoxic conditions. The metabolic profile of OE33 Cis R cells is significantly altered under moderate hypoxic conditions (0.5% O_2), where OE33 Cis R cells have a significantly lower oxygen consumption rate than parental OE33 Cis P cells. This result highlights the flexible nature of OE33 Cis R cells, whereby they are able to adapt to environmental conditions and reduce oxygen consumption rate in low oxygen conditions. Hypoxia plays a critical role in cisplatin resistance, and hypoxic tumours often display a high level of resistance to cisplatin [54,55]. Studies in lung cancer have reported that hypoxia can promote the activation of autophagy, resulting in chemoresistance [55]. In addition, cisplatin-resistant lung cancer cells display a hypoxia-induced upregulation of p53, resulting in the activation of p21 transcription, which results in the arrest of the cell cycle at the G0–G1 phase, ultimately reducing the effect of cisplatin [54]. As dynamic regions of hypoxia are found in most solid tumours, including OAC, it is critical to understand how OE33 Cis R cells adapt to their tumour microenvironment to determine the best method to target this cell population. The reduced OCR that is seen in OE33 Cis R under hypoxic conditions is something that needs to be further evaluated in future studies.

This study has investigated a number of key differences in an isogenic model of OAC cisplatin resistance. Importantly, OE33 Cis R cells have a significantly altered gene expression and inflammatory secretome profile compared to cisplatin-sensitive cells. In addition, cisplatin-resistant cells have an altered metabolic profile under normal and low oxygen conditions. The molecular differences identified in this study, including the increased sensitivity to radiation and 5-FU of cisplatin-resistant cells, provides novel insight into cisplatin resistance in OAC, and has identified molecular processes that could be targeted in the future as a means to overcome cisplatin resistance and improve therapeutic outcomes for OAC.

4. Materials and Methods

4.1. Generation of the OE33 Cis P and OE33 Cis R Cell Lines

The human OE33 oesophageal adenocarcinoma cell line was obtained from the European collection of cell cultures. The isogenic model of cisplatin-resistant OAC; Cis P (cisplatin-sensitive) and Cis R (cisplatin-resistant) cells was generated as previously described [20]. Briefly, the original OE33 cells were split to generate two passage-matched flasks of OE33 cells. One flask was mock treated, and the other was treated with a metronomic dosing of cisplatin. Both lines were developed side-by-side and treated identically, differing only in being treated with vehicle or cisplatin until cisplatin-resistant cells were developed.

4.2. Preparation of Chemotherapeutic Drugs

Stock solutions of cis-diamminedichloroplatinum (cisplatin) and 5-flurouracil (5-FU) were prepared in phosphate-buffered saline (PBS) and dimethyl sulfoxide (DMSO), respectively. Solutions were sterile filtered and then aliquoted and stored at −20 °C. Prior to use, the solution was incubated at 37 °C and mixed thoroughly.

4.3. Determining IC_{50} of Cisplatin for OE33 Cis P and OE33 Cis R Cells at Using Cell Counting kit-8 (CCK8) Assay

OE33 Cis P and OE33 Cis R cells were seeded at 5×10^3 cells/200 µL in complete Roswell Park Memorial Institute (RPMI) 1640 medium supplemented with 10% fetal calf serum (Lonza, Basal, Switzerland) and 1% penicillin-streptomycin (Lonza, Basal, Switzerland) in a 96-well flat-bottomed plate and incubated at 37 °C, 5% CO_2 overnight. Media was replaced with 180 µL of fresh complete RPMI and cells were treated with 20 µL of cisplatin at a range of increasing concentrations (0, 0.01, 1, 10, 50, 100, 200 µM). Cells were incubated for 48 h at 37 °C, 5% CO_2/95% air. 10 µL of cell counting kit-8 (CCK8) assay solution (Sigma-Aldrich, Missouri, USA) was added to each well after 48 h. Cells were incubated at 37 °C, 5% CO_2 for 1.5 to 2 h until appropriate colour development was observed. The absorbance was measured at 450 nm using a VersaMax microplate reader (Molecular Devices, Sunnyvale, CA, USA).

4.4. Clonogenic Assay

OE33 Cis P and OE33 Cis R cells were trypsinised, counted, and seeded at the optimised densities of 1–2.5 $\times 10^3$ in 1.5 mL of complete RPMI, in triplicate in six-well plates and allowed to adhere overnight. For chemosensitivity assays, cells were allowed to adhere for 24 h following which time they were treated with vehicle control or cisplatin. OE33 Cis P cells were treated with 1.3 µM of cisplatin, and OE33 Cis R cells were treated with either 1.3 µM or 2.8 µM of cisplatin. For radiosensitivity assays, cell were seeded and allowed to adhere for 48 h following which time OE33 Cis P and OE33 Cis R cells were either irradiated with 2 Gy (dose rate 1.73 Gy/min 195 KV 15 mA) or mock irradiated. Colonies were allowed to grow for 7 to 14 days, at which point they were fixed and stained with crystal violet (0.5%/ 25% v/v methanol) and allowed to air dry. Colonies consisting of 50 cells or more were counted using a colony counter (GelCount, Oxford Optronix, Oxford, UK). Plating efficiency (PE), which is the fraction of colonies formed by untreated cells, was calculated using the formula: PE = No. colonies/No. cells seeded. The surviving fraction (SF), which was the number of colonies formed following treatment, and was expressed in terms of PE, was calculated using the formula: SF = No. colonies/(No. cells seeded × PE).

4.5. Irradiation

Irradiation was performed using a XStrahl X-ray generator, (RS225), at a dose rate of 1.75 Gray per min.

4.6. RNA Extraction from Cell Lines

For total RNA extraction and purification, including miRNA, the RNeasy Mini Kit was used as per the manufacturer's instructions (Qiagen, UK). Sterile RNase and DNase-free filter tips were used throughout all of the RNA experiments (TipOne Starlab, UK). Cell pellets ($<5 \times 10^4$ cells) were resuspended in 350 µl of RLT lysis buffer and pellets >five × 104 cells were resuspended in 600 µL of RLT lysis buffer. One volume of 70% ethanol was added to the lysate and mixed well by pipetting. RNeasy mini columns were inserted into the top of two-mL collection tubes. Up to 700 µL of the lysate was added to the columns, which were then centrifuged at 8000× g for 15 seconds at room temperature (RT). A 700-µL volume of RW1 buffer was added to the column, and centrifuged 8000× g for 15 seconds at RT. The flow through was discarded, and 500 µL of RPE buffer was added to the column and centrifuged at 8000× *g* for 15 s at RT. The flow through was discarded, and 500 μL of buffer RPE was added to the column and centrifuged at 8000× *g* for 2 min at RT. The flow through was subsequently discarded, and the column was transferred to a new 1.5-mL collection tube. A 30 to 50-μL volume of RNase-free water was pipetted directly onto the column membrane and centrifuged for 1 min at 8000× *g* to elute the RNA from the silica membrane of the column. The concentration and purity of the eluted RNA was measured on the NanoDrop ND-1000 (Thermo Scientific, Delaware, USA). Then, RNA extracts were stored at −20 °C in the short term (<one month) or −80 °C in the long term (>one month).

4.7. Digital Gene Expression Sequencing

The gene expression sequencing was outsourced to LC Sciences (Texas, USA). Briefly, six μg total RNA from three biological replicates was prepared in 50-μL of DEPC (diethylpyrocarbonate) water, five μL of 3M of NaOAc, pH 5.2 and 150 μL of absolute ethanol to give a final volume of 205 μL. Samples were stored at −80 °C prior to shipping on dry ice. High-throughput sequencing was performed using Illumina sequencing by synthesis technology. LC Sciences provided analysed gene expression data and KEGG (Kyoto Encyclopaedia of Genes and Genomes) analysis. Gene expression abundance was normalised and evaluated in FPKM (Fragments Per Kilobase of transcript per Million reads) using the Cuffdiff module of Cufflinks_v2.2.1. The q-value was representative of a false discovery rate (FDR) adjusted p-value < 0.05. The fold change in gene expression was calculated from the equation: log2 (OE33 Cis R FPKM/OE33 Cis P PMK). Pathway analysis was performed with EASE (Expression Analysis Systematic Explorer). The KEGG pathway p-value is based on the EASE score: a modified Fisher exact p-value that measures if the probability of the (count/list total) is more than random chance compared to the background list (pop hits/pop total), where 'count' is the number of significant genes in a pathway, 'list total' is the number of genes in the submitted list associated with the category (e.g., KEGG pathway), 'pop hits' is the number of genes in the background list associated with the term, and 'pop total' is the number of genes in the background list associated with the category. Fold enrichment was calculated as (count/list total)/(pop hits/pop total). The lower the p-value, the more enrichment of the term. Gene expression changes were considered significant if the p value was <0.05. Heatmaps were generated using the 'pheatmap' package for the R project for statistical computing (version 3.5.1) [56,57].

4.8. Multiplex Enzyme Linked Immunosorbent Assay (ELISA)

Supernatant from OE33 Cis P and OE33 Cis R cells were defrosted on ice. The secretion of cytokines and angiogenic growth factors was analysed by ELISA as per the manufacturer's instructions. To assess angiogenic, vascular injury, inflammatory cytokine and chemokine secretions, a 47 multiplex kit spread across seven plates was used (Meso Scale Diagnostics, USA). The multiplex kit was used to quantify the secretions of CRP, Eotaxin, Eotaxin-3, GM-CSF, ICAM-1, IFN-γ, IL-10, IL-12/IL-23p40, IL-12p70, IL-13, IL-15, IL-16, IL-17A, IL-17A/F, IL-17B, IL-17C, IL-17D, IL-1RA, IL-1α, IL-1β, IL-2, IL-21, IL-22, IL-23, IL-27, IL-3, IL-31, IL-4, IL-5, IL-6, IL-7, IL-8, IL-8 (HA), IL-9, IP-10, MCP-1, MCP-4, MDC, MIP-1α, MIP-1β, MIP-3α, SAA, TARC, TNF-α, TNF-β, TSLP, VCAM-1, VEGF-A from OE33 Cis P and OE33 Cis R cell supernatants from cells that had been seeded at 250,000 cells per well for 48 h. Secretion data for all of the factors was normalised appropriately to cell lysate protein content using the BCA assay (Pierce).

4.9. OCR and ECAR Measurements in Cis P and Cis R Cells

OE33 Cis P and OE33 Cis R cells were seeded in five wells per treatment group at a density of 18,000 and 20,000 cells/well, respectively, in 24-well cell culture XFe24 microplates (Agilent Technologies, Santa Clara, CA, USA) at a volume of 100 μL and allowed to adhere at 37 °C in 5% CO_2/95% air. Five hours later, an additional 150 μL/well complete cell culture RPMI medium was added. Following 48 h of incubation, media was removed and cells were washed with unbuffered

Dulbecco's Modified Eagle's medium (DMEM) supplemented with 10 mM of glucose and 10 mM of sodium pyruvate, (pH 7.4) and incubated for one hour at 37 °C in a CO_2-free incubator. The oxygen consumption rate (OCR) and extracellular acidification rate (ECAR) were measured using a Seahorse Biosciences XFe24 Extracellular Flux Analyser (Agilent Technologies, Santa Clara, CA, USA). Three basal measurements of OCR and ECAR were taken over 24 min consisting of three repeats of mix (three min)/wait (2 min)/measurement (3 min) to establish basal respiration. Three additional measurements were obtained following the injection of three mitochondrial inhibitors including oligomycin (Sigma Aldrich, Missouri, USA), antimycin-A (Sigma Aldrich, Missouri, USA) and an uncoupling agent Carbonyl cyanide 4-(trifluoromethoxy)phenylhydrazone (FCCP) (Sigma Aldrich, Missouri, USA). ATP turnover was calculated by subtracting the OCR post oligomycin injection from baseline OCR prior to oligomycin addition. Proton leak was calculated by subtracting OCR post antimycin-A addition from OCR post oligomycin addition. Maximal respiration was calculated by subtracting OCR post antimycin addition from OCR post FCCP addition. Non-mitochondrial respiration was determined as the OCR value post antimycin-A addition. All of the measurements were normalised to cell number using the crystal violet assay, transferring the eluted stain to a 96-well plate before reading. For seahorse experiments carried out under (0.5% O_2) hypoxia, cells were seeded under normoxic conditions and allowed to adhere for 6 h at 37 °C 5% CO_2/95% air, following which time they were placed at 37 °C 0.5% O_2 5% CO_2 in the H35 Don whitley hypoxstation for 48 h, and seahorse measurements were carried out under hypoxia (0.5% O_2) in the i2 Whitley station using the same protocol for measuring rate as described for normoxic conditions.

4.10. Crystal Violet

Cells were fixed with 1% glutaraldehyde (Sigma-Aldrich, Missouri, USA) for 15 min at RT. The fixative was removed, and cells were washed with PBS and stained with 0.1% crystal violet for 30 min at RT. Plates were left to air dry and incubated with 50 µL of 1% Triton X-100 in PBS on a plate shaker for 30 min at RT. Absorbance was read at 595 nm on a VersaMax microplate reader (Molecular Devices, Sunnyvale, CA, USA).

4.11. Statistical Analysis

Statistical analysis was performed using GraphPad Prism version 5 software (GraphPad Software, CA, USA). Scientific data were expressed as mean ± standard error of the mean (SEM). SEM was calculated as the standard deviation of the original samples divided by the square root of the sample size. Specific statistical tests used are indicated in figure legends. For all of the statistical analysis, differences were considered statistically significant at $p < 0.05$.

Author Contributions: Conceptualisation, A.M.B., B.A.S.B., S.G.M. and J.O.S.; Data curation, A.M.B. and B.A.S.B.; Formal analysis, A.M.B., B.A.S.B., S.G.M. and J.O.S.; Funding acquisition, M.R.D. and J.O.S.; Investigation, A.M.B., B.A.S.B. and M.R.D.; Methodology, A.M.B., B.A.S.B. and M.R.D.; Software, S.A.K.; Supervision, B.N.K., S.G.M. and J.O.S.; Visualisation, S.A.K.; Writing—original draft, A.M.B.; Writing—review & editing, A.M.B., M.R.D., S.A.K., B.N.K., S.G.M. and J.O.S.

Abbreviations

5-FU	Fluorouracil
Cis	Cisplatin
ECAR	Extracellular Acidification Rate
ELISA	Enzyme Linked Immunosorbent assay

DMEM	Dulbecco's Modified Eagle's medium
IL-1α	Interleukin 1 alpha
IL-7	Interleukin 7
IL-8	Interleukin 8
ICAM-1	Intracellular Adhesion Molecule 1
KEGG	Kyoto Encyclopedia of Genes and Genomes
MiRNA	Micro ribonucleic acid
NeoCRT	Neoadjuvant Chemoradiation Therapy
NHEJ	Non Homologous end joining
OAC	Oesophageal Adenocarcinoma
OCR	Oxidative Phosphorylation
PE	Plating Efficiency
RMPI	Roswell Park Memorial Institute medium
SCC	Squamous Cell Carcinoma
SF	Surviving Fraction
TGF-β	Transforming Growth Factor Beta
VEGF	Vascular Endothelial Growth Factor

References

1. Arnold, M.; Soerjomataram, I.; Ferlay, J.; Forman, D. Global incidence of oesophageal cancer by histological subtype in 2012. *Gut* **2015**, *64*, 381–387. [CrossRef] [PubMed]
2. Ferlay, J.; Soerjomataram, I.; Dikshit, R.; Eser, S.; Mathers, C.; Rebelo, M.; Parkin, D.M.; Forman, D.; Bray, F. Cancer incidence and mortality worldwide: Sources, methods and major patterns in GLOBOCAN 2012. *Int. J. Cancer* **2015**, *136*, E359–E386. [CrossRef] [PubMed]
3. Abbas, G.; Krasna, M. Overview of esophageal cancer. *Ann. Cardiothorac. Surg.* **2017**, *6*, 131–136. [CrossRef] [PubMed]
4. Picardo, S.L.; Maher, S.G.; O'Sullivan, J.N.; Reynolds, J.V. Barrett's to oesophageal cancer sequence: A model of inflammatory-driven upper gastrointestinal cancer. *Digest. Surg.* **2012**, *29*, 251–260. [CrossRef] [PubMed]
5. Cools-Lartigue, J.; Spicer, J.; Ferri, L.E. Current status of management of malignant disease: Current management of esophageal cancer. *J. Gastrointest. Surg. Off. J. Soc. Surg. Aliment. Tract.* **2015**, *19*, 964–972. [CrossRef] [PubMed]
6. Donohoe, C.L.; Reynolds, J.V. Neoadjuvant treatment of locally advanced esophageal and junctional cancer: The evidence-base, current key questions and clinical trials. *J. Thorac. Dis.* **2017**, *9*, S697–S704. [CrossRef] [PubMed]
7. Walsh, T.N.; Noonan, N.; Hollywood, D.; Kelly, A.; Keeling, N.; Hennessy, T.P.J. A Comparison of Multimodal Therapy and Surgery for Esophageal Adenocarcinoma. *N. Engl. J. Med.* **1996**, *335*, 462–467. [CrossRef] [PubMed]
8. Jin, H.-L.; Zhu, H.; Ling, T.-S.; Zhang, H.-J.; Shi, R.-H. Neoadjuvant chemoradiotherapy for resectable esophageal carcinoma: A meta-analysis. *World J. Gastroenterol. WJG* **2009**, *15*, 5983–5991. [CrossRef] [PubMed]
9. Galluzzi, L.; Senovilla, L.; Vitale, I.; Michels, J.; Martins, I.; Kepp, O.; Castedo, M.; Kroemer, G. Molecular mechanisms of cisplatin resistance. *Oncogene* **2012**, *31*, 1869–1883. [CrossRef] [PubMed]
10. Reynolds, J.V.; Preston, S.R.; O'Neill, B.; Baeksgaard, L.; Griffin, S.M.; Mariette, C.; Cuffe, S.; Cunningham, M.; Crosby, T.; Parker, I.; et al. ICORG 10-14: NEOadjuvant trial in Adenocarcinoma of the oEsophagus and oesophagoGastric junction International Study (Neo-AEGIS). *BMC Cancer* **2017**, *17*, 401. [CrossRef]
11. Cunningham, D.; Allum, W.H.; Stenning, S.P.; Thompson, J.N.; Van de Velde, C.J.H.; Nicolson, M.; Scarffe, J.H.; Lofts, F.J.; Falk, S.J.; Iveson, T.J.; et al. Perioperative Chemotherapy versus Surgery Alone for Resectable Gastroesophageal Cancer. *N. Engl. J. Med.* **2006**, *355*, 11–20. [CrossRef]

12. Van Hagen, P.; Hulshof, M.C.C.M.; van Lanschot, J.J.B.; Steyerberg, E.W.; Henegouwen, M.I.V.B.; Wijnhoven, B.P.L.; Richel, D.J.; Nieuwenhuijzen, G.A.P.; Hospers, G.A.P.; Bonenkamp, J.J.; et al. Preoperative Chemoradiotherapy for Esophageal or Junctional Cancer. *N. Engl. J. Med.* **2012**, *366*, 2074–2084. [CrossRef] [PubMed]
13. Maher, S.G.; McDowell, D.T.; Collins, B.C.; Muldoon, C.; Gallagher, W.M.; Reynolds, J.V. Serum proteomic profiling reveals that pretreatment complement protein levels are predictive of esophageal cancer patient response to neoadjuvant chemoradiation. *Ann. Surg.* **2011**, *254*, 809–816. [CrossRef] [PubMed]
14. Cui, L.; Fu, J.; Pang, J.C.-S.; Qiu, Z.-K.; Liu, X.-M.; Chen, F.-R.; Shi, H.-L.; Ng, H.-K.; Chen, Z.-P. Overexpression of IL-7 enhances cisplatin resistance in glioma. *Cancer Biol. Therapy* **2012**, *13*, 496–503. [CrossRef] [PubMed]
15. Andrejeva, G.; Rathmell, J.C. Similarities and Distinctions of Cancer and Immune Metabolism in Inflammation and Tumors. *Cell Metabol.* **2017**, *26*, 49–70. [CrossRef] [PubMed]
16. Hanahan, D.; Weinberg, R.A. Hallmarks of cancer: The next generation. *Cell* **2011**, *144*, 646–674. [CrossRef] [PubMed]
17. Lynam-Lennon, N.; Maher, S.G.; Maguire, A.; Phelan, J.; Muldoon, C.; Reynolds, J.V.; O'Sullivan, J. Altered Mitochondrial Function and Energy Metabolism Is Associated with a Radioresistant Phenotype in Oesophageal Adenocarcinoma. *PLoS ONE* **2014**, *9*, e100738. [CrossRef] [PubMed]
18. Lynam-Lennon, N.; Reynolds, J.V.; Pidgeon, G.P.; Lysaght, J.; Marignol, L.; Maher, S.G. Alterations in DNA repair efficiency are involved in the radioresistance of esophageal adenocarcinoma. *Radiat. Res.* **2010**, *174*, 703–711. [CrossRef]
19. Wangpaichitr, M.; Theodoropoulos, G.; Wu, C.; You, M.; Feun, L.; Kuo, M.T.; Savaraj, N. The Relationship of Thioredoxin-1 and Cisplatin Resistance: Its Impact on ROS and Oxidative Metabolism in Lung Cancer Cells. *Mol. Cancer Ther.* **2012**. [CrossRef]
20. Lynam-Lennon, N.; Heavey, S.; Sommerville, G.; Bibby, B.A.S.; Ffrench, B.; Quinn, J.; Gasch, C.; O'Leary, J.J.; Gallagher, M.F.; Reynolds, J.V.; et al. MicroRNA-17 is downregulated in esophageal adenocarcinoma cancer stem-like cells and promotes a radioresistant phenotype. *Oncotarget* **2017**, *8*, 11400–11413. [CrossRef]
21. Buckley, A.M.; Lynam-Lennon, N.; Kennedy, S.A.; Dunne, M.R.; Aird, J.J.; Foley, E.K.; Clarke, N.; Ravi, N.; O'Toole, D.; Reynolds, J.V.; et al. Leukaemia inhibitory factor is associated with treatment resistance in oesophageal adenocarcinoma. *Oncotarget* **2018**, *9*, 33634–33647. [CrossRef] [PubMed]
22. Stordal, B.; Davey, M. Understanding cisplatin resistance using cellular models. *IUBMB Life* **2007**, *59*, 696–699. [CrossRef] [PubMed]
23. Hummel, R.; Sie, C.; Watson, D.I.; Wang, T.; Ansar, A.; Michael, M.Z.; Van der Hoek, M.; Haier, J.; Hussey, D.J. MicroRNA signatures in chemotherapy resistant esophageal cancer cell lines. *World J. Gastroenterol. WJG* **2014**, *20*, 14904–14912. [CrossRef] [PubMed]
24. Xie, X.-Q.; Zhao, Q.-H.; Wang, H.; Gu, K.-S. Dysregulation of mRNA profile in cisplatin-resistant gastric cancer cell line SGC7901. *World J. Gastroenterol.* **2017**, *23*, 1189–1202. [CrossRef]
25. Shen, D.W.; Pouliot, L.M.; Hall, M.D.; Gottesman, M.M. Cisplatin resistance: A cellular self-defense mechanism resulting from multiple epigenetic and genetic changes. *Pharmacol. Rev.* **2012**, *64*, 706–721. [CrossRef] [PubMed]
26. Adelstein, D.J.; Li, Y.; Adams, G.L.; Wagner, H., Jr.; Kish, J.A.; Ensley, J.F.; Schuller, D.E.; Forastiere, A.A. An Intergroup Phase III Comparison of Standard Radiation Therapy and Two Schedules of Concurrent Chemoradiotherapy in Patients With Unresectable Squamous Cell Head and Neck Cancer. *J. Clin. Oncol.* **2003**, *21*, 92–98. [CrossRef]
27. Keys, H.M.; Bundy, B.N.; Stehman, F.B.; Muderspach, L.I.; Chafe, W.E.; Suggs, C.L.; Walker, J.L.; Gersell, D. Cisplatin, Radiation, and Adjuvant Hysterectomy Compared with Radiation and Adjuvant Hysterectomy for Bulky Stage IB Cervical Carcinoma. *N. Engl. J. Med.* **1999**, *340*, 1154–1161. [CrossRef]
28. Tu, L.; Sun, L.; Xu, Y.; Wang, Y.; Zhou, L.; Liu, Y.; Zhu, J.; Peng, F.; Wei, Y.; Gong, Y. Paclitaxel and cisplatin combined with intensity-modulated radiotherapy for upper esophageal carcinoma. *Radiat. Oncol.* **2013**, *8*, 75. [CrossRef]
29. Ilson, D.H.; Minsky, B.; Kelsen, D. Irinotecan, cisplatin, and radiation in esophageal cancer. *Oncology* **2002**, *16*, 11–15.
30. Myint, W.K.; Ng, C.; Raaphorst, G.P. Examining the non-homologous repair process following cisplatin and radiation treatments. *Int. J. Radiat. Biol.* **2002**, *78*, 417–424. [CrossRef]

31. Boeckman, H.J.; Trego, K.S.; Henkels, K.M.; Turchi, J.J. Cisplatin sensitizes cancer cells to ionizing radiation via inhibition of non-homologous end joining. *Mol. Cancer Res. MCR* **2005**, *3*, 277–285. [CrossRef] [PubMed]
32. Eljack, N.D.; Ma, H.Y.; Drucker, J.; Shen, C.; Hambley, T.W.; New, E.J.; Friedrich, T.; Clarke, R.J. Mechanisms of cell uptake and toxicity of the anticancer drug cisplatin. *Metall. Integr. Biomet. Sci.* **2014**, *6*, 2126–2133. [CrossRef] [PubMed]
33. Kilari, D.; Guancial, E.; Kim, E.S. Role of copper transporters in platinum resistance. *World J. Clin. Oncol.* **2016**, *7*, 106–113. [CrossRef]
34. Baskar, R.; Dai, J.; Wenlong, N.; Yeo, R.; Yeoh, K.-W. Biological response of cancer cells to radiation treatment. *Front. Mol. Biosci.* **2014**, *1*, 24. [CrossRef] [PubMed]
35. Hummel, R.; Watson, D.I.; Smith, C.; Kist, J.; Michael, M.Z.; Haier, J.; Hussey, D.J. Mir-148a improves response to chemotherapy in sensitive and resistant oesophageal adenocarcinoma and squamous cell carcinoma cells. *J. Gastrointest. Surg. Off. J. Soc. Surg. Aliment. Tract.* **2011**, *15*, 429–438. [CrossRef] [PubMed]
36. Singh, A.; Settleman, J. EMT, cancer stem cells and drug resistance: An emerging axis of evil in the war on cancer. *Oncogene* **2010**, *29*, 4741–4751. [CrossRef]
37. Piskareva, O.; Harvey, H.; Nolan, J.; Conlon, R.; Alcock, L.; Buckley, P.; Dowling, P.; O'Sullivan, F.; Bray, I.; Stallings, R.L. The development of cisplatin resistance in neuroblastoma is accompanied by epithelial to mesenchymal transition in vitro. *Cancer Lett.* **2015**, *364*, 142–155. [CrossRef] [PubMed]
38. Katoh, M. Networking of WNT, FGF, Notch, BMP, and Hedgehog signaling pathways during carcinogenesis. *Stem Cell Rev.* **2007**, *3*, 30–38. [CrossRef] [PubMed]
39. Matsuoka, S.; Edwards, M.C.; Bai, C.; Parker, S.; Zhang, P.; Baldini, A.; Harper, J.W.; Elledge, S.J. p57KIP2, a structurally distinct member of the p21CIP1 Cdk inhibitor family, is a candidate tumor suppressor gene. *Genes Dev.* **1995**, *9*, 650–662. [CrossRef]
40. Vlachos, P.; Nyman, U.; Hajji, N.; Joseph, B. The cell cycle inhibitor p57(Kip2) promotes cell death via the mitochondrial apoptotic pathway. *Cell Death Differ.* **2007**, *14*, 1497–1507. [CrossRef]
41. Oshimori, N.; Oristian, D.; Fuchs, E. TGF-β Promotes Heterogeneity and Drug Resistance in Squamous Cell Carcinoma. *Cell* **2015**, *160*, 963–976. [CrossRef] [PubMed]
42. Bissey, P.-A.; Law, J.H.; Bruce, J.P.; Shi, W.; Renoult, A.; Chua, M.L.K.; Yip, K.W.; Liu, F.-F. Dysregulation of the MiR-449b target TGFBI alters the TGFβ pathway to induce cisplatin resistance in nasopharyngeal carcinoma. *Oncogenesis* **2018**, *7*, 40. [CrossRef]
43. Di Paolo, N.C.; Shayakhmetov, D.M. Interleukin 1α and the inflammatory process. *Nat. Immunol.* **2016**, *17*, 906. [CrossRef]
44. Benchekroun, M.N.; Parker, R.; Dabholkar, M.; Reed, E.; Sinha, B.K. Effects of interleukin-1 alpha on DNA repair in human ovarian carcinoma (NIH:OVCAR-3) cells: Implications in the mechanism of sensitization of cis-diamminedichloroplatinum(II). *Mol. Pharmacol.* **1995**, *47*, 1255–1260. [PubMed]
45. Webb, D.S.; Mostowski, H.S.; Gerrard, T.L. Cytokine-induced enhancement of ICAM-1 expression results in increased vulnerability of tumor cells to monocyte-mediated lysis. *J. Immunol.* **1991**, *146*, 3682–3686.
46. Jonjic, N.; Alberti, S.; Bernasconi, S.; Peri, G.; Jilek, P.; Anichini, A.; Parmiani, G.; Mantovani, A. Heterogeneous susceptibility of human melanoma clones to monocyte cytotoxicity: Role of ICAM-1 defined by antibody blocking and gene transfer. *Eur. J. Immunol.* **1992**, *22*, 2255–2260. [CrossRef] [PubMed]
47. Guo, P.; Huang, J.; Wang, L.; Jia, D.; Yang, J.; Dillon, D.A.; Zurakowski, D.; Mao, H.; Moses, M.A.; Auguste, D.T. ICAM-1 as a molecular target for triple negative breast cancer. *Proc. Natl. Acad. Sci. USA* **2014**, *111*, 14710–14715. [CrossRef]
48. Takizawa, K.; Kamijo, R.; Ito, D.; Hatori, M.; Sumitani, K.; Nagumo, M. Synergistic induction of ICAM-1 expression by cisplatin and 5-fluorouracil in a cancer cell line via a NF-κB independent pathway. *Br. J. Cancer* **1999**, *80*, 954. [CrossRef]
49. Tsai, S.T.; Wang, P.J.; Liou, N.J.; Lin, P.S.; Chen, C.H.; Chang, W.C. ICAM1 Is a Potential Cancer Stem Cell Marker of Esophageal Squamous Cell Carcinoma. *PLoS ONE* **2015**, *10*, e0142834. [CrossRef]
50. Xu, Y.; Gao, W.; Zhang, Y.; Wu, S.; Liu, Y.; Deng, X.; Xie, L.; Yang, J.; Yu, H.; Su, J.; et al. ABT737 reverses cisplatin resistance by targeting glucose metabolism of human ovarian cancer cells. *Int. J. Oncol.* **2018**, *53*, 1055–1068. [CrossRef]
51. Catanzaro, D.; Gaude, E.; Orso, G.; Giordano, C.; Guzzo, G.; Rasola, A.; Ragazzi, E.; Caparrotta, L.; Frezza, C.; Montopoli, M. Inhibition of glucose-6-phosphate dehydrogenase sensitizes cisplatin-resistant cells to death. *Oncotarget* **2015**, *6*, 30102–30114. [CrossRef] [PubMed]

52. Ippolito, L.; Marini, A.; Cavallini, L.; Morandi, A.; Pietrovito, L.; Pintus, G.; Giannoni, E.; Schrader, T.; Puhr, M.; Chiarugi, P.; et al. Metabolic shift toward oxidative phosphorylation in docetaxel resistant prostate cancer cells. *Oncotarget* **2016**, *7*, 61890–61904. [CrossRef]
53. Zhao, F.Q.; Keating, A.F. Functional properties and genomics of glucose transporters. *Curr. Genomics* **2007**, *8*, 113–128. [CrossRef] [PubMed]
54. Guo, Q.; Lan, F.; Yan, X.; Xiao, Z.; Wu, Y.; Zhang, Q. Hypoxia exposure induced cisplatin resistance partially via activating p53 and hypoxia inducible factor-1alpha in non-small cell lung cancer A549 cells. *Oncol. Lett.* **2018**, *16*, 801–808. [PubMed]
55. Wu, H.M.; Jiang, Z.F.; Ding, P.S.; Shao, L.J.; Liu, R.Y. Hypoxia-induced autophagy mediates cisplatin resistance in lung cancer cells. *Sci. Rep.* **2015**, *5*, 12291. [CrossRef] [PubMed]
56. Kolde, R. Pheatmap: Pretty Heatmaps. R Package Version 1.0.10. 2018. Available online: https://CRAN.R-project.org/package=pheatmap (accessed on 4 January 2019).
57. Team, R.C. *R: A Language and Environment for Statistical Computing*; R Foundation for Statistical Computing: Vienna, Austria, 2018.

8

Unveiling the Differential Antioxidant Activity of Maslinic Acid in Murine Melanoma Cells and in Rat Embryonic Healthy Cells Following Treatment with Hydrogen Peroxide

Khalida Mokhtari [1,2], Amalia Pérez-Jiménez [3], Leticia García-Salguero [1], José A. Lupiáñez [1] and Eva E. Rufino-Palomares [1,*]

1. Department of Biochemistry and Molecular Biology I, Faculty of Sciences, University of Granada, Avenida Fuentenueva, s/n, 18071 Granada, Spain; khalidafadoua@hotmail.com (K.M.); elgarcia@ugr.es (L.G.-S.); jlcara@ugr.es (J.A.L.)
2. Laboratory of Bioresources, Biotechnologies, Ethnopharmacology and Health, Department of Biology, Faculty of Sciences, Mohammed I University of Oujda, Oujda 60000, Morocco
3. Department of Zoology, Faculty of Sciences, University of Granada, Avenida Fuentenueva, s/n, 18071 Granada, Spain; calaya@ugr.es

* Correspondence: evaevae@ugr.es;

Academic Editor: Domenico Trombetta

Abstract: Maslinic acid (MA) is a natural triterpene from *Olea europaea* L. with multiple biological properties. The aim of the present study was to examine MA's effect on cell viability (by the MTT assay), reactive oxygen species (ROS levels, by flow cytometry) and key antioxidant enzyme activities (by spectrophotometry) in murine skin melanoma (B16F10) cells compared to those on healthy cells (A10). MA induced cytotoxic effects in cancer cells (IC_{50} 42 μM), whereas no effect was found in A10 cells treated with MA (up to 210 μM). In order to produce a stress situation in cells, 0.15 mM H_2O_2 was added. Under stressful conditions, MA protected both cell lines against oxidative damage, decreasing intracellular ROS, which were higher in B16F10 than in A10 cells. The treatment with H_2O_2 and without MA produced different responses in antioxidant enzyme activities depending on the cell line. In A10 cells, all the enzymes were up-regulated, but in B16F10 cells, only superoxide dismutase, glutathione S-transferase and glutathione peroxidase increased their activities. MA restored the enzyme activities to levels similar to those in the control group in both cell lines, highlighting that in A10 cells, the highest MA doses induced values lower than control. Overall, these findings demonstrate the great antioxidant capacity of MA.

Keywords: antioxidant activity; antioxidant enzymes; anti-proliferative activity; maslinic acid; melanoma; *Olea europaea* L.; ROS levels

---

1. Introduction

An imbalance between pro-oxidant and antioxidant molecules can lead to an oxidative stress situation that modifies normal cell physiology due to protein, lipid, carbohydrate and nucleic acid damage [1]. Many cellular processes depend on the variations in the levels of ROS and NADPH that take place during their development and that, fundamentally, are determined by the activity of the different production systems for this reduced coenzyme, especially those belonging to the pentose phosphate pathway (PPP), glucose-6-phosphate dehydrogenase (G6PDH), 6-phosphogluconate dehydrogenase (6PGDH) and, also, NADP-dependent isocitrate dehydrogenase (ICDH-NADP). The cellular redox state is key to interpreting the behavior of most of these key cellular processes for the vital development of organisms, such as cell differentiation [2–4], cellular growth [5–8], cell nutrition [6,9–11] and cell aging [12].

Reactive oxygen species (ROS) and reactive nitrogen species (RNS) are the most important endogenous pro-oxidants produced by normal cellular metabolism [13]. Under a normal physiological situation, an antioxidant defense system neutralizes ROS. This antioxidant system involves enzymes such as catalase (CAT), which reduces hydrogen peroxide; superoxide dismutase (SOD), which detoxifies the superoxide radical; glutathione peroxidase (GPX), which reduces hydrogen peroxide and other organic peroxides; S-transferase glutathione (GST), which detoxifies harmful molecules; glutathione reductase (GR), which regenerates glutathione (GSH) from its oxidized form (GSSG) by an NADPH-dependent pathway; and G6PDH, which produces NADPH for GR's mechanism. Beside enzymes, other molecules can also act as antioxidants, such as NADPH, GSH and different vitamins, among other molecules [14–16]. Despite this antioxidant system, an excessive production of ROS can lead to an oxidative stress situation inducing several types of damage to different biomolecules [17]. In cancer processes, an excessive production of ROS has been related to genomic instability due to the induction of DNA damage and to the alterations in signaling pathways involved in survival, proliferation and apoptosis resistance. Moreover, it has been demonstrated that ROS induce vascular endothelial growth factor (VEGF) expression, producing neovascularization and fast expansion of the cancer, modifying angiogenesis and metastasis, which induce the malignancy of cancer cells [17]. The use of natural compounds with antioxidant capacity that reduce ROS levels could decrease metastatic progression [15,17]. Furthermore, the immune defense system can be altered by ROS, since high levels of these molecules produced by NADPH oxidase can inhibit monocytes and macrophages and weaken the response of T-cells due to the down-regulation of several cytokines [17].

Hydrogen peroxide (H_2O_2) is originated from O_2 by SOD. It is not a free radical as such, but it is a reactive molecule, since it has the capacity to generate the hydroxyl radical in the presence of metals such as iron [1]. H_2O_2 is an important metabolite that arises mainly during aerobic metabolism, although it can derive from other sources [18]. H_2O_2 is a messenger molecule that diffuses through cells and tissues, inducing different effects that include deformations of the shapes of cells, the initiation of proliferation and the recruitment of immune cells. If not controlled, an excess of H_2O_2 can cause uncontrolled oxidative stress in cells, producing irreparable damage [19]. Therefore, cell death and survival processes can be modulated by controlling intracellular H_2O_2 levels by the use of antioxidants. Natural products are gaining interest due to their cost-effectiveness, few side effects and high availability. As such, products such as maslinic acid (MA) have received heightened interest.

MA, $C_{30}H_{48}O_4$ (2α,3β-dihydroxyolean-12-en-28-oic acid) is a natural pentacyclic triterpene, also known as crataegolic acid and derived from its structural analogue, oleanolic acid (Figure 1). It is formed by 30 carbon atoms grouped into five cycles that, as substituents, have two methyl groups each on the C-4 and C-21 carbons; single methyl groups on the C-8, C-10 and C-15 carbons; two hydroxyl groups each on the C-2 and C-3 carbons; one carboxyl group on the C-28 carbon; and a double bond on the C-12 and C-13 [20–23].

Maslinic acid is present in various plants, many of them common in the Mediterranean diet, such as eggplants, spinach, lentils, chickpeas, and even different aromatic herbs [24]. Moreover, it is especially abundant in *Crataegus oxyacantha*, in the surface wax of the fruits and leaves of *Olea europaea* L. and in the solid waste from olive oil extraction [25]. Furthermore, MA is among the main triterpenes present in olives and olive oil. Its concentration in the oil depends on the type of olive oil and the variety of olive tree [23].

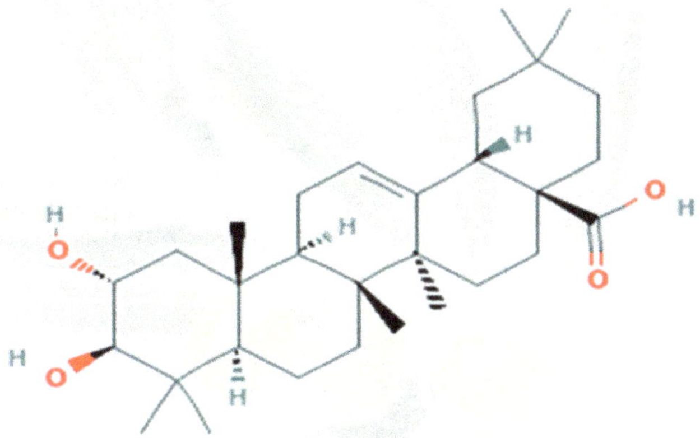

Figure 1. Schedule chemical structure of maslinic acid from pomace olive (*Olea europaea* L.) (PubChem).

MA enjoys high pharmacological interest, owing to its anti-tumor effect in certain types of cancer besides its anti-inflammatory, antioxidant, anti-diabetogenic, anti-hypertensive, anti-viral and cardioprotective effects, among others [1,23]. Among the bioactivities attributed to MA, its antioxidant effect is the most contradictory. It has been observed that the oxidative status induced by CCl_4 was decreased by MA treatment, which reduced lipid peroxides in the plasma and the susceptibility of lipids to peroxidation [26]. In the same way, the LDL oxidation in the plasma of rabbits produced by $CuSO^{4-}$ was decreased by MA obtained from *Punica granatum* [27]. In human plasma, MA showed peroxyl-radical scavenging and chelating capacities for copper but did not show a positive effect for the prevention of LDL oxidation [28]. Research in macrophages revealed that MA can act in a similar way to catalase, decreasing the generation of H_2O_2, but does not produce any direct inhibitory effects on NO and superoxide formation [29]. In a previous study, we concluded that MA produced an increase in the ROS level under stress conditions caused by the absence of FBS in melanoma cells [15]. Furthermore, in this same study, MA had an antioxidant effect at lower assayed levels; however, at higher dosages, MA induced cellular damage by apoptosis.

The aim of the present study was to evaluate MA's antioxidant effects in murine skin melanoma (B16F10) cells and in a healthy cell line derived from the thoracic aorta of an embryonic rat (A10), by analyzing the proliferation, ROS production and the activity of the main antioxidant enzymes under cellular stress conditions induced by H_2O_2.

2. Results

2.1. MA Decreases Proliferation of B16F10 Cells by a Dose-Dependent Mechanism

We evaluated MA's effect on B16F10 melanoma and A10 cell line proliferation using the MTT assay (Figure 2A,B). B16F10 and A10 cells were exposed to different doses of MA (0 to 212 μM) for 24 h. Then, cell survival was compared with that of untreated control cells. The percentage of living cells decreased as the dose of MA increased in cancer cells (B16F10), while in healthy cells (A10), MA did not produce any cytotoxic effect, even at the highest doses used (210 μM). In B16F10 cells, the growth inhibition values (IC_{50}) in response to MA were 42 μM after 24 h of addition of this compound. Based on this value, the rest of studies were performed with an exposure of cells to 10.6 μM ($IC_{50/4}$), 21.2 μM ($IC_{50/2}$), 42.3 μM (IC_{50}) and 84.6 μM ($2{\cdot}IC_{50}$) of MA for 24 h.

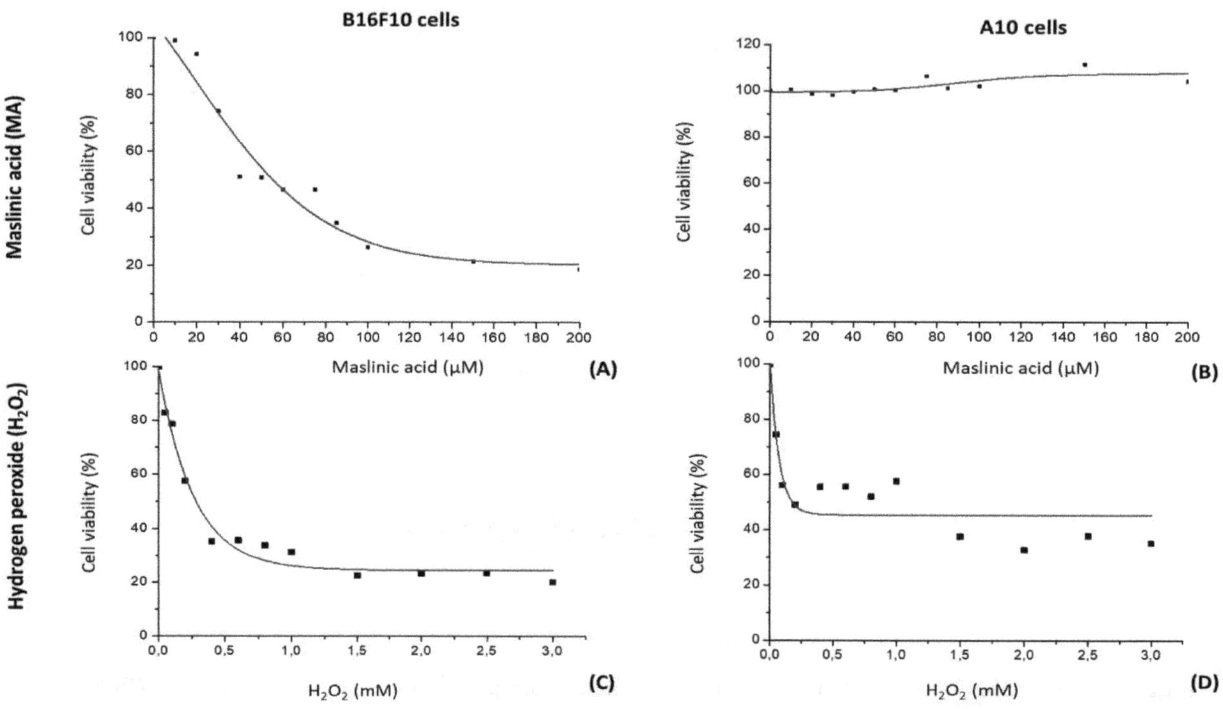

Figure 2. Cytotoxicity curves of maslinic acid (MA) for B16F10 murine melanoma cells (**A**) and A10 rat embryonic healthy cells (**B**) and of hydrogen peroxide (H_2O_2) for B16F10 murine melanoma cells (**C**) and A10 rat embryonic healthy cells (**D**). Cell proliferation was determined by the MTT assay. Values are expressed as means ± SEM ($n = 9$).

2.2. H_2O_2 Modifies Cell Viability

We examined H_2O_2's effects (0 to 3 mM of H_2O_2 for 24 h) on the cell viability of B16F10 and A10 cells to determine the optimal dose capable of producing stress without inducing cell death (Figure 2C,D). Cell survival was compared with that of untreated controls. The percentage of living cells decreased as the dose of H_2O_2 increased in both cell lines up to the concentration of 1.5 mM, beyoond which H_2O_2 had no cell viability effect. In both cell lines, we noticed an IC_{50} of 0.2 mM. In no case, with the doses used and the incubation time employed, was any mortality higher than 80% reached. Based on these results, the concentration of 0.15 mM of H_2O_2 was used to perform the rest of the studies.

2.3. Maslinic Acid's Influence on Mitochondrial-Membrane Potential

An assay of ROS production was performed to test the ROS levels that occurred over time in the presence of 0.150 mM H_2O_2 and different MA levels ($IC_{50/4}$, $IC_{50/2}$, IC_{50} and $2{\cdot}IC_{50}$). The results are shown in Figure 3. After 24 h of H_2O_2 treatment, ROS levels increased significantly in both cell lines, compared to those in the controls. The increment observed upon H_2O_2 addition was offset by MA supplementation, which resulted in decreased intracellular ROS levels at any MA level used ($IC_{50/4}$, $IC_{50/2}$, IC_{50} and $2{\cdot}IC_{50}$) in B16F10 and A10 cells. Moreover, in A10, ROS levels decreased below the value of control cells for all concentrations of MA tested.

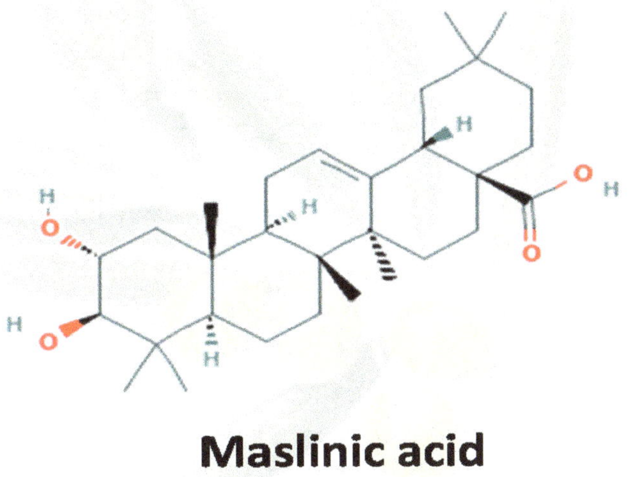

Figure 1. Schedule chemical structure of maslinic acid from pomace olive (*Olea europaea* L.) (PubChem).

MA enjoys high pharmacological interest, owing to its anti-tumor effect in certain types of cancer besides its anti-inflammatory, antioxidant, anti-diabetogenic, anti-hypertensive, anti-viral and cardioprotective effects, among others [1,23]. Among the bioactivities attributed to MA, its antioxidant effect is the most contradictory. It has been observed that the oxidative status induced by CCl_4 was decreased by MA treatment, which reduced lipid peroxides in the plasma and the susceptibility of lipids to peroxidation [26]. In the same way, the LDL oxidation in the plasma of rabbits produced by $CuSO^{4-}$ was decreased by MA obtained from *Punica granatum* [27]. In human plasma, MA showed peroxyl-radical scavenging and chelating capacities for copper but did not show a positive effect for the prevention of LDL oxidation [28]. Research in macrophages revealed that MA can act in a similar way to catalase, decreasing the generation of H_2O_2, but does not produce any direct inhibitory effects on NO and superoxide formation [29]. In a previous study, we concluded that MA produced an increase in the ROS level under stress conditions caused by the absence of FBS in melanoma cells [15]. Furthermore, in this same study, MA had an antioxidant effect at lower assayed levels; however, at higher dosages, MA induced cellular damage by apoptosis.

The aim of the present study was to evaluate MA's antioxidant effects in murine skin melanoma (B16F10) cells and in a healthy cell line derived from the thoracic aorta of an embryonic rat (A10), by analyzing the proliferation, ROS production and the activity of the main antioxidant enzymes under cellular stress conditions induced by H_2O_2.

2. Results

2.1. MA Decreases Proliferation of B16F10 Cells by a Dose-Dependent Mechanism

We evaluated MA's effect on B16F10 melanoma and A10 cell line proliferation using the MTT assay (Figure 2A,B). B16F10 and A10 cells were exposed to different doses of MA (0 to 212 μM) for 24 h. Then, cell survival was compared with that of untreated control cells. The percentage of living cells decreased as the dose of MA increased in cancer cells (B16F10), while in healthy cells (A10), MA did not produce any cytotoxic effect, even at the highest doses used (210 μM). In B16F10 cells, the growth inhibition values (IC_{50}) in response to MA were 42 μM after 24 h of addition of this compound. Based on this value, the rest of studies were performed with an exposure of cells to 10.6 μM ($IC_{50/4}$), 21.2 μM ($IC_{50/2}$), 42.3 μM (IC_{50}) and 84.6 μM ($2{\cdot}IC_{50}$) of MA for 24 h.

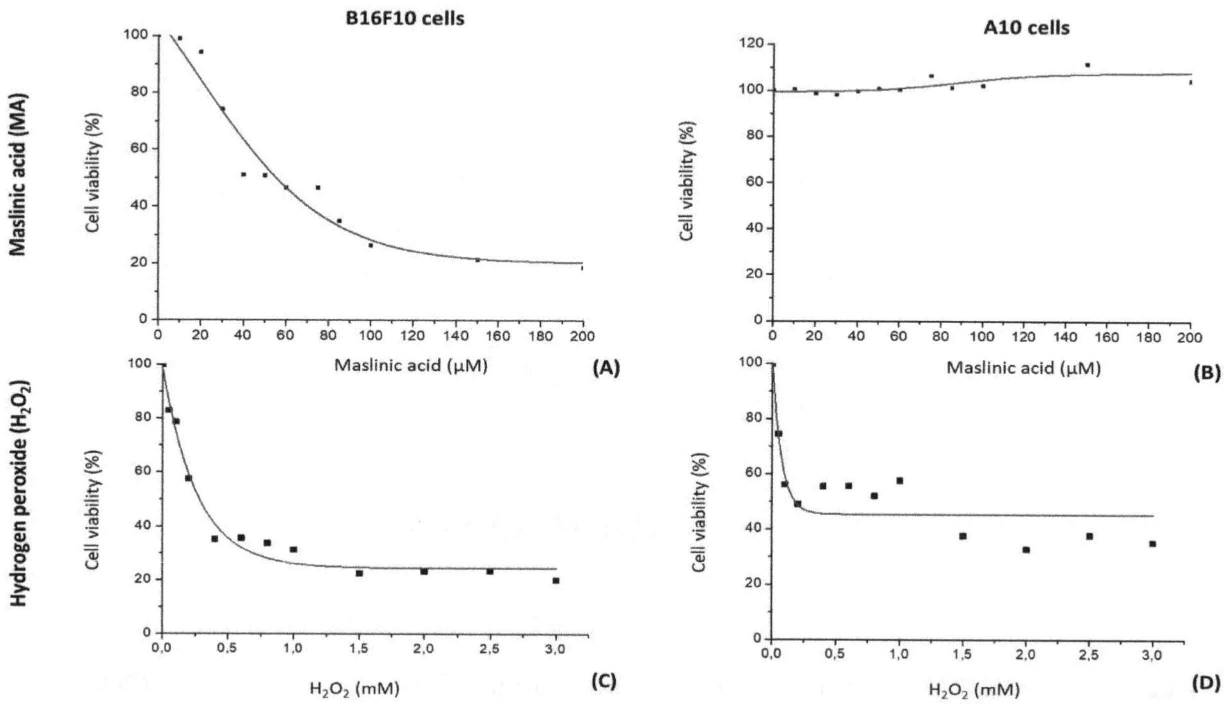

Figure 2. Cytotoxicity curves of maslinic acid (MA) for B16F10 murine melanoma cells (**A**) and A10 rat embryonic healthy cells (**B**) and of hydrogen peroxide (H_2O_2) for B16F10 murine melanoma cells (**C**) and A10 rat embryonic healthy cells (**D**). Cell proliferation was determined by the MTT assay. Values are expressed as means ± SEM ($n = 9$).

2.2. H_2O_2 *Modifies Cell Viability*

We examined H_2O_2's effects (0 to 3 mM of H_2O_2 for 24 h) on the cell viability of B16F10 and A10 cells to determine the optimal dose capable of producing stress without inducing cell death (Figure 2C,D). Cell survival was compared with that of untreated controls. The percentage of living cells decreased as the dose of H_2O_2 increased in both cell lines up to the concentration of 1.5 mM, beyoond which H_2O_2 had no cell viability effect. In both cell lines, we noticed an IC_{50} of 0.2 mM. In no case, with the doses used and the incubation time employed, was any mortality higher than 80% reached. Based on these results, the concentration of 0.15 mM of H_2O_2 was used to perform the rest of the studies.

2.3. *Maslinic Acid's Influence on Mitochondrial-Membrane Potential*

An assay of ROS production was performed to test the ROS levels that occurred over time in the presence of 0.150 mM H_2O_2 and different MA levels ($IC_{50/4}$, $IC_{50/2}$, IC_{50} and $2{\cdot}IC_{50}$). The results are shown in Figure 3. After 24 h of H_2O_2 treatment, ROS levels increased significantly in both cell lines, compared to those in the controls. The increment observed upon H_2O_2 addition was offset by MA supplementation, which resulted in decreased intracellular ROS levels at any MA level used ($IC_{50/4}$, $IC_{50/2}$, IC_{50} and $2{\cdot}IC_{50}$) in B16F10 and A10 cells. Moreover, in A10, ROS levels decreased below the value of control cells for all concentrations of MA tested.

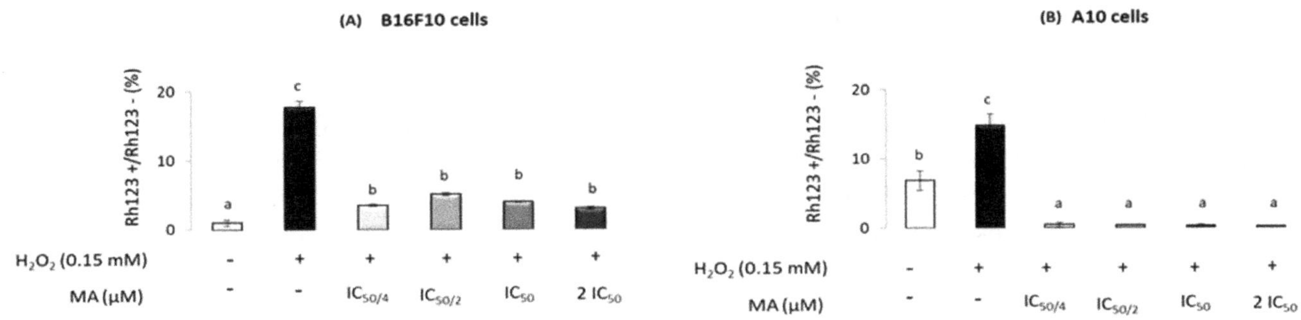

Figure 3. Positive fluorescent Rh123 on B16F10 cells (**A**) and A10 cells (**B**) with (+) or without (−) H_2O_2 and MA treatment at different doses: $IC_{50/4}$, $IC_{50/2}$, IC_{50} and $2{\cdot}IC_{50}$ (10.6, 21.6, 42.3 and 84.6 μM, respectively). Values are expressed as means ± SEM ($n = 9$). Different letters indicate significant differences ($p < 0.05$).

2.4. MA Exerts Antioxidant Activity, Modulating Enzymatic Defense System

The results obtained for SOD in B16F10 cells showed that H_2O_2 increased its activity and MA (at any level) decreased it, but without significant differences induced by different MA concentrations. In A10, H_2O_2 increased the SOD activity, an increment that was mitigated with MA addition. Moreover, 42.3 and 84.6 μM MA (IC_{50} and $2{\cdot}IC_{50}$, respectively) resulted in SOD activity levels lower than those found in the absence of H_2O_2 and MA (Figure 4A,B).

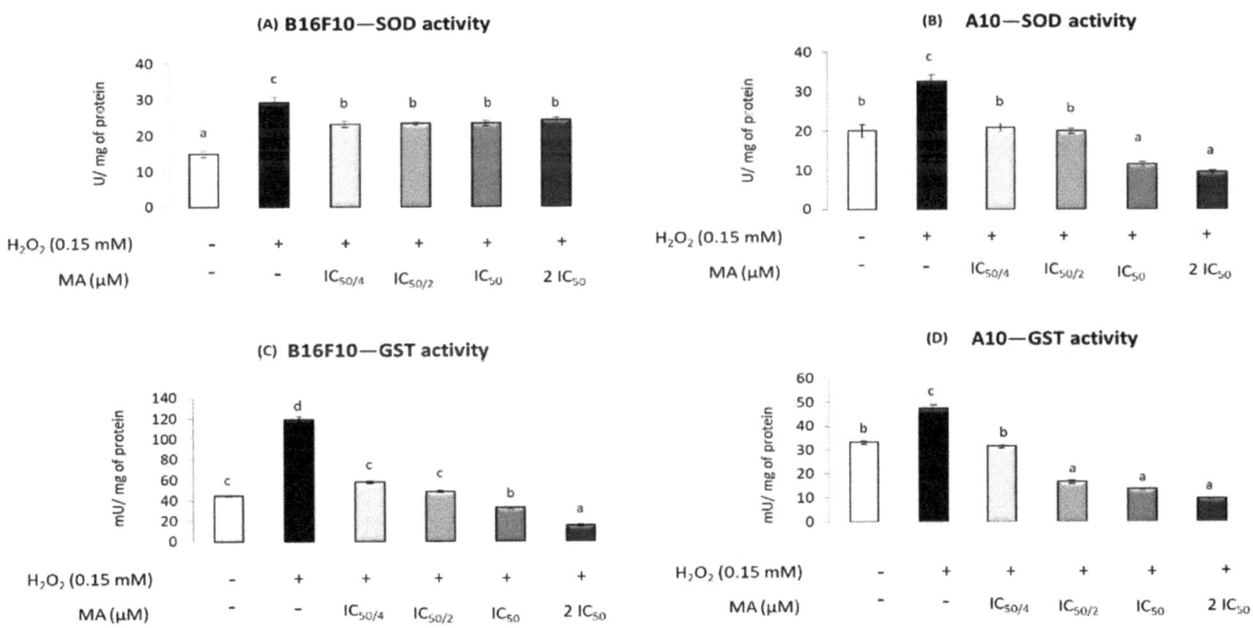

Figure 4. Effect of different maslinic acid doses—$IC_{50/4}$, $IC_{50/2}$, IC_{50} and $2{\cdot}IC_{50}$ (10.6, 21.6, 42.3 and 84.6 μM, respectively)—on the specific activity of superoxide dismutase (SOD) in cancer cells, B16F10 (**A**), and normal cells, A10 (**B**), and glutathione S-transferase (GST) in cancer cells, B16F10 (**C**), and normal cells, A10 (**D**), subjected to the presence of hydrogen peroxide. Symbols (+) and (−) indicate the presence or absence of incubation with H_2O_2, respectively. Enzyme activities (U or mU × mg $protein^{-1}$) are expressed as means ± SEM ($n = 9$). Different letters indicate significant differences ($p < 0.05$).

In B16F10 cells, GST activity increased in the presence of H_2O_2, whereas the incubation with the $IC_{50/4}$ and $IC_{50/2}$ of MA decreased the levels, making them equal to those in the control without H_2O_2 and MA. The use of the IC_{50} and $2{\cdot}IC_{50}$ MA concentrations induced GST activities lower than those in the control. Similar results were found in A10 for GST activity, with the exception of MA at $IC_{50/2}$, which also induced lower levels than control (Figure 4C,D).

In B16F10 cells, CAT activity decreased in the presence of H_2O_2 compared to that in the control, whereas MA increased the activity, inducing values higher than or similar to control when $IC_{50/4}$ or $IC_{50/2}$ were used. In A10 cells, H_2O_2 produced an increase in CAT activity, and its activity was not recovered until the highest doses of MA were used (IC_{50} and $2{\cdot}IC_{50}$) (Figure 5A,B).

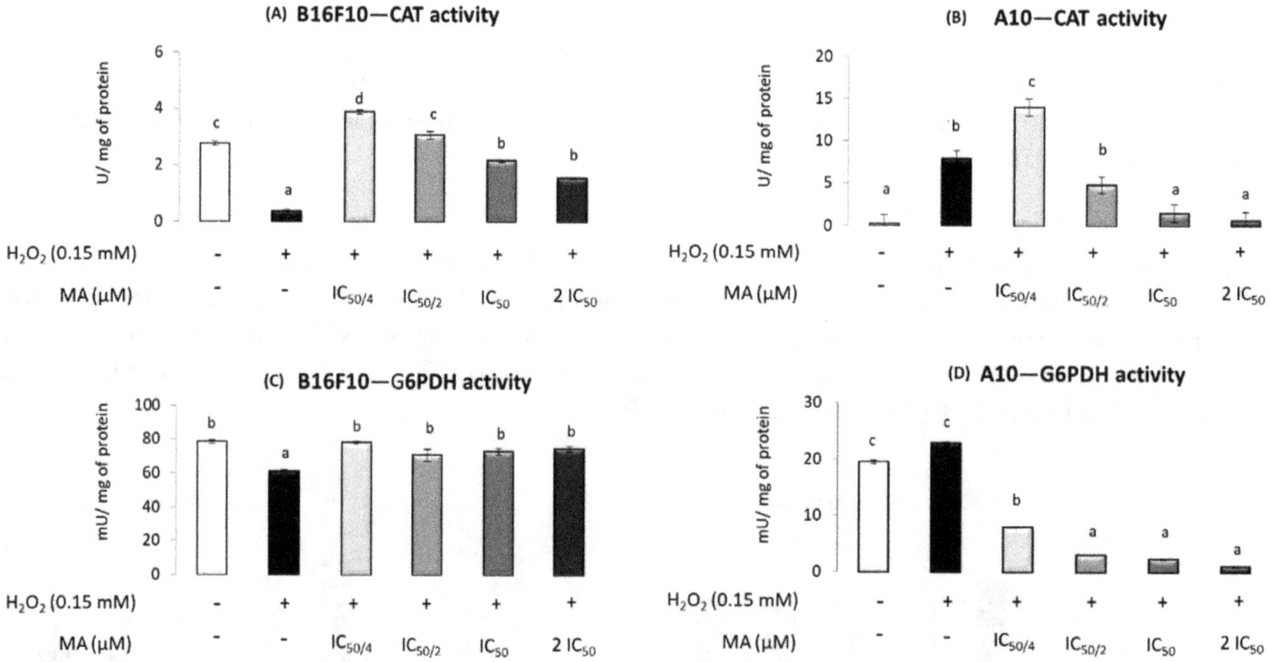

Figure 5. Effect of different maslinic acid doses—$IC_{50/4}$, $IC_{50/2}$, IC_{50} and 2 IC_{50} (10.6, 21.6, 42.3 and 84.6 μM, respectively)—on the specific activity of catalase (CAT) in cancer cells, B16F10 (**A**), and normal cells, A10 (**B**), and glucose 6-phosphate dehydrogenase (G6PDH) in cancer cells, B16F10 (**C**), and normal cells, A10 (**D**), subjected to the presence of hydrogen peroxide. Symbols (+) and (−) indicate the presence or absence of incubation with H_2O_2, respectively. Enzyme activities (U or mU × mg protein^{-1}) are expressed as means ± SEM (n = 9). Different letters indicate significant differences ($p < 0.05$).

Regarding G6PDH, the results indicated its activity decreased in the presence of H_2O_2 in B16F10 and MA at all the concentrations tested, with similar values to the control without H_2O_2 and MA. In A10 cells, no changes were induced by H_2O_2 in G6PDH, whereas MA decreased its activity at any tested level (Figure 5C,D).

GPX increased in the presence of H_2O_2 but no change was observed when MA was administrated in B16F10. In A10 cells, all concentrations of MA decreased the GPX activity increased by the H_2O_2, even below that in the control without H_2O_2 and MA (Figure 6A,B).

In B16F10, GR activity was decreased by H_2O_2 and no changes were observed at any MA level, with lower levels of activity maintained compared to the control. In A10, H_2O_2 increased GR activity, an increment that was mitigated with MA addition. Moreover, 42.3 and 84.6 μM MA induced values of GR activity lower than those found in the absence of H_2O_2 and MA (Figure 6C,D).

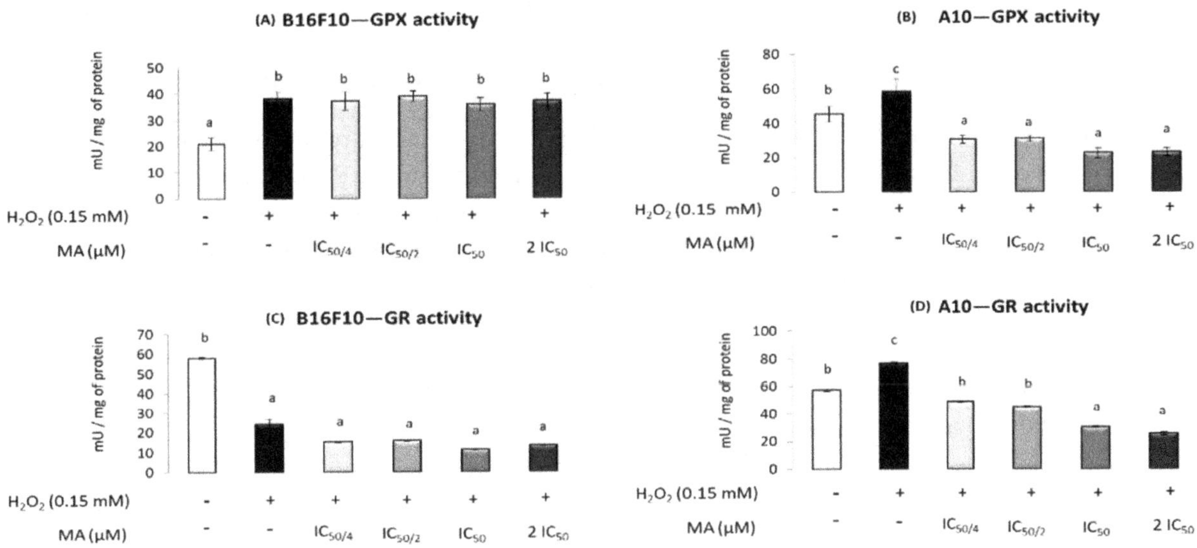

Figure 6. Effect of different maslinic acid doses—$IC_{50/4}$, $IC_{50/2}$, IC_{50} and $2{\cdot}IC_{50}$ (10.6, 21.6, 42.3 and 84.6 µM, respectively)—on the specific activity of glutathione peroxidase (GPX) in cancer cells, B16F10 (**A**), and normal cells, A10 (**B**), and glutathione reductase (GR) in cancer cells, B16F10 (**C**), and normal cells, A10 (**D**), subjected to the presence of hydrogen peroxide. Symbols (+) and (−) indicate the presence or absence of incubation with H_2O_2, respectively. Enzyme activity (mU × mg $protein^{-1}$) is expressed as means ± SEM ($n = 9$). Different letters indicate significant differences ($p < 0.05$)

3. Discussion

Maslinic acid (MA) is a pentacyclic triterpene abundant in the surface wax of fruits and leaves of *Olea europaea* L. with many demonstrated biological activities [23,30,31]. For this reason, MA is appreciated as a chemopreventive agent in different diseases such as cancer [23,28], cardiovascular and neurodegenerative pathologies, etc. [26].

In different cell lines, MA's cytotoxic effect has been studied, including in both cancer and healthy cells. In this sense, it has been shown that this triterpene affects cells in different ways depending on the kind of cells and the conditions of the experiment. In the present study, MA showed cytotoxic effects only in B16F10 cells, and this effect was important, as the IC_{50} of MA was 42 µM. In another study performed in melanoma cells by Kim et al. [32], the authors observed a lower MA cytotoxicity effect. Thus, they concluded that the IC_{50} for MA in SK-MEL-3 was also 42 µM, but in their study, the incubation period was 48 h versus the 24 h used in the present study. Other results obtained in our research group showed that in colon cancer cells, the IC_{50} value for MA was 30 µM in HT29 cells after 72 h of incubation [31,33,34], showing a higher cytotoxic effect in Caco-2 cells, in which the IC_{50} of MA was 10.82 µM, also after 72 h [35]. Other authors observed IC_{50} values for MA ranging between 32 and 64 µM in different cancer cells such as lung (A549), ovary (SK-OV-3), colon (HCT15) and glioma (XF498) cells after 48 h of incubation [32]. In several bladder cancer cell lines incubated with MA for 48 h, other authors found IC_{50} values between 20 and 300 µM [36]. Notwithstanding this, compared to in melanoma cells, a non-cytotoxic effect was found in A10 healthy cells in the present study. These results are relevant since they demonstrate the selective cytotoxic effect of this compound. Studies focused on the selective effect of MA are scarce. Reyes et al. [22] observed that epithelial intestinal cells incubated with 30 µM MA for 72 h (IC_{50} value for HT29) exhibited a survival rate of 78% for IEC-6 cells and 68% for IEC-18.

An intracellular redox balance is crucial to ensure viability, growth and the diversity of cell functions [15]. An excess of ROS is related to pathological processes producing oxidative damage when the antioxidant defense system is not able to counteract it. Hence, there is a growing interest of the scientific community and industry in obtaining substances of natural origin aimed at preventing these pathologies and alterations caused by ROS. In this context, it is important to characterize the protective biochemical functions of natural antioxidants and to study their intracellular pathway signaling. A large number of plant constituents, such as MA, have antioxidant properties [37].

The present study examined the antioxidant effects of MA in skin melanoma cancer cells (B16F10) and thoracic aorta of embryonic rat cells (A10). The major findings were that MA improves the oxidative stress caused by a H_2O_2 excess, decreasing the intracellular ROS levels in both cell lines. H_2O_2 was used in this study because it is known that when present in excess, it is one of the major compounds that can damage cells [38]. Other authors have clearly shown the effects of H_2O_2 on the viability and ROS production of different cell types that were subsequently treated with other antioxidant natural compounds that reversed the oxidative damage caused by the H_2O_2 [39,40]. Furthermore, studies similar to ours with other ROS-producing molecules (i.e., CCl_4) observed that MA counteracted the lipid peroxidation generated in the nucleus [26]. Similarly, MA prevented the $CuSO_4^-$-induced oxidation of rabbit plasma LDL [41]. Moreover, Yang et al. [42] evaluated the antioxidant effects of MA derivatives that showed radical-scavenging activity and inhibition of NO production in RAW 264.7 cells.

Regarding MA's effect on antioxidant enzymes in the B16F10 cell line, as expected, SOD, GST and GPX activities were increased in response to the H_2O_2 addition. However, H_2O_2 decreased CAT, G6PDH and GR activities. A H_2O_2 excess is responsible for cellular damage that includes an imbalance in membranes and biomolecule alterations. This fact supposes an extra energetic cost for the maintenance of cellular homeostasis in order to repair the damage produced. Both cellular damage and energy requirements could affect G6PDH activity, by either the impaired glucose transporters or enhanced glycolysis pathway, decreasing the glucose available for the pentose phosphate pathway. The regulation of NADPH levels is essential for understanding the behavior of numerous physiological processes, being especially important for growth and cell differentiation [2] but also for antioxidant processes, among others. NAPDH is mainly generated by the G6PDH enzyme and is required for the GPX and CAT activity involved in the H_2O_2 removal pathway. Thus, CAT is protected from inactivation by NADPH. Moreover, this reduction equivalent is used by GR to regenerate the oxidized glutathione to its reduced form required for GPX activity [43,44]. The lower G6PDH activity observed when H_2O_2 was added could result in a decrease in available NADPH levels, which might justify the reduction in CAT and GR activities. Similar results have been observed in previous studies in B16F10 cells subjected to stress conditions induced by FBS absence [15]. Mokhtari et al. [15] reported low activity levels for CAT that were produced by low NADPH levels due to an imbalance in cellular homeostasis.

It has been established that MA is a compound with antioxidant capacity [15,26,28]. When MA was added to the B16F10 cells, the changes induced by H_2O_2 excess in SOD and GST activities were counteracted. In this sense, the scavenger MA's effects reduced ROS levels and, subsequently, the need for the action of these antioxidant defenses. Moreover, the observed decrease in ROS levels due to MA would result in less cellular damage, which would reverse the possible mechanisms responsible for the decrease in G6PDH when H_2O_2 is added, raising its activity up to the control values. This recovered G6PDH activity would produce the NADPH level required to prevent and reverse the down-regulation of CAT [43]. Finally, a dose-response effect was observed for both GPX and CAT, highlighting the antioxidant behavior of MA in these cells.

The results found in this work, in A10 healthy cells, revealed that all the enzyme activities increased in the stressful conditions originated by the H_2O_2 addition, except for G6PDH, whose activity was slightly higher. MA, in these cells, restored the antioxidant enzyme activities, inducing values similar to those in the control group in cells treated with the lowest MA levels ($IC_{50/4}$). Furthermore, when cells were treated with the two highest doses of MA (IC_{50} and $2{\cdot}IC_{50}$), the activity of all antioxidant enzymes, with the exception of CAT, decreased below control levels. This fact confirms the relevant antioxidant effect of MA [15,28,43].

4. Materials and Methods

4.1. Compounds

Maslinic acid was obtained from olive pomace and kindly donated by Biomaslinic S.A., Granada, Spain. The extract is a chemically pure white powder composed of 98% maslinic acid and stable when stored at 4 °C. It was dissolved before use at 10 mg/mL in 50% dimethyl sulfoxide (DMSO) and 50% phosphate buffer solution (PBS). This solution was diluted in cell culture medium for assay purposes.

4.2. Cell Lines and Cultures

The mouse melanoma cell line B16F10 is a variant of the murine melanoma cell line B16. These cells show a higher metastatic potential than B16 cells [45]. A10 is a cell line derived from the thoracic aorta of an embryonic mouse, and it is used as a study model of smooth muscle cells (SMC). This cell type shows a great proliferative capacity and may be subcultured several times, allowing the rapid attainment of cell mass [46]. Both cell lines used were provided by the cell bank of the University of Granada (Spain). The cell lines were cultured in Dulbecco's modified Eagle's medium (DMEM) containing glucose (4.5 g/L) and L-glutamine (2 mM) from the commercial PAA brand, 10% heat-inactivated fetal bovine serum (FBS), and 0.5% gentamicin for B16F10 cells and 10,000 units/mL penicillin and 10 mg/mL streptomycin for A10 cells. The cell lines were maintained in a humidified atmosphere with 5% CO_2 at 37 °C. The cells were passaged at preconfluent densities by the use of a solution containing 0.05% trypsin and 0.5 mM EDTA. The cells were seeded in the culture dishes at the desired density. After 24 h, when the cells were attached to the dish, the cells were incubated with 0.15 mM hydrogen peroxide (H_2O_2), in order to produce a stress situation in the cells. Following that, the cells were incubated with several concentrations of MA as indicated below.

4.3. MTT Assay

The MTT assay was performed as described by Mokhtari et al. [15]. Briefly, a 200 μL cell suspension of B16F10 or A10 (1.5×10^3 cells/well) was cultured in 96-well plates. Subsequent to the adherence of the cells, different MA dilutions on a scale of 10 to 210 μM were added separately. The incubation times were 24 h for all cases. MTT was dissolved in the medium and added to the wells at a final concentration of 0.5 mg/mL. Following 2 h of incubation, the generated formazan was dissolved in DMSO. Absorbance was measured at 570 nm in a multiplate reader (Bio-tek®). The absorbance was proportional to the number of viable cells. The MA concentration leading to 50% inhibition of cell proliferation (IC_{50}) was determined. The results are expressed as the percentage of live cells compared with the control considered as 100% cell viability. Cell viability in B16F10 and A10 cells was also studied in the presence of H_2O_2 by the MTT assay. H_2O_2 was dissolved in the culture medium of the cell lines. The concentrations used were made extemporaneously and protected from light before use to prevent degradation of the compounds. After 24 h of incubation, the medium was removed; fresh medium was added with different concentrations of H_2O_2 per well—0, 0.05, 0.1, 0.2, 0.4, 0.6, 0.8, 1.1, 1.5, 2.0, 2.6 and 3 mM—to a final volume of 200 μL for 24 h.

4.4. Flow-Cytometry Analysis of the Mitochondrial-Membrane Potential

Changes in the mitochondrial-membrane potential can be examined by monitoring the cell fluorescence after double staining with rhodamine 123 (Rh123) and propidium iodide (PI). Rh123 is a membrane-permeable fluorescent cationic dye that is selectively taken up by mitochondria in direct proportion to the MMP (mitochondrial-membrane permeabilization) [47]. B16F10 and A10 cells (4×10^5 cells/well) were seeded on 12-well plates with 2 mL of medium and treated with 0.15 mM H_2O_2 for 24 h and MA at $IC_{50/4}$, $IC_{50/2}$, IC_{50} and $2{\cdot}IC_{50}$ (10.6, 21.6, 42.3 and 84.6 μM, respectively) concentrations for 24 h more. Following the treatment, the medium was removed and fresh medium with dihydrorhodamine (DHR), at a final concentration of 5 μg/mL, was added. After 30 min of incubation, the medium was removed and the cells were washed and resuspended in PBS with 5 μg/mL of PI. The intensity of fluorescence from Rh123 and PI was determined using an ACS flow cytometer (Coulter Corporation, Hialeah, FL, USA), at the excitation and emission wavelengths of 500 and 536 nm, respectively. The experiments were performed three times with two replicates per assay.

4.5. Antioxidant Enzyme Assays

In order to prepare the samples for analytic procedures, cells were homogenized in RIPA buffer. Immediately, the cells were sonicated on ice for 5 min and maintained under moderate shaking at 4 °C for 1 h. Every 15 min, the samples were moderately shaken in a vortex. The lysates were spun in a centrifuge at 10,000× *g* at 4 °C for 15 min. All the enzyme assays were carried out at 37 °C using a Power Wave X microplate scanning spectrophotometer (Bio-Tek Instruments, Winooski, VT, USA) and run in duplicate in 96-well microplates. The optimal substrate and protein concentrations for the measurement of maximal activity for each enzyme were established by preliminary assays. The enzymatic reactions were initiated by the addition of the cell extract, except for SOD, where xanthine oxidase was used. The millimolar extinction coefficients used for H_2O_2, NADH/NADPH and DTNB (5,5-dithiobis (2-nitrobenzoic acid)) were 0.039, 6.22 and 13.6, respectively. The assay conditions were as follows:

Superoxide dismutase (SOD; EC 1.15.1.1) activity was measured by the ferricytochrome c method using xanthine/xanthine oxidase as the source of superoxide radicals. The reaction mixture consisted of 50 mM potassium phosphate buffer (pH 7.8), 0.1 mM EDTA, 0.1 mM xanthine, 0.013 mM cytochrome c and 0.024 IU/mL xanthine oxidase. Activity is reported in units of SOD per milligram of protein. One unit of activity was defined as the amount of enzyme necessary to produce a 50% inhibition of the ferricytochrome c reduction rate [48].

Catalase (CAT; EC 1.11.1.6) activity was determined by measuring the decrease in hydrogen peroxide concentration at 240 nm according to Aebi [49]. The reaction mixture contained 50 mm potassium phosphate buffer (pH 7.0) and 10.6 mM freshly prepared H_2O_2.

Glucose-6-phosphate dehydrogenase (G6PDH; EC 1.1.1.49) activity was determined at pH 7.6 in a medium containing 50 mM HEPES buffer, 2 mM $MgCl_2$, 0.8 mM $NADP^+$ and glucose 6-phosphate used as substrate. The enzyme activity was determined by measuring the reduction of $NADP^+$ at 340 nm as previously described by Lupiáñez et al. [2] and Peragón et al. [50]. The change in absorbance at 340 nm was recorded and, after confirmation of no exogenous activity, the reaction started by the addition of substrate.

Glutathione S-transferase (GST; EC 2.5.1.18) activity was measured according to the method described by Habig et al. [51], using 1-chloro-2,4-dinitrobenzene as a substrate.

Glutathione peroxidase (GPX, EC 1.11.1.9) activity was determined using the method described by Flohe and Günzler [52], based on the oxidation of NADPH, which is used to regenerate the reduced glutathione (GSH) from oxidized glutathione (GS-SG) obtained by the action of glutathione peroxidase.

Glutathione reductase (GR, EC 1.8.1.7) was determined by the modified method of Carlberg and Mannervik [53]. We measured the decrease in absorbance produced by the oxidation of NADPH used by GR in the passage of oxidized glutathione (GS-SG) to reduced glutathione (GSH).

All enzyme activities (except for SOD) are expressed as units or milliunits per milligram of soluble protein (specific activity). One unit of enzyme activity was defined as the amount of enzyme required to transform 1 µmol of substrate per min under the above assay conditions.

Soluble protein concentrations were determined using the method of Bradford, with bovine serum albumin used as a standard.

4.6. Statistical Analysis

Data are shown as mean ± standard error mean (SEM). The statistical significance among different experimental groups was determined by one-way analysis of variance (ANOVA) tests. When *F* values ($p < 0.05$) were significant, means were compared using Tukey's HSD test. The SPSS version 15.0 for Windows software package was used for statistical analysis.

5. Conclusions

In conclusion, the results obtained in the present study demonstrate that MA exerts a selective anti-proliferative effect against the B16F10 cell line, whereas in A10 healthy cells, MA did not present a cytotoxic effect. This natural compound prevents the oxidative stress caused by H_2O_2 excess, decreasing the ROS production levels. Moreover, depending on the cell line, the antioxidant enzymatic responses were different in the presence of H_2O_2 and without MA. Thus, in healthy A10 cells, all enzymes up-regulated their activity, but in B16F10 cells, only SOD, GST and GPX increased it. In most cases, MA treatment restored the activities of enzymes to levels similar to those in the control group, highlighting that in A10 cells, the highest doses of MA (IC_{50} and $2 \cdot IC_{50}$) resulted in values below control. Overall, these findings demonstrate the great antioxidant capacity of maslinic acid.

Author Contributions: Conceptualization, J.A.L. and E.E.R.-P.; methodology, performing experiments, K.M., E.E.R.-P., A.P.-J. and L.G.-S.; data analysis, K.M. and E.E.R.-P.; results interpretation, E.E.R.-P. and A.P.-J.; writing—original draft preparation, K.M., E.E.R.-P. and A.P.-J.; writing—review and editing, J.A.L. and L.G.-S.; supervision, E.E.R.-P. and J.A.L.; project fund acquisition and administration, J.A.L. All authors have read and agreed to the published version of the manuscript.

References

1. Rodríguez-Rodríguez, R. Oleanolic acid and related triterpenoids from olives on vascular function: Molecular mechanisms and therapeutic perspectives. *Curr. Med. Chem.* **2015**, *22*, 1414–1425. [CrossRef] [PubMed]
2. Lupiáñez, J.A.; Adroher, F.J.; Vargas, A.M.; Osuna, A. Differential behaviour of glucose 6-phosphate dehydrogenase in two morphological forms of *Trypanosoma cruzi*. *Int. J. Biochem.* **1987**, *19*, 1085–1089. [CrossRef]
3. Adroher, F.J.; Osuna, A.; Lupiáñez, J.A. Differential energetic metabolism during *Trypanosoma cruzi* differentiation. I: Citrate synthase, NADP-isocitrate and succinate dehydrogenases. *Arch. Biochem. Biophys.* **1988**, *267*, 252–261. [CrossRef]
4. Adroher, F.J.; Osuna, A.; Lupiáñez, J.A. Differential energetic metabolism during *Trypanosoma cruzi* differentiation. II. Hexokinase, phosphofructokinase and pyruvate kinase. *Mol. Cell. Biochem.* **1990**, *94*, 71–82. [CrossRef] [PubMed]
5. Peragón, J.; Barroso, J.B.; de la Higuera, M.; Lupiáñez, J.A. Relationship between growth and protein turnover rates and nucleic acids in the liver of rainbow trout (*Oncorhynchus mykiss*) during development. *Can. J. Fish. Aquat. Sci.* **1998**, *55*, 649–657. [CrossRef]
6. Peragón, J.; Barroso, J.B.; García-Salguero, L.; Aranda, F.; de la Higuera, M.; Lupiáñez, J.A. Selective changes in the protein-turnover rates and nature of growth induced in trout liver by long-term starvation followed by re-feeding. *Mol. Cell. Biochem.* **1999**, *201*, 1–10. [CrossRef]
7. Peragón, J.; Barroso, J.B.; García-Salguero, L.; de la Higuera, M.; Lupiáñez, J.A. Dietary alterations in protein, carbohydrates and fat increase liver protein-turnover rate and decrease overall growth rate in the rainbow trout (*Oncorhynchus mykiss*). *Mol. Cell. Biochem.* **2000**, *209*, 97–104. [CrossRef]
8. Peragón, J.; Barroso, J.B.; García-Salguero, L.; de la Higuera, M.; Lupiáñez, J.A. Dietary-protein effects on growth and fractional protein-synthesis and degradation rates in liver and white muscle of rainbow-trout (*Oncorhynchus mykiss*). *Aquaculture* **1994**, *124*, 35–46. [CrossRef]
9. Barroso, J.B.; Peragón, J.; García-Salguero, L.; de la Higuera, M.; Lupiáñez, J.A. Carbohydrate deprivation reduces NADPH-production in fish liver but not in adipose tissue. *Int. J. Biochem. Cell Biol.* **2001**, *33*, 785–796. [CrossRef]
10. Peragón, J.; Barroso, J.B.; García-Salguero, L.; de la Higuera, M.; Lupiáñez, J.A. Growth, protein-turnover rates and nucleic-acid concentrations in the white muscle of rainbow trout during development. *Int. J. Biochem. Cell Biol.* **2001**, *33*, 1227–1238. [CrossRef]

11. Sánchez-Muros, M.J.; García-Rejón, L.; Lupiáñez, J.A.; de la Higuera, M. Long-term nutritional effects on the primary liver and kidney metabolism in rainbow trout (*Oncorhynchus mykiss*). II. Adaptive response of glucose 6-phosphate dehydrogenase activity to high-carbohydrate/low-protein and high-fat/on-carbohydrate diets. *Aquacult. Nutr.* **1996**, *2*, 193–200. [CrossRef]
12. Nóbrega-Pereira, S.; Fernández-Marcos, P.J.; Brioche, T.; Gómez-Cabrera, M.C.; Salvador-Pascual, A.; Flores, J.M.; Vina, J.; Serrano, M. G6PD protects from oxidative damage and improves healthspan in mice. *Nat. Commun.* **2016**, *7*, 10894. [CrossRef] [PubMed]
13. Brennan, J.P.; Southworth, R.; Medina, R.A.; Davidson, S.M.; Duchen, M.R.; Shattock, M.J. Mitochondrial uncoupling, with low concentration FCCP, induces ROS-dependent cardioprotection independent of KATP channel activation. *Cardiovas. Res.* **2006**, *72*, 313–321. [CrossRef]
14. Kurze, A.K.; Buhs, S.; Eggert, D.; Oliveira-Ferrer, L.; Muller, V.; Niendorf, A.; Wagener, C.; Nollau, P. Immature O-glycans recognized by the macrophage glycoreceptor CLEC10A (MGL) are induced by 4-hydroxy-tamoxifen, oxidative stress and DNA-damage in breast cancer cells. *Cell Commun. Signal.* **2019**, *17*, 107. [CrossRef] [PubMed]
15. Mokhtari, K.; Rufino-Palomares, E.E.; Pérez-Jiménez, A.; Reyes-Zurita, F.J.; Figuera, C.; García-Salguero, L.; Medina, P.P.; Peragón, J.; Lupiáñez, J.A. Maslinic acid, a triterpene from olive, affects the antioxidant and mitochondrial status of B16F10 melanoma cells grown under stressful conditions. *Evid.-Based Complement. Altern. Med.* **2015**, *2015*, 272457. [CrossRef]
16. Ahmad, K.; Hafeez, Z.B.; Bhat, A.R.; Rizvi, M.A.; Thakur, S.C.; Azam, A.; Athar, F. Antioxidant and apoptotic effects of *Callistemon lanceolatus* leaves and their compounds against human cancer cells. *Biomed. Pharmacother.* **2018**, *106*, 1195–1209. [CrossRef]
17. De Santiago-Arteche, R. Efecto de la Quimioterapia Antineoplásica en Pacientes con Cancer Colorectal Sobre Biomarcadores del Estrés Oxidativo y del Estado Redox Plasmático. Ph.D. Thesis, University of Burgos, Burgos, Spain, 2010; p. 262.
18. Zhang, Y.S.; Ning, Z.X.; Yang, S.Z.; Wu, H. Antioxidation properties and mechanism of action of dihydromyricetin from *Ampelopsis grossedentata*. *Acta Pharm. Sin.* **2003**, *38*, 241–244.
19. Yang, W.F.; Zhao, W.L. Determination of ginsenosides Re, Rb1 in Panax quinquefolius by micellar electrokinetic chromatography. *China J. Chin. Mater. Med.* **2003**, *28*, 1135–1137.
20. Reyes-Zurita, F.J.; Medina-O'Donnell, M.; Ferrer-Martín, R.M.; Rufino-Palomares, E.E.; Martín-Fonseca, S.; Rivas, F.; Martínez, A.; García-Granados, A.; Pérez-Jiménez, A.; García-Salguero, L.; et al. The oleanolic acid derivative, 3-O-succinyl-28-O-benzyl oleanolate, induces apoptosis in B16-F10 melanoma cells via the mitochondrial apoptotic pathway. *RSC Adv.* **2016**, *6*, 93590–93601. [CrossRef]
21. Reyes-Zurita, F.J.; Rufino-Palomares, E.E.; Lupiáñez, J.A.; Cascante, M. Maslinic acid, a natural triterpene from *Olea europaea* L., induces apoptosis in HT29 human colon-cancer cells via the mitochondrial apoptotic pathway. *Cancer Lett.* **2009**, *273*, 44–54. [CrossRef] [PubMed]
22. Reyes, F.J.; Centelles, J.J.; Lupiáñez, J.A.; Cascante, M. (2Alpha,3beta)-2,3-dihydroxyolean-12-en-28-oic acid, a new natural triterpene from *Olea europea*, induces caspase dependent apoptosis selectively in colon adenocarcinoma cells. *FEBS Lett.* **2006**, *580*, 6302–6310. [CrossRef] [PubMed]
23. Rufino-Palomares, E.E.; Pérez-Jiménez, A.; Reyes-Zurita, F.J.; García-Salguero, L.; Mokhtari, K.; Herrera-Merchán, A.; Medina, P.P.; Peragón, J.; Lupiáñez, J.A. Anti-cancer and anti-angiogenic properties of various natural pentacyclic tri-terpenoids and some of their chemical derivatives. *Curr. Org. Chem.* **2015**, *19*, 919–947. [CrossRef]
24. Juan, M.E.; Planas, J.M. Bioavailability and metabolism of maslinic acid, a natural pentacyclic triterpene. In *Recent Advances in Pharmaceutical Sciences VI*; Publisher: Kerala, India, 2016; pp. 131–145.
25. Siewert, B.; Csuk, R. Membrane damaging activity of a maslinic acid analog. *Eur. J. Med. Chem.* **2014**, *74*, 1–6. [CrossRef] [PubMed]
26. Montilla, M.P.; Agil, A.; Navarro, M.C.; Jiménez, M.I.; García-Granados, A.; Parra, A.; Cabo, M.M. Antioxidant activity of maslinic acid, a triterpene derivative obtained from *Olea europaea*. *Planta Med.* **2003**, *69*, 472–474. [PubMed]
27. Barroso, J.B.; García-Salguero, L.; Peragón, J.; de la Higuera, M.; Lupiáñez, J.A. The influence of dietary-protein on the kinetics of NADPH production systems in various tissues of rainbow-trout (*Oncorhynchus mykiss*). *Aquaculture* **1994**, *124*, 47–59. [CrossRef]

28. Allouche, Y.; Warleta, F.; Campos, M.; Sánchez-Quesada, C.; Uceda, M.; Beltrán, G.; Gaforio, J.J. Antioxidant, antiproliferative, and pro-apoptotic capacities of pentacyclic triterpenes found in the skin of olives on MCF-7 human breast cancer cells and their effects on DNA damage. *J. Agric. Food Chem.* **2011**, *59*, 121–130. [CrossRef]
29. Chen, J.C.; Zhang, G.H.; Zhang, Z.Q.; Qiu, M.H.; Zheng, Y.T.; Yang, L.M.; Yu, K.B. Octanorcucurbitane and cucurbitane triterpenoids from the tubers of *Hemsleya endecaphylla* with HIV-1 inhibitory activity. *J. Nat. Prod.* **2008**, *71*, 153–155. [CrossRef]
30. Reyes-Zurita, F.J.; Rufino-Palomares, E.E.; García-Salguero, L.; Peragón, J.; Medina, P.P.; Parra, A.; Cascante, M.; Lupiáñez, J.A. Maslinic acid, a natural T¡triterpene, induces a death receptor-mediated apoptotic mechanism in Caco-2 p53-deficient colon adenocarcinoma cells. *PLoS ONE* **2016**, *11*, e0146178. [CrossRef]
31. Rufino-Palomares, E.E.; Reyes-Zurita, F.J.; García-Salguero, L.; Mokhtari, K.; Medina, P.P.; Lupiáñez, J.A.; Peragón, J. Maslinic acid, a triterpenic anti-tumoural agent, interferes with cytoskeleton protein expression in HT29 human colon-cancer cells. *J. Proteom.* **2013**, *83*, 15–25. [CrossRef]
32. Kim, Y.K.; Yoon, S.K.; Ryu, S.Y. Cytotoxic triterpenes from stem bark of *Physocarpus intermedius*. *Planta Med.* **2000**, *66*, 485–486. [CrossRef] [PubMed]
33. Reyes-Zurita, F.J.; Pachón-Pena, G.; Lizarraga, D.; Rufino-Palomares, E.E.; Cascante, M.; Lupiáñez, J.A. The natural triterpene maslinic acid induces apoptosis in HT29 colon cancer cells by a JNK-p53-dependent mechanism. *BMC Cancer* **2011**, *11*, 154. [CrossRef] [PubMed]
34. Sánchez-Tena, S.; Reyes-Zurita, F.J.; Díaz-Moralli, S.; Vinardell, M.P.; Reed, M.; García-García, F.; Dopazo, J.; Lupiáñez, J.A.; Gunther, U.; Cascante, M. Maslinic acid-enriched diet decreases intestinal tumorigenesis in Apc(Min/+) mice through transcriptomic and metabolomic reprogramming. *PLoS ONE* **2013**, *8*, e59392. [CrossRef] [PubMed]
35. Reyes-Zurita, F.J.; Rufino-Palomares, E.E.; Medina, P.P.; García-Salguero, L.; Peragón, J.; Cascante, M.; Lupiáñez, J.A. Antitumour activity on extrinsic apoptotic targets of the triterpenoid maslinic acid in p53-deficient Caco-2 adenocarcinoma cells. *Biochimie* **2013**, *95*, 2157–2167. [CrossRef] [PubMed]
36. Zhang, S.; Ding, D.; Zhang, X.; Shan, L.; Liu, Z. Maslinic acid induced apoptosis in bladder cancer cells through activating p38 MAPK signaling pathway. *Mol. Cell. Biochem.* **2014**, *392*, 281–287. [CrossRef]
37. Medina, I.; Lois, S.; Lizarraga, D.; Pazos, M.; Tourino, S.; Cascante, M.; Torres, J.L. Functional fatty fish supplemented with grape procyanidins. Antioxidant and proapoptotic properties on colon cell lines. *J. Agric. Food Chem.* **2006**, *54*, 3598–3603. [CrossRef] [PubMed]
38. Sroka, Z.; Cisowski, W. Hydrogen peroxide scavenging, antioxidant and anti-radical activity of some phenolic acids. *Food Chem. Toxicol.* **2003**, *41*, 753–758. [CrossRef]
39. Choi, B.S.; Kim, H.; Lee, H.J.; Sapkota, K.; Park, S.E.; Kim, S.; Kim, S.J. Celastrol from 'Thunder God Vine' protects SH-SY5Y cells through the preservation of mitochondrial function and inhibition of p38 MAPK in a rotenone model of Parkinson's disease. *Neurochem. Res.* **2014**, *39*, 84–96. [CrossRef]
40. Rafatian, G.; Khodagholi, F.; Farimani, M.M.; Abraki, S.B.; Gardaneh, M. Increase of autophagy and attenuation of apoptosis by Salvigenin promote survival of SH-SY5Y cells following treatment with H_2O_2. *Mol. Cell. Biochem.* **2012**, *371*, 9–22. [CrossRef]
41. Baricevic, D.; Sosa, S.; Della Loggia, R.; Tubaro, A.; Simonovska, B.; Krasna, A.; Zupancic, A. Topical anti-inflammatory activity of *Salvia officinalis* L. leaves: The relevance of ursolic acid. *J. Ethnopharmacol.* **2001**, *75*, 125–132. [CrossRef]
42. Yang, Z.G.; Li, H.R.; Wang, L.Y.; Li, Y.H.; Lu, S.G.; Wen, X.F.; Wang, J.; Daikonya, A.; Kitanaka, S. Triterpenoids from *Hippophae rhamnoides* L. and their nitric oxide production-inhibitory and DPPH radical-scavenging activities. *Chem. Pharm. Bull.* **2007**, *55*, 15–18. [CrossRef]
43. Kirkman, H.N.; Rolfo, M.; Ferraris, A.M.; Gaetani, G.F. Mechanisms of protection of catalase by NADPH—Kinetics and stoichiometry. *J. Biol. Chem.* **1999**, *274*, 13908–13914. [CrossRef] [PubMed]
44. Pérez-Jiménez, A.; Abellán, E.; Arizcun, M.; Cardenete, G.; Morales, A.E.; Hidalgo, M.C. Dietary carbohydrates improve oxidative status of common dentex (*Dentex dentex*) juveniles, a carnivorous fish species. *Comp. Biochem. Physiol. A* **2017**, *203*, 17–23. [CrossRef] [PubMed]
45. Wang, W.; Xu, Z.; Yang, M.; Liu, R.; Wang, W.; Liu, P.; Guo, D. Structural determination of seven new triterpenoids from *Kadsura heteroclita* by NMR techniques. *Magn. Reson. Chem.* **2007**, *45*, 522–526. [CrossRef] [PubMed]

46. Rao, M.S.; Subbarao, V. Effect of dexamethasone on ciprofibrate-induced cell proliferation and peroxisome proliferation. *Fundam. Appl. Toxicol.* **1997**, *35*, 78–83. [CrossRef]
47. Rothe, G.; Oser, A.; Valet, G. Dihydrorhodamine 123: A new flow cytometric indicator for respiratory burst activity in neutrophil granulocytes. *Die Nat.* **1988**, *75*, 354–355. [CrossRef]
48. McCord, J.M.; Fridovich, I. Superoxide dismutase. An enzymic function for erythrocuprein (hemocuprein). *J. Biol. Chem.* **1969**, *244*, 6049–6055.
49. Aebi, H. Catalase in vitro. *Methods Enzymol.* **1984**, *105*, 121–126.
50. Peragón, J.; Aranda, F.; García-Salguero, L.; Corpas, F.J.; Lupiáñez, J.A. Stimulation of rat-kidney hexose-monophosphate shunt dehydrogenase-activity by chronic metabolic-acidosis. *Biochem. Int.* **1989**, *18*, 1041–1050.
51. Habig, W.H.; Pabst, M.J.; Jakoby, W.B. Glutathione S-transferases. The first enzymatic step in mercapturic acid formation. *J. Biol. Chem.* **1974**, *249*, 7130–7139.
52. Flohe, L.; Gunzler, W.A. Assays of glutathione peroxidase. *Methods Enzymol.* **1984**, *105*, 114–121.
53. Carlberg, I.; Mannervik, B. Purification by affinity chromatography of yeast glutathione reductase, the enzyme responsible for the NADPH-dependent reduction of the mixed disulfide of coenzyme A and glutathione. *Biochim. Biophys. Acta* **1977**, *484*, 268–274. [CrossRef]

9

Synthesis, Biological Evaluation and In Silico Studies of Novel Aminated Xanthones as Potential p53-Activating Agents

Agostinho Lemos [1], Ana Sara Gomes [2], Joana B. Loureiro [2], Pedro Brandão [1], Andreia Palmeira [1,3], Madalena M. M. Pinto [1,3], Lucília Saraiva [2,*] and Maria Emília Sousa [1,3,*]

1 Laboratory of Organic and Pharmaceutical Chemistry, Department of Chemical Sciences, Faculty of Pharmacy, University of Porto, Rua de Jorge Viterbo Ferreira, 228, 4050-313 Porto, Portugal; up201002662@ff.up.pt (A.L.); pedrocgbrandao@gmail.com (P.B.); andreiapalmeira@gmail.com (A.P.); madalena@ff.up.pt (M.M.M.P.)

2 UCIBIO/REQUIMTE, Laboratory of Microbiology, Department of Biological Sciences, Faculty of Pharmacy, University of Porto, Rua de Jorge Viterbo Ferreira, 228, 4050-313 Porto, Portugal; anasarag4@gmail.com (A.S.G.); up201407524@ff.up.pt (J.B.L.)

3 CIIMAR-Interdisciplinary Centre of Marine and Environmental Research, University of Porto, Novo Edificio do Terminal de Cruzeiros do Porto de Leixões, Avenida General Norton de Matos, S/N, 4450-208 Matosinhos, Portugal

* Correspondence: lucilia.saraiva@ff.up.pt (L.S.); esousa@ff.up.pt (M.E.S.);

Academic Editor: Qiao-Hong Chen

Abstract: Xanthone scaffold has been regarded as an attractive chemical tool in the search for bioactive molecules with antitumor activity, and in particular two xanthone derivatives, 12-hydroxy-2,2-dimethyl-3,4-dihydro-2*H*,6*H*-pyrano [3,2-*b*]xanthen-6-one (**4**) and 3,4-dimethoxy-9-oxo-9*H*-xanthene-1-carbaldehyde (**5**), were described as a murine double minute 2 (MDM2)-p53 inhibitor and a TAp73 activator, respectively. The xanthone **5** was used as a starting point for the construction of a library of 3,4-dioxygenated xanthones bearing chemical moieties of described MDM2-p53 inhibitors. Eleven aminated xanthones were successfully synthesized and initially screened for their ability to disrupt the MDM2-p53 interaction using a yeast cell-based assay. With this approach, xanthone **37** was identified as a putative p53-activating agent through inhibition of interaction with MDM2. Xanthone **37** inhibited the growth of human colon adenocarcinoma HCT116 cell lines in a p53-dependent manner. The growth inhibitory effect of xanthone **37** was associated with the induction of G1-phase cell cycle arrest and increased protein expression levels of p53 transcriptional targets. These results demonstrated the potential usefulness of coupling amine-containing structural motifs of known MDM2-p53 disruptors into a 3,4-dioxygenated xanthone scaffold in the design of novel and potent p53 activators with antitumor activity and favorable drug-like properties. Moreover, in silico docking studies were performed in order to predict the binding poses and residues involved in the potential MDM2-p53 interaction.

Keywords: antitumor activity; computational docking; MDM2-p53 interaction; xanthones; yeast-based assays

---

1. Introduction

The tumor suppressor p53 acts as a transcription factor, triggering the expression of multiple downstream target genes that play a pivotal role in the regulation of cell cycle arrest, apoptosis, senescence, and DNA repair [1–6]. Upon cellular stress stimuli, the activation of the p53 pathway may compromise the tumorigenesis, circumventing the proliferation of damaged cells with oncogenic potential. Inactivation of the p53 function represents one of the most common events in human cancers [7]. In approximately half of all human cancer cells, the p53 inactivation is caused by mutations within the p53 gene (*TP53*) or by post-translational modifications of its gene product [8]. In those tumors retaining the wild type (wt) p53 function, the tumor suppressor activity of p53 can be abolished by multiple mechanisms [9], mainly by direct interaction between p53 and its primary endogenous inhibitor, the murine double minute 2 (MDM2) protein [10,11]. The oncoprotein MDM2 physically interacts with the amino-terminal domain of p53 and negatively regulates its activity by blocking p53-mediated transactivation [12,13], by inducing the export of p53 from nucleus to the cytoplasm [14], and by promoting E3 ubiquitin ligase-mediated p53 degradation via the proteasomal pathway [15,16]. Targeting the MDM2-p53 interaction with small molecules has been regarded an attractive approach for the reactivation of the p53 pathway in wt p53-expressing tumors [17,18]. Since the seminal work of Vassilev et al. reporting the discovery of nutlin-3A (**1**, Figure 1) as the first inhibitor of MDM2-p53 interaction [19], an impressive number of MDM2-p53 disruptors from a huge diversity of chemical families have been identified in recent years, entering some of them into clinical trials [20,21].

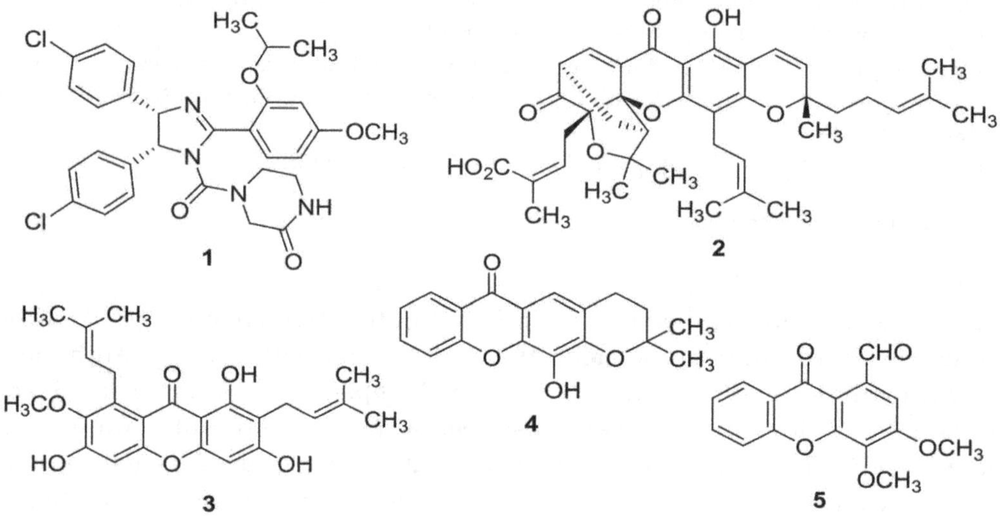

Figure 1. Chemical structures of nutlin-3A (**1**), gambogic acid (**2**), α-mangostin (**3**), 12-hydroxy-2,2-dimethyl-3,4-dihydro-2*H*,6*H*-pyrano[3,2-*b*]xanthen-6-one (**4**), and 3,4-dimethoxy-9-oxo-9*H*-xanthene-1-carbaldehyde (**5**).

Xanthones represent a privileged class of compounds with a multiplicity of biological activities, in particular with antitumor activity against several human tumor cell lines [22–36]. Intriguingly, our research group has demonstrated that the antitumor activity of some derivatives can be correlated to the disruption of the MDM2-p53 complex and the activation of a p53-dependent pathway [30,31]. In fact, implementing a yeast-based assay, the naturally occurring xanthones gambogic acid (**2**, Figure 1) and α-mangostin (**3**, Figure 1) were found to revert the inhibitory effect of MDM2 on p53-induced growth inhibition and on p53 transcriptional activity [30]. The synthetic xanthone 12-hydroxy-2,2-dimethyl-3,4-dihydro-2*H*,6*H*-pyrano [3,2-*b*]xanthen-6-one (**4**, Figure 1) was identified as a potential MDM2-p53 disruptor, using an in silico virtual screening strategy against MDM2 protein and a yeast-based assay [31]. Its molecular mechanism was corroborated in MDM2-overexpressing human tumor cell lines with wt p53. In fact, xanthone **4** selectively upregulated the p53 transcriptional activity, increasing the protein expression levels of p53-target genes in HCT116 human colon adenocarcinoma cells [31]. Nevertheless, xanthone **4** is highly hydrophobic and poorly water soluble, which could limit its in vivo use. Interestingly, Chen and co-workers explored the antitumor activity of xanthone **4** either in combination or hybridized with 5,6-dimethylxanthone-4-acetic acid (DMXAA) [37], a xanthone derivative with tumor-vascular disrupting activity. A very recent study reported the discovery of

3,4-dimethoxy-9-oxo-9*H*-xanthene-1-carbaldehyde (**5**, Figure 1) as a new TAp73 activator via disruption of its interaction with both MDM2 and mutant p53 [36].

Herein, based on the 3,4-oxygenated pattern of substitution of xanthones **4** and **5** (Figure 2A), and on chemical moieties derived from known MDM2-p53 disruptors, namely the molecules **1** [19], **6** [38], **7** [39], and **8** [40] (Figure 2B), we followed a molecular hybridization approach for the construction of novel 3,4-oxygenated xanthone derivatives (Figure 2D). In the present work, we opted to synthesize a library of aminated xanthones (Figure 2D) via a strategy of reductive amination of the xanthone **5** with a set of commercially available amine precursors (**9–19**) containing structural motifs of MDM2-p53 disruptors (Figure 2C). The introduction of amine moieties in the xanthone scaffold may contribute to a potential enhancement of drug-like properties, a critical parameter for the identification of promising drug candidates. The ability of the synthesized ligands to disrupt the MDM2-p53 interaction and to activate a p53-dependent pathway was further investigated using the previously established yeast-based assay and in human cancer cell lines. In silico docking studies were performed in order to predict the binding poses and residues involved in the potential MDM2-p53 interaction.

2. Results and Discussion

2.1. Chemistry

2.1.1. Synthesis of 3,4-dimethoxy-9-oxo-9*H*-xanthene-1-carbaldehyde (**5**)

In the present work, xanthone **5** was used as a starting precursor for the synthesis of a set of aminated xanthones with a 3,4-dioxygenated pattern of substitution. Recently, the multi-step synthesis of compound **5** has been reported [36] as consisting in: (i) a Friedel-Crafts acylation of 1,2,3-trimethoxybenzene (**20**) with the commercially available reagent 2-methoxybenzoyl chloride (**21**); (ii) an intramolecular nucleophilic aromatic substitution of (2-hydroxy-3,4-dimethoxyphenyl)(2-methoxyphenyl)methanone (**22**) and consecutive regioselective demethylation of the methoxy group at position C-4 under conventional heating; (iii) a Duff formylation at position C-1 of 4-hydroxy-3-methoxy-9*H*-xanthen-9-one (**23**); and (iv) a methylation of the hydroxyl group at position C-4 of 4-hydroxy-3-methoxy-9-oxo-9*H*-xanthene-1-carbaldehyde (**24**) (Scheme 1A). The difficulty in achieving a regioselective demethylation at position C-4 necessary for Duff formylation at position C-1 demanded the planning of an optimized synthetic route more appropriate for scaling-up. We hypothesized that the implementation of an analog precursor of **20** with a suitable substituent at position C-1 might provide a useful alternative for the synthesis of **5**, avoiding the troublesome demethylation and Duff formylation processes. Herein, the commercially available 1,2,3-trimethoxy-5-methylbenzene (**25**) was selected for the Friedel-Crafts acylation with the acyl chloride **21** and the Lewis acid aluminum chloride to furnish the intermediate (2-hydroxy-3,4-dimethoxy-6-methylphenyl)(2-methoxyphenyl)methanone (**26**). Subsequent intramolecular nucleophilic aromatic substitution followed by elimination of methanol under basic conditions and microwave (MW) irradiation provided the 3,4-dimethoxy-1-methyl-9*H*-xanthen-9-one (**27**) in good yield quantity. This two-step methodology for the construction of xanthone analogues of **27** has been previously described in the literature [32,41–43]. With the application of MW methodology in the basic cyclization of **26** instead of the conventional heating employed in the synthesis of **23**, the reaction time was reduced from 48 h to 6 h. Furthermore, xanthone **27** was obtained in higher reaction yield under MW irradiation (63% yield (**27**) vs. 38% yield (**23**)). Subsequently, the Vohl-Ziegler bromination of **27**, using dibenzoyl peroxide (DBP) and *N*-bromosuccinimide (NBS) as a radical initiator and a brominating agent, respectively, afforded the 1-(dibromomethyl)-3,4-dimethoxy-9*H*-xanthen-9-one (**28**) as the major product. A solvolytic displacement of bromine atoms of the xanthone **28** was effectively attained using 1-butyl-3-methylimidazolium tetrafluoroborate and water, under conventional heating, and furnished xanthone **5** in 64% yield quantity (Scheme 1B). Of note, the two-step procedure of Vohl-Ziegler bromination and subsequent solvolytic displacement required lower reaction times (4.5 h (2 steps from **27** to **5**) vs. 54 h (2 steps from **23** to **5**) and allowed the preparation of xanthone **5** in higher reaction yields (51% yield (2 steps from **27** to **5**) vs. 28% yield (2 steps from **23** to **5**)), compared to the Duff formylation/methylation pathway. Overall, the replacement of starting precursor **20** by the methylated derivative **25** at position C-1 of the aromatic ring was critical for the successful optimization of the preparation of xanthone **5**.

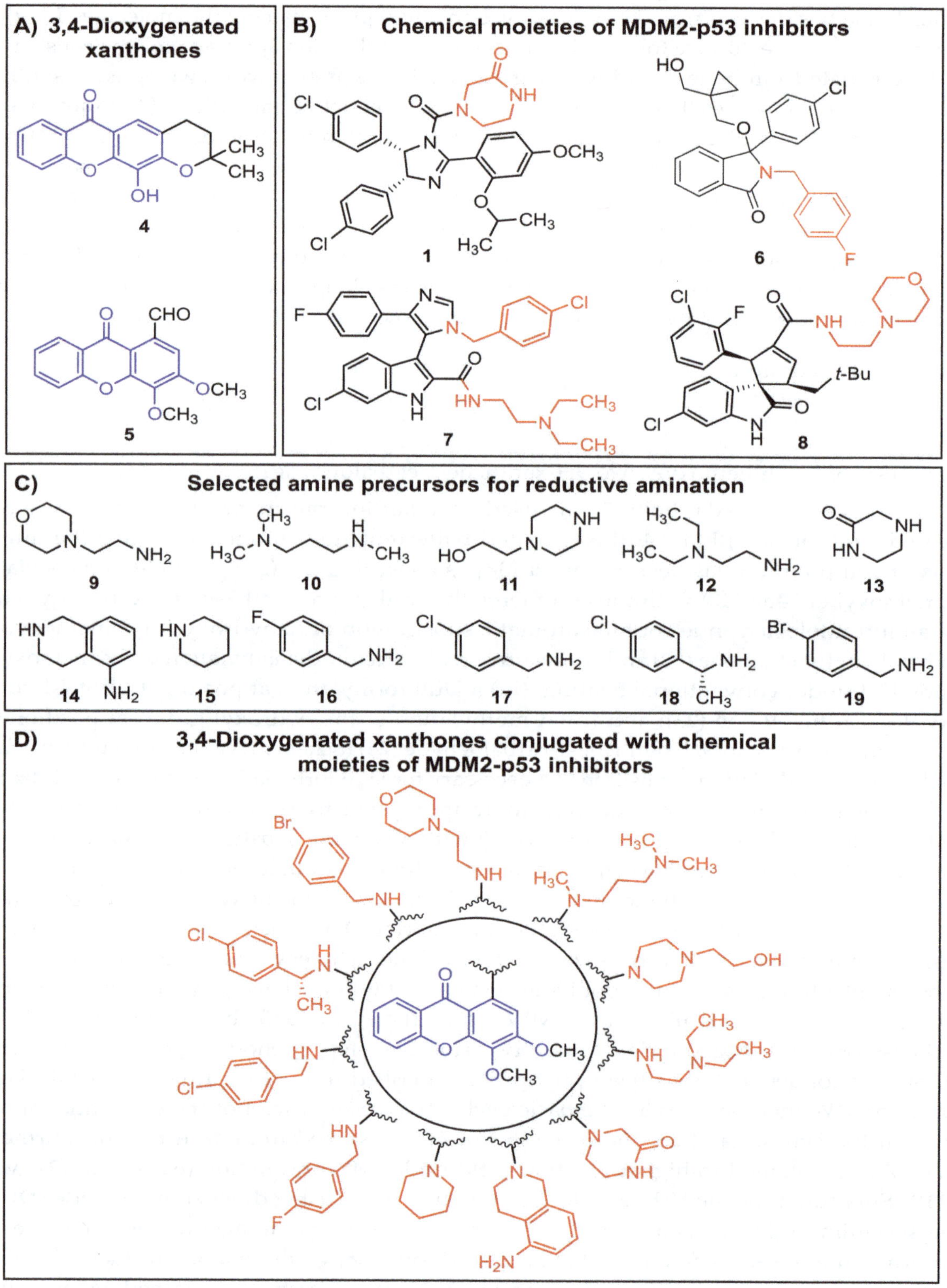

Figure 2. Strategy of molecular hybridization used for the construction of the library of aminated xanthones (**D**) by conjugation of the 3,4-dioxygenated substitution pattern of xanthones **4** and **5** (**A**) with the chemical moieties of known murine double minute 2 (MDM2)-p53 inhibitors (**C**), namely the molecules **1** (IC_{50} = 0.09 μM), **6** (IC_{50} = 2.6 μM), **7** (K_I = 0.656 μM), and **8** (K_I = 0.023 μM) (**B**).

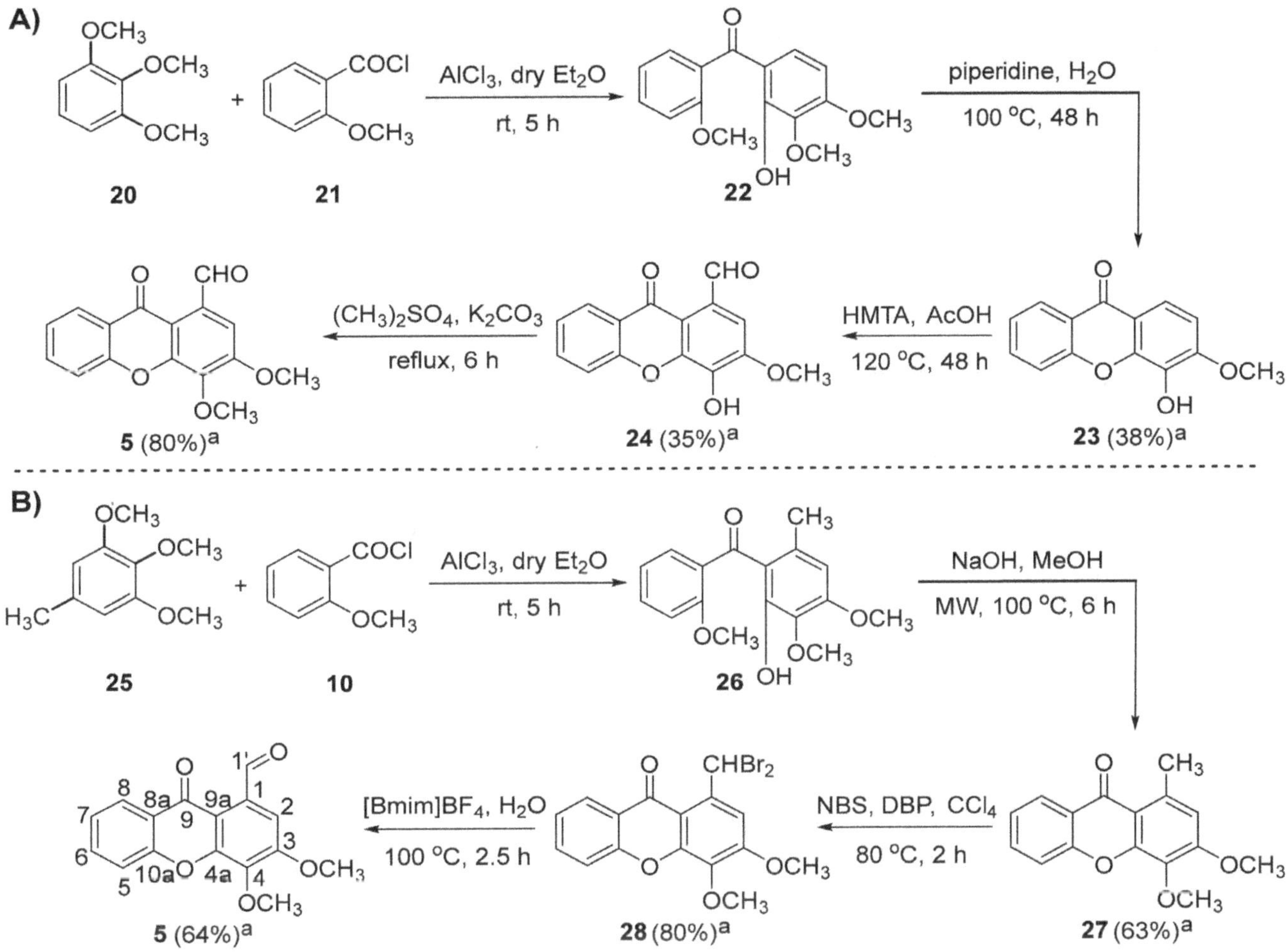

Scheme 1. (**A**) Synthetic route for the preparation of 3,4-dimethoxy-9-oxo-9*H*-xanthene-1-carbaldehyde (**5**) from 1,2,3-trimethoxybenzene (**20**). (**B**) Optimized synthetic route for the preparation of the xanthone **5** using the starting precursor 1,2,3-trimethoxy-5-methylbenzene (**25**). The compound numbering used concerns the nuclear magnetic resonance (NMR) assignments. Note: [BmIm]BF_4 = 1-butyl-3-methylimidazolium tetrafluoroborate; DBP = dibenzoyl peroxide; HMTA = hexamethylenetetramine; NBS = *N*-bromosuccinimide. [a] Isolated yields.

2.1.2. Synthesis of a Library of Aminated Xanthones (**30–40**)

A library of aminated xanthones **30–40** with a 3,4-dioxygenated pattern of substitution was obtained through a one-pot reductive amination of xanthone **5** with the appropriate amine precursors **9–19** (Scheme 2). In one-pot reductive aminations, the selection of the reducing agent is critical for their efficiency, since a suitable agent must reduce the Schiff base intermediate selectively over the carbonylated compounds. As an attempt to investigate the best reaction conditions, a solid-supported reactant containing borohydride (MP-BH_4) combined with methanol were initially employed, since it was successfully used in the reductive amination of a xanthone derivative (data not shown). When these conditions were applied to the reductive amination of **5**, the starting precursor was not completely consumed and the alcohol derivative 1-(hydroxymethyl)-3,4-dimethoxy-9*H*-xanthen-9-one (**29**) was the major product formed. The replacement of the above-mentioned conditions by the milder reducing agent sodium triacetoxyborohydride (STAB) and the solvent tetrahydrofuran allowed a total consumption of the xanthone **5**, favoring the one-pot amination/reduction pathway. Under the reaction conditions described in the Scheme 2, eleven aminated xanthones **30–40** were successfully synthesized in moderate to good yields (11 examples, 39–73% yields).

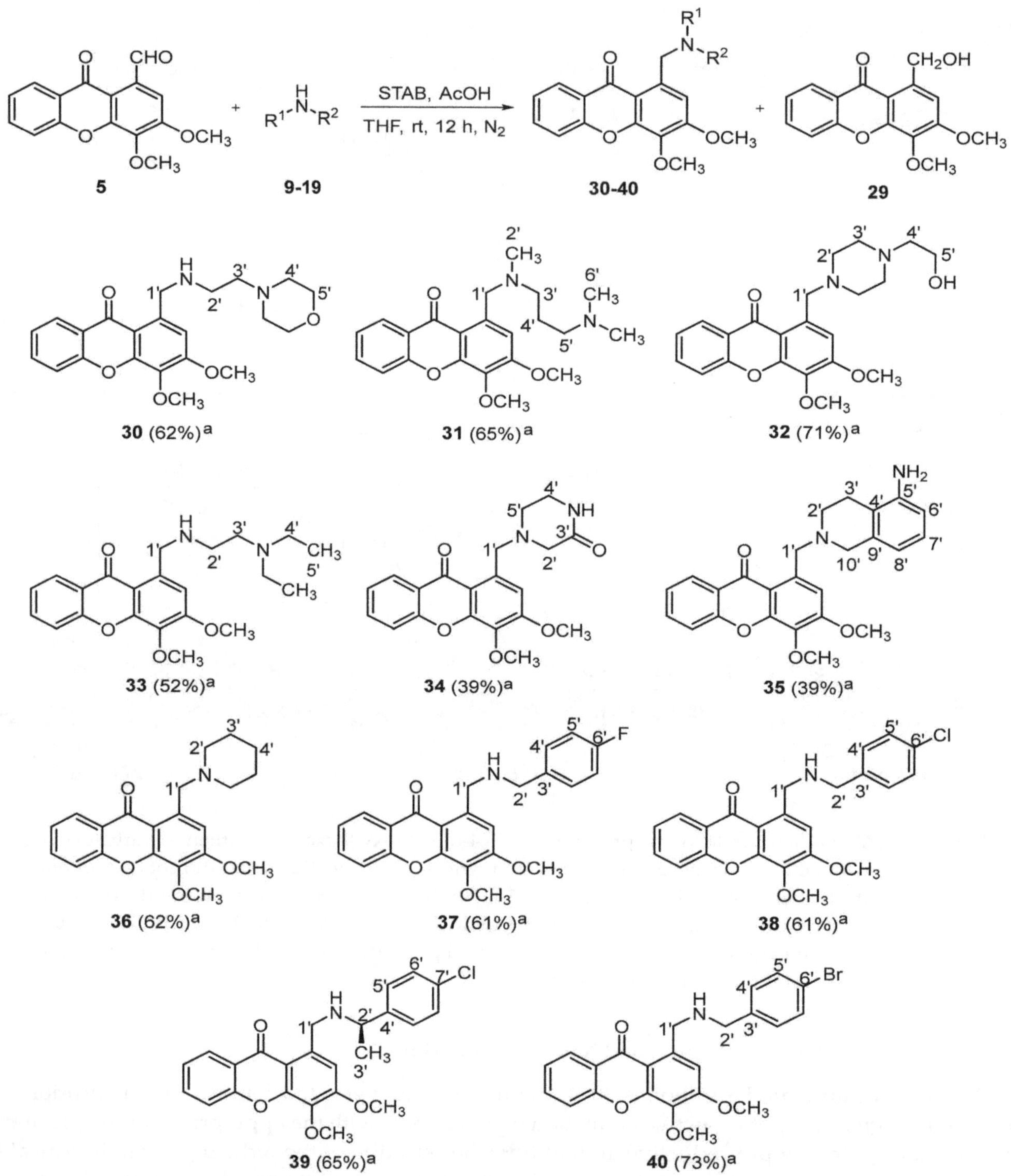

Scheme 2. Reductive amination of **5** with appropriate amine precursors **9–19** for the synthesis of aminated xanthones **30–40** with a 3,4-dioxygenated substitution pattern. The compound numbering used concerns the NMR assignments. [a] Isolated yields.

The structure elucidation of the xanthones **5** and **27–40** was established on the basis of high-resolution mass spectrometry (HRMS) (Figures S1–S15) and nuclear magnetic resonance (NMR) techniques (Figures S16–S45). The ^{13}C-NMR assignments were determined by bidimensional heteronuclear single quantum coherence (HSQC) and heteronuclear multiple bond correlation (HMBC) experiments (Supplementary Materials).

2.2. Biological Activity Evaluation

2.2.1. Effect of Synthesized Xanthone Derivatives **30–40** on the MDM2-p53 Interaction Using A Yeast-Based Screening Assay

Our group has previously developed a yeast-based screening assay to search for potential inhibitors of the MDM2-p53 interaction [30,31,44–46]. In this yeast cell system, the expression of human wt p53 induces a growth inhibition proportional to the degree of its activity (Figure 3, p53, dimethyl sulfoxide (DMSO)). On the other hand, this p53 inhibitory effect is reversed by yeast co-expression of human MDM2 (Figure 3, MDM2-p53, DMSO). This established yeast screening assay was used to study the potential inhibitory effect of 1-20 μM of xanthone derivatives **30–40** on the MDM2-p53 interaction. Figure 3 represents the maximal effect achieved with xanthone derivatives **30–40** at 10 μM. The results showed that only the xanthone **37** caused a significant reversion of the inhibitory effect of MDM2 on p53 (77.01 ± 7.35% of reversion, $n = 3$), with an almost complete reestablishment of the p53 growth inhibitory effect (63.55 ± 4.26% vs. 69.22 ± 2.23%; Figure 3, DMSO-treated p53-expressing yeast vs. xanthone **37**-treated MDM2-p53-expressing yeast). It should be noted that xanthone **37** did not interfere with the growth of control yeast (transformed with empty vectors) or yeast expressing human p53 alone (data not shown). As such, these results indicated that the xanthone **37** behaved as a potential p53-activating agent through inhibition of interaction with MDM2, and it was, therefore, selected for further investigation in human cancer cells.

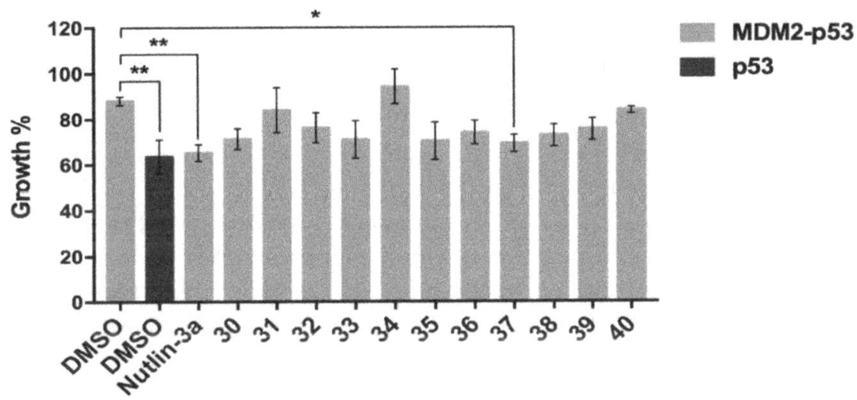

Figure 3. Effect of xanthones **30–40** on the MDM2-p53 interaction using a yeast-based assay. Effect of 10 μM xanthone derivatives **30–40** and nutlin-3A on the growth of yeast co-expressing p53 and MDM2 after 42 h treatment; results were plotted setting as 100% the growth of yeast transformed with the empty vector (control yeast); nutlin-3A (inhibitor of the MDM2-p53 interaction) was used as positive control. Data are mean ± standard error of the mean (SEM) of three independent experiments; mean values were statistically analyzed by one-way analysis of variance (ANOVA) with Tukey's multiple comparisons test, with significant differences from yeast co-expressing MDM2-p53 treated with DMSO. Note: * $p < 0.05$; ** $p < 0.01$.

2.2.2. Evaluation of the Antitumor Activity of Xanthone 37 in Human Cancer Cell Lines

Using the sulforhodamine B (SRB) assay, it was confirmed that xanthone **37** inhibited the growth of human HCT116 $p53^{+/+}$ colon cancer cells, with an IC_{50} (concentration that causes 50% growth inhibition) value of 8.67 ± 0.59 μM ($n = 4$), and of the MDM2-overexpressing human HepG2 liver carcinoma cells, with an IC_{50} value of 18.95 ± 0.39 μM ($n = 4$), after 48 h treatment.

To evaluate the dependency of the antitumor activity of xanthone **37** on the p53 pathway, we next determined the impact of xanthone **37** on the colony forming ability of HCT116 $p53^{+/+}$ cells and on the respective p53-knockout (HCT116 $p53^{-/-}$), using a colony formation assay (Figure 4A). The results showed a significant reduction of the growth inhibitory activity of xanthone **37**, at 3–5 μM in HCT116 $p53^{+/+}$ cells, demonstrating a p53-dependent antitumor effect of xanthone **37**. Accordingly, 10 and 20 μM of xanthone **37** caused a G1-phase cell cycle arrest in HCT116 $p53^{+/+}$ cells, but not in HCT116 p53$^{-/-}$ cells (Figure 4B) after 24 h treatment. It is of note that apoptosis analysis was also investigated by Annexin-V assay; nevertheless, apoptotic events were not detected at 10 and 20 μM of xanthone **37**, after 24 and 48 h treatment. In accordance with these results, we also observed that xanthone **37** upregulated the protein expression levels of MDM2, p53, and p21, in HCT116 p53$^{+/+}$ cells for 24 h treatment (Figure 4C).

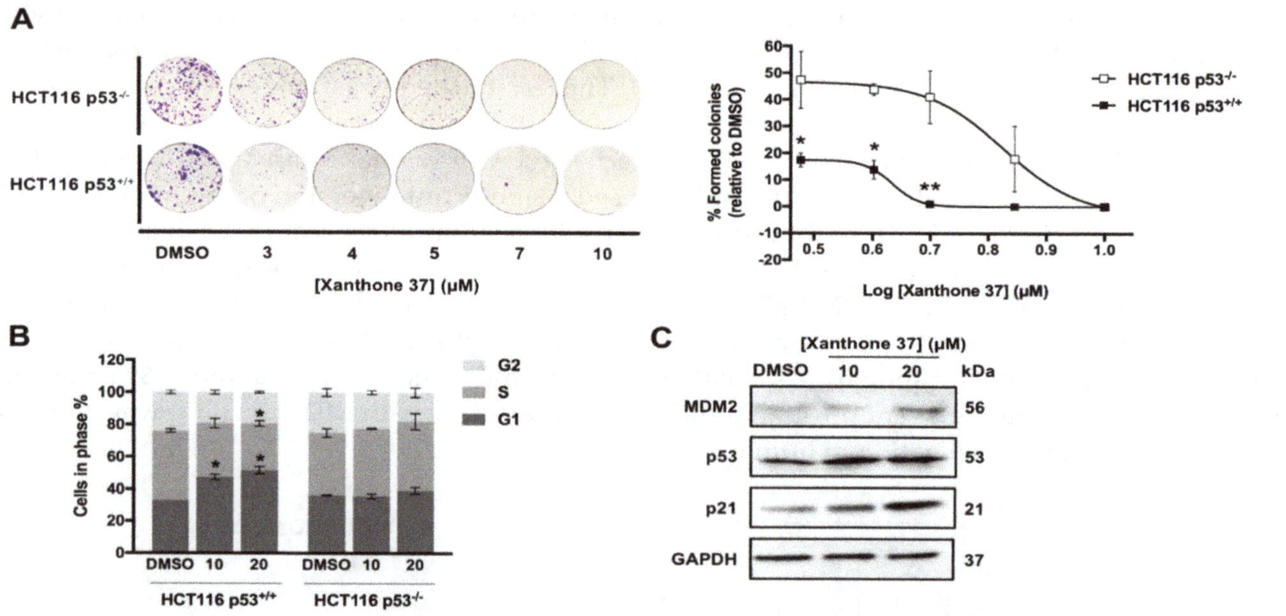

Figure 4. Xanthone **37** inhibits the colony forming capability of HCT116 cells through induction of cell cycle arrest and in a p53-dependent manner. (**A**) Evaluation of colony forming ability in HCT116 p53$^{+/+}$ and HCT116 p53$^{-/-}$ colon cancer cells after 11 days treatment with 3-10 μM of xanthone **37**; results were plotted setting as 100% the colonies formed after treatment with dimethyl sulfoxide (DMSO). (**B**) Effect of 10 and 20 μM of xanthone **37** on cell cycle progression of HCT116 p53$^{+/+}$ and HCT116 p53$^{-/-}$ cells, after 24 h treatment. (**C**) Effect of 10 and 20 μM of xanthone **37** on the expression levels of MDM2, p53, and p21 in HCT116 p53$^{+/+}$ cells analyzed by Western Blot after 24 h treatment. Immunoblots represent one of three independent experiments; Glyceraldehyde 3-phosphate dehydrogenase (GAPDH) was used as loading control. (**A**,**B**) Data are mean ± SEM of three independent experiments; values significantly different from HCT116 p53$^{-/-}$ cells using two-way ANOVA with Sidak's multiple comparisons test (**A**) or DMSO using Student's *t*-test (**B**) are indicated: * $p < 0.05$; ** $p < 0.01$.

Altogether, these results indicated that xanthone **37** had an in vitro p53-dependent antitumor activity mediated by induction of cell cycle arrest.

2.3. *In Slico Studies*

It is common knowledge that the amino-terminal (residues **18–26**) p53 α-helical peptide interacts with a deep hydrophobic cleft within the amino-terminal domain of MDM2 [47]. The MDM2 binding site consists of a large and a small pocket that interact with Phe19/Trp23 and Leu26 of p53, respectively (Figure 5A) [48]. The crystal structure of the MDM2 complexed with the transactivation domain of p53 (Protein Data Bank (PDB) id 1YCR [49]) allowed the visual inspection of the interactions between the Phe19, Trp23, and Leu26 residues of p53 and their respective pockets. Hydrogen-bonding interactions are established between the indole group of Trp23 and carbonyl backbone of Leu54, and between the NH backbone of Phe19 and the carbamoyl group of Gln72. Additional interactions are established between p53 and Leu57, Gly58, Ile61, Met62, Val75, Val93, and His96 residues of MDM2 (Figure 5B).

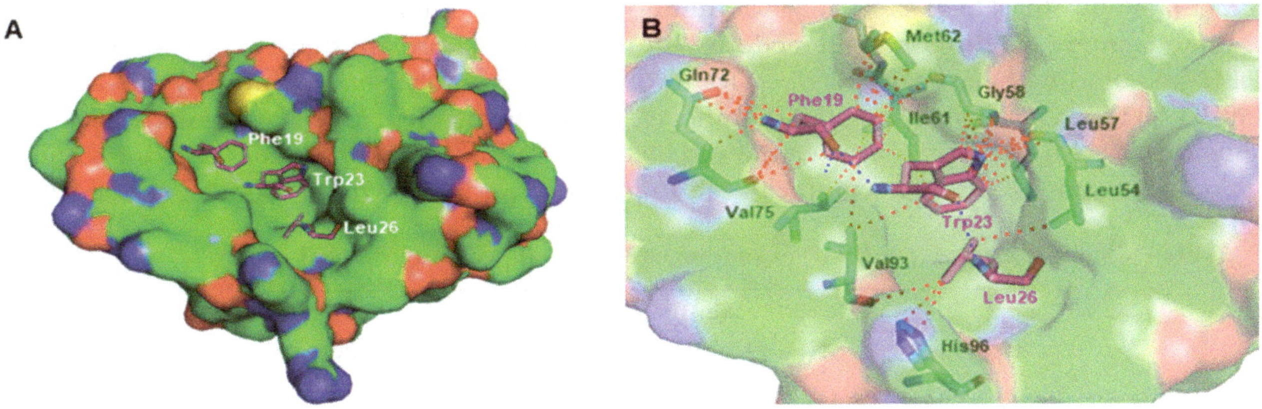

Figure 5. (**A**) Crystallographic p53 (for simplification, only Phe19, Trp23, and Leu26 residues are represented as purple sticks) bound to the three pockets of MDM2 (solid surface). (**B**) Binding mode of crystallographic p53 (for simplification, only residues Phe19, Trp23, and Leu26, are represented as purple sticks) in the hydrophobic cleft of MDM2 (transparent surface); MDM2 amino acid residues involved in interactions with p53 are represented as green sticks. Structural data were obtained from the X-ray crystal structure of MDM2-p53 complex (Protein Data Bank (PDB) id 1YCR). MDM2 is represented as surface, where carbon, oxygen, nitrogen, and sulfur are represented in green, red, blue, and yellow, respectively. Hydrogen-bonding interactions are depicted with a dashed blue line. Other types of interactions are represented as a dashed red line.

The 1.6 Å X-ray crystal structure of the small-molecule inhibitor of MDM2-p53 interaction **1** in complex with MDM2 (PDB id 4HG7 [50]) was selected for further molecular docking studies of the aminated xanthone derivatives **30–40** onto MDM2 protein, using the MDM2-p53 disruptors **1–4** as positive controls. In this work, AutoDock Vina [51] was the software chosen to predict docking conformations, as it has been described as being the best software in predicting crystallographic MDM2-p53 inhibitor poses (root-mean-square deviation (RMSD) < 1.0 Å) by redocking tests [52]. Docking scores for the most stable binding poses of xanthones **30–40** on MDM2 were determined using the AutoDock Vina software [51]. The predicted docking scores for known MDM2-p53 inhibitors (positive controls **1–4**) ranged from −7.7 to −8.0 kcal·mol^{-1} (Table 1). The most stable binding conformation of the synthesized xanthones **30–40** exhibited docking scores from −5.9 to 7.4 kcal· mol^{-1}, therefore being in the same range of binding affinity as the positive controls (Table 1).

Amongst the tested compounds, the xanthone **37** was identified as the most active compound in the yeast-based screening assay. In addition, the predicted free energy values for the most stable binding pose of xanthone **37** were more negative than the majority of the remaining ligands. Therefore, the xanthone **37** was further analyzed in terms of docking poses and residues potentially involved in the interaction with MDM2. Figure 6A shows the most stable conformation of xanthone **37** as suggested by the docking protocol. The xanthone **37** was predicted to interact within the p53-binding site, mimicking the key hydrophobic residues of p53 when bound to MDM2 (docking score of −7.3 kcal·mol^{-1}). Similarly to the binding mode of **1** within the p53-binding site (Figure 6B), no hydrogen-bonding interactions between the xanthone **37** and the MDM2 residues are predicted to be established. The *p*-fluorobenzylamino group of xanthone **37** occupies the Trp23 pocket and makes π-stacking interactions with Phe91 residue, amide-π interactions with the Leu57 and Gly58 residues, and CH-π interactions with the Leu54, Leu57, Gly58, Ile61, Val93, and Ile99 residues. Interestingly, the docking conformation of *p*-fluorobenzylamino group and the *p*-chlorophenyl ring of **1** are identical and superimposable (Figure 6A,B). The methoxy groups of the xanthone scaffold are oriented to the Leu26 pocket and make CH-CH interactions with the Leu54 residue. The adopted scaffold orientation of the xanthone **37** in the hydrophobic cleft where p53 is supposed to bind allows additional interactions to be formed, strengthening the binding of xanthone **37** to MDM2. For example, apart from the Gly58 residue of MDM2, the non-substituted aromatic ring of the xanthone scaffold is predicted to establish π-stacking interactions with the Phe55 residue, and amide-π and CH-π interactions with the Gln59 residue. The establishment of additional interactions within the MDM2 protein that are not observed in the MDM2-p53 binding have been described for a considerable number of high-affinity p53-activating agents [17]. The visual inspection of the xanthone **37** also suggests that an enhancement of its binding affinity towards MDM2 protein can be achieved by molecular modifications in the xanthone scaffold of **37** in order to optimize its interaction with the amino acid residues surrounding the Phe19 pocket.

Table 1. Docking scores (kcal·mol^{-1}) of xanthones **30–40** and positive controls **1–4** onto MDM2 target.

Xanthones 30–40	
Ligands	**Free Energy of the Ligand: MDM2 (kcal·mol^{-1})**
30	−6.6
31	−6.2
32	−6.6
33	−5.9
34	−6.9
35	−7.2
36	−6.6
37	−7.3
38	−7.1
39	−7.3
40	−7.4
Inhibitors of MDM2-p53 Interaction	
Ligands	**Free Energy of the Ligand: MDM2 (kcal·mol^{-1})**
1	−7.7
2	−8.0
3	−7.9
4	−8.0

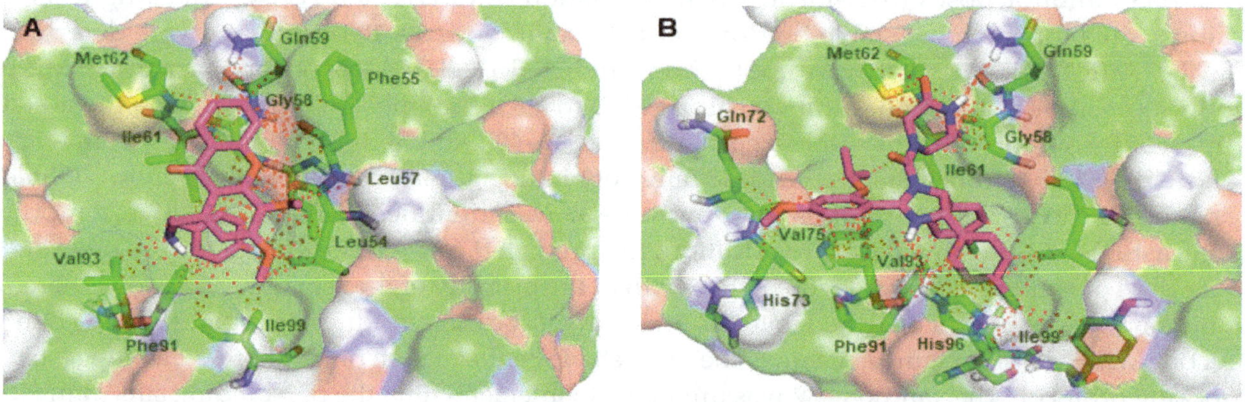

Figure 6. (**A**) Predicted binding pose of the xanthone **37** (purple sticks) in the binding site of MDM2. (**B**) MDM2 (transparent surface) in complex with the crystallographic nutlin-3A (**1**, purple sticks). MDM2 is represented as a transparent surface, where carbon, oxygen, nitrogen, and sulfur are represented in green, red, blue, and yellow, respectively. Small molecule-MDM2 interactions are depicted with a dashed red line. MDM2 residues involved in interactions with the ligands are represented as green sticks and labeled.

3. Materials and Methods

3.1. Chemistry

All reagents and solvents were purchased from Sigma Aldrich (Sigma-Aldrich Co. Ltd., Gillinghan, UK) and no further purification process was implemented. Solvents were evaporated using a rotary evaporator under reduced pressure, Buchi Waterchath B-480. Microwave (MW) reactions were performed using an Ethos MicroSYNTH 1600 Microwave Labstation from Milestone (Thermo Unicam, Portugal). The internal reaction temperature was controlled by a fiber optic probe sensor. All reactions were monitored by thin-layer chromatography (TLC) carried out on precoated plates with 0.2 mm of thickness using Merck silica gel 60 (GF_{254}) with appropriate mobile phases. Compounds **30–40** were easily detectable at 254 nm or 365 nm and after revelation with a solution of ninhydrin in ethanol 3 mg·mL^{-1} (activated by heat).

Flash column chromatography using silica gel 60 (0.040–0.063 mm, Merck, Darmstadt, Germany), flash cartridge chromatography (GraceResolv®, Grace Company, Deerfield, IL, USA), and Discovery® DSC-SCX SPE cationic exchange cartridge (Grace Company, Deerfield, IL, USA) were used in the purification of the synthesized compounds. Melting points (m.p.) were measured in a Köfler microscope (Wagner and Munz, Munich, Germany) and are uncorrected. ^{1}H- and ^{13}C-nuclear magnetic resonance (NMR) spectra were recorded at the University of Aveiro, Department of Chemistry in $CDCl_3$ or DMSO-d_6 (Deutero GmbH, Ely, UK) at room temperature on a Bruker Avance 300 spectrometer (300.13 MHz for ^{1}H and 75.47 MHz for ^{13}C, Bruker Biosciences Corporation, Billerica, MA, USA). Chemical shifts are expressed in δ (ppm) values relative to tetramethylsilane (TMS) as an internal reference. Coupling constants are reported in hertz (Hz). ^{13}C-NMR assignments were made by bidimensional heteronuclear single quantum coherence (HSQC) and heteronuclear multiple bond correlation (HMBC) NMR experiments (long-range C, H coupling constants were optimized to 7 Hz) or by comparison with the assignments of similar molecules. High-resolution mass spectroscopy (HRMS) spectra were measured on a Bruker FTMS APEX III mass spectrometer (Bruker Corporation, Billerica, MA, USA) and recorded as electrospray ionization (ESI) mode in Centro de Apoio Cientifico e Tecnolóxico á Investigación (CACTI, University of Vigo, Pontevedra, Spain). The following compounds were synthesized and purified by the described procedures.

3.1.1. Synthesis of 3,4-dimethoxy-1-methyl-9*H*-xanthen-9-one (**27**)

Xanthone **27** (9.34 g, 63% yield) was synthesized from 1,2,3-trimethoxy-5-methylbenzene (**25**) and characterized according to the previously described procedure [42].

3.1.2. Synthesis of 1-(dibromomethyl)-3,4-dimethoxy-9*H*-xanthen-9-one (**28**)

A mixture of **27** (2.52 g, 9.32 mmol), *N*-bromosuccinimide (3.32 g, 18.7 mmol), and dibenzoyl peroxide (0.68 g, 2.8 mmol) in carbon tetrachloride (25 mL) was refluxed (85 °C) for 2 h. The reaction was monitored using *n*-hexane/ethyl acetate in a proportion of 8:2. Once the reaction was completed, the resulting orange suspension was cooled at 0 °C and stirred for 30 min in an ice bath. The solid was filtered and washed with cold carbon tetrachloride. The filtrate was evaporated under reduced pressure and further purified by flash column chromatography (SiO_2, *n*-hexane/ethyl acetate in gradient) to obtain the **28** as a white powder.

For 1-(dibromomethyl)-3,4-dimethoxy-9*H*-xanthen-9-one (**28**): White powder (3.14 g, 80% yield); melting point (m.p.) 125–127 °C. ^{1}H-NMR ($CDCl_3$, 300.13 MHz): δ = 8.91 (1H, s, H-1), 8.30 (1H, dd, J = 8.0 and 1.6 Hz, H-8), 7.77 (1H, s, H-2), 7.73 (1H, ddd, J = 8.4, 7.0, and 1.6 Hz, H-6), 7.54 (1H, d, J = 8.4 Hz, H-5), 7.39 (1H, ddd, J = 7.5, H-7), 4.11 (3H, s, 4-OCH_3), 4.05 (3H, s, 3-OCH_3) ppm; ^{13}C-NMR ($CDCl_3$, 75.47 MHz): δ = 177.8 (C-9), 156.5 (C-3), 155.0 (C-10a), 150.4 (C-4a), 139.5 (C-4), 137.6 (C-1), 135.0 (C-6), 126.9 (C-8), 124.3 (C-7), 122.0 (C-8a), 117.6 (C-5), 111.9 (C-2), 110.8 (C-9a), 61.9 (3-OCH_3), 56.6 (4-OCH_3), 39.2 (C-1′) ppm. HRMS (ESI$^+$): m/z [$C_{16}H_{12}Br_2O_5$ + H]$^+$ calcd. for [$C_{16}H_{13}Br_2O_5$]: 426.91751; found: 426.91709.

3.1.3. Synthesis of 3,4-dimethoxy-9-oxo-9*H*-xanthene-1-carbaldehyde (**5**)

Xanthone **28** (3.14 g, 7.34 mmol) was added to a solution of 1-butyl-3-methylimidazolium tetrafluoroborate and water (6 mL, 5:1). The mixture was heated at 100 °C with stirring for 2.5 h. The reaction was monitored using *n*-hexane/ethyl acetate in a proportion of 7:3. After completion of the reaction, the resulting suspension was cooled at room temperature, diluted with water (10 mL), and extracted with ethyl acetate (5 × 100 mL). The combined organic layers were dried over anhydrous sodium sulfate, and after filtration of the solution, the solvent was evaporated under reduced pressure. The crude product was then purified by flash column chromatography (SiO_2, *n*-hexane/ethyl acetate in gradient). A light yellow powder corresponding to **5** was obtained.

For 3,4-dimethoxy-9-oxo-9*H*-xanthene-1-carbaldehyde (**5**): Light yellow powder (1.33 g, 64% yield); m.p. > 330 °C. ^{1}H-NMR ($CDCl_3$, 300.13 MHz): δ = 11.21 (1H, s, H-1′), 8.31 (1H, dd, *J* = 8.0 and 1.7 Hz, H-8), 7.77 (1H, ddd, *J* = 8.5, 7.0, and 1.7 Hz, H-6), 7.60 (1H, dd, *J* = 8.5 and 0.8 Hz, H-5), 7.56 (1H, s, H-2), 7.43 (1H, ddd, *J* = 8.0, 7.0, and 0.8 Hz, H-7), 4.11 (3H, s, 4-OCH_3), 4.07 (3H, s, 3-OCH_3) ppm; ^{13}C-NMR ($CDCl_3$, 75.47 MHz): δ = 192.8 (C-1′), 177.9 (C-9), 156.3 (C-3), 155.5 (C-10a), 150.9 (C-4a), 140.7 (C-4), 135.1 (C-6), 133.5 (C-1), 126.7 (C-8), 124.5 (C-7), 121.9 (C-8a), 117.8 (C-5), 116.1 (C-9a), 108.5 (C-2), 61.8 (4-OCH_3), 56.6 (3-OCH_3) ppm. HRMS (ESI$^+$): *m/z* $[C_{16}H_{12}O_5 + H]^+$ calcd. for $[C_{16}H_{13}O_5]$: 285.07575; found: 285.07598; $[C_{16}H_{12}O_5 + Na]^-$ calcd. for $[C_{16}H_{12}NaO_5]$: 307.05769; found 307.05750.

3.1.4. Synthesis of 1-(hydroxymethyl)-3,4-dimethoxy-9*H*-xanthen-9-one (**29**)

Xanthone **29** (52 mg, 52% yield) was synthesized from xanthone **5** and characterized according to the previously described procedure [36].

3.1.5. General Procedure for the Synthesis of Xanthones (**30–40**)

Xanthone **5** (40 mg, 0.141 mmol) was dissolved in tetrahydrofuran (3 mL) and the appropriate amine precursors **9–19** (0.197 mmol) were added to the solution under N_2 gas. After the addition of a 4.0 equimolar quantity of sodium triacetoxyborohydride (119 mg, 0.563 mmol), the resulting mixture was stirred at room temperature for 30 min. Subsequently, a 3.0 equimolar quantity of acetic acid (24 µL 0.423 mmol) was added to the solution, The reaction was carried out at room temperature for 12 h under N_2 gas. For monitoring the synthesis of xanthones **30–40** by TLC, two chromatographic systems were employed: (i) *n*-hexane/ethyl acetate (7:3) and methanol/triethylamine (10:0.1) for xanthones **30–36**; (ii) *n*-hexane/ethyl acetate (7:3) and chloroform/acetone/triethylamine (5:5:0.1) for xanthones **37–40**. Once completed of the reaction, three distinct work-up approaches were employed.

(a) For xanthones **30–32**: the solvent was evaporated under reduced pressure and the resulting crude product was basified with sodium hydroxide (10 mL, 5%, m/v) and extracted with chloroform (3 × 10 mL). The combined organic phases were then acidified and extracted with hydrochloric acid 5 M (3 × 30 mL). Afterwards, the aqueous phases were gathered and then basified with sodium hydroxide (100 mL, 20%, *m/v*). The crude product was extracted successively with chloroform (3 × 100 mL). The organic layers were gathered and dried over anhydrous sodium sulfate. After filtration, the solution was concentrated under reduced pressure, and the resulting crude product was purified by flash cartridge chromatography (SiO_2, chloroform/acetone/ammonium hydroxide, 90:10:1) to afford the xanthones 30, 31, and 32 as pure compounds.

For 3,4-dimethoxy-1-(((2-morpholinoethyl)amino)methyl)-9*H*-xanthen-9-one (**30**): Green powder (35 mg, 62% yield); m.p. 125–126 °C. ^{1}H-NMR ($CDCl_3$, 300.13 MHz): δ = 8.25 (1H, dd, *J* = 8.0 and 1.6 Hz, H-8), 7.72 (1H, ddd, *J* = 8.1, 7.0, and 1.6 Hz, H-6), 7.57 (1H, dd, *J* = 8.4 and 0.8 Hz, H-5), 7.38 (1H, ddd, *J* = 8.0, 7.1, and 0.9 Hz, H-7), 7.09 (1H, s, H-2), 4.34 (2H, s, H-1′); 4.04 (3H, s, 4-OCH_3), 4.01 (3H, s, 3-OCH_3), 3.66 (4H, t, *J* = 4.6 Hz, H-5′), 2.90 (2H, t, *J* = 6.1 Hz, H-2′), 2.60 (2H, t, *J* = 6.1 Hz, H-3′), 2.47 (4H, t, *J* = 4.3 Hz, H-4′) ppm; ^{13}C-NMR ($CDCl_3$, 75.47 MHz): δ = 178.0 (C-9), 156.5 (C-3), 155.3 (C-10a), 152.1 (C-4a), 137.0 (C-1), 136.0 (C-4), 134.6 (C-6), 126.5 (C-8), 124.1 (C-7), 122.1 (C-8a), 117.7 (C-5), 114.6 (C-9a), 111.6 (C-2), 67.0 (C-5′), 61.5 (4-OCH_3), 57.4 (C-2′), 56.4 (3-OCH_3), 53.7 (C-1′), 53.5 (C-4′), 45.3 (C-3′) ppm. HRMS (ESI$^+$): *m/z* $[C_{22}H_{26}N_2O_5 + H]^+$ calcd. for $[C_{22}H_{27}N_2O_5]$: 399.19145; found: 399.19060.

For 1-(((3-(dimethylamino)propyl)(methyl)amino)methyl)-3,4-dimethoxy-9*H*-xanthen-9-one (**31**): White powder (35 mg, 65% yield); m.p. 84–85 °C. ^{1}H-NMR ($CDCl_3$, 300.13 MHz): δ = 8.25 (1H, dd, *J* = 8.0 and 1.6 Hz, H-8), 7.69 (1H, ddd, *J* = 8.5, 7.0, and 1.6 Hz, H-6), 7.54 (1H, dd, *J*= 7.4 and 0.7, H-5), 7.53 (1H, s, H-2), 7.35 (1H, ddd, *J* = 8.0, 7.1, and 1.0 Hz, H-7), 4.36 (2H, s, H-1′); 4.05 (3H, s, 4-OCH_3),

4.02 (3H, s, 3-OCH_3), 2.65 (2H, t, J = 7.2 Hz, H-3′), 2.44 (2H, t, J = 7.5 Hz, H-5′), 2.39 (3H, s, H-2′), 2.28 (6H, s, H-6′), 1.82 (2H, m, J = 7.3 Hz, H-4′) ppm; ^{13}C-NMR ($CDCl_3$, 75.47 MHz): δ = 178.1 (C-9), 156.6 (C-3), 155.2 (C-10a), 151.9 (C-4a), 135.2 (C-1), 135.0 (C-4), 134.2 (C-6), 126.6 (C-8), 123.9 (C-7), 122.4 (C-8a), 117.6 (C-5), 114.5 (C-9a), 109.0 (C-2), 61.5 (4-OCH_3), 60.1 (C-1′), 57.8 (C-5′), 56.4 (3-OCH_3), 56.1 (C-3′), 45.3 (C-6′), 42.5 (C-2′), 25.3 (C-4′) ppm. HRMS (ESI$^+$): *m/z* [$C_{22}H_{28}N_2O_4$ + H]$^+$ calcd. for [$C_{22}H_{29}N_2O_4$]: 385.21218; found: 385.21139.

For 1-((4-(2-hydroxyethyl)piperazin-1-yl)methyl)-3,4-dimethoxy-9*H*-xanthen-9-one (**32**): Yellow powder (40 mg, 71% yield); m.p. 129–130 °C. ^{1}H-NMR ($CDCl_3$, 300.13 MHz): δ = 8.25 (1H, dd, J = 8.0 and 1.6 Hz, H-8), 7.68 (1H, ddd, J = 8.5, 7.0, and 1.6 Hz, H-6), 7.53 (1H, dd, J = 8.4 and 0.7 Hz, H-5), 7.48 (1H, s, H-2), 7.35 (1H, ddd, J = 8.0, 7.1, and 1.0 Hz, H-7), 4.32 (2H, s, H-1′), 4.03 (3H, s, 4-OCH_3), 4.01 (3H, s, 3-OCH_3), 3.63 (2H, t, J = 5.4 Hz), 2.58 (2H, t, J = 5.4 Hz) ppm; ^{13}C-NMR ($CDCl_3$, 75.47 MHz): δ = 178.1 (C-9), 156.5 (C-3), 155.2 (C-10a), 152.0 (C-4a), 138.8 (C-1), 134.8 (C-4), 134.2 (C-6), 126.6 (C-8), 123.9 (C-7), 122.5 (C-8a), 117.5 (C-5), 114.6 (C-9a), 108.2 (C-2), 61.5 (4-OCH_3), 60.2 (C-1′), 59.3 (C-5′), 57.7 (C-4′), 56.2 (3-OCH_3), 53.5 (C-3′), 53.2 (C-2′) ppm. HRMS (ESI$^+$): *m/z* [$C_{22}H_{26}N_2O_5$ + H]$^+$ calcd. for [$C_{22}H_{27}N_2O_5$]: 399.19145; found: 399.19059.

(b) For xanthones **33**–**36**: the solvent was evaporated under reduced pressure and the crude product was extracted with chloroform (3 × 10 mL). The organic phases were gathered, dried over anhydrous sodium sulfate, and after filtration, the resulting solution was concentrated under reduced pressure. Then, a solid phase extraction using a cation exchange cartridge Discovery® DSC-SCX was applied to further purify the crude product. Initially, an activation of the cartridge with methanol (100 mL) was carried out followed by loading the cartridge with the sample. Then, the elution was performed with the following solvents/solutions: (i) dichloromethane/methanol (5:5), (ii) methanol, and (iii) ammonium hydroxide/methanol (2%, *v/v*). The fractions obtained from the elution with ammonium hydroxide/methanol (2%, *v/v*) were gathered and the solvent was evaporated under reduced pressure. A flash cartridge chromatography with chloroform/acetone/ammonium hydroxide (90:10:1) was also performed to obtain the xanthones **33**, **34**, **35**, and **36** as pure compounds.

For 1-(((2-(diethylamino)ethyl)amino)methyl)-3,4-dimethoxy-9*H*-xanthen-9-one (**33**): Green powder (28 mg, 52% yield); m.p. 68–69 °C. ^{1}H-NMR ($CDCl_3$, 300.13 MHz): δ = 8.27 (1H, dd, J = 8.0 and 1.4 Hz, H-8), 7.71 (1H, ddd, J = 8.5, 7.0, and 1.6 Hz, H-6), 7.56 (1H, dd, J = 8.4 and 0.7 Hz, H-5), 7.37 (1H, ddd, J = 8.0, 7.1, and 1.0 Hz, H-7), 7.14 (1H, s, H-2), 4.39 (2H, s, H-1′); 4.05 (3H, s, 4-OCH_3), 4.01 (3H, s, 3-OCH_3), 2.87 (2H, t, J = 6.4 Hz, H-2′), 2.68 (2H, t, J = 6.4 Hz, H-3′), 2.55 (4H, m, J = 7.1 Hz, H-4′), 1.01 (6H, t, J = 7.1 Hz, H-5′) ppm; ^{13}C-NMR ($CDCl_3$, 75.47 MHz): δ = 178.1 (C-9), 156.5 (C-3), 155.3 (C-10a), 152.1 (C-4a), 137.4 (C-1), 135.8 (C-4), 134.5 (C-6), 126.6 (C-8), 124.0 (C-7), 122.2 (C-8a), 117.7 (C-5), 114.5 (C-9a), 111.1 (C-2), 61.5 (4-OCH_3), 56.4 (3-OCH_3), 53.4 (C-3′), 52.4 (C-1′), 46.9 (C-4′), 46.8 (C-2′), 11.6 (C-5′) ppm. HRMS (ESI$^+$): *m/z* [$C_{22}H_{28}N_2O_4$ + H]$^+$ calcd. for [$C_{22}H_{29}N_2O_4$]: 385.21218; found: 385.21150.

For 4-((3,4-dimethoxy-9-oxo-9*H*-xanthen-1-yl)methyl)piperazin-2-one (**34**): Orange powder (20 mg, 39% yield); m.p. 245–247 °C. ^{1}H-NMR (DMSO-d_6, 300.13 MHz): δ = 8.13 (1H, dd, J = 8.0 and 1.5 Hz, H-8), 7.82 (1H, ddd, J = 8.5, 7.0, and 1.6 Hz, H-6), 7.65 (1H, dd, J = 8.4 and 0.6, H-5), 7.45 (1H, ddd, J = 8.0, 7.1, and 1.0 Hz, H-7), 7.36 (1H, s, H-2), 4.24 (2H, s, H-1′); 3.98 (3H, s, 4-OCH_3), 3.90 (3H, s, 3-OCH_3), 3.20 (2H, t, J = 5.3 Hz, H-5′), 3.13 (2H, s, H-2′), 2.66 (2H, t, J = 5.3 Hz, H-4′) ppm; ^{13}C-NMR (DMSO-d_6, 75.47 MHz): δ = 176.7 (C-9), 168.0 (C-3′), 156.2 (C-3), 154.6 (C-10a), 151.8 (C-4a), 136.9 (C-1), 135.0 (C-4), 134.7 (C-6), 126.1 (C-8), 124.3 (C-7), 121.8 (C-8a), 117.7 (C-5), 113.7 (C-9a), 109.2 (C-2), 60.9 (4-OCH_3), 58.5 (C-1′), 57.2 (C-5′), 56.3 (3-OCH_3), 48.7 (C-2′), 30.7 (C-4′) ppm. HRMS (ESI$^+$): *m/z* [$C_{20}H_{20}N_2O_5$ + H]$^+$ calcd. for [$C_{20}H_{21}N_2O_5$]: 369.14450; found: 369.14369.

For 1-((5-amino-3,4-dihydroisoquinolin-2(1*H*)-yl)methyl)-3,4-dimethoxy-9*H*-xanthen-9-one (**35**): White powder (23 mg, 39% yield); m.p. 171–172 °C. ^{1}H-NMR ($CDCl_3$, 300.13 MHz): δ = 8.26 (1H, dd, J = 8.0 and 1.4 Hz, H-8), 7.69 (1H, ddd, J = 8.5, 7.0, and 1.6 Hz, H-6), 7.57 (1H, s, H-2), 7.54 (1H, dd, J = 8.4 and 0.7 Hz, H-5), 7.35 (1H, ddd, J = 8.0, 7.1, and 1.0 Hz, H-7), 6.99 (1H, t, J = 7.7 Hz, H-7′), 6.57 (1H, d, J = 7.8 Hz, H-6′), 6.53 (1H, d, J = 7.6 Hz, H-8′), 4.48 (2H, s, H-1′); 4.02 (3H, s, 4-OCH_3), 3.97

(3H, s, 3-OCH_3), 3.81 (2H, s, H-10′), 2.93 (2H, t, J = 5.9 Hz, H-2′), 2.66 (2H, t, J = 5.9 Hz, H-3′) ppm; ^{13}C-NMR ($CDCl_3$, 75.47 MHz): δ = 178.2 (C-9), 156.7 (C-3), 155.2 (C-10a), 151.9 (C-4a), 144.1 (C-5′), 139.3 (C-1), 136.3 (C-9′), 134.8 (C-4), 134.2 (C-6), 126.6 (C-8), 126.4 (C-7′), 123.8 (C-7), 122.5 (C-8a), 119.5 (C-4′), 117.6 (C-5), 117.1 (C-8′), 114.5 (C-9a), 112.7 (C-6′), 108.0 (C-2), 61.5 (4-OCH_3), 60.1 (C-1′), 56.7 (C-10′), 56.3 (3-OCH_3), 51.0 (C-2′), 24.9 (C-3′) ppm. HRMS (ESI$^+$): *m/z* [$C_{25}H_{24}N_2O_4$ + H]$^+$ calcd. for [$C_{25}H_{25}N_2O_4$]: 417.18088; found: 417.18018.

For 3,4-dimethoxy-1-(piperidin-1-ylmethyl)-9*H*-xanthen-9-one (**36**): Yellow powder (31 mg, 62% yield); m.p. 108-109 °C. ^{1}H-NMR ($CDCl_3$, 300.13 MHz): δ = 8.25 (1H, dd, J = 8.0 and 1.6 Hz, H-8), 7.66 (1H, ddd, J = 8.5, 8.0, and 1.6 Hz, H-6), 7.56 (1H, s, H-2), 7.52 (1H, dd, J = 8.3 and 0.7 Hz, H-5), 7.33 (1H, ddd, J = 7.9, 7.1, and 0.9 Hz, H-7), 4.26 (2H, s, H-1′); 4.03 (3H, s, 4-OCH_3), 4.01 (3H, s, 3-OCH_3), 2.57 (4H, t, J = 4.6 Hz, H-2′), 1.65 (4H, m, J = 5.5 Hz, H-3′), 1,50 (2H, m, J = 5.5 Hz, H-4′) ppm; ^{13}C-NMR ($CDCl_3$, 75.47 MHz) ppm: δ = 177.5 (C-9), 156.1 (C-3), 154.7 (C-10a), 151.3 (C-4a), 138.9 (C-4), 134.2 (C-1), 133.8 (C-6), 126.0 (C-8), 123.3 (C-7), 121.9 (C-8a), 117.1 (C-5), 113.9 (C-9a), 107.8 (C-2), 60.8 (4-OCH_3), 56.1 (3-OCH_3), 55.7 (C-2′), 54.3 (C-1′), 25.7 (C-3′), 23.8 (C-4′) ppm. HRMS (ESI$^+$): *m/z* [$C_{21}H_{23}NO_4$ + H]$^+$ calcd. for [$C_{21}H_{24}NO_4$]: 354.16998; found: 354.16939.

(c) For xanthones **37**–**40**: the solvent was evaporated under reduced pressure and the resulting crude product was basified with sodium hydroxide (10 mL, 5%, *m/v*) and extracted with chloroform (3 × 10 mL). The combined organic phases were then acidified and extracted with hydrochloric acid 5 M (3 × 30 mL). The resulting organic phase was dried over anhydrous sodium sulfate and, after filtration, the solution was concentrated under reduced pressure. Then, a solid phase extraction using a cation exchange cartridge Discovery® DSC-SCX was applied to further purify the crude product. Initially, an activation of the cartridge with methanol (100 mL) was carried out followed by loading the cartridge with the sample. Then, the elution was performed with the following solvents/solutions: (i) dichloromethane/methanol (5:5), (ii) methanol, and (iii) ammonium hydroxide/methanol (2%, *v/v*). The fractions obtained from the elution with ammonium hydroxide/methanol (2%, *v/v*) were gathered and the solvent was evaporated under reduced pressure to furnish the xanthones **37**, **38**, **39**, and **40** as pure compounds.

For 1-(((4-fluorobenzyl)amino)methyl)-3,4-dimethoxy-9*H*-xanthen-9-one (**37**): White powder, (34 mg, 61% yield); m.p. 163–165 °C. ^{1}H-NMR ($CDCl_3$, 300.13 MHz): δ = 8.28 (1H, dd, J = 8.0 and 1.6 Hz, H-8), 7.71 (1H, ddd, J = 8.5, 7.0, and 1.6 Hz, H-6), 7.55 (1H, dd, J = 8.5 and 0.8 Hz, H-5), 7.40 (1H, ddd, J = 8.0, 7.0, and 0.8 Hz, H-7), 7.36 (2H, m, H-5′), 7.01 (2H, m, H-4′), 6.96 (1H, s, H-2), 4.30 (2H, s, H-1′), 4.01 (3H, s, 4-OCH_3), 4.01 (3H, s, 3-OCH_3), 3.85 (2H, s, H-2′) ppm; ^{13}C-NMR ($CDCl_3$, 75.47 MHz): δ = 178.1 (C-9), 160.3 (C-6′), 156.3 (C-3), 155.3 (C-10a), 152.2 (C-4a), 138.6 (C-4), 135.9 (C-3′), 135.7 (C-1), 134.5 (C-6), 129.8 (C-5′), 126.7 (C-8), 124.0 (C-7), 122.2 (C-8a), 117.7 (C-5), 115.3 (C-4′), 114.7 (C-9a), 110.9 (C-2), 61.5 (4-OCH_3), 56.3 (3-OCH_3), 53.3 (C-1′), 52.5 (C-2′) ppm. HRMS (ESI$^+$): *m/z* [$C_{23}H_{20}FNO_4$ + H]$^+$ calcd. for [$C_{23}H_{21}FNO_4$]: 394.14491; found: 394.14410.

For 1-(((4-chlorobenzyl)amino)methyl)-3,4-dimethoxy-9*H*-xanthen-9-one (**38**): Light yellow powder (35 mg, 61% yield); m.p. 162–163 °C. ^{1}H-NMR ($CDCl_3$, 300.13 MHz): δ = 8.25 (1H, dd, J = 8.0 and 1.6 Hz, H-8), 7.79 (1H, ddd, J = 8.5, 7.0, and 1.6 Hz, H-6), 7.66 (2H, m, H-5′), 7.60 (1H, dd, J = 8.5 and 0.9 Hz, H-5), 7.43 (1H, ddd, J = 8.0, 7.0, and 0.9 Hz, H-7), 7.39 (1H, s, H-2), 7.38 (2H, m, H-4′), 4.53 (2H, s, H-2′); 4.33 (2H, s, H-1′), 4.07 (3H, s, 4-OCH_3), 4.01 (3H, s, 3-OCH_3) ppm; ^{13}C-NMR ($CDCl_3$, 75.47 MHz): δ = 179.6 (C-9), 157.0 (C-3), 155.5 (C-10a), 152.0 (C-4a), 137.7 (C-4), 135.8 (C-1), 135.6 (C-6), 131.7 (C-5′), 129.5 (C-4′), 129.4 (C-3′), 127.3 (C-6′), 126.6 (C-8), 124.6 (C-7), 121.3 (C-8a), 117.9 (C-5), 115.5 (C-2), 114.8 (C-9a), 61.6 (4-OCH_3), 57.1 (3-OCH_3), 51.3 (C-1′), 50.7 (C-2′) ppm. HRMS (ESI$^+$): *m/z* [$C_{23}H_{20}ClNO_4$ + H]$^+$ calcd. for [$C_{23}H_{21}ClNO_4$]: 410.11536; found: 410.11466.

For (*R*)-1-(((1-(4-chlorophenyl)ethyl)amino)methyl)-3,4-dimethoxy-9*H*-xanthen-9-one (**39**): White powder (39 mg, 65% yield); m.p. 163–164 °C. ^{1}H-NMR ($CDCl_3$, 300.13 MHz): δ = 8.26 (1H, dd, J = 8.0 and 1.6 Hz, H-8), 7.79 (1H, ddd, J = 8.5, 7.0, and 1.6 Hz, H-6), 7.70 (2H, m, H-6′), 7.59 (1H, dd, J = 8.5 and 0.8 Hz, H-5), 7.43 (1H, ddd, J = 8.0, 7.0, and 0.8 Hz, H-7), 7.42 (2H, m, H-5′), 7.25 (1H, s, H-2), 4.54 (2H, s, H-1′); 4.27 (1H, q, J = 6.8 Hz, H-1′), 4.04 (3H, s, 4-OCH_3), 4.01 (3H, s, 3-OCH_3),

1.83 (3H, d, $J = 6.8$ Hz, H-3′) ppm; ^{13}C-NMR ($CDCl_3$, 75.47 MHz): $\delta = 179.6$ (C-9), 156.8 (C-3), 155.4 (C-10a), 151.9 (C-4a), 137.6 (C-4), 135.5 (C-6), 134.5 (C-1), 131.8 (C-7′), 129.8 (C-6′), 129.5 (C-5′), 127.3 (C-4′), 126.6 (C-8), 124.6 (C-7), 121.3 (C-8a), 117.9 (C-5), 115.6 (C-2), 114.9 (C-9a), 61.6 (4-OCH_3), 58.9 (C-2′), 57.0 (3-OCH_3), 50.2 (C-1′), 20.2 (C-3′) ppm. HRMS (ESI$^+$): *m/z* [$C_{24}H_{22}ClNO_4$ + H]$^+$ calcd. for [$C_{24}H_{23}ClNO_4$]: 424.13101; found: 424.13018.

For 1-(((4-bromobenzyl)amino)methyl)-3,4-dimethoxy-9*H*-xanthen-9-one (**40**): White powder (47 mg, 73% yield); m.p. 161–162 °C. ^{1}H-NMR ($CDCl_3$, 300.13 MHz): $\delta = 8.27$ (1H, dd, $J = 8.0$ and 1.6 Hz, H-8), 7.73 (1H, ddd, $J = 8.5$, 7.0, and 1.6 Hz, H-6), 7.58 (1H, dd, $J = 8.5$ and 0.8 Hz, H-5), 7.48 (2H, m, H-5′), 7.39 (2H, m, H-4′), 7.38 (1H, ddd, $J = 8.0$, 7.0, and 0.8 Hz, H-7), 7.08 (1H, s, H-2), 4.31 (2H, s, H-1′); 4.01 (3H, s, 4-OCH_3), 4.01 (3H, s, 3-OCH_3), 3.88 (2H, s, H-2′) ppm; ^{13}C-NMR ($CDCl_3$, 75.47 MHz): $\delta = 178.6$ (C-9), 156.5 (C-3), 155.3 (C-10a), 152.2 (C-4a), 136.4 (C-4), 136.2 (C-1), 134.9 (C-6), 131.8 (C-5′), 130.7 (C-4′), 128.4 (C-3′), 126.6 (C-8), 124.2 (C-7), 121.9 (C-8a), 121.8 (C-6′), 117.7 (C-5), 114.7 (C-9a), 112.5 (C-2), 61.6 (4-OCH_3), 56.7 (3-OCH_3), 52.7 (C-1′), 52.0 (C-2′) ppm. HRMS (ESI$^+$): *m/z* [$C_{23}H_{20}BrNO_4$ + H]$^+$ calcd. for [$C_{23}H_{21}BrNO_4$]: 454.06485; found: 454.06385.

3.2. *Biological Evaluation*

3.2.1. Yeast Strains and Growth Conditions

For the yeast assay, the previously obtained *Saccharomyces cerevisiae* cells co-expressing human p53 or human MDM2, as well as yeast control (transformed with empty vectors) [30,31], were used. To induce expression of human proteins, yeast cells were grown in selective induction medium with 2% (*w/w*) galactose and 2% (*w/w*) raffinose, in the presence of 1–20 μM of xanthones **30–40** or 0.1% DMSO, at 30 °C under continuous orbital shaking (200 rpm) for approximately 42 h, as described [30,31]. Yeast cell growth was analyzed by counting the number of colony-forming units (CFU) after 2 days incubation at 30 °C on Sabouraud Dextrose Agar plates from Liofilchem (Frilabo, Porto, Portugal). Results were estimated considering 100% growth as the number of CFU obtained with untreated yeast co-expressing p53 and MDM2.

3.2.2. Human Cancer Cell Lines and Culture Conditions

Human colon adenocarcinoma HCT116 cell lines expressing wt p53 (HCT116 p53$^{+/+}$) and its p53-null isogenic derivative (HCT116 p53$^{-/-}$) were provided by B. Vogelstein (The Johns Hopkins Kimmel Cancer Center, Baltimore, MD, USA). Human liver HepG2 carcinoma cell lines were purchased from ATCC (Rockville, MD, USA). Cancer cells were cultured in RPMI-1640 medium with ultraglutamine (Lonza, VWR, Carnaxide, Portugal), and supplemented with 10% fetal bovine serum (FBS; Merck Millipore, VWR). Cells were maintained at 37 °C in a humidified atmosphere of 5% CO_2.

3.2.3. Cell Proliferation Assay

Cell proliferation was determined using the SRB assay, as described [30,31]. Briefly, cells were seeded in 96-well plates at 5.0×10^3 cells/well for HCT116 p53$^{+/+}$ cells and 4.0×10^3 cells/well for HepG2 and 24 h later treated with serial dilutions (3.13–50 μM) of xanthone **37** or 0.25% DMSO for 48 h. IC_{50} values were determined from the concentration-response curves.

3.2.4. Colony Formation Assay

HCT116 p53$^{+/+}$ and HCT116 p53$^{-/-}$ cells were seeded in a 6-well plate at 1.0×10^3 cells/well and treated with 3, 4, 5, 7, and 10 μM of xanthone **37** or DMSO at the time of seeding. After 11 days incubation, colonies were fixed using 10% of methanol and 10% acetic acid for 10 min and stained with 0.5% crystal violet (Sigma-Aldrich) in 1:1 methanol/water for 15 min. Colonies with more than 20 cells were counted.

3.2.5. Cell Cycle Analysis

HCT116 p53$^{+/+}$ and HCT116 p53$^{-/-}$ cells were seeded in a 6-well plate at 1.5×10^5 cells/well for 24 h and treated with 10 and 20 μM of xanthone **37** or DMSO for 24 h. Cells were collected, fixed, and stained with propidium iodide (Fluka, Sigma-Aldrich). Cell cycle was analyzed by flow cytometry, as described [45].

3.2.6. Western Blot Analysis

HCT116 p53$^{+/+}$ were seeded in a 6-well plate at 1.5×10^5 cells/well for 24 h and treated with 10 and 20 μM of xanthone **37** or DMSO for 24 h. Total protein extracts of cancer cells were obtained and analyzed by Western blot, as described [45]. Membranes were probed with a mouse monoclonal anti-p53 (DO-1), anti-MDM2 (D-12), or with a rabbit polyclonal anti-p21 (C-19), followed by an anti-mouse or anti-rabbit horseradish-peroxidase (HRP)-conjugated secondary antibody. For loading control, membranes were stripped and re-probed with mouse monoclonal anti-GAPDH (6C5). All antibodies were purchased from Santa Cruz Biotechnology (Frilabo, Porto, Portugal). The signal was detected with enhanced chemiluminescence (ECL) Amersham Kit from GE Healthcare (VWR) and with Molecular Imager® ChemiDoc™ XRS+ System, using Image Lab™ software.

3.2.7. Statistical Analysis

Data's statistical analysis was performed using the Prism 7 program (GraphPad Software Inc., California, USA). Differences between means were tested for significance using one-way ANOVA with Tukey's multiple comparisons test, two-way ANOVA with Sidak's multiple comparisons test, and Student's *t*-test (* $p < 0.05$; ** $p < 0.01$).

3.3. In Silico Studies onto MDM2

The chemical structures of gambogic acid (**2**), α-mangostin (**3**), 12-hydroxy-2,2-dimethyl-3,4-dihydro-2*H*,6*H*-pyrano[3,2-*b*]xanthen-6-one (**4**), and the xanthones **30–40** were drawn using ChemSketch (Advanced Chemistry Development, Inc. (ACD/Labs), Canada); the structure of known MDM2-p53 inhibitor nutlin-3A (**1**) was obtained from PubChem [53]. The three-dimensional (3D) structures of the xanthones and **1** were minimized using the ArgusLab version 4.0.1 software for Windows by Hamiltonian (quantum mechanics) using the Parameterized Model number 3 (PM3) semi-empirical method [54]. The 3D structure of MDM2 was extracted from Protein Data Bank (PDB id 4HG7) [50]. Docking simulations involving MDM2 and the small molecules were undertaken in AutoDock Vina (Scripps Research Institute, USA) [51]. AutoDock Vina considered the macromolecular target conformation as a rigid unit, while the ligands were allowed to be flexible and adaptable to the target. Vina explored the lowest binding affinity conformations and returned nine different conformations for each ligand. AutoDock Vina was run using an exhaustiveness of 8 and a grid box with the dimensions of 19.7 Å, 26.1 Å, and 14.1 Å, engulfing the binding cavity occupied by the crystallographic nutlin-3A (PDB id 4HG7). Ligand conformations and interactions with the binding cavity were visualized using PyMOL version 1.3 [55]. In order to validate the docking approach for the macromolecular target structure used, nutlin-3A was docked onto the binding cavity of MDM2 using AutoDock Vina, and the obtained docking conformation was compared to crystallographic nutlin-3A (PDB id 4HG7) using RMSD (not shown). Docking scores of xanthones and positive controls were compared.

4. Conclusions

An alternative and efficient strategy for the preparation of carbaldehydic xanthones was successfully developed. The use of a precursor with a methyl substituent at position C-1 revealed to be crucial for the optimization of the synthesis of **5**. The newly described approach required lower reaction times and enabled the preparation of xanthone **5** in a higher global yield. In this work, a series of eleven aminated xanthones (**30–40**) possessing a 3,4-dioxygenated pattern of substitution was efficiently constructed in moderate to good yields. From this group of compounds, xanthone **37** was identified for the first time as a putative p53-activating agent, using a yeast-based screening assay. Xanthone **37** was revealed to inhibit the growth of human HCT116 $p53^{+/+}$ colon cancer cells, being that this effect is associated with cell cycle arrest through activation of the p53 pathway. Nevertheless, further studies are required to confirm the mechanism of action of **37**, which may lead to the identification of a novel xanthone derivative with promising antitumor activity.

These results demonstrated the potential usefulness of coupling amine-containing structural motifs of known MDM2-p53 disruptors into the 3,4-dioxygenated xanthone scaffold as a starting point for the design of novel and improved p53-activating agents with antitumor activity and drug-like properties.

Author Contributions: A.L. performed the in silico studies and the synthesis of xanthones and wrote the manuscript. A.L., A.S.G., and J.B.L. performed biological experiments and analyzed the data. P.B. contributed to the experimental synthetic work. M.E.S. and L.S. conceived and designed the study, coordinated the experimental work, and wrote the manuscript. A.P. coordinated the in silico studies. M.M.M.P., M.E.S., and L.S. provided financial support for the study, analyzed the data, and wrote the manuscript.

References

1. Lane, D.P. Cancer. p53, guardian of the genome. *Nature* **1992**, *358*, 15–16. [CrossRef]
2. Shaw, P.H. The role of p53 in cell cycle regulation. *Pathol. Res. Pract.* **1996**, *192*, 669–675. [CrossRef]
3. Toledo, F.; Wahl, G.M. Regulating the p53 pathway: In vitro hypotheses, in vivo *veritas*. *Nat. Rev. Cancer* **2006**, *6*, 909–923. [CrossRef] [PubMed]
4. Vazquez, A.; Bond, E.E.; Levine, A.J.; Bond, G.L. The genetics of the p53 pathway, apoptosis and cancer therapy. *Nat. Rev. Drug Discov.* **2008**, *7*, 979–987. [CrossRef] [PubMed]
5. Rufini, A.; Tucci, P.; Celardo, I.; Melino, G. Senescence and aging: The critical roles of p53. *Oncogene* **2013**, *32*, 5129–5143. [CrossRef] [PubMed]
6. Williams, A.B.; Schumacher, B. p53 in the DNA-damage-repair process. *Cold Spring Harb. Perspect. Med.* **2016**, *6*, a026070. [CrossRef]
7. Vogelstein, B.; Lane, D.; Levine, A.J. Surfing the p53 network. *Nature (London, U.K.)* **2000**, *408*, 307–310. [CrossRef] [PubMed]
8. Hainaut, P.; Hollstein, M. p53 and human cancer: The first ten thousand mutations. *Adv. Cancer Res.* **1999**, *77*, 81–137.
9. Wang, X. p53 regulation: Teamwork between RING domains of MDM2 and MDMX. *Cell Cycle* **2011**, *10*, 4225–4229. [CrossRef] [PubMed]
10. Wu, X.; Bayle, J.H.; Olson, D.; Levine, A.J. The p53-MDM2 autoregulatory feedback loop. *Genes Dev.* **1993**, *7*, 1126–1132. [CrossRef] [PubMed]
11. Momand, J.; Wu, H.H.; Dasgupta, G. MDM2 - master regulator of the p53 tumor suppressor protein. *Gene* **2000**, *242*, 15–29. [CrossRef]
12. Momand, J.; Zambetti, G.P.; Olson, D.C.; George, D.; Levine, A.J. The MDM2 oncogene product forms a complex with the p53 protein and inhibits p53-mediated transactivation. *Cell* **1992**, *69*, 1237–1245. [CrossRef]
13. Oliner, J.D.; Pietenpol, J.A.; Thiagalingam, S.; Gyuris, J.; Kinzler, K.W.; Vogelstein, B. Oncoprotein MDM2 conceals the activation domain of tumor supressor p53. *Nature (London, U.K.)* **1993**, *362*, 857–860. [CrossRef]
14. Roth, J.; Dobbelstein, M.; Freedman, D.A.; Shenk, T.; Levine, A.J. Nucleo-cytoplasmic shuttling of the HDM2 oncoprotein regulated the levels of the p53 protein via a pathway used by the human immunodeficiency vírus ver protein. *EMBO J.* **1998**, *17*, 554–564. [CrossRef]
15. Haupt, Y.; Maya, R.; Kazaz, A.; Oren, M. MDM2 promotes the rapid degradation of p53. *Nature* **1997**, *387*, 296–299. [CrossRef] [PubMed]

16. Pant, V.; Lozano, G. Limiting the power of p53 through the ubiquitin proteasome pathway. *Genes Dev.* **2014**, *28*, 1739–1751. [CrossRef] [PubMed]
17. Zhao, Y.; Aguilar, A.; Bernard, D.; Wang, S. Small-molecule inhibitors of the MDM2-p53 protein-protein interaction (MDM2 inhibitors) in clinical trials for cancer treatment: Miniperspective. *J. Med. Chem.* **2014**, *58*, 1038–1052. [CrossRef] [PubMed]
18. Wang, S.; Zhao, Y.; Aguilar, A.; Bernard, D.; Yang, C.Y. Targeting the MDM2-p53 protein-protein interaction for new cancer therapy: Progress and challenges. *Cold Spring Harb. Perspect. Med.* **2017**, *7*, a026245. [CrossRef]
19. Vassilev, L.T.; Vu, B.T.; Graves, B.; Carvajal, D.; Podlaski, F.; Filipovic, Z.; Kong, N.; Kammlott, U.; Lukacs, C.; Klein, C.; Fotouhi, N.; Liu, E.A. In vivo activation of the p53 pathway by small-molecule antagonists of MDM2. *Science* **2004**, *303*, 844–848. [CrossRef]
20. Lemos, A.; Leão, M.; Soares, J.; Palmeira, A.; Pinto, M.; Saraiva, L.; Sousa, M.E. Medicinal chemistry strategies to disrupt p53-MDM2/MDMX interaction. *Med. Res. Rev.* **2016**, *36*, 789–844. [CrossRef]
21. Tisato, V.; Voltan, R.; Gonelli, A.; Secchiero, P.; Zauli, G. MDM2/X inhibitors under clinical evaluation: Perspectives for the management of hematological malignancies and pediatric cancer. *J. Hematol. Oncol.* **2017**, *10*, 133. [CrossRef] [PubMed]
22. Pinto, M.M.M.; Sousa, M.E.; Nascimento, M.S. Xanthone derivatives: New insights in biological activities. *Curr. Med. Chem.* **2005**, *12*, 2517–2538. [CrossRef] [PubMed]
23. Pouli, N.; Marakos, P. Fused xanthone derivatives as antiproliferative agents. *Anticancer Agents Med. Chem.* **2009**, *9*, 77–98. [CrossRef]
24. Pedro, M.; Cerqueira, F.; Sousa, M.E.; Nascimento, M.S.J.; Pinto, M. Xanthones as inhibitors of growth of human cancer cell lines and their effects on the proliferation of human lymphocytes in vitro. *Bioorg. Med. Chem.* **2002**, *10*, 3725–3730. [CrossRef]
25. Sousa, E.P.; Silva, A.M.S.; Pinto, M.M.M.; Pedro, M.M.; Cerqueira, F.A.M.; Nascimento, M.S.J. Isomeric kielcorins and dihydroxyxanthones: Synthesis, structure elucidation, and inhibitory activities of growth of human cancer cell lines and on the proliferation of human lymphocytes in vitro. *Helv. Chim. Acta* **2002**, *85*, 2862–2876. [CrossRef]
26. Castanheiro, R.A.; Pinto, M.M.; Silva, A.M.; Cravo, S.M.; Gales, L.; Damas, A.M.; Nazareth, N.; Nascimento, M.S.J.; Eaton, G. Dihydroxyxanthones prenylated derivatives: Synthesis, structure elucidation, and growth inhibitory activity on human tumor cell lines with improvement of selectivity for MCF-7. *Bioorg. Med. Chem.* **2007**, *15*, 6080–6088. [CrossRef]
27. Sousa, E.; Paiva, A.; Nazareth, N.; Gales, L.; Damas, A.M.; Nascimento, M.S.J.; Pinto, M. Bromoalkoxyxanthones as promising antitumor agents: Synthesis, crystal structure and effect on human tumor cell lines. *Eur. J. Med. Chem.* **2009**, *44*, 3830–3835. [CrossRef]
28. Palmeira, A.; Paiva, A.; Sousa, E.; Seca, H.; Almeida, G.M.; Lima, R.T.; Fernandes, M.X.; Pinto, M.; Vasconcelos, M.H. Insights into the in vitro antitumor mechanism of action of a new pyranoxanthone. *Chem. Biol. Drug Des.* **2010**, *76*, 43–58. [CrossRef]
29. Paiva, A.M.; Sousa, M.E.; Camoes, A.; Nascimento, M.S.J.; Pinto, M.M.M. Prenylated xanthones: Antiproliferative effects and enhancement of the growth inhibitory action of 4-hydroxytamoxifen in estrogen receptor-positive breast cancer cell line. *Med. Chem. Res.* **2012**, *21*, 552–558. [CrossRef]
30. Leão, M.; Gomes, S.; Pedraza-Chaverri, J.; Machado, N.; Sousa, E.; Pinto, M.; Inga, A.; Pereira, C.; Saraiva, L. α-Mangostin and gambogic acid as potential inhibitors of the p53-MDM2 interaction revealed by a yeast-based approach. *J. Nat. Prod.* **2013**, *76*, 774–778. [CrossRef]
31. Leão, M.; Pereira, C.; Bisio, A.; Ciribilli, Y.; Paiva, A.M.; Machado, N.; Palmeira, A.; Fernandes, M.X.; Sousa, E.; Pinto, M.; Inga, A.; Saraiva, L. Discovery of a new small-molecule inhibitor of p53-MDM2 interaction using a yeast-based approach. *Biochem. Pharmacol.* **2013**, *85*, 1234–1245. [CrossRef]
32. Fernandes, C.; Masawang, K.; Tiritan, M.E.; Sousa, E.; de Lima, V.; Afonso, C.; Bousbaa, H.; Sudprasert, W.; Pedro, M.; Pinto, M. New chiral derivatives of xanthones: Synthesis and investigation of enantioselectivity as inhibitors of growth of human tumor cell lines. *Bioorg. Med. Chem.* **2014**, *22*, 1049–1062. [CrossRef]
33. Barbosa, J.; Lima, R.T.; Sousa, D.; Gomes, A.S.; Palmeira, A.; Seca, H.; Choosang, K.; Pakkong, P.; Bousbaa, H.; Pinto, M.M.; et al. Screening a small library of xanthones for antitumor activity and identification of a hit compound which induces apoptosis. *Molecules* **2016**, *21*, 81. [CrossRef]

34. Cidade, H.; Rocha, V.; Palmeira, A.; Marques, C.; Tiritan, M.E.; Ferreira, H.; Lobo, J.S.; Almeida, I.F.; Sousa, M.E.; Pinto, M. In silico and in vitro antioxidant and cytotoxicity evaluation of oxygenated xanthone derivatives. *Arab. J. Chem.* **2017**. [CrossRef]
35. Alves, A.; Correia-da-Silva, M.; Nunes, C.; Campos, J.; Sousa, E.; Silva, P.M.A.; Bousbaa, H.; Rodrigues, F.; Ferreira, D.; Costa, P.C.; et al. Discovery of a new xanthone against glioma: Synthesis and development of (pro)liposome formulations. *Molecules* **2019**, *24*, 409. [CrossRef]
36. Gomes, S.; Raimundo, L.; Soares, J.; Loureiro, J.B.; Leão, M.; Ramos, H.; Monteiro, M.N.; Lemos, A.; Moreira, J.; Pinto, M.; et al. New inhibitor of the TAp73 interaction with MDM2 and mutant p53 with promising antitumor activity against neuroblastoma. *Cancer Lett.* **2019**, *446*, 90–102. [CrossRef]
37. Liu, J.; Zhou, F.; Zhang, L.; Wang, H.; Zhang, J.; Zhang, C.; Jiang, Z.; Li, Y.; Liu, Z.; Chen, H. DMXAA-pyranoxanthone hybrids enhance inhibition activities against human cancer cells with multi-target functions. *Eur. J. Med. Chem.* **2018**, *143*, 1768–1778. [CrossRef]
38. Hardcastle, I.R.; Liu, J.; Valeur, E.; Watson, A.; Ahmed, S.U.; Blackburn, T.J.; Bennaceur, K.; Clegg, W.; Drummond, C.; Endicott, J.A.; et al. Isoindolinone inhibitors of the murine double minute 2 (MDM2)-p53 protein-protein interaction: Structure-activity studies leading to improved potency. *J. Med. Chem.* **2011**, *54*, 1233–1243. [CrossRef]
39. Twarda-Ciapa, A.; Krzanik, S.; Kubica, K.; Guzik, K.; Labuzek, B.; Neochoritis, C.G.; Khoury, K.; Kowalska, K.; Czub, M.; Dubin, G.; et al. 1,4,5-Trisubstituted imidazole-based p53-MDM2/MDMX antagonists with aliphatic linkers for conjugation with biological carriers. *J. Med. Chem.* **2017**, *60*, 4234–4244. [CrossRef]
40. Gicquel, M.; Gomez, C.; Alvarez, M.C.G.; Pamlard, O.; Guérineau, V.; Jacquet, E.; Bignon, J.; Voituriez, A.; Marinetti, A. Inhibition of p53-murine double minute 2 (MDM2) interactions with 3,3′-spirocyclopentene oxindole derivatives. *J. Med. Chem.* **2018**, *61*, 9386–9392. [CrossRef]
41. Quillinan, A.J.; Schelnmann, F. Studies in the xanthone series. Part XII. A general synthesis of polyoxygenated xanthones from benzophenone precursors. *J. Chem. Soc. Perkin Trans.* **1973**, *1*, 1329–1337. [CrossRef]
42. Resende, D.I.S.P.; Pereira-Terra, P.; Inácio, Â.S.; da Costa, P.M.; Pinto, E.; Sousa, E.; Pinto, M.M.M. Lichen xanthones as models for new antifungal agents. *Molecules* **2018**, *23*, 2617. [CrossRef]
43. Martins, E.; Silva, V.; Lemos, A.; Palmeira, A.; Puthongking, P.; Sousa, E.; Rocha-Pereira, C.; Ghanem, C.I.; Carmo, H.; Remião, F.; et al. Newly synthesized oxygenated xanthones as potential P-glycoprotein activators: In vitro, ex vivo, and in silico studies. *Molecules* **2019**, *24*, 707. [CrossRef]
44. Soares, J.; Espadinha, M.; Raimundo, L.; Ramos, H.; Gomes, A.S.; Gomes, S.; Loureiro, J.B.; Inga, A.; Reis, F.; Gomes, C.; et al. DIMP53-1: A novel small-molecule dual inhibitor of p53-MDM2/X interactions with multifunctional p53-dependent anticancer properties. *Mol. Oncol.* **2017**, *11*, 612–627. [CrossRef]
45. Soares, J.; Pereira, N.A.; Monteiro, Â.; Leão, M.; Bessa, C.; dos Santos, D.J.; Raimundo, L.; Queiroz, G.; Bisio, A.; Inga, A.; et al. Oxazoloisoindolinones with in vitro antitumor activity selectively activate a p53-pathway through potential inhibition of the p53-MDM2 interaction. *Eur. J. Pharm. Sci.* **2015**, *66*, 138–147. [CrossRef]
46. Soares, J.; Raimundo, L.; Pereira, N.A.; dos Santos, D.J.; Pérez, M.; Queiroz, G.; Leão, M.; Santos, M.M.M.; Saraiva, L. A tryptophanol-derived oxazolopiperidone lactam is cytotoxic against tumors via inhibition of p53 interaction with murine double minute proteins. *Pharmacol. Res.* **2015**, *95–96*, 42–52. [CrossRef]
47. Chen, L.; Yin, H.; Farooqi, B.; Sebti, S.; Hamilton, A.D.; Chen, J. p53 α-helix mimetics antagonize p53/MDM2 interaction and activate p53. *Mol. Cancer Ther.* **2005**, *4*, 1019–1025. [CrossRef]
48. Kalid, O.; Ben-Tal, N. Study of MDM2 binding to p53-analogues: Affinity, helicity, and applicability to drug design. *J. Chem. Inf. Model.* **2009**, *49*, 865–876. [CrossRef]
49. Kussie, P.H.; Gorina, S.; Marechal, V.; Elenbaas, B.; Moreau, J.; Levine, A.J.; Pavletich, N.P. Structure of the MDM2 oncoprotein bound to the p53 tumor suppressor transactivation domain. *Science* **1996**, *274*, 948–953. [CrossRef]
50. Anil, B.; Riedinger, C.; Endicott, J.A.; Nobie, M.E. The structure of an MDM2-nutlin-3a complex solved by the use of a validated MDM2 surface-entropy reduction mutant. *Acta Crystallogr. D Biol. Crystallogr.* **2013**, *69*, 1358–1366. [CrossRef]
51. Trott, O.; Olson, A.J. AutoDock Vina: Improving the speed and the accuracy of docking with a new scoring function, efficient optimization and multithreading. *J. Comput. Chem.* **2010**, *31*, 455–461. [CrossRef] [PubMed]

52. Bharatham, N.; Bharatham, K.; Shelat, A.A.; Bashford, D. Ligand binding mode prediction by docking: MDM2/MDMX inhibitors as a case study. *J. Chem. Inf. Model.* **2014**, *54*, 648–659. [CrossRef] [PubMed]
53. Wang, Y.; Xiao, J.; Sujek, T.O.; Zhang, J.; Wang, J.; Bryant, S.H. PubChem: A public information system for analyzing bioactivities of small molecules. *Nucleic Acids Res.* **2009**, *37*, 623–633. [CrossRef] [PubMed]
54. Kini, R.M.; Evans, H.J. Molecular modeling of proteins: A strategy for energy minimization by molecular mechanics in the AMBER force field. *J. Biomol. Struct. Dyn.* **1991**, *9*, 475–488. [CrossRef] [PubMed]
55. Seeliger, D.; de Groot, B.L. Ligand docking and binding site analysis with PyMOL and AutoDock/Vina. *J. Comput. Aided Mol. Des.* **2010**, *24*, 417–422. [CrossRef] [PubMed]

10

Synthesis of New Derivatives of Benzofuran as Potential Anticancer Agents

Mariola Napiórkowska [1,*], Marcin Cieślak [2,*], Julia Kaźmierczak-Barańska [2], Karolina Królewska-Golińska [2] and Barbara Nawrot [2]

1 Chair and Department of Biochemistry, Medical University of Warsaw, 1 Banacha Str., 02-097 Warsaw, Poland
2 Centre of Molecular and Macromolecular Studies, Polish Academy of Sciences, 112 Sienkiewicza Str., 90-363 Łódź, Poland; julia@cbmm.lodz.pl (J.K.-B.); kkrolews@cbmm.lodz.pl (K.K.-G.); bnawrot@cbmm.lodz.pl (B.N.)
* Correspondence: mariola.napiorkowska@wum.edu.pl (M.N.); marcin@cbmm.lodz.pl (M.C.);

Academic Editor: Qiao-Hong Chen

Abstract: The results of our previous research indicated that some derivatives of benzofurans, particularly halogeno-derivatives, are selectively toxic towards human leukemia cells. Continuing our work with this group of compounds we here report new data on the synthesis as well as regarding the physico-chemical and biological characterization of fourteen new derivatives of benzofurans, including six brominated compounds. The structures of all new compounds were established by spectroscopic methods (^{1}H- and, ^{13}C-NMR, ESI MS), and elemental analyses. Their cytotoxicity was evaluated against K562 (leukemia), MOLT-4 (leukemia), HeLa (cervix carcinoma), and normal cells (HUVEC). Five compounds (**1c, 1e, 2d, 3a, 3d**) showed significant cytotoxic activity against all tested cell lines and selectivity for cancer cell lines. The SAR analysis (structure-activity relationship analysis) indicated that the presence of bromine introduced to a methyl or acetyl group that was attached to the benzofuran system increased their cytotoxicity both in normal and cancer cells.

Keywords: benzofurans; chemical synthesis; cytotoxic properties; HeLa; MOLT-4; K562

1. Introduction

Benzofuran skeleton holds an important position in organic chemistry and it is considered to be one of the most important heterocyclic systems because of its diverse profile of biological activity. This structural unit is a central part of a variety of biologically active compounds. Natural and synthetic benzofuran derivatives have been reported to possess wide therapeutic properties, including antiviral, immunosuppressive, antioxidant, antifungal, anti-inflammatory, antimicrobial, analgesic, antihyperglycemic, and antitumor activities [1–6]. *Cicerfuran*, *Conocarpan*, and *Ailanthoidol* are the best known biologically active natural benzofurans (Figure 1). Specifically, the *Cicerfuran* shows antifungal activity, *Conocarpan* has been reported as an antifungal and antitrypanosomal agent, and *Ailanthoidol* exhibits anticancer, antiviral, immunosuppressive, antioxidant, and antifungal activity [1,2,7]. The synthetic benzofuran derivatives are represented by *Amiodarone* (Figure 1), being used in the treatment of ventricular and supraventricular arrhythmias, and by *Bufuralol*, which is a non-specific β-adrenergic blocker with an affinity for β1 and β2-adrenergic receptors [3,4,7].

Nowadays, when cancer, after cardiovascular diseases, is the second most common cause of death and still constitutes an unresolved problem of clinical medicine and pharmacology, extensive research regarding new anticancer compounds is especially important. These new drugs should possess improved pharmacokinetics and specifically destroy cancer cells, without causing negative side effects. Research in the group of benzofuran derivatives is justified, especially by the fact that one can find many examples of data in the literature on benzofurans with anticancer activity. In many cases, the benzofuran skeleton is fused with other heterocyclic or aromatic moieties (Figure 2).

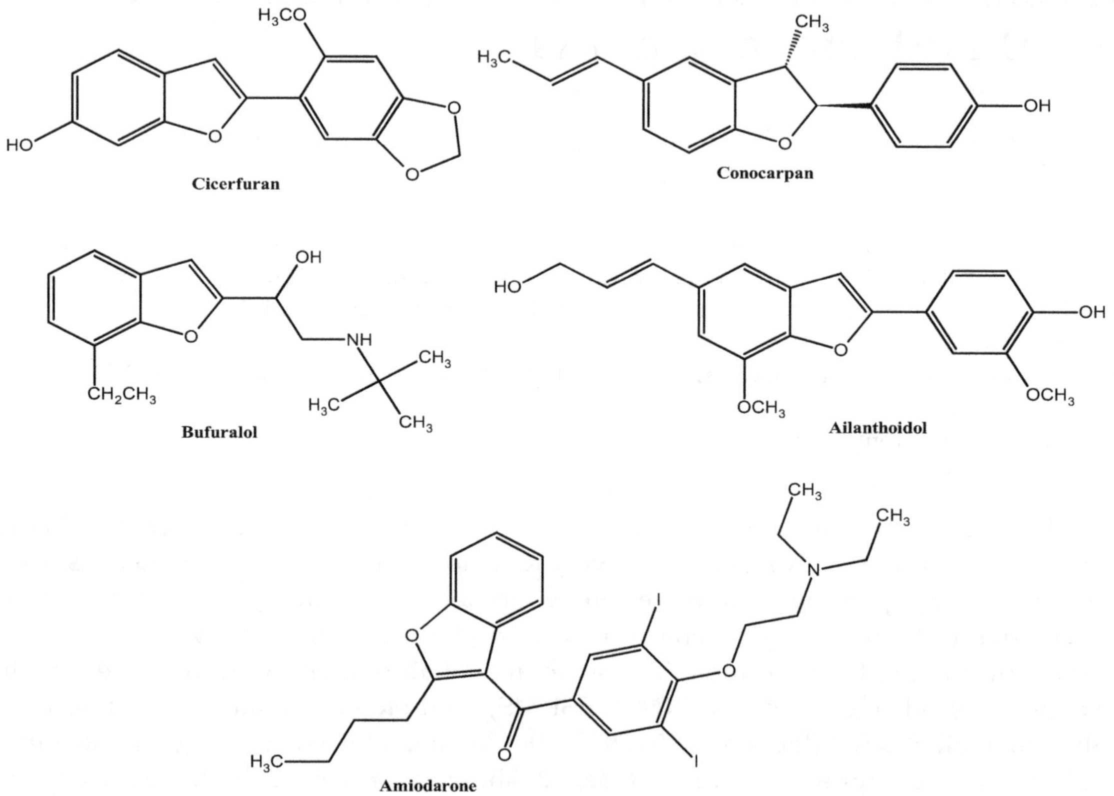

Figure 1. Structures of natural and synthetic benzofuran derivatives with biological activity.

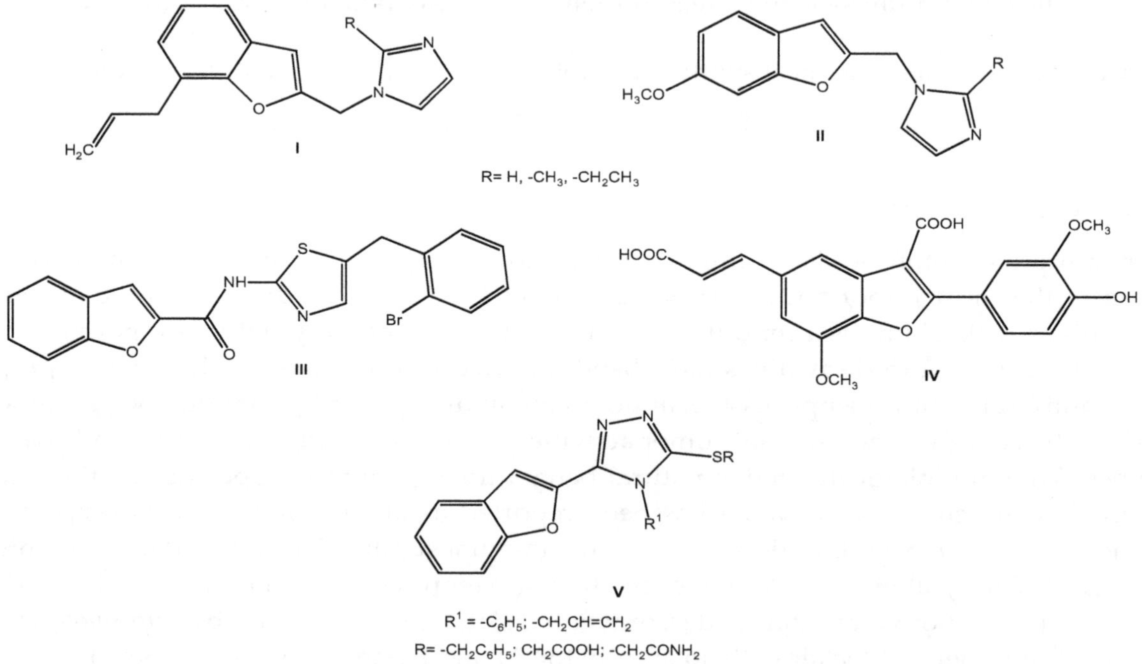

Figure 2. Structures of synthetic benofuran derivatives **I–V** with anticancer activity [7].

There are several benzofuranyl imidazole derivatives among them (**I** and **II**), which were found to be cytotoxic towards an ovarian carcinoma cell line (Skov-3). The study of *N*-(5-(2-bromobenzyl) thiazole-2-yl) benzofuran-2-carboxamide (**III**) showed that this compound inhibited the growth of HCC (human hepatocellular carcinoma) cells and induced their apoptosis. The synthetic derivative **IV** was found to have antitumor activity and it was an effective chemopreventive and chemotherapeutic agent against malignant T cells. Moreover, a series of triazole derivatives **V** showed moderate antitumor activity. Recent data reported this type of benzofuran derivatives as potential therapeutic agents for breast cancer [7].

These are only a few examples from a large group of benzofurans with anticancer activity. Moreover, examples of compounds with cytotoxic activity were found among the simple derivatives of benzofuran like 2- and 3-benzofuranocarboxylic acid derivatives **VI–VII** (Figure 3). The above-mentioned compounds exhibit significant cytotoxic activity against human cancer cell lines [8].

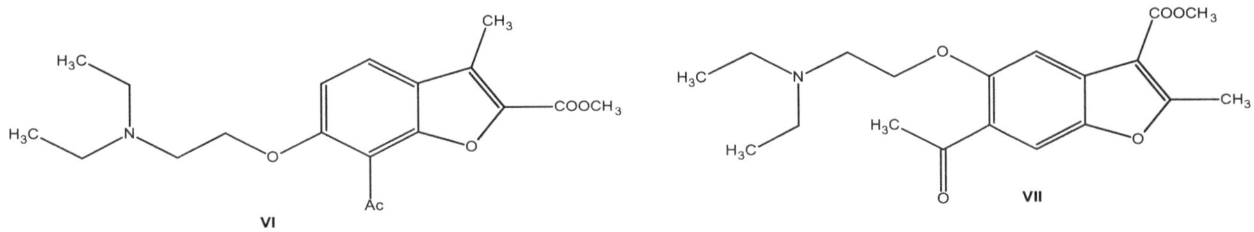

Figure 3. Structures of 2- and 3-benzofurancarboxylic acid derivatives **VI–VII** with cytotoxic activity.

The literature survey shows that benzofurans containing halogens in their structure constitute an important group of compounds, with antitumor, cytotoxic, spasmolytic, antiarrhythmic, and antifungal activity [9–20]. Thus, this group of compounds is interesting for researchers, especially because the presence of halogen can increase the activity and selectivity of derivatives. This is probably related to the ability of halogens to create a "halogen bond", which results from the formation of the σ-hole. Although the halogen bonds are weaker than hydrogen bonds, they have specific effects and can lead to significant gains in binding affinity. These interactions can be found in protein-receptor complexes as well as in small molecules [21–24].

Furthermore, we have identified three bromo derivatives **VIII–X** (Figure 4) that showed selective toxicity towards human leukemia cells in our previous studies [25,26]. Compound **VIII** is especially cytotoxic towards K562 and HL-60 leukemic cell lines (IC_{50} 5.0 and 0.1 μM, respectively), however it is not toxic towards HeLa cancer cells and healthy endothelial cells (HUVEC) (IC_{50} > 1 mM). Moreover, the observed remarkable cytotoxicity of **VIII** towards K562 cells resulted from cells apoptosis. Compounds **IX** and **X** proved to be highly toxic towards cancer cells (IC_{50} in a few μM range) and non-toxic towards endothelial cells (HUVEC) [25–27]. Unfortunately, these compounds are poorly soluble in water, which limits their use in the cell culture or animal studies.

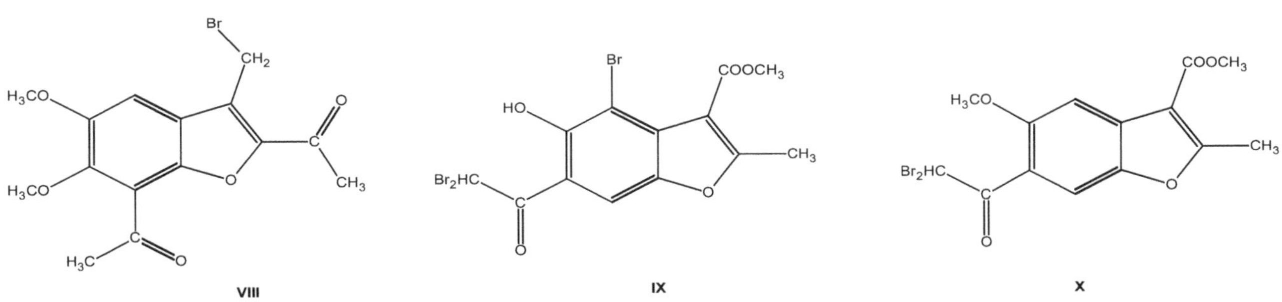

Figure 4. Structures of the benzofuran derivatives **VIII–X**, lead compounds used in the present studies.

Using **VIII–X** as the lead compounds, we designed and synthesized fourteen new derivatives with hopes for their better solubility in aqueous solutions (of lower lipophilicity when compared to **VIII–X**). The biological activity (i.e., cytotoxicity, activation of apoptosis, interaction with DNA) of these new derivatives was also evaluated.

2. Results

2.1. Synthesis

Our goal was to obtain a small library of new, less lipophilic derivatives/analogs of lead compounds **VIII–X**. We designed the synthesis of a set of compounds containing a carboxyl (**1**), formamide (**1a**), and methoxycarbonyl groups (**1b**), instead of an acetyl group in the position 2 of the parent benzofuran ring to obtain new benzofuran **VIII** analogs.

Thus, the starting acid **1**, which was obtained by the multistep synthesis according to the previously reported procedures [28] was submitted either to oxalyl chloride and ammonium solution treatment or methylated with dimethyl sulphate, delivering the amide derivative **1a** and methyl ester **1b**, respectively (Scheme 1). In the next step, compounds **1** and **1b** were submitted to bromination. For this purpose, ester **1b** was reacted with molecular bromine in chloroform. Under these conditions, hydrogen in the methyl group at position 3 was substituted by a bromine atom to give compound **1c**, which only differed by the substituent in position 2 (methoxycarbonyl versus acetyl). During bromination of the acid **1** using bromine in chloroform or NBS in CCl_4, a mixture of products was obtained, which was difficult to separate. Thus, the reaction conditions were changed and ethanol, instead of CCl_4, was used as a solvent in bromination reaction that was carried out in the presence of the NBS, while acetic acid was used as a solvent in the respective reaction that was carried out in the presence of bromine. Under these conditions, we managed to isolate the bromo-derivative **1d**, with satisfactory yield. Moreover, bromo-derivative **1e** was also obtained, but only in the reaction that was facilitated by NBS. The analyses of nuclear magnetic resonance spectra (^{1}H- and ^{13}C-NMR), mass spectra, and elemental analysis showed that the structures of the received compounds were different from the assumed ones (bromination of the methyl group at position 3). Instead, the derivatives in which the carboxyl group was replaced by the bromine atom at the position 2 were isolated. Moreover, we confirmed the formation of **1e**, in which one bromine atom substituted the hydrogen atom in the acetyl group of the benzene moiety of benzofuran ring. The use of polar protic solvents (acetic acid, ethanol) could explain this substitution.

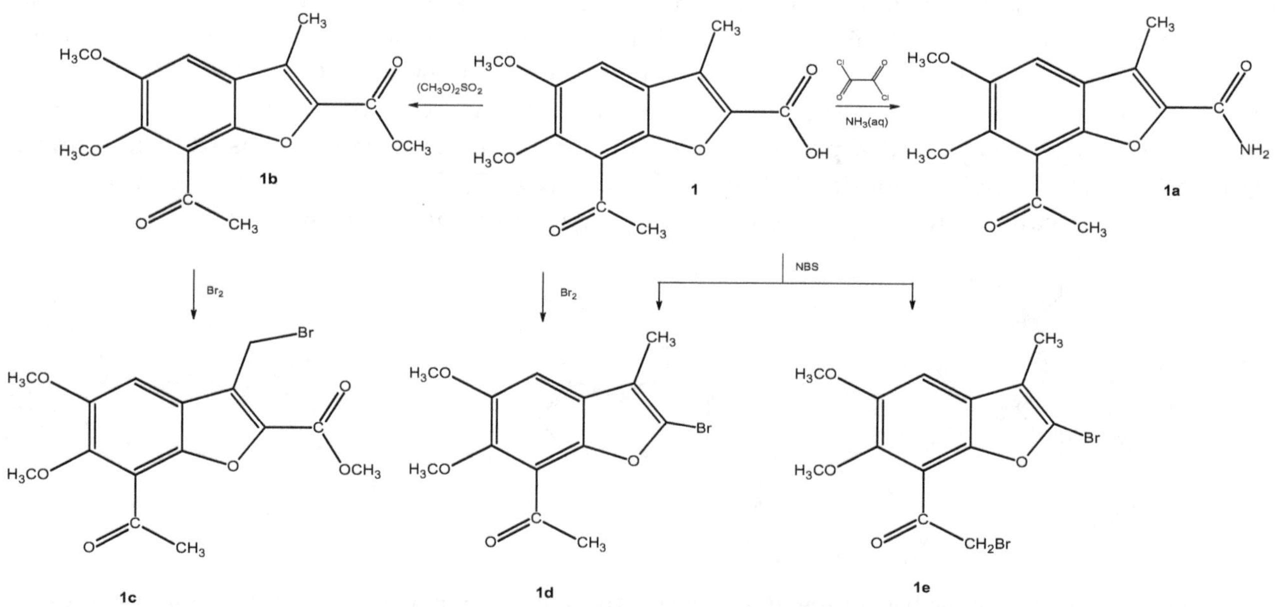

Scheme 1. Synthesis of analogues of compound **VIII**.

Analysis of the calculated log*P* values (Table 1) has shown that carboxyl and formamide analogs of lead compound **VIII** (**1** and **1a**, respectively) are much less lipophilic, while methoxycarbonyl analogs **1b** and **1c** exhibit similar properties as **VIII**. In contrast, an introduction of the bromine atom at position 2 of the furane ring resulted in significant increase of the benzofuran system hydrophobicity.

Table 1. Theoretical log*P* values (clog*P*) for obtained compounds calculated by the OSIRIS Property Explorer program.

Compound	clog*P*
VIII	2.4327
1	1.7254
1a	1.3276
1b	2.1533
1c	2.4745
1d	3.0089
1e	3.3301
IX	3.5663
2a	1.1219
2b	1.8471
2d	2.2688
2e	2.2449
X	3.1168
3a	2.9350
3b	1.7954
3c	1.3972
3d	2.5445

Schemes 2 and 3 show the syntheses of analogs of compounds **IX** and **X**, respectively. The starting material in both cases was 6-acetyl-5-hydroxy-2-methylbenzofuran-3-carboxylic acid (**2**), which was subjected to multidirectional transformations (Scheme 2). In the first approach, the amide-derivative **2a** was obtained in the reaction of the acid **2** with oxalyl chloride and ammonium hydroxide. Next, the bromo-derivative **2b** was obtained by the bromination of **2a** with bromine in acetic acid as a solvent. The nuclear magnetic resonance (^{1}H- and ^{13}C-NMR), mass spectrometry and elemental analyses confirmed the substitution of hydrogen by bromine in aromatic ring in the position 4. We assume that the presence of the OH group in position 5 of the benzene ring assisted in the electrophilic substitution of bromide cation in its ortho position. In the second path, the acid **2** was brominated in the same conditions and the bromo-derivative **2e**, also with a bromine substitution to the benzene ring, was obtained. In the third approach, an ester-derivative **2c**, which was obtained in the reaction of the acid **2** with dimethyl sulphate, was brominated by using NBS in CCl_4 to give the derivative **2d**, with a bromomethyl group in the position 2. Interestingly, all of the obtained derivatives **2** (**2a**–**2e**) exhibited lower clog*P* values, confirming the better water solubility of derivatives compared to lead compound **IX**, and the most pronounced occurred primary carboxamides **2a** and **2b**.

To obtain analogs of compound **X**, the starting acid **2** was reacted with an excess of dimethyl sulphate and the obtained derivative **3** was subjected to a multidirectional synthesis (Scheme 3). In the first case, bromine was introduced into the methyl group to give a compound **3d**, by reaction with NBS in CCl_4. In the reaction of the compound **3** with a bromine in acetic acid, the lead compound **X** was obtained and then finally reduced to provide a hydroxyl-derivative **3a**. In the third path, ester **3** was hydrolyzed in alkaline conditions to acid **3b**, and finally this derivative was converted to an amide **3c** by reaction with oxalyl chloride and ammonium hydroxide. Importantly, all of the new benzofuran derivatives related to **X** are characterized by lower clog*P* values when compared to the lead compound, indicating their improved solubility in aqueous media (Table 1).

The introduced substituents significantly affected the lipophilicity of the obtained benzofurans. In most cases, the new derivatives had a lower clog*P* value in comparison with the lead compounds. The exception are three derivatives **1c**, **1d**, **1e**, where the substitution of bromine in the furan ring (compounds **1d** and **1e**) or in the methyl group caused the clog*P* to increase (Table 2).

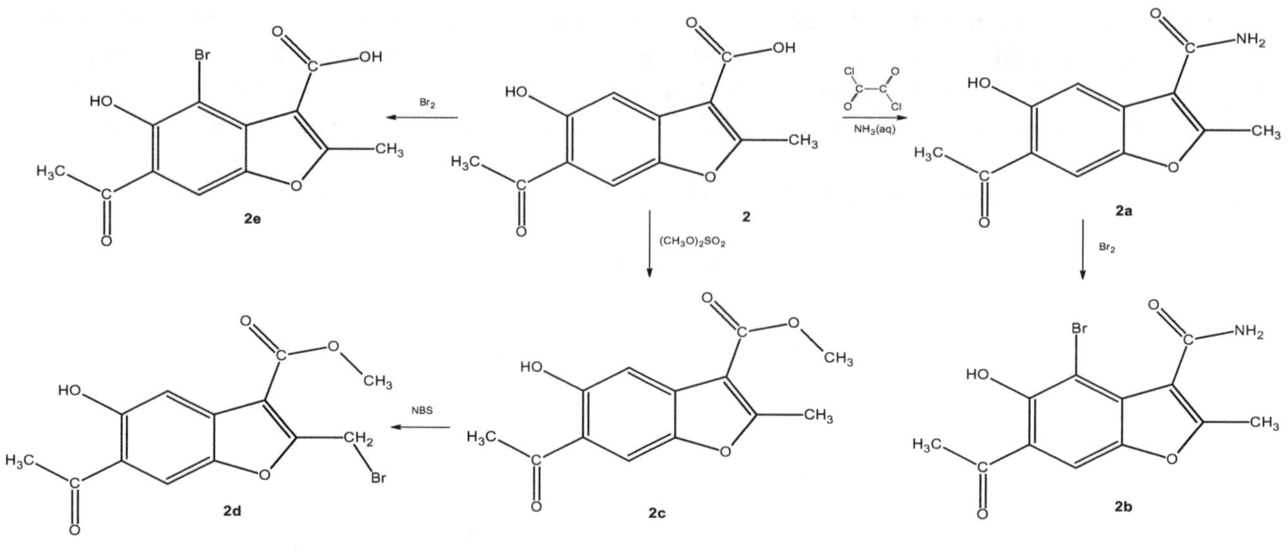

Scheme 2. Synthesis of analogues of compound **IX**.

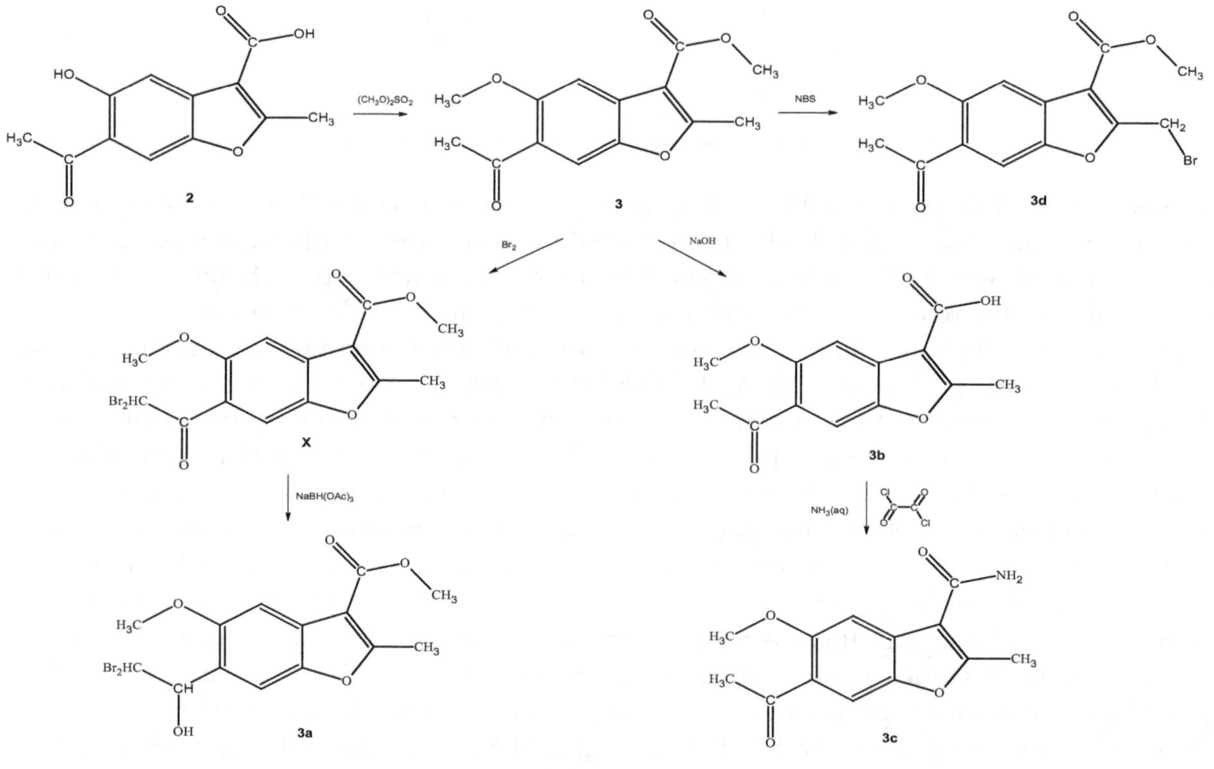

Scheme 3. Synthesis of analogues of compound **X**.

2.2. MTT Cytotoxicity Studies

Fourteen new benzofuran derivatives were tested for their cytotoxic properties in K562, MOLT-4 (leukemia, suspension cells), HeLa (cervix carcinoma, adherent cells), and normal endothelial cells (HUVEC). First, we measured the viability of cells after 48 h incubation with the given compound at the concentration of 100 μM. Next, for compounds that reduced cancer cells survival for more than 50%, we determined IC_{50} values. Cells that were exposed to 1% DMSO (a vehicle) served as the control with 100% survival. Cells treated with 1 μM staurosporine served as the internal control of the cytotoxicity experiments.

We have identified five compounds **1c**, **1e**, **2d**, **3a**, and **3d** in the initial screening, which, at the concentration of 100 μM, reduced the viability of all tested cancer cells K562, HeLa and MOLT-4 for more than 50% (data not shown). These compounds were also cytotoxic against human normal endothelial cells, so these compounds did not show any selectivity between the cancer and normal cells.

Next, for compounds **1c**, **1e**, **2d**, **3a**, and **3d**, the IC_{50} values were calculated (data given in Table 2). The test compounds were similarly toxic toward both cancer and normal cells, with IC_{50} values in the range of 20–85 μM. The exceptions were compounds **1c** and **3d**, which show IC_{50} out of this range (180 μM for MOLT-4 and 6 μM for HUVEC cells, respectively). We did not observe any significant differences in susceptibility between adherent and suspension cell lines.

Table 2. The IC_{50} values [μM] after 48 h incubation with cells.

Compound	HeLa	K562	MOLT-4	HUVEC
1c	50	25	180	30
1e	28	41	70	30
2d	35	20	35	30
3a	80	85	85	67
3d	35	28	55	6

For compounds **1c**, **1e**, **2d**, and **3d**, that exhibited the highest toxicity for K562 leukemia cells (IC_{50} below 50 μM), we investigated whether they induce apoptosis in these cells. We have measured the activity of caspases 3 and 7 (caspase 3/7), which are markers of programmed cell death. The K562 cells were treated with 1% DMSO (negative control), 1 μM staurosporine (positive control), or a test compound at the concentration of $5 \times IC_{50}$ for 18 h. The activity of caspase 3/7 was measured using pro-fluorescent peptide substrate.

As shown in Figure 5, staurosporine, which is a strong inducer of apoptosis significantly increased the activity of caspase 3/7 in K562 cells. On the other hand, 1% DMSO had no effect on the activation of caspases. Interestingly, the incubation of cells with compound **1e** resulted in nearly five-fold increase in the activity of caspase 3/7, while compounds **1c** and **2d** activated caspase 3/7 to a lesser extent (about two-fold increase). In the presence of compound **3d**, the activation of caspases was minimal, if any. Altogether, this result suggests that the cytotoxic activity of test benzofurans **1c**, **1e**, and **2d** in K562 cells may be due to the induction of death by apoptosis.

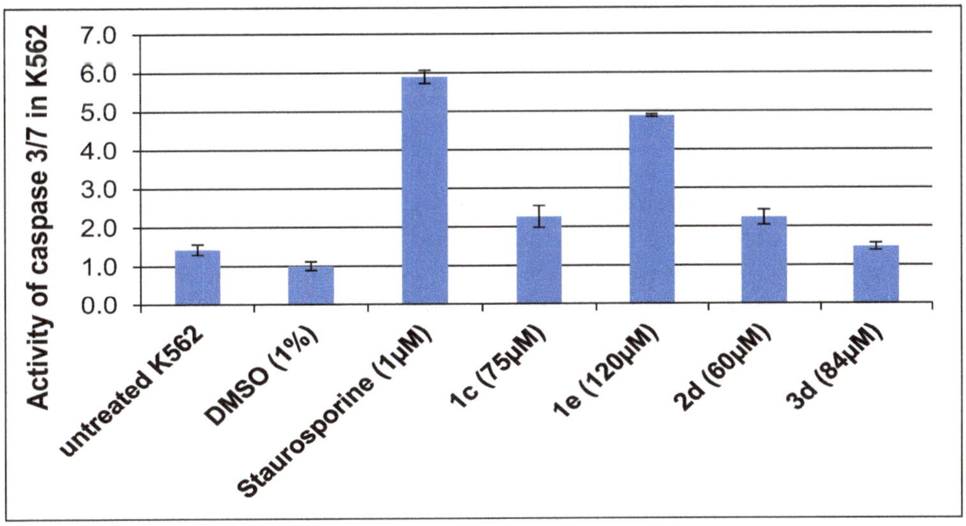

Figure 5. Activity of caspase 3 and 7 in K562 cells treated with the test benzofurans **1c**, **1e**, **2d**, **3d**, or staurosporine for 18 h. Apoptosis was determined by Apo-ONE® Homogeneous Caspase-3/7 Assay (Promega, Madison, WI, USA). Abbreviations: DMSO—K562 cells treated with 1% DMSO. The caspase activation level in cells exposed to 1% DMSO was normalized to 1.0. Mean values +/− SD are shown.

2.3. Interaction with DNA

The results of MTT cytotoxicity experiments indicated that compounds **1c**, **1e**, **2d**, and **3d** were highly toxic towards the used cell lines. We hypothesized that a possible explanation of observed cytotoxicity might be due to an interaction of test benzofurans with genomic DNA (e.g., by intercalation). To verify this hypothesis, we investigated whether the test benzofurans have any effect on digestion of a plasmid DNA (pcDNA3.1 HisC) with endonuclease *BamH1*. pcDNA3.1 HisC contains a unique *BamH1* restriction site which allows for plasmid linearization. Plasmid DNA exists in linear, superhelical, and circular forms that differ in electrophoretic mobility (Figure 6 lane 1). Plasmid DNA was converted to a linear form upon digestion with *BamH1* (lane 2). Daunorubicin, which is a strong intercalator to double-stranded DNA, was used as a control in this experiment and it completely inhibited the digestion of plasmid DNA with *BamH1* (lane 3). In the presence of test compounds, pcDNA3.1 HisC was partially digested with *Bam H1* restriction enzyme (Figure 6 lanes 4–7). Most of the plasmid DNA was converted to a linear form, however there is a circular form still present. These results suggest that test benzofurans, to some extent, interact with DNA (especially compounds **1c**, **1e**, **2d**), and this interaction inhibits the digestion of double stranded DNA chain with restriction endonuclease.

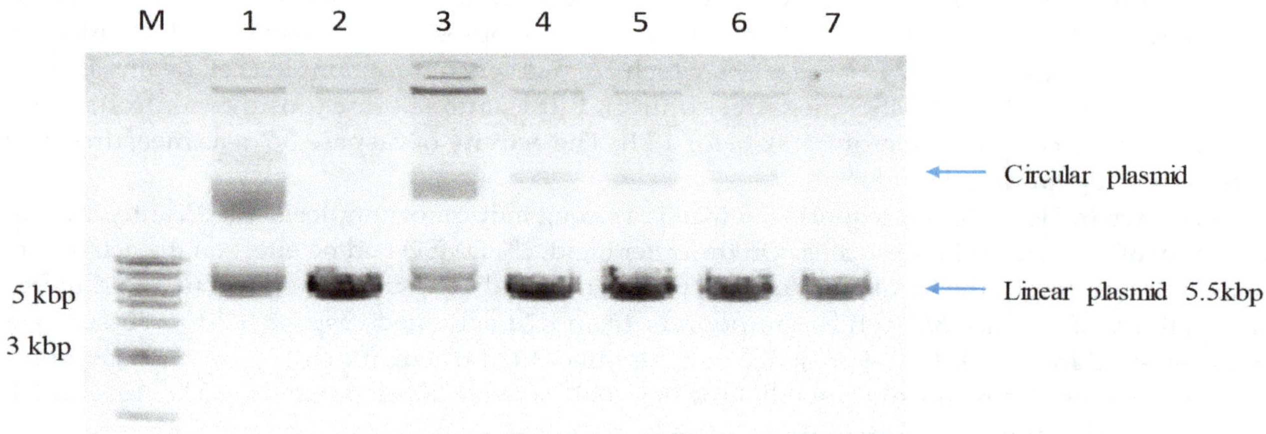

Figure 6. Digestion of pcDNA3.1HisC (total length 5.5kbp) with *BamH1* endonuclease. M—marker DNA; 1—not digested plasmid DNA; 2—plasmid DNA digested with *BamH1* (DNA present in linear form); 3—plasmid DNA + daunorubicin + *BamH1*; 4—plasmid DNA + **1c** + *BamH1*; 5—plasmid DNA + **2d** + *BamH1*; 6—plasmid DNA + **1e** + *BamH1*; and, 7—plasmid DNA + **3d** + *BamH1*.

3. Discussion

We have previously identified benzofurans **VIII**, **IX**, and **X** (lead benzofurans), which efficiently killed cancer cells and were not toxic toward normal endothelial cells [25–27]. Moreover, lead compound **VIII** demonstrated selective toxicity toward leukemia cell lines. However, these compounds were poorly soluble in aqueous solutions. Based on their structure, we have synthesized 14 new derivatives with decreased lipophilicity. The polarity of new compounds was predicted based on the calculated log*P* values. We tested their cytotoxic properties in human cells of cancer and normal origin. Five compounds, **1c**, **1e**, **2d**, **3a**, and **3d**, displayed the highest cytotoxicity toward cancer cell lines. However, these compounds were less toxic than lead compounds **VIII**, **IX**, **X**, and did not demonstrate any selectivity toward leukemia cells (Table 2). Moreover, new derivatives exhibited significant toxicity in normal endothelial cells. Cells death is usually carried out in one of the two major mechanisms: apoptosis or necrosis. Apoptosis is a highly regulated and controlled process that does not elicit an inflammation response at the site of cell death. Necrosis leads to sudden and uncontrolled cell disintegration that is associated with release of the cellular content and massive inflammation [29]. Therefore, in the next experiments, we investigated whether the cellular toxicity of new benzofurans is the result of apoptosis or necrosis. Our data demonstrate that the activity of caspase 3/7 (an apoptosis marker) is significantly increased (1.5- to 5-fold) in the presence of benzofurans (Figure 5). It suggests that these derivatives induce apoptosis in cancer cells. In the search of cellular targets for testing benzofurans, we examined whether DNA may be such a target. Using biochemical assay, we found out that the incubation of test compounds with plasmid DNA inhibited its cleavage with selected endonuclease (*BamH1*). A similar result was obtained with daunorubicin, which is a strong DNA intercalating agent. The presence of undigested plasmid DNA suggests that benzofurans intercalate to DNA (or bind DNA in other way). However, a comparison of DNA digestion products clearly indicates that the binding of benzofurans to DNA is much weaker than daunorubicin (Figure 6).

The presence of a bromine substituent in the alkyl chain attached to the furan ring is most likely to be responsible for cytotoxic activity of compounds **1c**, **2d**, and **3d**. The activity of compound **1e** is probably related to the presence of a bromoacetyl substituent in a benzene ring. Whilst the presence of a halogen (bromine) directly substituted to the benzene ring or the furan skeleton does not seem to increase the cytotoxic activity of the tested compounds, for example, **2e**, **2b**, and **1d**. The amide derivatives of benzofurans (compounds **2a**, **3c**, **1a**) that lack halogen-containing alkyl substituents (a bromine atom) did not show the cytotoxic properties toward cancer cell lines. A similar effect is observed for derivatives with a free acidic group (compounds **1**, **3b**) and ester derivatives (**1b**).

We can observe a marked decrease in the activity and selectivity of these derivatives when comparing the activity of bromo-derivatives **1c** and **1e** with the activity of the lead compound **VIII**. This effect is probably due to the absence of the acetyl group at the 2-position of the furan ring. The derivative **1c** has an ester group and the compound **1e** a bromine atom in this position. Thus, it can be concluded that the arrangement of substituents: the acetyl group at the 2-position and the bromomethyl at the three-position determines the activity and selectivity of the lead compound.

Analysis of the results for the active **2d** derivative in comparison to its lead compound **IX** also indicates that the structural modifications of **2d** resulted in a loss of selectivity and decreased activity. In this case, the derivatives differ in the location of the halogen atom. The **2d** derivative contains the bromomethyl substituent in the two-position and the acetyl group in the six-position of the benzofuran system, while the **IX** contains the methyl group in the two-position and the bromoacetyl substituent in the six-position of the benzofuran system. It can again be assumed that the presence of a halogen atom substituted to an alkyl/acetyl moiety determines the activity of the derivatives, but the appropriate positioning of substituents is important in their selectivity. Finally, by comparing the active derivatives **3a** and **3d** with their lead compound **X**, we also observe a decrease in activity and selectivity. The **3a** compound differs from the leading compound by the presence of a hydroxyl group. It can be hypothesized that the reduction of the keto group and the possibility of creating additional hydrogen bonds, as well as an increase in the hydrophilicity could affect the activity of this derivative.

Compound **3d** contains a bromomethyl substituent at the two-position and an acetyl group at the six-position, while **X** contains a bromoacetyl group at the six-position and a methyl at the two-position. Both of the compounds exhibit cytotoxicity, but the absence of the bromoacetyl substituent in compound **3d** eliminated its selectivity and decreased cytotoxicity to the cancer cells.

4. Materials and Methods

4.1. Chemistry

All of the solvents, reagents, and chemicals used in these studies were purchased from Aldrich Chemical (Saint Louis, MO, USA) and Merck AG (Saint Louis, MO, USA). The melting points were determined with Electrothermal 9100 capillary apparatus and they are uncorrected. The nuclear magnetic resonance spectra (University of Warsaw, Warsaw, Poland) were recorded in DMSO-d_6 or $CDCl_3$ on VMNRS300 operating at 300 MHz (^{1}H-NMR) and 75 MHz (^{13}C-NMR). Chemical shifts (δ) are expressed in parts per million relative to tetramethylsilane used as the internal reference. The coupling constants (J) values are given in hertz (Hz) and spin multiples are given as s (singlet), d (dublet), t (triplet), and m (multiplet). Mass spectral ESI (Electrospray Ionization) measurements were carried out on a MicrOTOF II, Bruker instrument with a TOF detector (Jagiellonian Univeristy in Krakov, Poland). The spectra were obtained in the positive ion mode. Elemental analyses were recorded with CHNS micro analyzer elementary model Vario Micro Cube with electronic microbalance (Jagiellonian Univeristy in Krakow, Poland). Flash chromatography was performed on Merck Kieselgel 0.05–0.2 mm reinst (70–325 mesh ASTM, Saint Louis, MO, USA) silica gel using chloroform as eluent. TLC monitored progress of the reactions described in the experimental section on silica gel (plates with fluorescent indicator 254 nm, layer thickness 0.2 mm, Kieselgel G. Merck, Saint Louis, MO, USA), using chloroform-methanol as an eluent system at the *v*/*v* ratio of 9.8:0.2 or 9.5:0.5.

4.2. General Synthetic Procedures

Procedure 1. Procedure for Synthesis of Amides.

An appropriate carboxylic acid (0.004 mol) was suspended in anhydrous dichlorometane (DCM) (10 mL). Next, oxalyl chloride (0.43 mL, 0.005 mol) and the one drop of dimethylformamide (DMF) were added to the solution. The reaction mixture was stirred at room temperature for 24 h. Then, ammonium solution (aq. 30%, 5 mL) was added drop by drop and the mixture was stirred at room temperature for additional 12 h. When the reaction was complete (TLC control) the resulting mixture was diluted with water (50 mL) and extracted with DCM (3 × 50 mL). The organic extracts were dried with magnesium sulfate and concentrated under reduced pressure. The resulting solid was purified by a silica gel column chromatography (eluent: chloroform or chloroform:methanol; 50:0.2, *v*/*v*).

Procedure 2. Procedure for the Preparation of Methyl ester.

Procedure according to the method described earlier [11]. Thus, a mixture of appropriate carboxylic acid (0.02 mol), K_2CO_3 (0.1 mol) and $(CH_3O)_2SO_2$ (0.02 mol) in acetone was refluxed for 48 h. When the reaction was complete, the mixture was filtered and the solvent was removed on rotary evaporator [11]. The residue was purified by a silica gel column chromatography (eluent: chloroform or chloroform:methanol; 50:0.2 *v*/*v*).

Procedure 3. Procedure for Bromination by Using N-Bromosuccinimide (NBS).

In this method, the procedure was used, as described earlier [11]. Briefly, *N*-bromosuccinimide (NBS) (0.02 mol) and the catalytic amount of benzoyl peroxide were added to a solution of the appropriate ester or acid (0.02 mol) in dry carbon tetrachloride or alternatively in ethanol (50 mL). The reaction mixture was refluxed for 24 h. When the reaction was complete (TLC monitoring), the mixture was filtered and the solvent was removed under reduced pressure. Silica gel column chromatography purified the residue (eluent: chloroform or chloroform:methanol; 50:0.2 *v*/*v*).

Procedure 4. Procedure for Bromination by Using Br_2.

Method a. Procedure according to the method that was described earlier [11]. Thus, an appropriate ester, amide, or acid (0.02 mol) was dissolved in $CHCl_3$ (20 mL), and then a solution of bromine in $CHCl_3$ (0.02 mol in 10 mL) was added dropwise with stirring for 1 h. The obtained mixture was stirred at room temperature for 24 h. When the reaction was finished, the solvent was removed under reduced pressure. The residue was purified by a silica gel column chromatography (eluent: chloroform or chloroform:methanol; 50:0.2 *v*/*v*).

Method b. Procedure according to the method described earlier [11]. Thus, an appropriate ester, amide, or acid (0.02 mol) was dissolved in CH_3COOH (80%, 20 mL), and then a solution of bromine in CH_3COOH (0.02 mol in 10 mL) was added dropwise with stirring for 1 h. The obtained mixture was stirred at room temperature for 24 h. When the reaction was complete, the resulting mixture was diluted by $Na_2S_2O_3$ solution (10 mL) and extracted with DCM (3 × 50 mL). The obtained organic extracts were dried with calcium chloride, filtered, and concentrated under reduced pressure. Silica gel column chromatography purified the residue (eluent: chloroform or chloroform:methanol; 50:0.2 *v*/*v*).

Procedure 5. Procedure for Reduction.

A starting ketone (0.0024 mol) was dissolved in the peroxides-free dioxane (20 mL), and then $NABH(OAc)_3$ (0.0048 mol) was added. The mixture was stirred at room temperature for 24–48 h. When the reaction was complete, the solvent was removed under reduced pressure. The solid residue was dissolved in $CHCl_3$ (50 mL) and then washed with water (3 × 20 mL). The organic solution was dried with magnesium sulfate, filtered, and concentrated under reduced pressure. Finally, silica gel column chromatography purified the residue (eluent: chloroform or chloroform:methanol; 50:0.2 *v/v*).

4.2.1. Synthesis of Analogues of Compound **VIII**

Synthesis of 7-Acetyl-5,6-Dimethoxy-3-Methylbenzofuran-2-Carboxylic Acid (**1**)

7-Acetyl-5,6-dimethoxy-3-methylbenzofuran-2-carboxylic acid was obtained in the multistep reaction according to the method described earlier [28].

M.W. = 278.2573; $C_{14}H_{14}O_6$; Yield: 30%; white powder, m.p. 212–214 °C; ^{1}H-NMR (300 MHz, DMSO, δ/ppm): 2.50 (3H, s, -CH_3), 2.62 (3H, s, -$COCH_3$), 3.84 (3H, s, -OCH_3), 3.92 (3H, s, -OCH_3), 7.47 (1H, s, Ar-H), 13.41 (1H, br.s, -COOH); ^{13}C-NMR: δ 9.15, 32.13, 56.43, 61.755, 105.50, 119.64, 124.39, 124.68, 142.19, 144.27, 147.40, 150.07, 160.76, 197.33;.HRMS (*m/z*): calculated value for [M + Na] 100% = 301.0683; found 100% = 301.0681$^+$; Anal. Calc. for $C_{14}H_{14}O_6$: 60.43% C; 5.07% H, found 59.25% C; 4.92% H.

Synthesis of 7-Acetyl-5,6-Dimethoxy-3-Methylbenzofuran-2-Carboxamide (**1a**)

7-Acetyl-5,6-dimethoxy-3-methylbenzofuran-2-carboxamide was obtained according to Procedure 1.

M.W. = 277.2726; $C_{14}H_{15}NO_5$, Yield: 37%; white powder, m.p. 203–205 °C; ^{1}H-NMR (300 MHz, $CDCl_3$, δ/ppm): 2.50 (3H, s, -CH_3), 2.68 (3H, s, -$COCH_3$), 3.80 (3H, s, -OCH_3), 3.90 (3H, s, -OCH_3), 7.41 (1H, s, Ar-H), 7.70 (2H, br.m, -NH_2); ^{13}C-NMR: δ 8.73, 32.47, 56.04, 61.85, 104.99, 120.02, 121.07, 125.07, 143.14, 144.08, 146.34, 150.07, 160.93, 197.55; HRMS (*m/z*): calculated value for [M + Na] 100% = 300.0842, found 100% = 300.0842$^+$. Anal. Calc. for $C_{14}H_{15}NO_5$: 60.64% C; 5.45% H, 5.05% N, found 60.04% C; 4.537% H, 4.81% N.

Synthesis of Methyl 7-Acetyl-5,6-Dimethoxy-3-Methylbenzofuran-2-Carboxylate (**1b**)

Methyl 7-acetyl-5,6-dimethoxy-3-methyl-1-benzofuran-2-carboxylate was obtained according to Procedure 2. M.W. = 292.2839; $C_{15}H_{16}O_6$; Yield: 60%; white powder, m.p. 98–100 °C; ^{1}H-NMR (300 MHz, $CDCl_3$, δ/ppm): 2.55 (3H, s, -CH_3), 2.73 (3H, s, -$COCH_3$), 3.94 (3H, s, -OCH_3), 3.95 (3H, s, -OCH_3), 3.95 (3H, s, -$COOCH_3$), 7.10 (1H, s, Ar-H); ^{13}C-NMR: δ 9.22, 32.34, 51.84, 56.38, 62.40, 104.42, 120.28, 124.84, 125.43, 141.68, 145.57, 148.67, 150.58, 160.41, 197.50; HRMS (*m/z*): calculated value for [M + Na] 100% = 315.0839, found 100% = 315.0839. Anal. Calc. for $C_{15}H_{16}O_6$: 61.64% C; 5.52% H, found 61.35% C; 5.516% H.

Synthesis of Methyl 7-Acetyl-3-(Bromomethyl)-5,6-Dimethoxybenzofuran-2-Carboxylate (**1c**)

Methyl 7-acetyl-3-(bromomethyl)-5,6-dimethoxybenzofuran-2-carboxylate was obtained according to Procedure 4 (method a). M.W. = 371.1800; $C_{15}H_{15}BrO_6$; Yield: 20%; white powder, m.p. 124–125 °C; ^{1}H-NMR (300 MHz, $CDCl_3$, δ/ppm): 2.72 (3H, s, -$COCH_3$), 3.97 (9H, m, -OCH_3, -OCH_3, -$COOCH_3$), 4.90 (2H, -CH_2Br), 7.33 (1H, s, Ar-H); ^{13}C-NMR: δ 20.46, 32.30, 52.35, 56.43, 62.41, 104.32, 120.53, 122.56, 124.99, 141.66, 145.71, 149.11, 151.01, 159.61, 197.15; HRMS (*m/z*): calculated value for [M + Na] 100% = 392.9944, 99% = 394.9927, found 100% = 392.9945, 99% = 394.9926. Anal. Calc. for $C_{15}H_{14}$ BrO_6: 48.54% C; 4.07% H, found 48.82% C; 4.15% H.

Synthesis of 1-(2-Bromo-5,6-Dimethoxy-3-Methylbenzofuran-7-yl)ethanone (**1d**)

1-(2-Bromo-5,6-dimethoxy-3-methylbenzofuran-7-yl)ethanone was obtained according to Procedure 3 (in ethanol) as well as Procedure 4 (method b). Yield: M.W. = 313.1439; $C_{13}H_{13}BrO_4$; Yield: 27%; white powder, m.p. 94–95 °C; ^{1}H-NMR (300 MHz, $CDCl_3$, δ/ppm): 2.16 (3H, s, -CH_3), 2.69 (3H, s, -$COCH_3$), 3.90 (3H, s, -OCH_3), 3.93 (3H, s, -OCH_3), 6.98 (1H, s, Ar-H); ^{13}C-NMR: δ 8.69, 32.26, 56.47, 62.38, 103.39, 114.99, 119.83, 125.37, 126.39, 145.20, 1454.74, 150.22, 197.82; HRMS (*m/z*): calculated value for [M + Na] 100% = 334.9889, 99% = 336.9870, found 100% = 334.9897, 99% = 336.9869. Anal. Calc. for $C_{13}H_{13}BrO_4$: 49.86% C; 4.18% H, found 49.76% C; 4.159% H.

Synthesis of 2-Bromo-1-(2-Bromo-5,6-Dimethoxy-3-Methylbenzofuran-7-yl]ethanone (**1e**)

2-Bromo-1-(2-bromo-5,6-dimethoxy-3-methylbenzofuran-7-yl)ethanone was obtained according to Procedure 3 (in ethanol). M.W. = 392.0399; $C_{13}H_{12}Br_2O_4$; Yield: 27%; white powder, m.p. 128–129 °C; ^{1}H-NMR (300 MHz, $CDCl_3$, δ/ppm): 2.17 (3H, s, $-CH_3$), 3.94 (6H, s, $-OCH_3$, $-OCH_3$), 4.58 (2H, s, $-COCH_2Br$), 7.03 (1H, s, Ar-H); ^{13}C-NMR: δ 8.69, 36.49, 56.53, 62.49, 104.60, 115.16, 116.09, 125.46, 126.66, 145.84, 145.95, 150.10, 190.29; HRMS (*m/z*): calculated value for [M + Na] 50% = 412.8995, 100% = 414.8975, 49% = 416.8956, found 50% = 412.8991, 100% = 414.8973, 49% = 416.8944. Anal. Calc. for $C_{13}H_{12}$ Br_2O_4: 39.83% C; 3.09% H, found 40.21% C; 3.066% H.

4.2.2. Synthesis of Analogues of Compound **IX**

Synthesis of 6-Acetyl-5-Hydroxy-2-Methylbenzofuran-3-Carboxamide (**2a**)

6-Acetyl-5-hydroxy-2-methylbenzofuran-3-carboxamide was obtained according to Procedure 1. M.W. = 233.2200; $C_{12}H_{11}NO_4$; Yield: 50%; white powder, m.p. 268–267 °C; ^{1}H-NMR (300 MHz, DMSO, δ/ppm): 2.65 (3H, s, $-COCH_3$), 2.68 (3H, s, $-CH_3$), 7.22 (1H, s, Ar-H), 7.48 (2H, br.s, $-NH_2$), 8.11 (1H, s, Ar-H), 11.97 (1H, s, -OH); ^{13}C-NMR: δ 14.20, 27.52, 107.03, 112.69, 112.74, 116.38, 133.39, 146.00, 157.39, 163.86, 164.22, 204.26; HRMS (*m/z*): calculated value for [M + Na] 100% = 256.0580, found 100% = 256.0582. Anal. Calc. for $C_{12}H_{11}NO_4$: 61.80% C; 4.75% H, 6.01% N, found 60.85% C; 4.766% H, 5.83% N.

Synthesis of 6-Acetyl-4-Bromo-5-Hydroxy-2-Methylbenzofuran-3-Carboxamide (**2b**)

6-Acetyl-4-bromo-5-hydroxy-2-methylbenzofuran-3-carboxamide was obtained according to Procedure 4 (method b). M.W. = 312.1161; $C_{12}H_{10}BrNO_4$; Yield: 40%; white powder, m.p. 249–248 °C; ^{1}H-NMR (300 MHz, DMSO, δ/ppm): 2.50 (3H, s, $-COCH_3$), 2.68 (3H, s, $-CH_3$), 7.69 (1H, br.s, $-NH_2$), 7.94 (1H, br.s, $-NH_2$), 8.23 (1H, s, Ar-H), 12.88 (1H, s, -OH); ^{13}C-NMR: δ 13.20, 27.05, 99.21, 112.59, 115.82, 115.86, 133.19, 145.62, 154.37, 160.33, 163.79, 204.99; HRMS (*m/z*): calculated value for [M + Na] 100% = 333.9685, 98% = 335.9666, found 100% = 333.9685, 98% = 335.9669. Anal. Calc. for $C_{12}H_{10}BrNO_4$: 46.18% C; 3.23% H, 4.49% N, found 46.33% C; 3.265% H, 4.35% N.

Synthesis of Methyl 6-Acetyl-5-Hydroxy-2-Methylbenzofuran-3-Carboxylate (**2c**)

Methyl 6-acetyl-5-hydroxy-2-methylbenzofuran-3-carboxylate (**2c**) was obtained according to the method described previously [11].

Synthesis of Methyl 6-Acetyl-2-(Bromomethyl)-5-Hydroxybenzofuran-3-Carboxylate (**2d**)

Methyl 6-acetyl-2-(bromomethyl)-5-hydroxybenzofuran-3-carboxylate was obtained according to Procedure 3 (in CCl_4). M.W. = 327.1274; $C_{13}H_{11}BrO_5$; Yield: 30%; white powder, m.p. 94–95 °C (chyba 138–140); ^{1}H-NMR (300 MHz, $CDCl_3$, δ/ppm): 2.70 (3H, s, $-COCH_3$), 3.99 (3H, s, $-COOCH_3$), 4.94 (2H, s, $-CH_2Br$), 7.53 (1H, s, Ar-H), 7.88 (1H, s, Ar-H), 12.11 (1H, s, -OH); ^{13}C-NMR: δ 14.19, 26.80, 52.08, 110.51, 112.63, 117.59, 132.64, 146.73, 155.99, 161.21, 162.63, 164.00, 203.35; HRMS (*m/z*): calculated value for [M + Na] 100% = 348.9682, 99% = 350.9663, found 100% = 348.9683, 99% = 350.9663. Anal. Calc. for $C_{13}H_{11}BrO_5$: 47.73% C; 3.39% H, found 47.33% C; 3.265% H.

Synthesis of 6-Acetyl-4-Bromo-5-Hydroxy-2-Methylbenzofuran-3-Carboxylic Acid (**2e**)

6-Acetyl-4-bromo-5-hydroxy-2-methylbenzofuran-3-carboxylic acid was obtained according Procedure 4 (method b). M.W. = 313.1008; $C_{12}H_9BrO_5$; Yield: 30%; white powder, m.p. 196–197 °C; ^{1}H-NMR (300 MHz, $CDCl_3$, δ/ppm): 2.48 (3H, s, $-COCH_3$), 2.69 (3H, s, $-CH_3$), 7.72 (1H, s, Ar-H), 12.89 (1H, s, -OH); ^{13}C-NMR: δ 13.20, 26.70, 94.45, 100.68, 111.33, 116.11, 132.08, 145.99, 155.30, 159.72, 203.35;

HRMS (*m/z*): calculated value for [M + Na] 100% = 334.9526, 99% = 336.9506, found 100%= 334.9525, 99% = 336.9505. Anal. Calc. for $C_{12}H_9BrO_5$: 46.03% C; 2.90% H, found 46.33% C; 2.265% H.

4.2.3. Synthesis of Analogues of Compound **X**

Synthesis of Methyl 6-Acetyl-5-Methoxy-2-Methylbenzofuran-3-Carboxylate (**3**) and Methyl 6-(Dibromoacetyl)-5-Methoxy-2-Methyl-1-Benzofuran-3-Carboxylate (**X**)

Methyl 6-acetyl-5-methoxy-2-methylbenzofuran-3-carboxylate (**3**) and methyl 6-(dibromoacetyl)-5-methoxy-2-methylbenzofuran-3-carboxylate (**X**) were obtained according to the method described previously [11].

Synthesis of Methyl 6-(2,2-Dibromo-1-Hydroxyethyl)-5-Methoxy-2-Methylbenzofuran-3-Carboxylate (**3a**)

Methyl 6-(2,2-dibromo-1-hydroxyethyl)-5-methoxy-2-methylbenzofuran-3-carboxylate (**3a**) was obtained according to Procedure 5. M.W. = 422.0659; $C_{14}H_{14}Br_2O_5$; Yield: 70%; white powder, m.p. 170–172 °C; ^{1}H-NMR (300 MHz, DMSO, δ/ppm): 2.74 (3H, s, -$COOCH_3$), 3.18 (1H, br.s, -CH-), 3.93 (3H, s, -OCH_3), 3.94 (3H, s, -CH_3), 5.34 (1H, br.s, –OH), 6.14 (1H, d, -CH-, J = 3 Hz), 7.41 (1H, s, Ar-H), 7.59 (1H, s, Ar-H); ^{13}C-NMR: δ 14.73, 51.46, 51.77, 55.93, 75.00, 102.26, 108.96, 110.78, 123.97, 126.92, 148.14, 153.17, 164.71, 164.75; HRMS (*m/z*): calculated value for [M + Na] 50% = 442.9100, 100% = 444.9081, 50% = 446.9063, found 50% = 442.9094, 100% = 444.9079, 50% = 446.9065. Anal. Calc. for $C_{14}H_{14}Br_2O_6$: 39.84% C; 3.34% H, found 40.20% C; 3.37% H.

Synthesis of 6-Acetyl-5-Methoxy-2-Methylbenzofuran-3-Carboxylic Acid (**3b**)

A mixture of methyl 6-acetyl-5-methoxy-2-methylbenzofuran-3-carboxylate (0.0008 mol) and 2 M NaOH (0.6 mL, 0.0012 mol) in ethanol (1.2 mL) was heated for 1 h. The bulk of the solvent was evaporated and the residue was acidified with 2 M HCl (1.2 mL) to give a fine precipitate. Next, the mixture was cooled to room temperature and then filtered to give the product. M.W. = 248.2313; $C_{13}H_{12}O_5$; Yield: 30%; white powder, m.p. 249–250 °C; ^{1}H-NMR (300 MHz, DMSO, δ/ppm): 2.55 (3H, s, -$COCH_3$), 2.71 (3H, s, -CH_3), 3.90 (3H, s, -OCH_3), 7.45 (1H, s, Ar-H), 7.69 (1H, s, Ar-H); ^{13}C-NMR: δ 14.41, 31.61, 56.03, 103.27, 109.23, 111.32, 124.90, 130.79, 147.06, 155.84, 164.66, 166.58, 197.99; HRMS (*m/z*): calculated value for [M + Na] 100% = 271.0577, found 100% = 270.0737. Anal. Calc. for $C_{13}H_{12}O_5$* $\frac{1}{2}$ H_2O: 60.50% C; 5.07% H, found 60.05% C; 4.715% H.

Synthesis of 6-Acetyl-5-Methoxy-2-Methylbenzofuran-3-Carboxamide (**3c**)

6-Acetyl-5-methoxy-2-methylbenzofuran-3-carboxamide was obtained according to Procedure 1.

M.W. = 247.2466; $C_{13}H_{13}NO_4$; Yield: 30%; white powder, m.p. 223–224 °C; ^{1}H-NMR (300 MHz, DMSO, δ/ppm): 2.55 (3H, s, -$COCH_3$), 2.68 (3H, s, -CH_3), 3.98 (3H, s, -OCH_3), 7.22 (1H, s, Ar-H), 7.53 (2H, br.s, -NH_2), 7.70 (1H, s, Ar-H); ^{13}C-NMR: δ 14.11, 31.61, 56.17, 103.10, 111.14, 112.81, 124.65, 130.56, 146.94, 155.49, 162.02, 164.42, 198.08; HRMS (*m/z*): calculated value for [M + Na] 100% = 270.0737, found 100% = 270.0737. Anal. Calc. for $C_{13}H_{13}NO_4$: 63.15% C; 5.30% H, 5.67% N, found 62.90% C; 5.245% H, 5.63% N.

Synthesis of Methyl 6-Acetyl-2-(Bromomethyl)-5-Methoxybenzofuran-3-Carboxylate (**3d**)

Methyl 6-acetyl-2-(bromomethyl)-5-methoxybenzofuran-3-carboxylate was obtained according to Procedure 3 (in CCl_4). M.W. = 341.1540; $C_{14}H_{13}BrO_5$; Yield: 30%; white powder, m.p. 148–150 °C; ^{1}H-NMR (300 MHz, $CDCl_3$, δ/ppm): 2.65 (3H, s, -$COCH_3$), 3.98 (3H, s, -OCH_3), 4.01 (3H, s, -COOCH3), 4.91 (2H, s, -CH2Br), 7.50 (1H, s, Ar-H), 7.86 7.70 (1H, s, Ar-H); ^{13}C-NMR: δ 20.94, 31.08, 52.07, 56.03, 103.76, 110.48, 112.98, 127.44, 129.80, 148.49, 156.56, 161.91, 163.30, 199.04; HRMS (*m/z*): calculated value for [M + Na] 100% = 362.9839, 99% = 364.9820, found 100% = 362.9839, 99% = 364.9820. Anal. Calc. for $C_{14}H_{13}BrO_5$: 49.29% C; 3.84% H, found 48.87% C; 3.755% H.

4.3. Anticancer Activity

4.3.1. Cells and Cytotoxicity Assay

Human umbilical vein endothelial cells (Life Technologies, Waltham, MA, USA) were cultured (according to the manufacturer instructions) in Medium 200 supplemented with Low Serum Growth Supplement. 1×10^4 HUVEC cells were seeded on each well on a 96-well plate (Nunc). The HeLa (human cervix carcinoma) K562 and MOLT-4 (leukemia) cells were cultured in RPMI 1640 medium supplemented with antibiotics and 10% fetal calf serum (HeLa, K562) in a 5% CO_2-95% air atmosphere. 7×10^3 HeLa, K562, or MOLT-4 cells were seeded on each well on 96-well plate (Nunc). 24 h later cells were treated with the test compounds and then incubated for an additional 48 hours. Stock solutions of test compounds were freshly prepared in DMSO (dimethylsulfoxide). The final concentrations of compounds that were tested in the cell cultures were: 2×10^{-1}, 1×10^{-1}, 5×10^{-2}, 1×10^{-2}, 1×10^{-3} and 1×10^{-4} mM. The concentration of DMSO in the cell culture medium was 1%.

The values of IC_{50} (the concentration of test compound that is required to reduce the cell survival fraction to 50% of the control) were calculated from dose-response curves and used as a measure of cellular sensitivity to a given treatment.

The MTT [3-(4,5-dimethylthiazol-2-yl)-2,5-diphenyltetrazolium bromide; Sigma, St. Louis, MO, USA] assay determined the cytotoxicity of all the compounds, as described previously [30]. Briefly, after 24 h or 48 h of incubation with the drug, the cells were treated with the MTT reagent, and incubation was continued for 2 h. MTT-formazan crystals were dissolved in 20% SDS and 50% DMF at pH 4.7 and absorbance was read at 570 and 650 nm on an ELISA-PLATE READER (FLUOstar Omega, BMG LABTECH GmbH, Ortenberg, Germany). As a control (100% viability), cells that were grown in the presence of medium vehicle only with 1% DMSO were used.

4.3.2. Induction of Cell Apoptosis Analyzed by Caspase-3/7 Assay

20×10^3 K562 cells were seeded on each well of 96-well plate in RPMI 1640 medium supplemented with 10% fetal calf serum and antibiotics. Cells were grown for 24 h at 37 °C and 5% CO_2. The test compounds were dissolved in DMSO and added to the cell culture. The concentration of tested benzo[b]furans in cell culture was $5 \times IC_{50}$.

Cells treated with 1% DMSO served as a negative control, while cells incubated with staurosporine (a strong inducer of apoptosis) were used as a positive control. Cells were exposed to test compounds for 18 h at 37 °C and 5% CO_2. Subsequently, Apo-ONE® Homogeneous Caspase-3/7 Assay (Promega, Madison, WI, USA) measured the activity of caspase 3 and 7, according to the manufacturer's instructions. Briefly, the cells were lysed and incubated for 1.5 h with profluorescent substrate for caspase 3 and 7. Next, fluorescence was read at an excitation wavelength of 485 nm and emission of 520 nm with FLUOStar Omega plate reader (BMG-Labtech, Ortenberg, Germany).

4.3.3. Digestion of Plasmid DNA with BamHI Restriction Nuclease

0.5 μg of plasmid DNA (pcDNAHisC, total length 5.5 kbp) containing a unique *BamHI* restriction site was dissolved in a 1× *BamHI* reaction buffer and then incubated overnight at 37 °C with the test compounds or daunorubicin, a strong intercalating agent, which was used as a positive control. The concentration of the test compounds and daunorubicin samples was 100 μM. In the next step, the reaction mixtures were digested with *BamHI* restriction endonuclease (2 U/μL) for 3 h at 37 °C. The total reaction volume was 10 μL. Products of the reaction were subjected to the 1% agarose gel electrophoresis in TBE buffer. The gel was stained with ethidium bromide and DNA fragments were visualized under a UV lamp (GBox, Syngene, Cambridge, UK).

5. Conclusions

We synthesized and tested a group of new benzofuran derivatives. The presence of bromine in the alkyl group in the furan ring is most likely responsible for the cytotoxic properties of the tested derivatives (compounds **1c**, **2d**, **3d**). Compound **1e** shows the cytotoxic property, and contains an acetyl halide substituent (bromine) in the benzene ring and a bromine atom that is directly attached to the furan ring. The most active compounds **2d** and **3d**, showed increased polarity when compared to the lead compounds **VIII-X**, but their cytotoxicity against human cancer cells decreased by 5–10 folds and the toxicity against normal cells increased. The formation of amide derivatives of benzofurans (compounds **1a**, **2a**, **2b**, **3c**) and the lack of a halogen-containing alkyl substituent in their structure resulted in better water solubility but loss of cytotoxic properties towards the cancer cells studied. A reduction of the bromoacetyl group in compound **X** increased its polarity but also eliminated the selectivity of the compound and diminished its toxicity towards tumor cells.

Author Contributions: Conceptualization, M.N.; Methodology, M.N. and M.C.; Performed the experiments M.N., M.C., J.K.-B., K.K.-G. Writing—Original Draft Preparation, M.N.; Writing—Review & Editing, M.N., M.C. and B.N.; Visualization, M.N. and M.C.; Supervision, B.N.; Project Administration, M.N. and M.C.; Funding Acquisition, M.N. and B.N.

Acknowledgments: The cytotoxicity, activation of caspases and DNA interaction studies were performed in the Screening Laboratory at the Division of Bioorganic Chemistry, Centre of Molecular and Macromolecular Studies of the Polish Academy of Sciences.

References

1. Habtemarian, S. Antiinflammatory activity of the antirheumatic herbal drug, gravel root (Eupatorium purpureum): Further biological activities and constituents. *Phytoter. Res.* **2001**, *15*, 687–690. [CrossRef] [PubMed]
2. Pauletti, M.P.; Araujo, A.R.; Young, M.C.; Giesbrecht, A.M.; Bolzani, V.D. nor-Lignans from the leaves of Styrax ferrugineus (Styracaceae) with antibacterial and antifungal activity. *Phytochemistry* **2000**, *55*, 597–601. [CrossRef]
3. Masubuchi, M.; Kawasaki, K.; Ebiike, H.; Ikeda, Y.; Tsujii, S.; Sogabe, S.; Fujii, T.; Sakata, K.; Shiratori, Y.; Aoki, Y.; et al. Design and synthesis of novel benzofurans as new class of antifungal agents targeting fungal N-myristoyltransferase. Part 1. *Bioorg. Med. Chem. Lett.* **2001**, *11*, 1833–1837. [CrossRef]
4. Wróbel, J.E.; Dietrich, A.J.; Antane, M.M. Benzotiophenes, Benzofurans, and Indoles useful in the treatment of insulin resistance and hyperglycemia. U.S. Patent 6,251,936, 26 June 2001.
5. Kayser, O.; Chen, M.; Kharazmi, A.; Kiderlen, A.F. Aurones Interfere with *Leismania major* mitochondrial fumarate reductase. *Z. Naturforsch. C* **2002**, *57*, 717–720. [CrossRef]
6. Hayakawa, I.; Shioya, R.; Agatsuma, T.; Furukawa, H.; Naruto, S.; Sugano, Y. 4-Hydroxy-3-methyl-6-phenylbenzofuran-2-carboxylic acid ethyl ester derivatives as potent anti-tumor agents. *Bioorg. Med. Chem. Lett.* **2004**, *14*, 455–458. [CrossRef] [PubMed]
7. Dawood, K.M. Benzofuran derivatives: A patent review. *Expert Opin. Ther. Pat.* **2013**, *23*, 1133–1156. [CrossRef] [PubMed]
8. Kossakowski, J.; Ostrowska, K.; Hejchman, E.; Wolska, I. Synthesis and structural characterization of derivatives of 2- and 3-benzo[b]furan carboxylic acids with potential cytotoxic activity. *Il Farmaco* **2005**, *60*, 519–527. [CrossRef] [PubMed]
9. Graves, A.P.; Brenk, R.; Shoichet, B.K. Decoys for Docking. *J. Med. Chem.* **2005**, *48*, 3714–3728. [CrossRef]
10. Repolles, M.J.; Pubill, C.F.; Cabeza, L.L.; Carbo, B.M.; Cerda, R.J.A.; Negrie, R.C. Benzofuran, dihydrobenzofuran, dihydrobenzopyran and benzopyran derivatives as antidepressant agents. Spanish Patent ES2131020 A1, 1 July 1999.
11. Kossakowski, J.; Krawiecka, M.; Kuran, B.; Stefańska, J.; Wolska, I. Synthesis and preliminary evaluation of the antimicrobial activity of selected 3-benzofurancarboxylic acid derivatives. *Molecules* **2010**, *15*, 4737–4749. [CrossRef]
12. Kossakowski, J.; Ostrowska, K. Synthesis of new derivatives of 2,3-dihydro-7-benzo[b]furanol with potential pharmacological activity. *Acta Pol. Pharm.* **2006**, *63*, 271–275.

13. Kossakowski, J.; Ostrowska, K.; Struga, M.; Stefańska, J. Synthesis of new derivatives of 2,2-dimethyl-2,3-dihydro-7-benzo[b]furanol with potential antimicrobial activity. *Med. Chem. Res.* **2009**, *18*, 555–565. [CrossRef]
14. Kodama, I.; Kamiya, K.; Toyama, J. Amiodarone: Ionic and cellular mechanisms of action of the most promising class III agent. *Am. J. Cardiol.* **1999**, *84*, 20R–28R. [CrossRef]
15. Courchesne, W.E. Characterization of novel, broad-based fungicidal activity for anti-arrhythmic drug amiodarone. *J. Pharmacol. Exp. Ther.* **2002**, *300*, 195–199. [CrossRef]
16. Courchesne, W.E.; Ozturk, S. Amiodarone induces a caffeine-inhibited, MID1-dependent rise in free cytoplasic calcium in *Saccharomyces cerevisiae*. *Mol. Microbiol.* **2003**, *47*, 223–234. [CrossRef]
17. Gill, J.; Heel, R.C.; Fitton, A. Amiodarone. An overview of its pharmacological properties, and review of its therapeutic use in cardiac arrhythmias. *Drugs* **1992**, *43*, 69–110. [CrossRef]
18. Pizzichini, M.; Aleo, M.F.; Marcolongo, R.; Marinello, E. The mechanism of benziodarone activity. *Quad. Sclavo. Diagn.* **1982**, *18*, 203–208.
19. Heel, R.C.; Brogden, R.N.; Speight, T.M.; Avery, G.S. Benzbromarone: A review of its pharmacological properties and therapeutic use in gout and hyperuricaemia. *Drugs* **1977**, *14*, 349–366. [CrossRef]
20. Masbernard, A.; Giudicelli, C.P. Ten years' experience with benzbromarone in the management of gout and hyperuricaemia. *S. Afr. Med. J.* **1981**, *59*, 701–706.
21. Lu, Y.; Shi, T.; Wang, Y.; Yang, H.; Yan, X.; Luo, X.; Jiang, H.; Zhu, W. Halogen Bonding-A Novel Interaction for Rational Drug Design? *J. Med. Chem.* **2009**, *52*, 2584–2862. [CrossRef]
22. Bissantz, C.; Kuhn, B.; Stahl, M. A Medicinal Chemist's Guide to Molecular Interaction. *J. Med. Chem.* **2010**, *53*, 5061–5084. [CrossRef]
23. Wilcken, R.; Zimmermann, M.O.; Lange, A.; Joerger, A.C.; Boeckler, F.M. Principles and Applications of Halogen Bonding in Medicinal Chemistry and Chemical Biology. *J. Med. Chem.* **2013**, *56*, 1363–1388. [CrossRef]
24. Ford, C.M.; Shing, H.P. Computational Tools To model Halogen Bonds in Medicinal Chemistry. *J. Med. Chem.* **2016**, *59*, 1655–1670. [CrossRef] [PubMed]
25. Krawiecka, M.; Kuran, B.; Kossakowski, J.; Cieślak, M.; Kazmierczak-Barańska, J.; Królewska, K.; Nawrot, B. Synthesis and cytotoxic properties of halogen and aryl-/heteroarylpiperazinyl derivatives of benzofurans. *Anti Cancer Agents Med. Chem.* **2015**, *15*, 115–121. [CrossRef]
26. Kossakowski, J.; Kuran, B.; Kazmierczak-Baranska, J.; Królewska, K.; Nawrot, B.; Krawiecka, M.; Cieslak, M. Halogen derivatives of benzo[b]furans useful as anti-neoplastic or anti-proliferative drugs. Spanish Patent EP 2631232 A1, 9 January 2013.
27. Królewska-Golińska, K.; Cieślak, M.J.; Sobczak, M.; Dolot, R.; Radzikowska-Cieciura, E.; Napiórkowska, M.; Wybrańska, I.; Nawrot, B. Novel benzo[b]furans with anti-microtubule activity upregulate expression of apoptotic genes and arrest leukemia cells in G2/M phase. *Anticancer Agents Med. Chem.* **2018**. [CrossRef] [PubMed]
28. Zawadowski, T.; Suski, S.; Rump, S.; Borkowska, G. Synthesis of new aminoalkanoles derivatives of benzofurans with an expected β-adrenolityc activity. *Acta Polon. Pharm.* **1989**, *XLVI*, 201–208.
29. Fink, S.L.; Cookson, B.T. Apoptosis, Pyroptosis, and Necrosis: Mechanistic Description of Dead and Dying Eukaryotic Cells. *Infect. Immun.* **2005**, *73*, 1907–1916. [CrossRef]
30. Maszewska, M.; Leclaire, J.; Cieslak, M.; Nawrot, B.; Okruszek, A.; Caminade, A.M.; Majoral, J.P. Water-soluble polycationic dendrimers with a phosphoramidothioate backbone: Preliminary studies of cytotoxicity and oligonucleotide/plasmid delivery in human cell culture. *Oligonucleotides* **2003**, *13*, 193–205. [CrossRef]

11

Polish Propolis—Chemical Composition and Biological Effects in Tongue Cancer Cells and Macrophages

Joanna Wezgowiec [1,*], Anna Wieczynska [2,3], Wlodzimierz Wieckiewicz [4,*], Julita Kulbacka [5], Jolanta Saczko [5], Natalia Pachura [6], Mieszko Wieckiewicz [1], Roman Gancarz [2] and Kazimiera A. Wilk [2]

1 Department of Experimental Dentistry, Wroclaw Medical University, 50-425 Wroclaw, Poland; m.wieckiewicz@onet.pl
2 Department of Engineering and Technology of Chemical Processes, Wroclaw University of Science and Technology, 50-370 Wroclaw, Poland; anna.wieczynska@pwr.edu.pl (A.W.); roman.gancarz@pwr.edu.pl (R.G.); kazimiera.wilk@pwr.edu.pl (K.A.W.)
3 Institute of Genetics and Microbiology, University of Wroclaw, 51-148 Wroclaw, Poland
4 Department of Prosthetic Dentistry, Wroclaw Medical University, 50-425 Wroclaw, Poland
5 Department of Molecular and Cellular Biology, Wroclaw Medical University, 50-556 Wroclaw, Poland; julita.kulbacka@umed.wroc.pl (J.K.); jolanta.saczko@umed.wroc.pl (J.S.)
6 Department of Chemistry, Wroclaw University of Environmental and Life Sciences, 50-375 Wroclaw, Poland; natalia.pachura@upwr.edu.pl
* Correspondence: joanna.wezgowiec@umed.wroc.pl (J.W.); wlodzimierz.wieckiewicz@umed.wroc.pl (W.W.)

Academic Editors: José Antonio Lupiáñez, Amalia Pérez-Jiménez and Eva E. Rufino-Palomares

Abstract: The purpose of this study was to compare the chemical composition and biological properties of Polish propolis. Ethanol, ethanol-hexane, hexane and hexane-ethanol extracts of propolis from three different regions of Poland were prepared. On the basis of the evaluation of their chemical composition as well as the extraction yield and free radical scavenging activity, the ethanol and hexane-ethanol extractions were proposed as the most effective methods. Subsequently, the biological properties of the extracts were evaluated to investigate the selectivity of an anticancer effect on tongue cancer cells in comparison to normal gingival fibroblasts. The obtained products demonstrated anticancer activity against tongue cancer cells. Additionally, when the lowest extract concentration (100 μg/mL) was applied, they were not cytotoxic to gingival fibroblasts. Finally, a possible anti-inflammatory potential of the prepared products was revealed, as reduced mitochondrial activity and proliferation of macrophages exposed to the extracts were observed. The results obtained indicate a potential of Polish propolis as a natural product with cancer-selective toxicity and anti-inflammatory effect. However, further studies are still needed to thoroughly explain the molecular mechanisms of its action and to obtain the promising health benefits of this versatile natural product.

Keywords: total phenolic content; total flavonoid content; GC-MS; DPPH; antioxidant; anticancer agent; anti-inflammatory agent; gingival fibroblasts; oral cancer; natural extract

---

1. Introduction

Nature, as an immemorial source of diverse active molecules, continues to serve as a major inspiration for drug development. Therapeutic applications of natural products offer great opportunities for modern medicine, while being simultaneously a huge challenge due to the problem of standardization procedures and the chemical complexity of these substances. On the other hand, such complexity is inevitable and a final therapeutic effect of a whole extract in general is better than effects of individual compounds since it results from the synergistic activity of the extract components [1].

One of the most attractive natural products is propolis—the resinous substance collected by bees from plants and mixed with wax and enzymes. It is then used to strengthen and protect their hives as well as to prevent decomposition of intruders' carcasses. People have also widely used propolis in folk medicine, as it is known for a broad spectrum of biological properties including antibacterial, antifungal, antiviral, anti-inflammatory, antioxidant and anticancer activity [2]. Nowadays, it is used in the cosmetics industry, i.e., as a component of anti-acne creams and products for oral hygiene [3]. However, the therapeutic potential of propolis is still untapped and many research groups continue investigation of a chemical composition and biological properties of this material. The studies revealed a variability in propolis composition depending on the geographical region of collection and the plant sources. For instance, bud exudates of different poplar buds are the main source of propolis collected in the temperate zone, including Europe [4]. Silva-Carvalho et al. reported that poplar propolis is mainly composed of flavonoids, phenolic acids and its esters [3].

In particular, contemporary oral medicine may benefit from the wide spectrum of propolis activities. Many dental specialties which make use of this natural product have been reported [5]. Research on Polish propolis is mainly focused on its antimicrobial properties [6–11]. Interestingly, no research on the use of Polish propolis against oral cancer has been published so far. There is little research concerning the antiproliferative effect of Polish propolis on glioblastoma cells [12], colon, lung and breast cancer cells [13], as well as prostate cancer cells [14]. On the other hand, taking into account global data, the problem of oral cancer treatment is still unsolved. In 2018, new cases of oral cancer occurred globally in approximately 355,000 people and caused 177,000 deaths. The most common oral cancer type is tongue squamous cell carcinoma (TSCC), characterized by high lymphatic metastasis, recurrence and drug resistance. The current treatment approaches include surgery, which may be followed by radiotherapy and/or chemotherapy. However, there is still no effective therapeutic strategy and the death toll linked to this disease is still increasing [15].

The purpose of this study was to evaluate the anticancer properties of three different types of propolis from different regions of Poland on the in vitro model of tongue cancer cells. For this reason, ethanol, ethanol-hexane, hexane and hexane-ethanol extracts of Polish propolis were prepared. Normal human gingival fibroblasts were used as a control group of non-cancer cells and a murine macrophage-like cell line was used to evaluate anti-inflammatory potential of the prepared products. Additionally, chemical composition and antioxidant activity of the prepared extracts were compared.

2. Results

2.1. Extraction Yield

The extraction yields of the propolis extracts were calculated and are presented in Table 1. The extraction yield values of the ethanol extracts of propolis (EEP) were higher than the hexane extracts of propolis (HEP) and the highest values of extraction yield were obtained for propolis from Masovia (P2) and West Pomerania Province (P3). Therefore, the results indicated that ethanol was a better solvent than *n*-hexane. In addition, the hexane-ethanol extracts of propolis (HEEP) had the second highest extraction yields among all the propolis extracts analyzed.

2.2. Total Polyphenol Content

The total polyphenol content (TPC) was determined with the Folin–Ciocalteu method (Table 2). The statistical analysis revealed that there was not strong variation between the TPC of all propolis harvested in different provinces of Poland ($F(2, 109) = 0.86794$; $p = 0.42270$). However, regardless of a type of propolis, there were statistically significant differences of TPC ($F(3, 108) = 1178.4$; $p = 0.0000$) between different extracts, such as ethanol extract of propolis (EEP), ethanol-hexane extract of propolis (EHEP), hexane extract of propolis (HEP) and hexane-ethanol extract of propolis (HEEP). The TPC for

EEP and HEEP was above 220 mg GAE (gallic acid equivalent)/g of the propolis extract, while the TPC for EHEP and HEP was below 50 mg GAE/g. Tukey's post-hoc test revealed that all differences of TPC between each type of propolis extract tested were statistically significant at $p < 0.05$. Interestingly, when only EEP and HEEP were considered, the strong differences among TPC of the propolis harvested in different provinces were observed ($F(2, 51) = 31.058$; $p = 0.00000$). Thus, the propolis extracts from West Pomerania Province (P3) had the highest TPC, while the lowest TPC was obtained for propolis extracts from Podlasie (P1).

Table 1. Extraction yields of the prepared extracts; P1—propolis from Podlasie, P2—propolis from Masovia, P3—propolis from West Pomerania Province, EEP—ethanol extract of propolis, EHEP—ethanol-hexane extracts of propolis, HEP—hexane extract of propolis, HEEP—hexane-ethanol extracts of propolis.

Symbol	Sequence of Solvents	Extraction Yield [%]		
		P1	P2	P3
EEP	ethanol	33.4	57.5	63.7
EHEP	ethanol–hexane	24.2	8.4	13.3
HEP	hexane	28.2	17.5	14.5
HEEP	hexane–ethanol	32.9	42.7	47.9

Table 2. Total polyphenol content and total flavonoid content of the prepared extracts; the results are expressed as mean ± SD; P1—propolis from Podlasie, P2—propolis from Masovia, P3—propolis from West Pomerania Province, EEP—ethanol extract of propolis, EHEP—ethanol-hexane extracts of propolis, HEP—hexane extract of propolis, HEEP—hexane-ethanol extracts of propolis, GAE—gallic acid equivalent, QE—quercetin equivalent.

Propolis Extract	P1	P2	P3
	Total Polyphenol Content [mg GAE/g]		
EEP	222.05 ± 14.29	259.63 ± 11.73	275.79 ± 13.42
EHEP	16.36 ± 1.12	19.60 ± 1.07	18.02 ± 1.09
HEP	20.45 ± 4.08	45.02 ± 7.22	38.84 ± 6.40
HEEP	249.92 ± 8.64	277.19 ± 14.28	308.92 ± 15.85
	Total Flavonoid Content [mg QE/g]		
EEP	18.76 ± 0.66	22.19 ± 0.44	19.79 ± 0.19
EHEP	11.10 ± 0.06	10.87 ± 0.03	12.99 ± 0.07
HEP	12.23 ± 0.21	13.49 ± 0.13	14.45 ± 0.19
HEEP	19.00 ± 0.57	22.46 ± 0.40	21.63 ± 0.25

2.3. *Total Flavonoid Content*

The total flavonoid content (TFC), evaluated via aluminum chloride method, was presented in Table 2. Similarly to the measurement results of TPC, this analysis also revealed no statistically significant differences among propolis of different origin ($F(2, 133) = 3.3270$; $p = 0.03891$). On the other hand, differences among various extracts—EEP, EHEP, HEP and HEEP—were statistically significant ($F(3, 132) = 360.77$; $p = 0.0000$). Tukey's post-hoc test revealed that all differences of TFC between each extract type tested were statistically significant at $p < 0.05$, except for the differences between EEP and HEEP samples ($p = 0.122385$). For all the ethanol and hexane-ethanol extracts (EEP and HEEP) analyzed, TFC was above 18.76 mg QE (quercetin equivalent)/g of the propolis extract, while ethanol-hexane and hexane extracts (EHEP and HEP) were characterized by significantly lower TFC. The highest TFC among all samples tested was found for propolis extracts from Masovia (EEP_P2 and HEEP_P2).

2.4. *GC-MS Analysis*

The chemical composition of EEP from different regions of Poland (Podlasie, Masovia and West Pomerania Province) was determined using gas chromatography–mass spectrometry (GC-MS) and is presented in Appendix A, Table A1. Briefly, the analysis of EEP revealed the presence of seventy-two components, out of which sixty-two were identified. The main components of the material analyses were TMS derivatives of 4-coumaric acid, D-fructose, D-glucose, D-mannopyranose, benzoic acid, lignoceric acid, ferulic acid and naringenin. GC-MS analysis of the ethanol extracts of propolis from Podlasie (EEP_P1) and Masovia (EEP_P2) showed a higher concentration of aromatic acids than the ethanol extract of propolis from West Pomerania Province (EEP_P3). The concentration of the compounds selected is presented in Table A1. The results indicate that the highest concentration of 4-coumaric acid and caffeic acid was measured in EEP_P2, while the lowest one was found in EEP_P3. Furthermore, the highest concentration of ferulic acid and benzoic acid was measured in EEP_P1, while the lowest one was found in EEP_P3.

The chemical composition of HEP from different regions of Poland is presented in Appendix A, Table A2. The profile of the compounds of the n-hexane extracts of propolis, determined by GC-MS, contains forty-one compounds (out of which forty were identified). The results showed domination of waxes and fatty acids derivatives of TMS. The main compounds of HEP_P1 and HEP_P2 were methyl triacontyl ether, heptacosane, pentacosane and lignoceric acid. The main compounds of HEP_P3 were heptacosane, lignoceric acid, 13-octadecanoic acid and methyl triacontyl ether. In addition, HEPs contained around two times more (HEP_P1: 8.10%, HEP_P2: 8.47%) or four times more (HEP_P3: 13.19%) benzoic acid than EEP.

The chemical composition of HEEP harvested from different regions of Poland is presented in Appendix A, Table A3. The profile of the compounds of the hexane-ethanol extracts of propolis contained sixty-five compounds (out of which sixty-two were identified). High similarity of the content of EEP and HEEP was observed. The dominant compounds in HEEP were 4-coumaric acid, D-fructose, D-glucose, D-mannopyranose and ferulic acid.

Fatty Acids Composition

The complete chemical composition of fatty acids in HEP from different regions of Poland is presented in Appendix A, Table A4. Fourteen compounds were identified when analyzing fatty acids contained in propolis of different origins. The main components found in the HEP fraction are: hexadecanoic acid methyl ester, heptadecanoic acid methyl ester, oleic acid methyl ester and tetracosanoic acid methyl ester.

2.5. DPPH Free Radical Scavenging Activity

A 2,2-diphenyl-1-picrylhydrazyl (DPPH) assay was used to measure antioxidant activity of the propolis extracts, with the results presented in Figure 1.

As shown in the Figure 1a–c, all the tested ethanol-hexane and hexane extracts (EHEP and HEP) obtained from propolis harvested in different regions of Poland (P1, P2, P3) had only minimal DPPH free radical scavenging activity compared to the standard. Therefore, they were assumed as having no effect at all. In contrast, for EEP and HEEP, the free radical scavenging activity increased with the increase of the extracts' concentration from 0 to 200 μg/mL. For these active extracts their IC_{50} were calculated (the concentration of extracts that inhibits the formation of DPPH free radicals by 50%) and showed in Table 3. Statistically significant differences among IC_{50} of propolis from different regions of Poland were demonstrated ($F(2, 55) = 43.365$; $p = 0.00000$). Tukey's post-hoc test revealed that all differences of IC_{50} between each type of propolis tested (P1, P2, P3) were statistically significant at $p < 0.05$. Regardless of the type of propolis studied, the type of extract did not significantly influence the obtained values of IC_{50} ($F(1, 56) = 0.09896$; $p = 0.75425$). The lowest IC_{50} values were calculated for propolis extracts from West Pomerania Province (P3), indicating the highest antioxidant potential of these preparations among all the extracts tested.

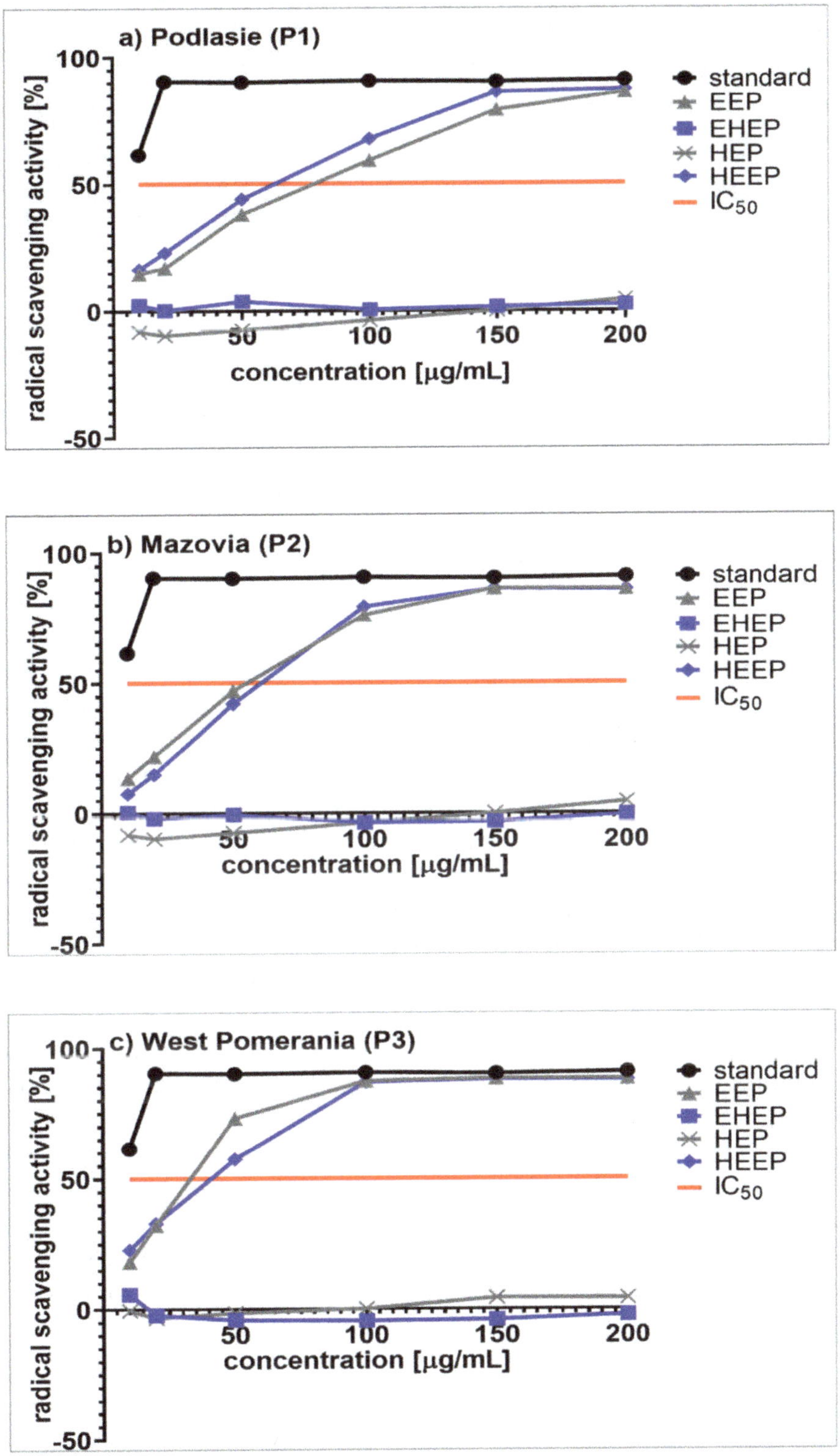

Figure 1. DPPH free radical scavenging activity of the prepared propolis extracts from: (**a**) Podlasie (P1); (**b**) Masovia (P2); (**c**) West Pomerania Province (P3); EEP— ethanol extract of propolis, EHEP—ethanol-hexane extracts of propolis, HEP—hexane extract of propolis, HEEP—hexane-ethanol extracts of propolis.

Table 3. The concentration of extracts that inhibits the formation of DPPH free radicals by 50% (IC_{50}); P1—propolis from Podlasie, P2—propolis from Masovia, P3—propolis from West Pomerania Province, EEP—ethanol extract of propolis, HEEP—hexane-ethanol extracts of propolis.

Propolis Extract	IC_{50} [μg/mL]		
	P1	P2	P3
EEP	78.02 ± 4.86	55.07 ± 7.39	33.01 ± 2.73
HEEP	62.84 ± 14.59	60.72 ± 2.89	40.92 ± 7.55

2.6. *Anticancer Activity*

The anticancer activity of the selected Polish propolis extracts was evaluated on human squamous cell carcinoma derived from tongue (SCC-25) after incubation for 5 min and 24 h. For this purpose, 3-(4,5-dimethyl-2-thiazolyl)-2,5-diphenyl-2*H*-tetrazolium bromide assay (MTT assay) and sulforhodamine B assay (SRB assay) were performed. In addition, for both methods, 24 h incubation with human gingival fibroblasts (HGFs) was used as a control model to investigate the effects of propolis in normal, i.e., non-cancer cells. The cytotoxicity values of EEP and HEEP harvested from three different regions in Poland and applied at three concentrations (100, 500 and 1000 μg/mL) are presented in Figure 2 (MTT assay results) and in Figure 3 (SRB assay results).

2.6.1. MTT Assay

When 5 min of incubation with the propolis extracts was applied, mitochondrial activity of SCC-25 cells was only slightly reduced (Figure 2a). Moreover, when concentrations of all the extracts tested were increased, the mitochondrial activity was still above 80% compared to the control. However, the prolonged 24 h incubation period affected the cell viability significantly (Figure 2b). Three-way ANOVA revealed that for all tested extracts of Polish propolis the differences between groups based on the propolis type or extraction type were not statistically significant ($p = 0.093920$ and $p = 0.493920$, respectively). The only factor determining significant differences between groups was the extract concentration ($p = 0.000000$). For tongue cancer cells, incubation with each of the tested propolis extract at a concentration of 500 and 1000 μg/mL resulted in a decrease of mitochondrial activity to ca. 20% of the control. When the concentration of the propolis extracts applied was 100 μg/mL, the mitochondrial activity was most reduced for EEP_P3 (33% of the control) and least reduced for EEP_P1 (59% of the control), therefore, EEP_P1 was less active. The results obtained for HGFs treated with propolis indicated that the tested propolis extracts impaired also the viability of normal cells (Figure 2c). Incubation of HGFs with each tested propolis extract at a concentration of 500 and 1000 μg/mL reduced the mitochondrial activity to ca. 40% compared to the control. In addition, when the propolis extract concentration of 100 μg/mL was applied, EEP_P3 was the most active propolis extract, which reduced the mitochondrial activity to 52% of the control. Furthermore, HEEP_P2 reduced the mitochondrial activity to 76% compared to the control and therefore it was the least active propolis extract. Three-way ANOVA results for HGFs revealed that all the factors studied (type of propolis, type of extract and extract concentration) were source of significant variation at $p < 0.05$.

2.6.2. SRB Assay

When SCC-25 cells were incubated with Polish propolis for 5 min, for all the concentrations of all the extracts tested the total protein content of cells was above 93% compared to the control (Figure 3a). Therefore, no cytotoxic effect of propolis extracts after a short-time incubation was revealed. However, the prolonged incubation, i.e., 24 h, affected the cellular proliferation significantly (Figure 3b). The results showed that 24 h incubation of tongue cancer cells with increasing concentration of propolis extract resulted in a decrease of total protein content. For example, when the concentrations of 100 and 500 μg/mL of all Polish propolis extracts were applied, cellular protein content was reduced to ca. 55% of the control. Notably, the least activity was observed at 100 μg/mL of EEP_P1, that reduced the cellular protein content to 72% compared to the control. However, for 500 µg/mL of HEEP_P1 the cellular protein content was reduced to 45% of the control. Finally, when tongue cancer cells were incubated with each of the Polish propolis extracts tested at a concentration of 1000 µg/mL, it resulted in a decrease in total protein content to ca. 45% compared to the control. The results for HGFs indicated that the analyzed propolis extracts at concentrations of 500 and 1000 µg/mL impaired the proliferation of normal cells (Figure 3c). Incubation of HGFs with 1000 µg/mL propolis extracts reduced total protein content to ca. 30% compared to the control. Incubation of HGFs with 1000 µg/mL of HEEP_P2 resulted in the lowest level of protein content, reduced to 20% of the control. On the other hand, incubation of HGFs with 1000 µg/mL of EEP_P1 resulted in the highest level of total protein content, i.e., 40% of the control. Additionally, incubation of HGFs with 500 µg/mL propolis extracts also induced a significant cytotoxicity. In contrast, for the concentration of 100 µg/mL, the lowest level of total protein content, i.e., 79% of the control, was observed when HGFs were incubated with EEP_P3 and HEEP_P3. The three-way ANOVA of results both for SCC-25 and HGFs revealed that all the factors studied (type of propolis, type of extract and extract concentration) were sources of significant variation at $p < 0.05$.

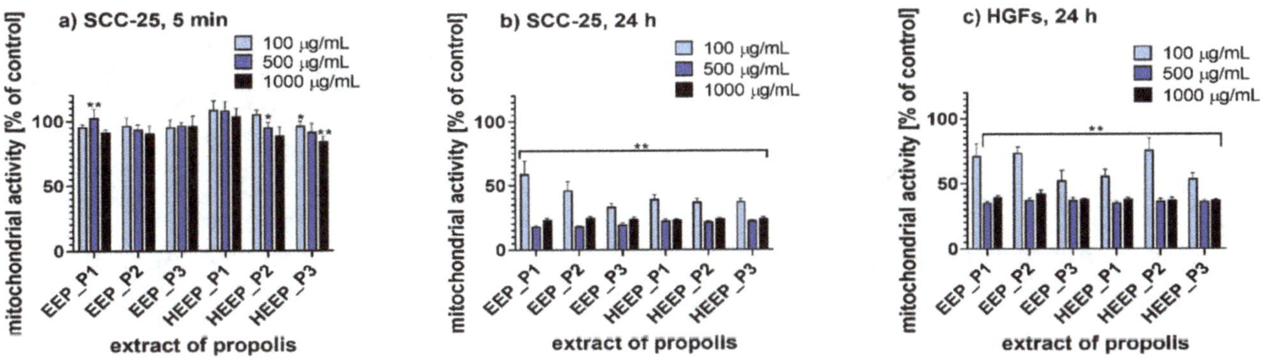

Figure 2. MTT assay results for: (**a**) tongue cancer cells (SCC-25) incubated for 5 min with propolis extracts; (**b**) tongue cancer cells (SCC-25) incubated for 24 h with propolis extracts; (**c**) human gingival fibroblasts (HGFs) incubated for 24 h with propolis extracts; * $p < 0.05$, ** $p < 0.005$; P1—propolis from Podlasie, P2—propolis from Masovia, P3—propolis from West Pomerania Province, EEP—ethanol extract of propolis, HEEP—hexane-ethanol extracts of propolis.

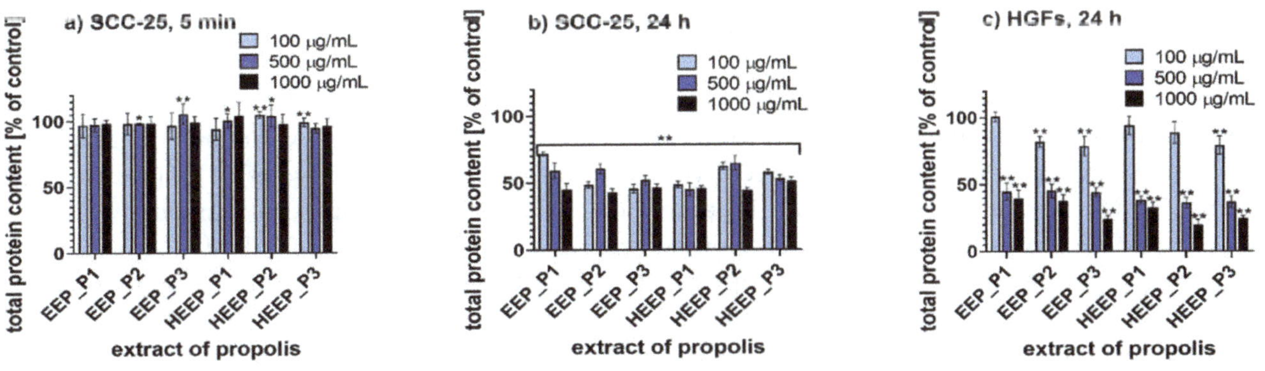

Figure 3. Sulforhodamine B (SRB) assay results for: (**a**) tongue cancer cells (SCC-25) incubated for 5 min with propolis extracts; (**b**) tongue cancer cells (SCC-25) incubated for 24 h with propolis extracts; (**c**) human gingival fibroblasts (HGFs) incubated for 24 h with propolis extracts; * $p < 0.05$, ** $p < 0.005$; P1—propolis from Podlasie, P2—propolis from Masovia, P3—propolis from West Pomerania Province, EEP—ethanol extract of propolis, HEEP—hexane-ethanol extracts of propolis.

2.7. Anti-Inflammatory Potential

Anti-inflammatory potential of the propolis extracts selected was evaluated on murine macrophage-like cell line (P388-D1) via MTT assay (Figure 4a) and SRB assay (Figure 4b) after 24 h of incubation. For all the analyzed concentrations of all the extracts tested it was observed that the prolonged 24 h incubation period affected the cellular mitochondrial activity and proliferation significantly. Incubation with each tested propolis extract at a concentration of 1000 μg/mL resulted in a decrease in mitochondrial activity of P388-D1 cells to ca. 19% of the control (Figure 4a) and a decrease in total protein content to ca. 38% of the control (Figure 4b). When the lowest concentration of extracts (100 μg/mL) was applied, the cellular mitochondrial activity was reduced to 48% and the cellular protein content to ca. 55% of the control.

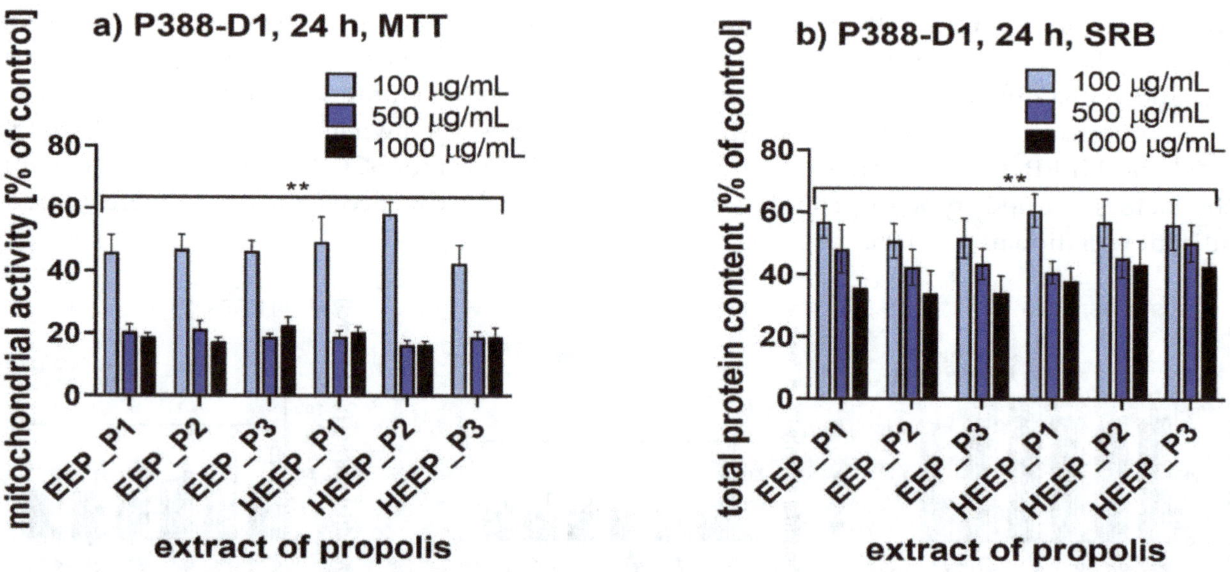

Figure 4. Results for murine macrophage cells (P388-D1) incubated for 24 h with propolis extracts; (**a**) MTT assay; (**b**) SRB assay; ** $p < 0.005$; P1—propolis from Podlasie, P2—propolis from Masovia, P3—propolis from West Pomerania Province, EEP—ethanol extract of propolis, HEEP—hexane-ethanol extracts of propolis.

3. Discussion

Propolis demonstrated antiproliferative activity on various cancer cell lines. It was reported that this natural product can block specific oncogene signaling pathways, leading to a decrease in cell proliferation. It can also increase apoptosis, exert antiangiogenic effects, and modulate the tumor microenvironment [3,16].

In spite of these beneficial properties, research on the anticancer activity of propolis on human tongue cancer cells is very limited. Antiproliferative activity of the ethanol extract of Chilean propolis on human mouth epidermoid carcinoma cells (KB) was demonstrated by Russo et al. [17]. Furthermore, Yen et al. and Chiu et al. showed an anti-inflammatory effect of various propolis extracts by inhibiting one of the inflammatory markers—COX-2—in KB cell line [18]. The study of Salehi et al. determined the chemopreventive effect of Iranian propolis on dysplastic changes in the rats' tongue epithelium after administration of carcinogens (DMBA). The results have showed that propolis can prevent DMBA-induced dysplasia of the oral mucosa in animal model [19]. A similar effect was obtained for hydroalcoholic extract of Brazilian red propolis (HERP) on oral squamous cell carcinoma (OSCC) in rodents. The research revealed that HERP inhibited tumor growth and progression [20].

The anticancer effect of propolis is often attributed to one of its active components—caffeic acid phenethyl ester (CAPE). It can be considered as a potential support for therapy of patients with oral squamous cell carcinoma due to the ability to inhibit cellular proliferation and to prevent cancer metastasis [21–23]. On the other hand, the other approach to the clarification of the natural drug's mechanisms of action is more comprehensive and takes into account a complexity of the product rather than the effect of its individual components. The study of Czyżewska et al. suggested that the synergistic effect of different polyphenols (chrysin, galangin, pinocembrin, caffeic acid, p-coumaric acid and ferulic acid) is responsible for the propolis' ability to inhibit the growth of human tongue cancer cells through apoptosis [24]. Another study indicated the synergistic effect of the main components of Iranian propolis on mouth epidermoid carcinoma (KB) cells. MTT assay revealed that IC_{50} values of EEP and its main component, quercetin (Q) were 40 µg/mL and 195 µg/mL respectively after 48 h of incubation [25].

In this study, the whole extracts of Polish propolis were evaluated in terms of the selectivity of their anticancer effect on the tongue cancer cells in comparison to the normal gingival fibroblasts. Chemical analyses revealed that ethanolic and hexane-ethanol extraction were the most effective methods of raw propolis extraction to receive the most chemically complex product. This conclusion confirms the findings of the other studies indicating ethanol extraction as the most common method of raw propolis processing [26–28]. The second proposed method—ethanol–hexane extraction—may be an interesting alternative allowing the wax content removal [29]. Both spectroscopic and chromatographic methods enabled determination of a chemical character of the extracts obtained. The chemical compounds identified in the prepared propolis extracts are analogous to the results described by Sahinler and Kaftanogl [30] as well as by Anjum et al. [31], showing high concentration of the aromatic acids, hydrocarbons, alcohols, polyphenols and fatty acids. The presence of phenolic compounds in the propolis extracts is particularly promising when its anticancer activity is considered [32].

The biological analysis of the selected systems showed that the prolonged 24 h incubation of cells with propolis significantly affected the cell viability measured via MTT and SRB assays. Differences between groups, based on the propolis type or extraction type, were not statistically significant. This may confirm the hypothesis that differences in the chemical composition of the extracts obtained did not influence the general biological effect induced by them. It should be emphasized that higher concentrations of the propolis extracts (500 and 1000 µg/mL) significantly affected the viability of normal HGFs as well. For this reason, only the extract concentration of 100 µg/mL could be considered as effective selectively in cancer cells. Similar results demonstrating the cytotoxic effect of propolis on normal human fibroblasts were obtained by Tyszka-Czochara et al. [33], Popova et al. [13] and in our previous study [10]. Moreover, the study presented by Popova et al. revealed the similar chemical profile of the propolis sample (mainly flavanones and dihydroflavonols, as well as a series of esters of p-coumaric acid, ferulic acid, benzoic acid and fatty acids (palmitic acid, linoleic acid, oleic acid) compared to the extracts analyzed in our study [13]).

Additionally, due to the polyphenolic content of propolis, the anti-inflammatory activity of the extracts prepared was verified on macrophage models commonly used in case of natural compounds [34,35]. Szliszka et al. suggested that phenolic compounds may be responsible for a crucial contribution of Brazilian green propolis in the modulation of chemokine-mediated inflammation [34]. In our study, the impairment of the cellular proliferation and mitochondrial activity observed in macrophage-like cell line (P388-D1) suggested a possible anti-inflammatory activity of the prepared extracts. Here we have observed that the effect was dependent on the cytotoxic effect of propolis extracts applied.

In the future, the preliminary results reported in this research should be used to select the ethanol and hexane-ethanol extraction as the most effective methods of propolis extraction to obtain chemically complex and biologically active products. The prepared extracts should become a subject of an in-depth analysis aimed at the identification of the most active components and at the investigation of a precise molecular mechanism of their anticancer and anti-inflammatory action. In addition, the selected natural extracts could be combined with conventional chemotherapeutic regimens in order to propose safer and more effective treatment of cancer [36]. Finally, functional polymer microparticles for encapsulation of biologically active compounds could be designed and manufactured [37].

4. Materials and Methods

4.1. Material

The research materials were propolis samples originating from three different regions in Poland (Table 4). Raw propolis was collected from beehives manually. Before processing it was stored at room temperature under dark conditions.

Table 4. Geographical origin of the Polish propolis examined.

Symbol	Region of Origin	The Most Abundant Plants in the Region	Bee Species
P1	Podlasie (Hajnowka)	spruce (*Picea abies L.*)—30%, pine (*Pinus sylvestris L.*)—27%, alder (*Alnus glutinosa L.*)—20%, sessile oak (*Quercus petraea L.*)—10%, silver birch (*Betula pendula L.*)—7%	*Apis mellifera carnica x Apis mellifera caucasica*
P2	Mazovia (Ciechanow)	pine (*Pinus sylvestris L.*)—70%, alder (*Alnus glutinosa L.*)—10%, sessile oak (*Quercus petraea L.*)—10%, silver birch (*Betula pendula L.*)—7%	*Apis mellifera carnica*
P3	West Pomerania (Miedzyzdroje)	pine (*Pinus sylvestris L.*)—75%, alder (*Alnus glutinosa L.*)—5%, beech (*Fagus sylvatica L.*)—5%, sessile oak (*Quercus petraea L.*)—5%, silver birch (*Betula pendula L.*)—4%	*Apis mellifera mellifera*

4.2. Extraction

Ethanol, ethanol-hexane, hexane and hexane-ethanol extracts of Polish propolis were prepared according to the procedure illustrated in Figure 5. For this purpose, 5 g of raw propolis was cut into small pieces, dissolved in 50 mL of 70% ethanol (POCH, Poland) or 50 mL of hexane (POCH, Poland) and stirred for 48 h at room temperature under dark conditions, using a magnetic stirrer (Big-squid, IKA, Germany). Subsequently, the samples were centrifuged at 10,500 rpm for 10 min at room temperature, using a 5804 centrifuge (Eppendorf, Germany). The supernatant obtained was named ethanol extract of propolis (EEP) and hexane extract of propolis (HEP). Then, the residue was extracted one more time with ethanol or hexane to obtain EEP_II or HEP_II, respectively. Subsequently, the residue left after ethanol extraction was treated twice with hexane to obtain ethanol-hexane extracts (EHEP and EHEP_II). The residue left after hexane extraction was dissolved twice with 70% ethanol to obtain hexane-ethanol extracts (HEEP and HEEP_II). Non-dissolved residues were discarded.

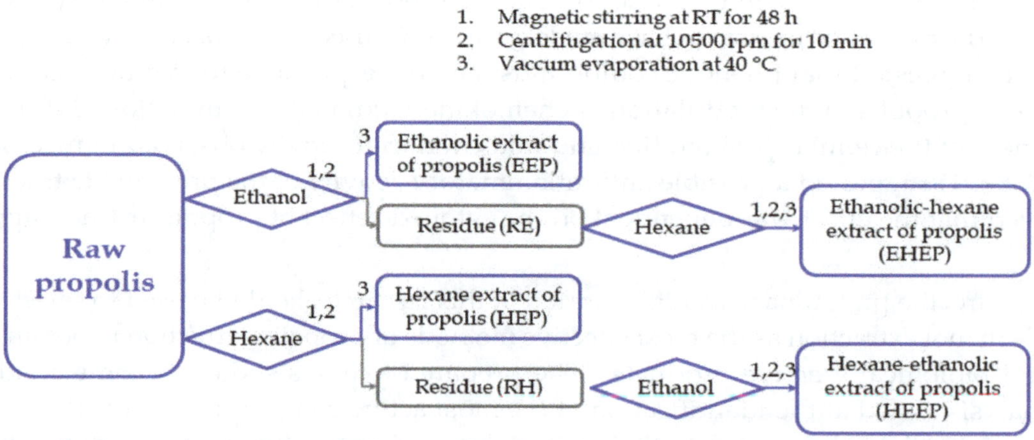

Figure 5. Schematic illustration of procedure for propolis extract preparation; EEP—ethanol extract of propolis, EHEP—ethanol-hexane extracts of propolis, HEP—hexane extract of propolis, HEEP—hexane-ethanol extracts of propolis, RE—residue after extraction with ethanol, RH—residue after extraction with hexane.

The extracts were evaporated to dryness at 40 °C using a RV 10 rotary vacuum evaporator (IKA, Germany) and stored at 4 °C under dark conditions. After evaporation, the samples obtained were weighted using an analytical balance: WPS 510/C/2 (Radwag, Poland); extraction yields were expressed in percentage as a ratio of the mass of the sample after evaporation to the mass of the propolis material before extraction. The samples obtained after second extraction with the same solvent (EEP_II, HEP_II, EHEP_II, HEEP_II) were not subjected to further analysis due to their small quantity. Then, the samples were dissolved in methanol (POCH, Poland) at a concentration of 1 mg/mL (for chemical studies) or in DMSO (POCH, Poland) at a concentration of 100 mg/mL (for biological studies).

4.3. Total Polyphenol Content

The total soluble phenolic compounds in the samples were determined using the Folin–Ciocalteu colorimetric method [38]. For this purpose, 100 µL of analyzed propolis extract was dissolved in methanol (1 mg/mL) and then mixed with 900 µL of distilled water and 100 µL of Folin and Ciocalteu's phenol reagent (Sigma-Aldrich, Poland). After 5 min of incubation, 1 mL of 7% Na_2CO_3 (POCH, Poland) and 400 µL of distilled water were added. Subsequently, the mixture was incubated for 2 h and the absorbance was measured at 765 nm using a UV-Vis spectrophotometer: SP 8001 (Metertech, Norway). Gallic acid (Sigma-Aldrich, Poland) was used as a standard. The results were expressed in mg of gallic acid equivalent per g of propolis extract (mg GAE/g). The minimum number of measurements for each extract was n = 9.

4.4. Total Flavonoid Content

The total flavonoid contents in the samples were determined using an aluminum chloride method [39]. Briefly, 100 µL of propolis extract dissolved in methanol (1 mg/mL) was mixed with 100 µL of 2% $AlCl_3$ (Sigma-Aldrich, Poland). After 15 min of incubation, the absorbance was measured at 435 nm using a UV-Vis spectrophotometer: SP 8001 (Metertech, Norway). Quercetin (Sigma-Aldrich, Poland) was used as a standard. The results were expressed in mg of quercetin equivalent per g of propolis extract (mg QE/g). The minimum number of measurements for each extract was n = 9.

4.5. GC-MS Analysis

The propolis extracts obtained (EEP, HEP and HEEP) were evaluated in terms of a low-molecular-weight compound content by means of derivatization with N,O-bis (trimethylsilyl) trifluoroacetamide (BSTFA) silylation approach on gas chromatography, coupled with mass spectrometry (Shimadzu GC-MS QP 2020, Shimadzu, Kyoto, Japan). Each of the extracts was evaporated under reduced pressure. Then, 500 µL of pyridine and 50 µL of BSTFA were added to all samples. The mixture was placed in a vial and heated for 15 min at 70 °C. Separation was achieved using Zebron ZB-5 capillary column with a length of 30 m, inner diameter of 0.25 mm, and film thickness of 0.25 µm (Phenomenex, Torrance, CA, USA). The GC-MS analysis was performed according to the following parameters: scan mode with mass range from 40 to 1050 *m/z* in electronic impact (EI) mode at 70 eV; mode at 10 scan s^{-1} mode. Analyses were conducted using helium as a carrier gas at a flow rate of 1.0 mL min^{-1} in a split ratio of 1:20 and the following program: (a) 100 °C for 1 min; (b) rate of 2.0 °C min^{-1} from 100 to 190 °C; (c) rate of 5 °C min^{-1} from 190 to 300 °C. An injector was held at 280 °C, respectively. Compounds were identified by using two different analytical methods that compare: retention times with authentic chemicals (Supelco C7-C40 Saturated Alkanes Standard), and obtained mass spectra with available library data (Willey NIST 17, match index >90%).

Fatty Acids Composition

The lipid fraction was obtained according to the previously described method [40]. In the next step, the extracted nonpolar fraction, approx. 30 mg, was saponified (10 min at 75 °C) with 2 mL of 0.5 M KOH/MeOH solution and subjected to methylation (10 min at 75 °C) using 2 mL of 14% (*v/v*) BF3/MeOH (Sigma-Aldrich, St. Louis, MO, USA). Subsequently, water was added to reaction mixture and methyl esters of fatty acids were extracted with 10 mL of hexane (UQF Wroclaw, Poland), then washed with 10 mL 10% sodium bicarbonate (UQF Wroclaw, Poland) and desiccated with anhydrous sodium sulphate. The organic phase was evaporated under reduced pressure and stored at −27 °C until chromatographical analysis. The FAME profile was assessed using gas chromatograph coupled with a mass spectrometer (Shimadzu GCMS QP 2020, Shimadzu, Kyoto, Japan). Separation was achieved using Zebron ZB-FAME capillary column with a length of 60 m, inner diameter of 0.20 mm, and film thickness of 0.20 μm (Phenomenex, Torrance, CA, USA). The GC-MS analysis was according to the following parameters: scan mode with mass range from 40 to 400 *m/z* in electronic impact (EI) mode at 70 eV; mode at 3 scan s^{-1} mode. Analyses were conducted using helium as a carrier gas at a flow rate of 1.8 mL min^{-1} in a split ratio of 1:10 and the following program: (a) 80 °C for 2 min; (b) rate of 3.0 °C min^{-1} from 80 to 180 °C; (c) rate of 8 °C min^{-1} from 180 to 240 °C. An injector was held at 280 °C, respectively. Compounds were identified by using two different analytical methods that compare: retention times with authentic chemicals (Supelco 37 Component FAME Mix), and obtained mass spectra with available library data (Willey NIST 17, match index >90%).

4.6. DPPH Free Radical Scavenging Activity

The 2,2-diphenyl-1-picrylhydrazyl (DPPH) free radical scavenging activity was determined using a method described by Yang et al. [39]. For this purpose, 100 μL of propolis extract dissolved in methanol (10, 20, 50, 100, 150, 200 μg/mL) was placed into a 96 well plate (Nunc, Denmark) and 100 μL of 0.2 mM DPPH solution (Sigma-Aldrich, Poland) was added. After 15 min of incubation, the absorbance was measured at 517 nm using a multiwell-plate reader (EnSpire Multimode Reader, Perkin Elmer, USA). Ascorbic acid (P.P.H. STANLAB Sp.J., Poland) was used as a standard. The percentage inhibition capacity was calculated from the following equation:

$$\text{percentage inhibition} = (A_0 - A_1)/(A_0 \times 100),$$

where A_0 is the absorbance of the control group and A_1 is the absorbance of the extracts.

4.7. Biological Characterisation

Taking into account the results of the chemical analyses, hexane extracts (HEP) and ethanol-hexane extracts (EHEP) were excluded from further studies. Biological analyses were conducted only for ethanol extracts (EEP) and hexane-ethanol extracts (HEEP), which were characterized by the highest TPC, TFC and DPPH free radical scavenging activity.

4.7.1. Cell Culture

Human squamous cell carcinomas derived from tongue (SCC-25 cell line, ATCC CRL-1628, ATCC, USA) were cultured in a 1:1 mixture of Dulbecco's Modified Eagle's Medium (DMEM) and Ham's F12 medium (Lonza, Switzerland) supplemented with 10% fetal bovine serum (FBS, Sigma-Aldrich, Poland), and antibiotics: penicillin/streptomycin (Sigma-Aldrich, Poland), as recommended by ATCC.

Human gingival fibroblasts (HGFs) were mechanically isolated from a fragment of gingival tissue (1–2 mm) in healthy patients, according to the procedure described by Dominiak and Saczko [41]. The biopsies were provided by the Department of Dental Surgery at the Wroclaw Medical University in accordance with the requirements of the Bioethics Commission of Wroclaw Medical University (Bioethical Committee approval, No.: KB-8/2010). The fragment of tissue was taken by a scalpel and immediately placed on Petri dishes (60 mm, Nunc, Denmark) with DMEM (Sigma-Aldrich, Poland) containing 10% FBS (Sigma-Aldrich, Poland) and antibiotics: penicillin/streptomycin (Sigma-Aldrich, Poland).

Murine macrophage-like cells (P388-D1 cell line, ATCC CCL-46, ATCC, USA) were cultured in a 1:1 mixture of DMEM and RPMI 1640 medium (Lonza, Switzerland) supplemented with 10% FBS (Sigma-Aldrich, Poland) and antibiotics: penicillin/streptomycin (Sigma-Aldrich, Poland).

All cell lines were incubated in a humidified atmosphere at 37 °C and 5% CO_2. After trypsinization with 0.25% trypsin-EDTA (Sigma-Aldrich, Poland), the cells were passaged and grown in 25 cm^2 flasks (Equimed, Poland). In order to evaluate cytotoxicity of the extracts tested, cells were seeded into a 96-well plate (Nunc, Denmark). After 24 h, the culture medium was removed and then propolis extracts, diluted with an appropriate culture medium (100, 500 and 1000 µg/mL), were added for 5 min or 24 h. MTT and SRB assays were performed 24 h later. All results were referred to the untreated control cells.

4.7.2. MTT Assay

To evaluate cytotoxicity of propolis extracts (EEP and HEEP) on the basis of differences in mitochondrial function, 3-(4,5-dimethyl-2-thiazolyl)-2,5-diphenyl-2*H*-tetrazolium bromide (MTT) assay was performed. Cells were incubated for 90 min with 100 µL of the MTT reagent (Sigma-Aldrich, Poland) at 37 °C. Then, formazan crystals were dissolved by addition of 100 µL of acidic isopropanol and by mixing. The absorbance was measured at 570 nm using a multiwell plate reader (EnSpire Multimode Reader, Perkin Elmer, USA). The results were expressed as the percentage of treated cells with altered mitochondrial function in relation to untreated control cells with normal mitochondrial activity, considered as 100%.

4.7.3. SRB Assay

To evaluate cytotoxicity of propolis extracts on the basis of differences in total protein content in cells, sulforhodamine B (SRB) assay was performed. The protocol was based on the procedure described in [42]. Cell monolayers were fixed with 10% (vol/vol) trichloroacetic acid (Roth, Poland) for 1 h at 4 °C, subsequently washed (five times) in cold water and desiccated. Cell staining was performed for 30 min using 0.4% SRB (Sigma-Aldrich, Poland) in 1% acetic acid (Sigma-Aldrich, Poland) at room temperature. After incubation, the excess of dye was removed by means of washing with 1% (*v*/*v*) acetic acid (four times). Plates were desiccated and the protein-bound dye was dissolved in 10 mM Tris base solution (pH 10.5) (BioShop, Canada). The absorbance was measured at 490 nm using a multiwell plate reader (GloMax Discover, Promega, USA). The results were expressed as the percentage of total protein content in treated cells in relation to untreated control cells.

4.8. Statistical Analysis

The results are presented as means ± standard deviation (SD) values for minimum $n = 9$ repeats. The results were analyzed by one-way ANOVA and $\alpha = 0.05$ using Statistica ver. 13.3 software (StatSoft, Poland). F-values and p-values were determined, the values $p \leq 0.05$ were considered as statistically significant. Tukey's HSD test was performed when ANOVA indicated statistically significant results. Additionally, for the MTT and SRB assays, the statistical significance of the differences between mean values of different groups and the untreated control group was evaluated by Student's t-test. The values $p \leq 0.05$ were marked with an asterisk and considered as statistically significant. Finally, for MTT and SRB assay results, three–way ANOVA test was performed to indicate, which factor (type of propolis, type of extract, extract concentration) determines significant differences between groups, $p \leq 0.05$ were considered as statistically significant.

5. Conclusions

This study has revealed differences in chemical composition and antioxidant activity of the extracts of three different types of Polish propolis obtained after extraction with ethanol, hexane and combinations of both. The products selected (EEP and HEEP) demonstrated anticancer activity in the tongue cancer cells and cytotoxicity towards murine macrophages. In addition, EEP and HEEP did not have any cytotoxic effect in the normal gingival fibroblasts when the lowest concentration was applied.

The following conclusions can be drawn on the basis of the results obtained:

- The highest total extraction yields were obtained for ethanol and hexane-ethanol extracts (EEP and HEEP);
- Total polyphenol content (TPC) and total flavonoid content (TFC) of ethanol and hexane-ethanol extracts (EEP and HEEP) were much higher than TPC and TFC of ethanol-hexane and hexane extracts (EHEP and HEP);
- Antioxidant potential of ethanol and hexane-ethanol extracts (EEP and HEEP) was much higher than that of ethanol-hexane and hexane extracts (EHEP and HEP);
- The extracts selected (EEP and HEEP) demonstrated anticancer activity in the tongue cancer cells; 24 h incubation affected cell viability and cellular proliferation significantly;
- The propolis extracts tested at higher concentrations (500 and 1000 μg/mL) impaired the proliferation of normal cells as well;
- The observed cytotoxicity of the extracts prepared towards murine macrophages requires further investigation to evaluate their possible anti-inflammatory potential.

As a final conclusion, we can select the minimal dose of 100 μg/mL of the extracts applied, which caused anticancer effect on human tongue cancer cells with limited cytotoxic effect on normal mucosal cells and simultaneous anti-inflammatory potential. However, further studies on Polish propolis are still necessary in order to thoroughly explain the molecular mechanisms of its action and to obtain promising health benefits of this versatile natural product.

Author Contributions: Conceptualization, J.W., W.W. and K.A.W.; methodology, J.W. and A.W.; validation, J.K., J.S., R.G. and K.A.W.; formal analysis, J.W., A.W. and N.P.; investigation, J.W., A.W. and N.P.; resources, J.W., W.W., J.K., J.S., M.W. and K.A.W.; writing—original draft preparation, J.W.; writing—review and editing, A.W., J.K., J.S., M.W., R.G. and K.A.W.; visualization, J.W.; supervision, J.K., J.S., R.G. and K.A.W.; project administration, J.W.; funding acquisition, J.W., W.W., M.W. and K.A.W. All authors have read and agreed to the published version of the manuscript.

Acknowledgments: A. Szumny from Department of Chemistry, Wroclaw University of Environmental and Life Sciences, is acknowledged for his supervision of GC-MS analysis and for a critical revision of the manuscript.

Appendix A

Table A1. GC-MS profile of ethanol extracts of propolis (EEP) from different regions of Poland: *EEP_P1*—Podlasie (Hajnowka), *EEP_P2*—Masovia (Ciechanow), *EEP_P3*—West Pomerania Province (Miedzyzdroje).

	Substances	RT	RI_{exp}	RI_{lit}	EEP_P1[%]	EEP_P2[%]	EEP_P3[%]
1	Benzyl alcohol, TMS derivative	6.110	1155	1152	0.12	0.15	0.1
2	Benzoic Acid, TMS derivative	8.795	1246	1249	4.35	3.8	3.15
3	Glycerol, TMS	10.162	1287	1289	0.78	0.99	1.55
4	Butanedioic acid, 2TMS derivative	11.445	1320	1321	0.12	0.04	0.13
5	1-Monoacetin, 2O-TMS	11.740	1326	1324	0.13	0.07	0.08
6	4-Hydroxybenzaldehyde, TMS derivative	13.737	1373	1383	0.22	0.16	0.08
7	Hydroquinone, 2TMS derivative	15.308	1409	1408	0.24	0.2	0.08
8	Malic acid, 3TMS derivative	20.278	1511	1497	0.09	0.06	1.1
9	5-Oxoproline, TMS derivative	20.680	1521	1527	0.1	0.09	-
10	Vanillin, TMS derivative	21.622	1536	1530	1.48	0.5	0.37
11	Cinnamic acid, TMS derivative	22.048	1545	1542	0.12	0.14	0.25
12	4-Hydroxybenzoic acid, 2TMS derivative	26.623	1634	1635	0.27	0.22	0.08
13	Dodecanoic acid, TMS	27.858	1658	1655	0.13	0.09	-
14	β-D-Xylopyranose, 4TMS derivative	34.330	1784	1777	0.17	-	-
15	o-Coumaric acid, 2TMS derivative	34.975	1797	1815	0.26	0.26	0.09
16	D-Psicofuranose	37.465	1848	1837	1.28	1.2	0.76
17	D-Fructose, 5TMS derivative	37.855	1856	1867	7.4	9.55	8.51
18	D-Sorbitol, 6TMS derivative	41.075	1922	1920	0.22	0.09	7.15
19	D-Glucose, 5TMS derivative	41.635	1934	1928	4.82	8.5	-

Table A1. *Cont.*

	Substances	RT	RI exp	RI lit	EEP_P1[%]	EEP_P2[%]	EEP_P3[%]
20	4-Coumaric acid, 2TMS derivative	42.223	1947	1949	10.74	13.68	1.34
21	D-Glucitol, 6TMS derivative	43.902	1982	1980	0.44	0.34	0.18
22	Gallic acid, 4TMS derivative	44.118	1986	1987	0.39	0.1	0.21
23	Salicylic acid, trimethylsilyl ether, benzyl ester	45.910	2028	2025	0.55	0.49	0.11
24	D-Mannopyranose, 5TMS derivative	46.347	2038	2037	4.87	8.84	7.8
25	D-Gluconic acid, 6TMS derivative	46.875	2052	2043	0.16	0.16	0.09
26	Palmitic Acid, TMS derivative	47.070	2057	2050	0.85	0.7	0.69
27	Isoferulic acid, 2TMS derivative	48.435	2090	2081	0.17	0.67	2.7
28	Ferulic acid, 2TMS derivative	48.950	2103	2103	4.79	2.95	2.69
29	Myo-Inositol, 6TMS derivative	49.822	2132	2129	0.18	0.1	1.17
30	Phtalic acid derivative*	50.387	2150	-	1.07	1.19	4.02
31	Caffeic acid, 3TMS derivative	50.548	2157	2155	1.06	2.15	-
32	Unknown	51.908	2202	-	1.54	2.48	0.19
33	13-Octadecenoic acid, (E)-, TMS derivative	52.383	2222	2228	0.59	0.72	0.88
34	3,7,11,15-Tetramethyl-2,6,10,14-hexadecatetraene-1-ol trimethylsilyl ether	52.697	2236	2234	1.65	2.7	0.25
35	Tricosane	54.272	2300	2300	1.14	0.42	0.08
36	Unknown	55.733	2370	-	-	-	1.21
37	Unknown	56.810	2424	-	-	-	2.4
38	Pterostilbene, trimethylsilyl ether	57.507	2462	-	0.39	0.48	0.82
39	Pentacosane	58.223	2501	2506	0.83	0.26	0.64
40	Unknown	58.548	2519	-	4.41	4.32	1.5
41	Ethyl trans-caffeate, bis(tert-butyldimethylsilyl) ether	58.675	2527	2547	0.11	0.08	0.16
42	Bisphenol C*	59.085	2551	-	1.47	3.58	5.2
43	1-Docosanol, TMS derivative	59.220	2558	2557	0.25	0.48	0.67
44	Unknown	59.577	2579	-	0.3	0.19	0.45
45	Butanoic acid, 4-methoxy-2-nitro-, 2,6-bis(1,1-dimethylethyl)-4-methoxyphenyl ester	59.990	2604	2595	0.6	0.25	3.25
46	Unknown	60.465	2635	-	0.45	0.71	0.56
47	Behenic acid, TMS derivative	60.650	2645	2644	1.05	0.37	-
48	Unknown	60.938	2664	-	0.82	1.22	2.59
49	Unknown	61.132	2675	-	0.27	0.59	1.51
50	Unknown	61.280	2685	-	2.12	0.96	0.9
51	Maltose, 8TMS derivative, isomer 2	61.415	2693	2693	1.56	2.96	5.33
52	n-Heptacosane	61.527	2700	2700	0.82	0.2	-
53	Sucrose, 8TMS derivative	61.700	2712	2712	2.38	0.43	0.23
54	D-(+)-Turanose, octakis(trimethylsilyl) ether, methyloxime (isomer 1)	61.925	2727	2724	0.53	1.96	4.92
55	Maltose, OTMS	62.035	2735	2733	0.38	0.18	0.11
56	D-Cellobiose, (isomer 2), 8TMS derivative	62.258	2749	2762	1.7	2.64	0.43
57	Naringenin, O,O′-bis(trimethylsilyl)-	62.612	2772	2778	1.07	3.48	6.06
58	Unknown	63.180	2813	-	-	-	2.08
59	Isosakuranetin, TMS derivative	63.345	2821	2818	0.74	1.43	0.2
60	Lignoceric acid, TMS derivative	63.648	2842	2838	7.82	3.45	0.35
61	Sakuranetin, TMS derivative	64.200	2882	2877	0.96	0.58	0.26
62	Catechine, 5TMS derivative	64.872	2932	2938	0.17	0.13	-
63	Gettibiose, TMS derivative	65.712	2991	2989	0.39	0.38	0.29
64	Triacontane	65.933	3009	3003	0.44	0.36	0.27
65	Pectolinaringenin, TMS derivative	66.108	3021	3037	0.54	0.41	0.38
66	Hexacosanoic acid, TMS derivative	66.367	3041	3039	0.7	0.18	1.84
67	Nonacosan-10-ol, O-TMS	66.840	3078	3048	2.59	0.64	-
68	Nonacosan-9-ol, O-TMS	66.925	3085	3053	2.13	1.06	0.91
69	Hentriacontane	67.132	3100	3103	0.36	0.2	0.83
70	Kaempferol, 4TMS	67.298	3114	3112	0.29	0.86	0.77
71	Trimethylsilyl octacosanoate, TMS derivative	69.220	3256	3229	0.52	0.2	0.52
72	Methyl triacontyl ether	69.512	3275	3233	8.38	0.97	0.44

RI (retention time); RI_{exp}. and RI_{lit}. indicate retention indices based on experiments and literature, respectively.

Table A2. GC-MS profile of hexane extracts of propolis (HEP) from different regions of Poland: *HEP_P1*—Podlasie (Hajnowka), *HEP_P2*—Masovia (Ciechanow), *HEP_P3*—West Pomerania Province (Miedzyzdroje).

	Substances	RT	RI exp	RI lit	HEP_P1[%]	HEP_P2[%]	HEP_P3[%]
1	Benzoic Acid, TMS derivative	8.765	1246	1249	8.1	8.47	13.19
2	Glycerol, TMS	10.137	1287	1289	0.82	0.47	0.6
3	Decanoic acid, TMS derivative	17.830	1460	1450	0.15	1.5	0.14
4	Vanillin, TMS derivative	21.590	1536	1530	0.79	0.36	0.27
5	Cinnamic acid, TMS derivative	21.998	1545	1542	0.17	0.26	0.87
6	Dodecanoic acid, TMS	27.828	1658	1655	0.31	0.37	0.36
7	β-D-Xylopyranose, 4TMS derivative	34.300	1784	1777	0.25	1.36	-
8	D-Fructose, 5TMS derivative	37.770	1856	1867	0.36	0.36	0.38
9	4,7,10-Hexadecatrienoic acid, methyl ester	40.008	1899	1902	0.36	0.13	-
10	D-Sorbitol, 6TMS derivative	41.032	1922	1920	0.2	-	-
11	4-Coumaric acid, 2TMS derivative	42.122	1947	1949	0.33	0.19	0.21
12	Salicylic acid, trimethylsilyl ether, benzyl ester	45.865	2028	2025	0.87	1.84	0.63
13	Palmitic Acid, TMS derivative	47.035	2057	2050	2.48	3.06	2.96
14	Ferulic acid, 2TMS derivative	48.887	2103	2103	1.2	0.76	3.01
15	Phtalic acid derivative*	50.357	2150		1.04	1.31	0.21
16	Methyl caffeate, 2TMS derivative	51.882	2201	1997	1.02	1.67	0.07
17	13-Octadecenoic acid, (E)-, TMS derivative	52.365	2222	2228	1.7	4.3	8.05
18	3,7,11,15-Tetramethyl-2,6,10,14-hexadecatetraene-1-ol trimethylsilyl ether	52.677	2236	2234	0.77	1.21	-
19	Stearic acid, TMS derivative	53.047	2249	2246	0.55	0.89	1.15
20	Tricosane	54.255	2300	2300	3.55	2.67	3.05
21	Arachidic acid, TMS derivative	57.212	2446	2447	0.43	0.4	0.63
22	Pterostilbene, trimethylsilyl ether	57.723	2462	-	0.34	0.28	0.13
23	Pentacosane	58.200	2501	2506	5.24	4.6	4.00
24	Ethyl trans-caffeate, bis(tert-butyldimethylsilyl) ether	58.518	2527	2547	0.84	1.54	1.2
25	Bisphenol C*	59.043	2551		0.3	0.52	1.28
26	Behenic acid, TMS derivative	60.617	2643	2644	2.11	1.42	2.19
27	Unknown	61.255	2683	-	2.02	1.56	1.77
28	n-Heptacosane	61.512	2700	2700	14.11	14.31	12.45
29	Maltose, OTMS	62.007	2735	2733	0.38	0.19	0.1
30	D-Cellobiose, (isomer 2), 8TMS derivative	62.290	2749	2762	0.37	1.16	0.55
31	Octacosane	63.003	2798	2800	0.56	1.09	0.68
32	Lignoceric acid, TMS derivative	63.620	2842	2838	7.72	5.88	12.02
33	Sakuranetin, TMS derivative	64.170	2882	2877	0.53	-	0.23
34	Nonacosane	64.438	2899	2900	7.15	9.24	7.34
35	Hexacosanoic acid, TMS derivative	66.345	3041	3039	0.63	0.67	2.21
36	Nonacosan-10-ol, O-TMS	66.817	3078	3048	5.01	3.31	3.27
37	Nonacosan-9-ol, O-TMS	66.907	3085	3053	4.36	3.24	2.7
38	Hentriacontane	67.115	3100	3103	4.25	6.66	4.62
39	Myristic acid, 9-hexadecenyl ester, (Z)-	68.128	3177	3130	0.6	0.34	0.17
40	Trimethylsilyl octacosanoate, TMS derivative	69.188	3256	3229	1.21	1.01	0.5
41	Methyl triacontyl ether	69.493	3276	3233	16.8	11.36	6.82

RI (retention time); RI_{exp}. and RI_{lit}. indicate retention indices based on experiments and literature, respectively.

Table A3. GC-MS profile of hexane-ethanol extracts of propolis (HEEP) from different regions of Poland: *HEEP_P1*—Podlasie (Hajnowka), *HEEP_P2*—Masovia (Ciechanow), *HEEP_P3*—West Pomerania Province (Miedzyzdroje).

	Substances	RT	RI exp	RI lit	HEEP_P1[%]	HEEP_P2[%]	HEEP_P3[%]
1	Benzyl alcohol, TMS derivative	6.112	1155	1152	0.09	0.04	0.08
2	Benzoic Acid, TMS derivative	8.797	1246	1249	3.16	1.24	1.27
3	Cinnamaldehyde	9.905	1272	1274	0.04	0.08	0.06
4	Glycerol, TMS	10.170	1287	1289	0.87	1.05	1.8
5	Butanedioic acid, 2TMS derivative	11.465	1320	1321	0.12	0.05	0.18
6	1-Monoacetin, 2O-TMS	11.748	1326	1324	0.14	0.06	0.09
7	4-Hydroxybenzaldehyde, TMS derivative	13.748	1373	1383	0.26	0.19	0.14
8	Hydroquinone, 2TMS derivative	15.325	1409	1408	0.4	0.22	0.13
9	Cinnamyl alcohol, trimethylsilyl ether	16.273	1422	1428	-	0.02	0.03
10	Malic acid, 3TMS derivative	20.282	1511	1497	0.12	0.12	0.81
11	5-Oxoproline, TMS derivative	20.693	1521	1527	0.12	0.06	0.05
12	Vanillin, TMS derivative	21.640	1537	1530	1.82	0.46	0.27
13	Cinnamic acid, TMS derivative	22.043	1545	1542	0.07	0.05	0.15
14	3,4-Dihydroxybenzaldehyde,	26.045	1622	1612	-	0.13	0.27

Table A3. *Cont.*

	Substances	RT	RI $_{exp}$	RI $_{lit}$	HEEP_P1[%]	HEEP_P2[%]	HEEP_P3[%]
15	4-Hydroxybenzoic acid, 2TMS derivative	26.638	1634	1635	0.48	0.22	0.18
16	Dodecanoic acid, TMS	27.668	1658	1655	0.14	0.02	0.08
17	β-D-Xylopyranose, 4TMS derivative	34.563	1784	1777	0.13	0.03	0.03
18	o-Coumaric acid, 2TMS derivative	34.968	1797	1815	0.28	0.25	0.09
19	4-Methoxycinnamic acid, TMS derivative	36.602	1830	1833	-	0.08	0.26
20	D-Psicofuranose	37.475	1848	1837	1.46	1.59	2.24
21	D-Fructose, 5TMS derivative	37.865	1856	1866	12.58	11.92	2.03
22	D-Sorbitol, 6TMS derivative	41.092	1922	1920	0.16	0.1	-
23	D-Glucose, 5TMS derivative	41.658	1934	1928	7.14	11.9	8.27
24	4-Coumaric acid, 2TMS derivative	42.252	1947	1949	16.74	13.52	10.74
25	D-Glucitol, 6TMS derivative	43.917	1982	1980	0.43	0.25	0.44
26	Gallic acid, 4TMS derivative	44.125	1987	1987	0.68	0.13	-
27	Salicylic acid, trimethylsilyl ether, benzyl ester	45.932	2028	2025	0.1	0.08	0.2
28	D-Mannopyranose, 5TMS derivative	46.353	2038	2037	6.33	13.13	9.13
29	D-Gluconic acid, 6TMS derivative	46.885	2052	2043	0.15	0.2	0.08
30	Palmitic Acid, TMS derivative	47.083	2057	2050	0.49	0.18	0.09
31	Isoferulic acid, 2TMS derivative	48.453	2090	2081	0.09	0.78	2.95
32	Ferulic acid, 2TMS derivative	48.965	2103	2103	7.93	3.02	3.86
33	Myo-Inositol, 6TMS derivative	49.845	2132	2129	0.09	0.13	1.3
34	Phtalic acid derivative*	50.403	2150	-	0.7	0.24	0.03
35	Caffeic acid, 3TMS derivative	50.565	2157	2155	0.89	0.83	0.03
36	Linoleic acid, TMS	51.922	2203	2212	1.31	2.48	4.6
37	13-Octadecenoic acid, (E)-, TMS derivative	52.392	2222	2228	0.17	1.77	0.06
38	3,7,11,15-Tetramethyl-2,6,10,14-hexadecatetraene-1-ol trimethylsilyl ether	52.703	2236	2234	1.01	0.07	0.07
39	2′,6′-Dihydroxy 4′-methoxydihydrochalcone, trimethylsilyl ether	52.717	2418	2405	-	1.99	0.1
40	Pterostilbene, trimethylsilyl ether	57.520	2462	-	0.43	0.77	2.58
41	Pentacosane	58.563	2501	2506	5.85	0.44	0.87
42	Ethyl trans-caffeate, bis(tert-butyldimethylsilyl) ether	58.560	2527	2547	-	3.55	2.22
43	Bisphenol*	59.088	2551		1.65	0.13	0.12
44	1-Docosanol, TMS derivative	59.223	2558	2557	0.19	4.51	4.76
45	Butanoic acid, 4-methoxy-2-nitro-, 2,6-bis(1,1-dimethylethyl)-4-methoxyphenyl ester	59.998	2604	2595	0.72	0.32	0.67
46	Unknown	60.475	2635		0.99	0.84	3.44
47	Behenic acid, TMS derivative	60.550	2645	2644	0.31	0.94	0.83
48	Unknown	60.947	2664		0.95	1.73	2.77
49	Unknown	61.285	2685		3.22	0.69	1.67
50	Maltose, 8TMS derivative, isomer 2	61.422	2693	2693	1.83	3.42	5.26
51	n-Heptacosane	61.537	2700	2700	0.21	0.11	0.31
52	Sucrose, 8TMS derivative	61.705	2712	2712	5.88	0.52	2.61
53	D-(+)-Turanose, octakis(trimethylsilyl) ether, methyloxime (isomer 1)	61.937	2727	2724	0.71	2.66	4.98
54	Maltose, OTMS	62.040	2735	2733	0.29	0.13	0.12
55	D-Cellobiose, (isomer 2), 8TMS derivative	62.262	2749	2762	1.51	0.32	1.3
56	Naringenin, O,O′-bis(trimethylsilyl)-	62.617	2772	2778	1.14	4.1	5.95
57	Isosakuranetin, TMS derivative	63.352	2821	2818	0.94	1.37	2.13
58	Lignoceric acid, TMS derivative	63.650	2842	2838	1.22	1.68	0.44
59	Sakuranetin, TMS derivative	64.215	2882	2877	1.75	0.64	0.11
60	Catechine, 5TMS derivative	64.880	2932	2938	0.33	0.11	0.07
61	Gettibiose, TMS derivative	65.720	2991	2989	0.76	0.36	0.66
62	Triacontane	65.948	3009	3003	0.78	0.4	0.35
63	Hexacosanoic acid, TMS derivative	66.375	3041	3039	0.5	0.69	2.04
64	Unknown	66.975	3085	-	0.66	0.61	0.74
65	Hentriacontane	67.137	3100	3103	0.49	0.23	0.77

RI (retention time); RI_{exp}. and RI_{lit}. indicate retention indices based on experiments and literature, respectively.

Table A4. Percentage of fatty acids in hexane extracts of propolis (HEP) from different regions of Poland: *HEP_P1*—Podlasie (Hajnowka), *HEP_P2*—Masovia (Ciechanow), *HEP_P3*—West Pomerania Province (Miedzyzdroje).

	Substances	RT	RI $_{exp}$	RI $_{lit}$	HEP_P1[%]	HEP_P2[%]	HEP_P3[%]
1	Benzoic acid, methyl ester	15.055	1623	1612	0.69	2.73	0.92
2	Lauric acid, methyl ester	18.820	1877	1804	1.85	2.32	1.28
3	cis-9-Tetradecenoic acid, methyl ester	25.410	2116	2026	5.16	1.94	2.30
4	Pentadecanoic acid, methyl ester	27.530	2194	2108	1.75	0.79	0.70
5	Hexadecanoic acid, methyl ester	29.590	2271	2208	31.17	27.63	20.54
6	Heptadecanoic acid, methyl ester	32.790	2666	2309	9.68	7.67	6.34
7	Octadecanoic acid, methyl ester	34.345	2394	2418	6.40	5.28	4.23
8	Oleic acid, methyl ester	35.050	2488	2434	18.18	25.30	25.90
9	cis-11-Octadecenoic acid, methyl ester	35.565	2512	2468	1.19	0.48	0.81
10	Linolenic acid, methyl ester	37.775	2625	2571	0.95	2.38	5.86
11	Eicosanoic acid, methyl ester	38.180	2651	2639	1.02	1.86	1.89
12	Docosanoic acid, methyl ester	40.790	2844	2835	4.70	5.71	5.00
13	Me. C20:4n3; Eicosa-(8,11,14,17)-tetraenoate <methyl>	41.060	2866	2865	2.48	2.37	2.75
14	Tetracosanoic acid, methyl ester	42.805	3067	3039	14.79	13.91	21.49

RI (retention time); $RI_{exp.}$ and $RI_{lit.}$ indicate retention indices based on experiments and literature, respectively.

References

1. Thomford, N.E.; Senthebane, D.A.; Rowe, A.; Munro, D.; Seele, P.; Maroyi, A.; Dzobo, K. Natural Products for Drug Discovery in the 21st Century: Innovations for Novel Drug Discovery. *Int. J. Mol. Sci.* **2018**, *19*, 1578. [CrossRef]
2. Sforcin, J.M. Biological Properties and Therapeutic Applications of Propolis. *Phytotherapy Res.* **2016**, *30*, 894–905. [CrossRef] [PubMed]
3. Carvalho, R.; Baltazar, F.; Aguiar, C.A.A. Propolis: A Complex Natural Product with a Plethora of Biological Activities That Can Be Explored for Drug Development. *Evid.-Based Complement. Altern. Med.* **2015**, *2015*, 1–29. [CrossRef] [PubMed]
4. Giannopoulou, E.; De Castro, S.L.; Marcucci, M.C. Propolis: Recent advances in chemistry and plant origin. *Apidologie* **2000**, *31*, 3–15. [CrossRef]
5. Więckiewicz, W.; Miernik, M.; Więckiewicz, M.; Morawiec, T. Does Propolis Help to Maintain Oral Health? *Evid.-Based Complement. Altern. Med.* **2013**, *2013*, 1–8. [CrossRef] [PubMed]
6. Przybyłek, I.; Karpiński, T.M. Antibacterial Properties of Propolis. *Molecules* **2019**, *24*, 2047. [CrossRef]
7. Grecka, K.; Kuś, P.M.; Okińczyc, P.; Worobo, R.; Walkusz, J.; Szweda, P. The Anti-Staphylococcal Potential of Ethanolic Polish Propolis Extracts. *Molecules* **2019**, *24*, 1732. [CrossRef]
8. Pobiega, K.; Kraśniewska, K.; Derewiaka, D.; Gniewosz, M. Comparison of the antimicrobial activity of propolis extracts obtained by means of various extraction methods. *J. Food Sci. Technol.* **2019**, *56*, 5386–5395. [CrossRef]
9. Piekarz, T.; Mertas, A.; Wiatrak, K.; Rój, R.; Kownacki, P.; Śmieszek-Wilczewska, J.; Kopczyńska, E.; Wrzoł, M.; Cisowska, M.; Szliszka, E.; et al. The Influence of Toothpaste Containing Australian Melaleuca alternifolia Oil and Ethanolic Extract of Polish Propolis on Oral Hygiene and Microbiome in Patients Requiring Conservative Procedures. *Molecules* **2017**, *22*, 1957. [CrossRef]
10. Wieczynska, A.; Wezgowiec, J.; Wieckiewicz, W.; Czarny, A.; Kulbacka, J.; Nowakowska, D.; Gancarz, R.; Wilk, K.A. Antimicrobial Activity, Cytotoxicity and Total Phenolic Content of Different Extracts of Propolis from the West Pomeranian Region in Poland. *Acta Pol. Pharm.-Drug Res.* **2017**, *74*, 715–722.
11. Wojtyczka, R.D.; Dziedzic, A.; Idzik, D.; Kępa, M.; Kubina, R.; Kabała-Dzik, A.; Smoleń-Dzirba, J.; Stojko, J.; Sajewicz, M.; Wąsik, T.J. Susceptibility of Staphylococcus aureus Clinical Isolates to Propolis Extract Alone or in Combination with Antimicrobial Drugs. *Molecules* **2013**, *18*, 9623–9640. [CrossRef]
12. Borawska, M.; Naliwajko, S.; Moskwa, J.; Markiewicz-Żukowska, R.; Puścion-Jakubik, A.; Soroczyńska, J. Anti-proliferative and anti-migration effects of Polish propolis combined with Hypericum perforatum L. on glioblastoma multiforme cell line U87MG. *BMC Complement. Altern. Med.* **2016**, *16*, 367. [CrossRef] [PubMed]

13. Popova, M.; Giannopoulou, E.; Skalicka-Woźniak, K.; Graikou, K.; Widelski, J.; Giannopoulou, E.; Kalofonos, H.P.; Sivolapenko, G.; Gaweł-Bęben, K.; Antosiewicz, B.; et al. Characterization and Biological Evaluation of Propolis from Poland. *Molecules* **2017**, *22*, 1159. [CrossRef] [PubMed]
14. Szliszka, E.; Sokół-Łętowska, A.; Kucharska, A.Z.; Jaworska, D.; Czuba, Z.; Krol, W. Ethanolic Extract of Polish Propolis: Chemical Composition and TRAIL-R2 Death Receptor Targeting Apoptotic Activity against Prostate Cancer Cells. *Evid.-Based Complement. Altern. Med.* **2013**, *2013*, 1–12. [CrossRef]
15. Yu, X.; Li, Z. MicroRNA expression and its implications for diagnosis and therapy of tongue squamous cell carcinoma. *J. Cell. Mol. Med.* **2015**, *20*, 10–16. [CrossRef] [PubMed]
16. Chan, G.C.; Cheung, K.-W.; Sze, D.M.-Y. The Immunomodulatory and Anticancer Properties of Propolis. *Clin. Rev. Allergy Immunol.* **2012**, *44*, 262–273. [CrossRef]
17. Russo, A.; Cardile, V.; Sánchez, F.; Troncoso, N.; Vanella, A.; Garbarino, J. Chilean propolis: Antioxidant activity and antiproliferative action in human tumor cell lines. *Life Sci.* **2004**, *76*, 545–558. [CrossRef]
18. Yen, C.-H.; Chiu, H.-F.; Wu, C.-H.; Lu, Y.-Y.; Han, Y.-C.; Shen, Y.; Venkatakrishnan, K.; Wang, C.-K. Beneficial efficacy of various propolis extracts and their digestive products by in vitro simulated gastrointestinal digestion. *LWT* **2017**, *84*, 281–289. [CrossRef]
19. Salehi, M.; Motallebnejad, M.; Moghadamnia, A.A.; Seyemajidi, M.; Khanghah, S.N.; Ebrahimpour, A.; Molania, T. An Intervention Airing the Effect of Iranian Propolis on Epithelial Dysplasia of the Tongue: A Preliminary Study. *J. Clin. Diagn. Res.* **2017**, *11*, ZC67–ZC70. [CrossRef]
20. Ribeiro, D.R.; Alves Ângela, V.F.; Dos Santos, E.P.; Padilha, F.F.; Gomes, M.Z.; Rabelo, A.S.; Cardoso, J.; Massarioli, A.P.; Alencar, S.M.; De Albuquerque-Júnior, R.L.C.; et al. Inhibition of DMBA-induced Oral Squamous Cells Carcinoma Growth by Brazilian Red Propolis in Rodent Model. *Basic Clin. Pharmacol. Toxicol.* **2015**, *117*, 85–95. [CrossRef]
21. Lee, Y.-T.; Don, M.-J.; Hung, P.-S.; Shen, Y.-C.; Lo, Y.-S.; Chang, K.-W.; Chen, C.-F.; Ho, L.-K. Cytotoxicity of phenolic acid phenethyl esters on oral cancer cells. *Cancer Lett.* **2005**, *223*, 19–25. [CrossRef] [PubMed]
22. Kuo, Y.-Y.; Jim, W.-T.; Su, L.-C.; Chung, C.-J.; Lin, C.-Y.; Huo, C.; Tseng, J.-C.; Huang, S.-H.; Lai, C.-J.; Chen, B.-C.; et al. Caffeic Acid Phenethyl Ester Is a Potential Therapeutic Agent for Oral Cancer. *Int. J. Mol. Sci.* **2015**, *16*, 10748–10766. [CrossRef] [PubMed]
23. Kuo, Y.-Y.; Lin, H.-P.; Huo, C.; Su, L.-C.; Yang, J.; Hsiao, P.-H.; Chiang, H.-C.; Chung, C.-J.; Wang, H.-D.; Chang, J.-Y.; et al. Caffeic Acid Phenethyl Ester Suppresses Proliferation and Survival of TW2.6 Human Oral Cancer Cells via Inhibition of Akt Signaling. *Int. J. Mol. Sci.* **2013**, *14*, 8801–8817. [CrossRef] [PubMed]
24. Czyżewska, U.; Siemionow, K.; Zaręba, I.; Miltyk, W. Proapoptotic Activity of Propolis and Their Components on Human Tongue Squamous Cell Carcinoma Cell Line (CAL-27). *PLOS ONE* **2016**, *11*, e0157091. [CrossRef]
25. Asgharpour, F.; Moghadamnia, A.A.; Zabihi, E.; Kazemi, S.; Namvar, A.E.; Gholinia, H.; Motallebnejad, M.; Nouri, H.R. Iranian propolis efficiently inhibits growth of oral streptococci and cancer cell lines. *BMC Complement. Altern. Med.* **2019**, *19*, 266–268. [CrossRef]
26. Sawaya, A.C.; Cunha, I.B.D.S.; Marcucci, M.C. Analytical methods applied to diverse types of Brazilian propolis. *Chem. Central J.* **2011**, *5*, 1–10. [CrossRef]
27. Rassu, G.; Cossu, M.; Langasco, R.; Carta, A.; Cavalli, R.; Giunchedi, P.; Gavini, E. Propolis as lipid bioactive nano-carrier for topical nasal drug delivery. *Colloids Surfaces B Biointerfaces* **2015**, *136*, 908–917. [CrossRef]
28. Kubilienė, L.; Laugaliene, V.; Pavilonis, A.; Maruska, A.; Majiene, D.; Barčauskaitė, K.; Kubilius, R.; Kasparaviciene, G.; Savickas, A. Alternative preparation of propolis extracts: Comparison of their composition and biological activities. *BMC Complement. Altern. Med.* **2015**, *15*, 156. [CrossRef]
29. Maciejewicz, W. Isolation of Flavonoid Aglycones from Propolis by A Column Chromatography Method and Their Identification By Gc-Ms And Tlc Methods. *J. Liq. Chromatogr. Relat. Technol.* **2001**, *24*, 1171–1179. [CrossRef]
30. Anjum, S.I.; Ullah, A.; Khan, K.A.; Attaullah, M.; Khan, H.; Ali, H.; Bashir, M.A.; Tahir, M.; Rana, R.M.; Ghramh, H.A.; et al. Composition and functional properties of propolis (bee glue): A review. *Saudi J. Boil. Sci.* **2019**, *26*, 1695–1703. [CrossRef] [PubMed]
31. Sahinler, N.; Kaftanoglu, O. Natural product propolis: Chemical composition. *Nat. Prod. Res.* **2005**, *19*, 183–188. [CrossRef] [PubMed]
32. Roleira, F.M.F.; Da Silva, E.J.T.; Varela, C.; Costa, S.; Silva, T.; Garrido, J.; Borges, F. Plant derived and dietary phenolic antioxidants: Anticancer properties. *Food Chem.* **2015**, *183*, 235–258. [CrossRef] [PubMed]

33. Tyszka-Czochara, M.; Paśko, P.; Reczyński, W.; Szlósarczyk, M.; Bystrowska, B.; Opoka, W. Zinc and propolis reduces cytotoxicity and proliferation in skin fibroblast cell culture: Total polyphenol content and antioxidant capacity of propolis. *Boil. Trace Element Res.* **2014**, *160*, 123–131. [CrossRef] [PubMed]
34. Szliszka, E.; Kucharska, A.Z.; Sokół-Łętowska, A.; Mertas, A.; Czuba, Z.; Krol, W. Chemical Composition and Anti-Inflammatory Effect of Ethanolic Extract of Brazilian Green Propolis on Activated J774A.1 Macrophages. *Evid.-Based Complement. Altern. Med.* **2013**, *2013*, 1–13. [CrossRef] [PubMed]
35. Bueno-Silva, B.; Rosalen, P.L.; Alencar, S.M.; Mayer, M.P.A. Anti-inflammatory mechanisms of neovestitol from Brazilian red propolis in LPS-activated macrophages. *J. Funct. Foods* **2017**, *36*, 440–447. [CrossRef]
36. Parashar, K.; Sood, S.; Mehaidli, A.; Curran, C.; Vegh, C.; Nguyen, C.; Pignanelli, C.; Zhang, Z.; Liang, G.; Wang, Y.; et al. Evaluating the Anti-cancer Efficacy of a Synthetic Curcumin Analog on Human Melanoma Cells and Its Interaction with Standard Chemotherapeutics. *Molecules* **2019**, *24*, 2483. [CrossRef]
37. Tsirigotis-Maniecka, M.; Szyk-Warszynska, L.; Michna, A.; Warszyński, P.; Wilk, K.A. Colloidal characteristics and functionality of rationally designed esculin-loaded hydrogel microcapsules. *J. Colloid Interface Sci.* **2018**, *530*, 444–458. [CrossRef]
38. Makhafola, T.J.; Elgorashi, E.; McGaw, L.J.; Verschaeve, L.; Jn, E. The correlation between antimutagenic activity and total phenolic content of extracts of 31 plant species with high antioxidant activity. *BMC Complement. Altern. Med.* **2016**, *16*, 490. [CrossRef]
39. Yang, H.; Dong, Y.; Du, H.; Shi, H.; Peng, Y.; Li, X. Antioxidant Compounds from Propolis Collected in Anhui, China. *Molecules* **2011**, *16*, 3444–3455. [CrossRef]
40. Zali, A.G.; Ehsanzadeh, P.; Szumny, A.; Matkowski, A. Genotype-specific response of Foeniculum vulgare grain yield and essential oil composition to proline treatment under different irrigation conditions. *Ind. Crop. Prod.* **2018**, *124*, 177–185. [CrossRef]
41. Dominiak, M.; Saczko, J. Method of Primary Culture of Human Fibroblasts for Autologous Augmentation. Patent No. PL209784B1, 31 October 2011.
42. Houghton, P.; Fang, R.; Techatanawat, I.; Steventon, G.; Hylands, P.J.; Lee, C. The sulphorhodamine (SRB) assay and other approaches to testing plant extracts and derived compounds for activities related to reputed anticancer activity. *Methods* **2007**, *42*, 377–387. [CrossRef] [PubMed]

12

A Comparative Study of the Anticancer Activity and PARP-1 Inhibiting Effect of Benzofuran–Pyrazole Scaffold and Its Nano-Sized Particles in Human Breast Cancer Cells

Manal M. Anwar [1], Somaia S. Abd El-Karim [1], Ahlam H. Mahmoud [1], Abd El-Galil E. Amr [2,3,*] and Mohamed A. Al-Omar [2]

1 Department of Therapeutic Chemistry, National Research Centre, Dokki, Cairo 12622, Egypt
2 Pharmaceutical Chemistry Department, Drug Exploration & Development Chair (DEDC), College of Pharmacy, King Saud University, Riyadh 11451, Saudi Arabia
3 Applied Organic Chemistry Department, National Research Center, Cairo, Dokki 12622, Egypt
* Correspondence: aamr@ksu.edu.sa;

Academic Editor: Qiao-Hong Chen

Abstract: Breast cancer is considered the most common and deadly cancer among women worldwide. Nanomedicine has become extremely attractive in the field of cancer treatment. Due to the high surface to volume ratio and other unique properties, nanomaterials can be specifically targeted to certain cells and tissues to interact with the living systems. The strategic planning of this study is based on using the nanoprecipitation method to prepare nanoparticles **BZP-NPs** (3.8–5.7 nm) of the previously prepared benzofuran–pyrazole compound (**IV**) **BZP** which showed promising cytotoxic activity. The capacity of **BZP** and **BZP-NPs** to suppress the growth of human breast tumor MCF-7 and MDA-MB-231 cells was evaluated using MTT assay. The IC_{50} doses of **BZP** and **BZP-NPs** targeting normal breast cells MCF-12A exceeded those targeting the cancer cells by >1000-fold, demonstrating their reasonable safety profiles in normal cells. Furthermore, cell cycle analysis, apoptosis induction detection, assessment of p53, Bcl-2, caspase-3, and PARP-1 levels of **BZP** and its nano-sized-**BZP-NPs** particles were also evaluated. Although the obtained results were in the favor of compound **IV** in its normal sized particles, **BZP-NPs** appeared as a hit compound which showed improved cytotoxicity against the tested human breast cancer cells associated with the induction of pre-G1 apoptosis as well as cell cycle arrest at G2/M phase. The increase in caspase-3 level, upregulation of p53, and downregulation of Bcl-2 protein expression levels confirmed apoptosis. Furthermore, ELISA results exhibited that **BZP-NPs** produced a more favorable impact as a PARP-1 enzyme inhibitor than the parent **BZP**.

Keywords: breast cancer; benzofuran–pyrazole; nanoparticles; cytotoxic activity; apoptosis; PARP-1 inhibition

---

1. Introduction

Breast cancer is the most common malignancy in women, accounting for about 18% of female cancers and over half a million new cases are diagnosed worldwide each year. Its incidence increases with age and is currently rising. Although earlier diagnosis has improved the survival rates, saving lives and elevating treatment rates, metastatic breast cancer is still considered as the major factor of breast cancer-related mortality [1–4]. Despite the continuous development in the treatment of cancer disease, the strategy for cancer management has remained essentially unchanged: surgical resection of the malignant tumor followed by either chemotherapeutic administration, radiotherapy, or a combination of the two. In fact, both of these therapies cause unselective and undesirable damage to the healthy tissues. In addition, a number of factors can lead to treatment failure, such as the remaining of some residual cells after the surgery, resistance to chemotherapies, physiological obstacles against the treatments, such as the blood–brain barrier and cellular barriers which hamper the access to drug targets, debilitating systemic toxicities, and poor pharmacokinetics of the chemotherapeutic [5–7].

Nanomedicine is defined as the use of nanotechnology for different medical purposes. Nanotechnology deals with research of materials of dimensions ranges between 1 to 100 nm (National Nanotechnology Initiative). This active protocol is applied in various science applications including cancer chemotherapeutics [8]. Deep studies have shed light on the combination of nanotechnology with cancer biology advances to gain novel techniques for cancer care. The concept that the strategy of nanomedicines is based on improving the therapeutic index of anticancer drugs by optimizing their pharmacokinetics and tissue distribution to facilitate and fasten delivery to the site of action is well known and has been investigated clinically [9–11]. Smaller (sub-100 nm) nanomedicine systems and lower molecular weight macromolecules have been shown to extravasate to a greater extent and/or penetrate farther from the vasculature than larger systems. This size effect has also been associated with improved efficacy [11,12]. Because of their sizes, the chemical properties and biodistribution of the nanomaterials are different from bulky materials. Thus, in recent years, nanomedicine has been considered as one of the most promising and important tools to defeat the problems obtained due to the administration of the traditional antitumor drugs. In addition, nanoparticle formulations can reduce or prevent systemic toxicities by specific delivery of the drugs to the cancer cells via size-mediated passive targeting and physiologically mediated active targeting. They can overcome drug resistance by the delivery of complimentary treatments and they can improve early detection of the disease using targeted delivery of molecular imaging agents to tumors in order to improve the diagnostic imaging of the tumor tissues, thus beginning the treatment before the onset of metastasis [13,14].

Inspired by the literature studies mentioned above and in continuation with our previous efforts in developing new effective agents of significant anticancer activity [15–17], this study deals with generating the previously prepared 1-(5-(3-(benzofuran-2-yl)-1-phenyl-1*H*-pyrazol-4-yl)-4,5-dihydro-3-(1*H*-pyrrol-2-yl)pyrazol-1-yl)ethanone **(IV) BZP** in nanoparticles **BZP-NPs** of sizes 3.8–5.7 nm (Figure 1).

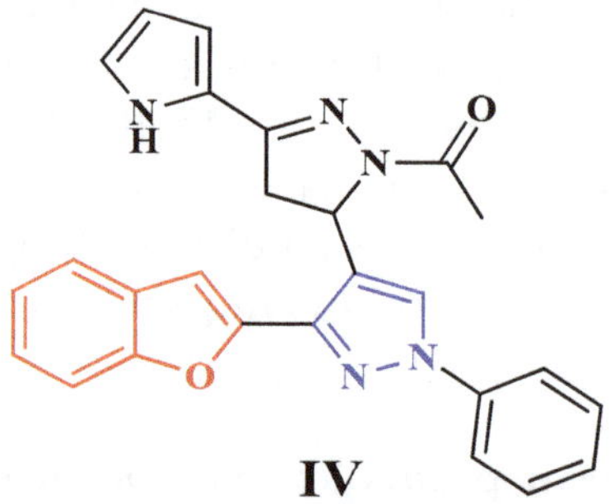

IV

Figure 1. The chemical structure of the benzofuran-pyrazole compound **IV** (**BZP**).

In our previous research, compound **IV (BZP)** was subjected, among other eight different benzofuran-pyrazole derivatives, to NCI for *in vitro* anticancer evaluation targeting full 60 human cancer cell lines using a single high dose concentration (10^{-5} M) under the drug discovery program of the NCI [15]. The derivatives were chosen depending upon the degree of structural variations and computer modeling techniques in NCI. Fortunately, compound **IV (BZP)** exhibited promising cytotoxic potency against various cancer cell lines, so it was further evaluated by NCI team at five different minimal concentrations (0.01, 0.1, 1, 10, and 100 μM). It displayed cell growth inhibition of different breast cancer lines in the range of 45.95–55.44%. These data motivated the authors to convert compound **IV** (**BZP**) to nano-sized **BZP-NPs** to study the influence of the nanorange and whether nano-sized particles enhance the cytotoxic potency of the benzofuran compound.

The anticancer activity of **BZP** compound **IV** was assessed in comparison with its nano-sized **BZP-NPs** against MCF-7 and MDA-MB-231cancer cell lines. Various cellular mechanisms of action were also studied, such as apoptosis, cell cycle analysis, detection of caspase-3, p53, and Bcl-2 intensities, in addition to the efficiency of PARP-1 enzyme inhibition in the two types of the tested breast cancer cell lines

2. Results and Discussion

2.1. Chemistry

The preparation approach of the benzofuran–pyrazole derivative **IV** was outlined in Scheme 1 according to the reported method [15]. Using the Vilsmeier–Haach reaction, the key starting 1-(benzofuran-2-yl)ethanone (**I**) was converted to the intermediate pyrazole-4-carbaldehyde (**II**). The chalcone analogue **III** was obtained in a good yield by Claisen–Schmidt condensation of **II** with 2-acetylpyrrole in ethanolic sodium hydroxide solution. Cyclocondensation of **III** with hydrazine hydrate in acetic acid yielded the target compound **IV** in 85% yield (Scheme 1).

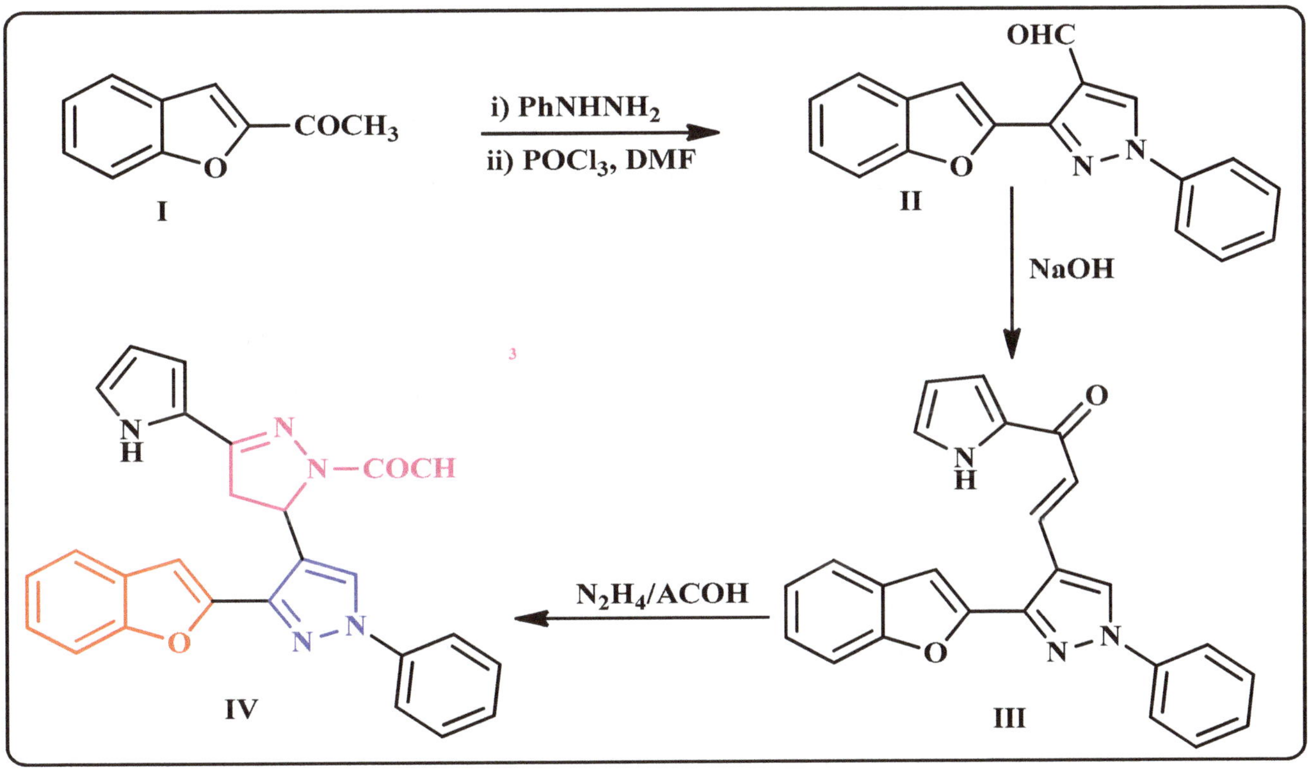

Scheme 1. Synthetic route of the benzofuran–pyrazole derivative (**IV**).

The nano-sized benzofuran–pyrazole **BZP-NPs** of different sizes (3.8–5.7 nm) were synthesized using the nanoprecipitation method [18]. The sizes and morphology of the nanobenzofuran–pyrazole hybrid **BZP-NPs** were examined by dynamic light scattering (DLS) and transmission electron microscopy (TEM). The results showed that nanoparticles were spherical in shape and their average size was 3.8–5.7 nm (Figure 2). The stability of the **BZP-NPs** was further investigated by X-ray diffraction (XRD) using a Pananalylical Empyrean X-ray Diffractometer and thermal analysis using a SDT Q600 V20.9 Build 20 thermal gravimetric instrument (Figures S1 and S2, Supplementary material).

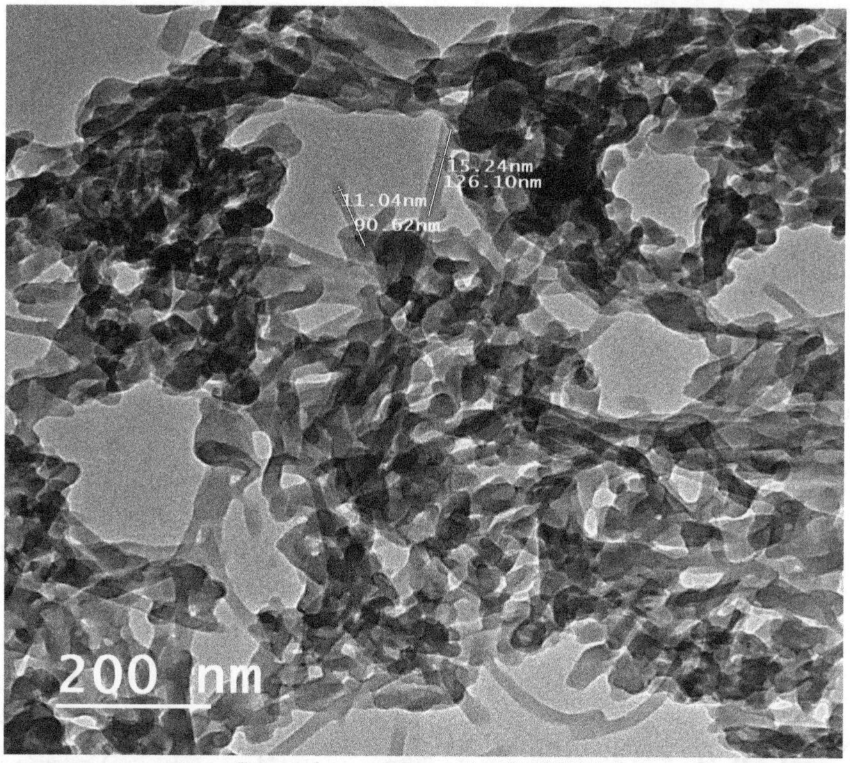

Benzofuran–pyrazole **IV** (**BZP**)

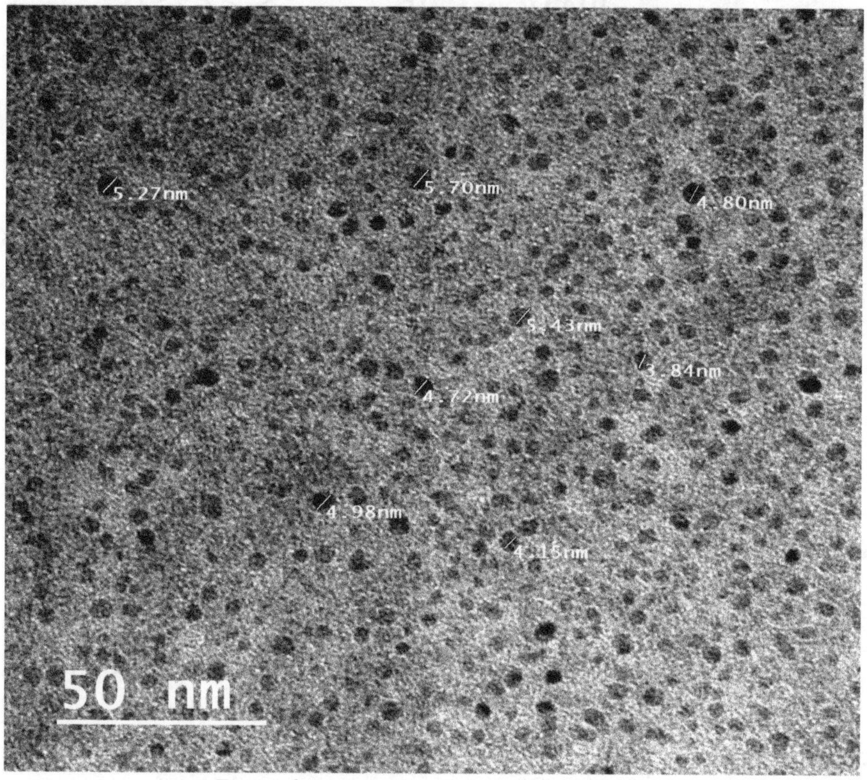

Benzofuran–pyrazole **IV** (**BZP-NPs**)

Figure 2. Electron micrograph of the **BZP** and **BZP-NPs**. The bar marker represents 50 nm.

Surface charge and stability of the nanoparticles were analyzed using the Malvern Zetasizer nano Zs instrument (MAL1074157) and the zeta potential was −27.3 mV with a polydispersity index (PDI) of 0.77 (Figure 3).

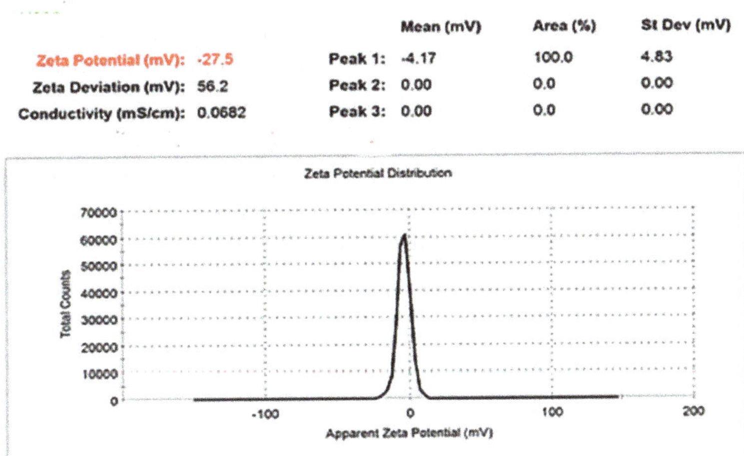

Figure 3. Zeta potential distribution of **BZP-NPs**.

2.2. *Biological Analysis*

2.2.1. In Vitro Anticancer Activity

The sensitivity of two human breast cancer cell lines, MCF-7 and MDA-MB-231, was evaluated against the benzofuran–pyrazole compound **BZP** and the target nano-sized benzofuran–pyrazole nanoparticles **BZP-NPs** using MTT assay. Doxorubicin served as a standard drug [17]. The resultant data were expressed as IC_{50} (nM) values which are the average of at least three independent experiments and are tabulated in Table 1. The obtained results showed that compound **IV** (**BZP**) produced significant cytotoxic activity against both breast cancer cell lines, with about 85- and 62-fold, respectively, greater potency than that of doxorubicin. Dramatic increase in the activity was observed by about 620 and 1000-fold for targeting both types of cancer cells by **BZP-NPs** compared to the reference drug doxorubicin. It could be detected that MDA-MB-231 cancer cells represented significant sensitivity against the nano-sized particles **BZP-NPs** more than their sensitivity against **BZP**.

Table 1. In vitro cytotoxic activity of compound **IV** (**BZP**) and **BZP-NPs**.

Compound Name	IC_{50} (nM)		
	MCF-7	MDA-MB-231	MCF-12A
Compound IV (**BZP**)	7 ± 1	10 ± 1	87600 ± 335
Compound IV (**BZP-NPs**)	1 ± 0.4	0.6 ± 0.1	21540 ± 66
Doxorubicin	620 ± 31	620 ± 31	

Despite the obvious benefits of chemotherapeutic drugs, there are several treatment-related damages to the normal cells that should be considered before finalizing the cancer treatment strategy. This study investigated the impact of compound **IV** (**BZP**) and **BZP-NPs** on normal breast cells (MRC-12A) using MTT assay [16]. Interestingly, a significant increase in the IC_{50} doses of **IV BZP** and **BZP-NPs** against the normal breast cells was detected when compared to their IC_{50} doses against both cancer cell lines (>1000-fold) (Table 1). This result confirmed the significant safety profile of the benzofuran-pyrazole compound **IV** either in the normal size particles or in its nano-sized particles **BZP-NPs**.

2.2.2. Cell Cycle Analysis

Due to the antiproliferative efficacy of compound **IV** (**BZP**) and **BZP-NPs**, it was of interest to study its modes of action in both tested types of cancer cells, including cell cycle progression and apoptosis induction. Cell death occurs via different pathways, including apoptosis or type I cell-death, and autophagy or type II cell-death, which are both forms of programmed cell death, whereas necrosis is a nonphysiological process resulting from an infection or injury [19,20]. Apoptosis rate in MCF-7 and MDA-MB-231 cells was detected by flow cytometry, using propidium iodide (PI) and an annexin-V–FITC double staining assay [21]. After incubation of both types of the tested cancer cells for 24 h with BZP and BZP-NPs at their IC_{50} concentrations of 7 nM and 1 nM for MCF-7 cells and at 10 nM and 0.6 nM for MDA-MB-231 cells, they were labeled with the two dyes. The corresponding red (PI) and green (FITC) fluorescence was detected using flow cytometry and the results were compared to DMSO-treated cells which served as a negative control. Marked alterations in cell cycle phases have occurred. There was a great enhancement in the percentage of apoptotic cells at the pre-G phase. The tested particles (**BZP**) and (**BZP-NPs**) induced total apoptotic cells (annexin V^+/PI^- and annexin V^+/PI^+) of percentages 9.18%, 21.54%, respectively, in MCF-7 cells vs. 2.64% in the control MCF-7 cells. They also induced total apoptotic percentages of 11.09% and 23.17%, respectively, in MDA-MB-231 cells vs. 2.82% in the control MDA-MB-231cells. It is observable that the **BZP-NPs** produced a more favorable impact about two-fold more potent than **BZP** particles against both types of the tested cancer cells, especially MDA-MB-231 cells, which was consistent with the cytotoxicity assay results (Figures 4 and 5). Also, exposure of MCF-7 and MDA-MB-231 cells to **BZP** and **BZP-NPs** led to an interference with the cell cycle distribution, inducing a pronounced elevation in the percentage of cells at the G2/M phase, reaching 11.26% and 17.52%, respectively, in MCF-7 vs. 6.28% in the control cells and to 12.11% and 19.24% in MDA-MB-231 cells, respectively, vs. 4.92% in the negative control (Table 2). Accordingly, it can be concluded that the compound **IV** (**BZP**) inhibits the cancer cells' proliferation with a synchronous significant arrest at the G2/M phase. The inhibition potency was signified by the **BZP-NPs** (Figures 6 and 7). Accumulation of cells at G2/M phase is a remarkable hallmark of the apoptotic role of **BZP** and **BZP-NPs** in both tested cancer cell lines.

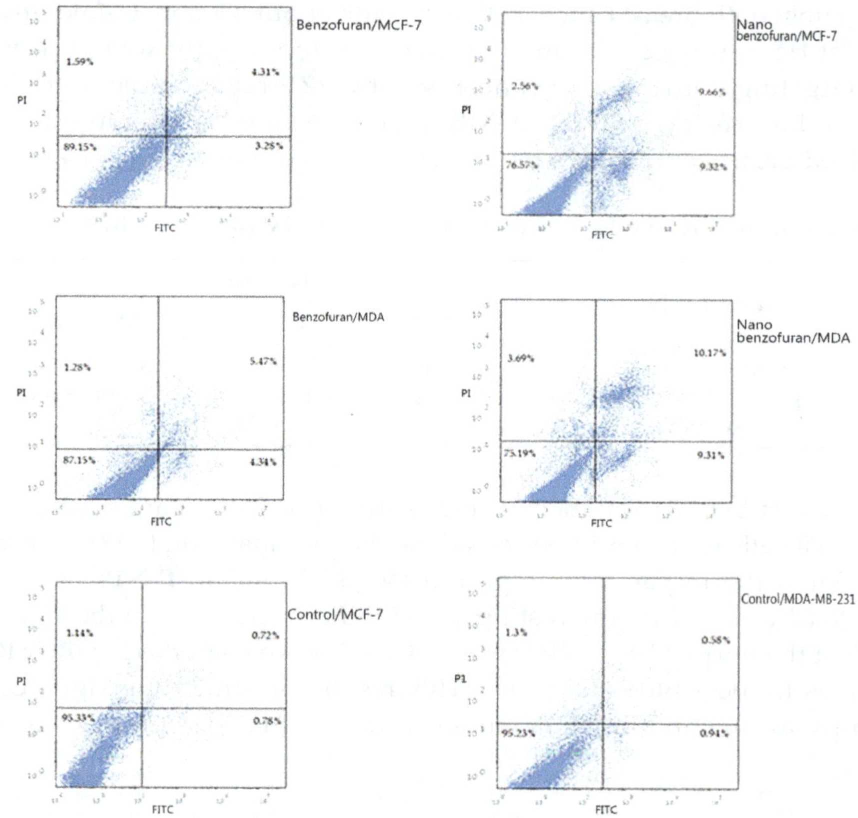

Figure 4. Representative dot plots of MCF-7 and MDA-MB-231 cells treated with compound **IV** (**BZP**) and **BZP-NPs** at their IC_{50} (μM) for 24 h, analyzed by flow cytometry after double staining of the cells with annexin-V FITC and PI.

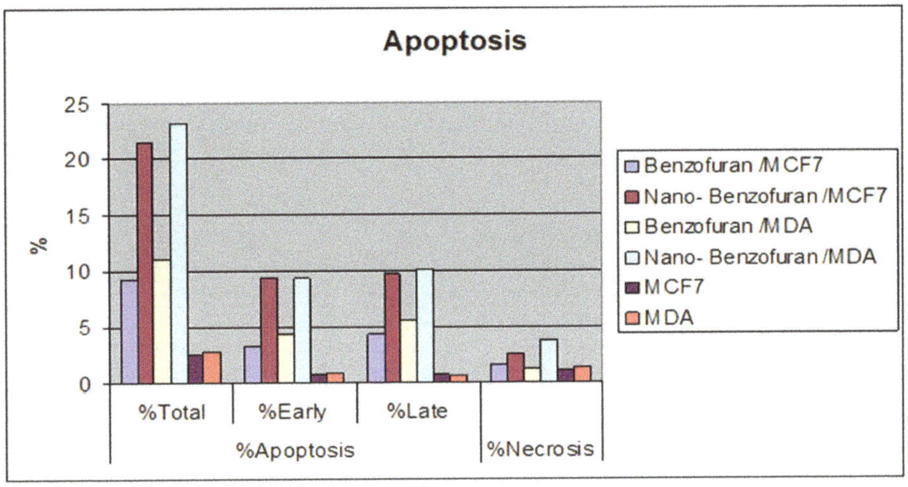

Figure 5. Percentage of compound **IV** (**BZP**) and **BZP-NPs** in MCF-7 and MDA-MB-231 cancer cells.

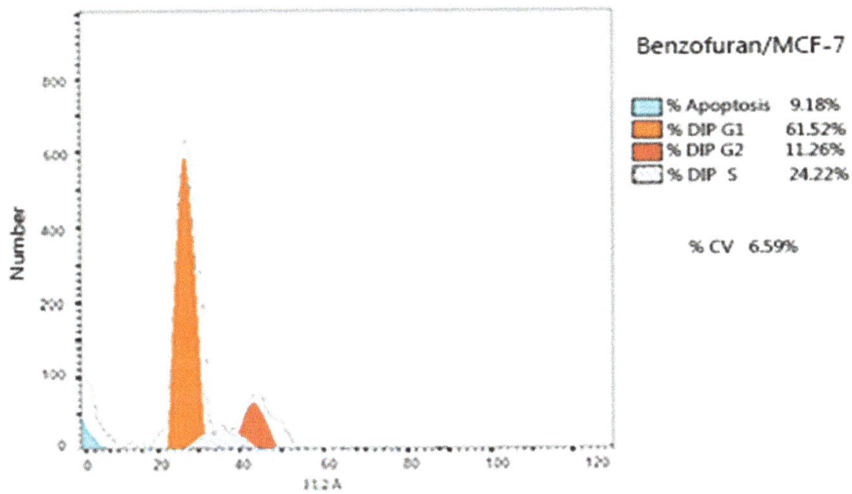

(**A**): The effect of compound **IV** (**BZP**) on MCF-7 cancer cells

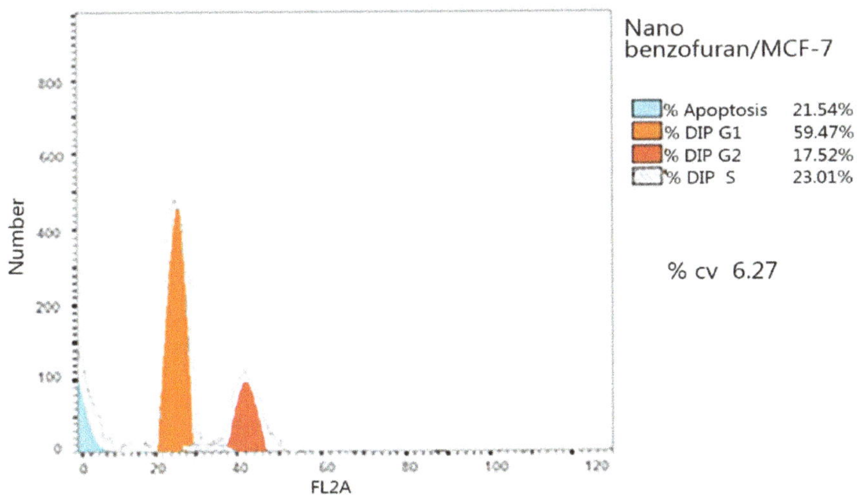

(**B**): The effect of compound **IV** (**BZP-NPs**) on MCF-7 cancer cells

Figure 6. *Cont.*

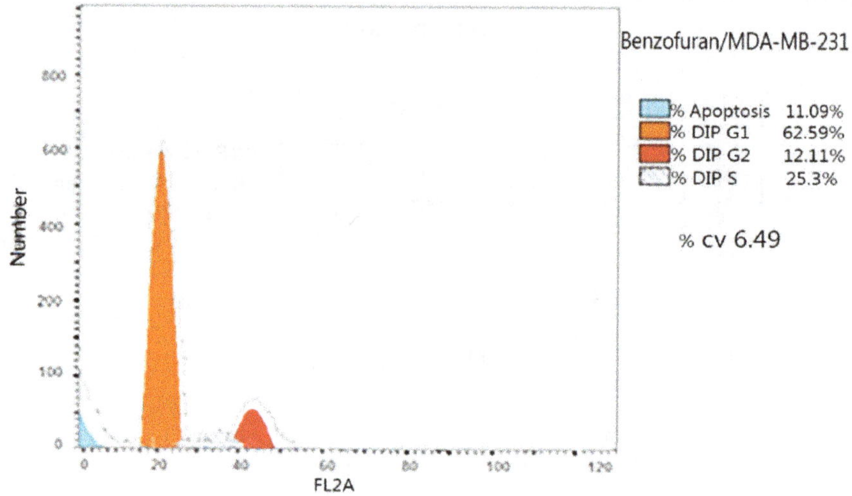

(**C**): The effect of compound **IV** (**BZP**) on MDA-MB-231cancer cells

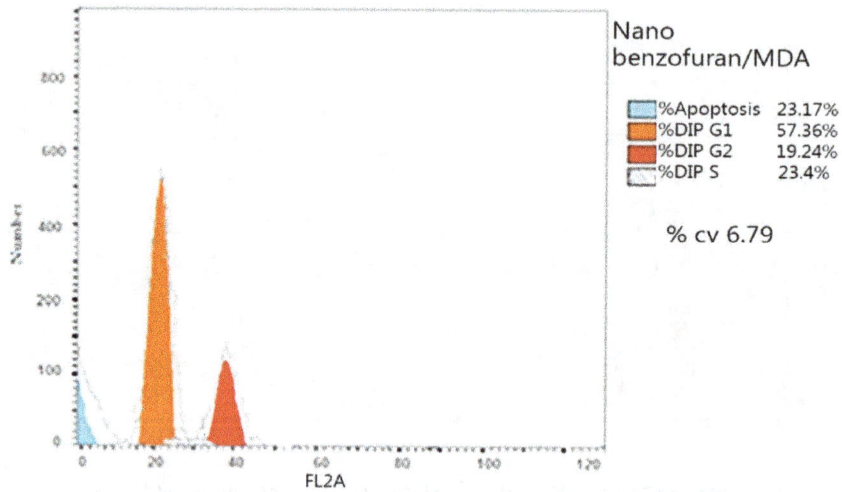

(**D**): The effect of compound **IV** (**BZP-NPs**) on MDA-MB-231cancer cells

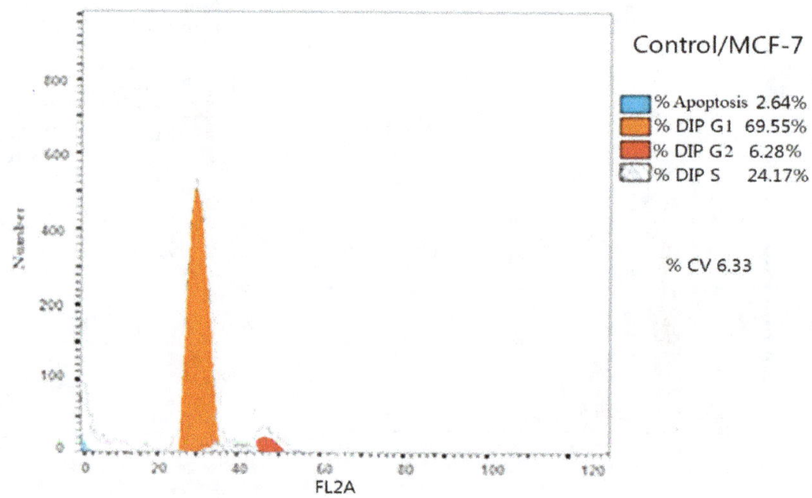

(**E**): The negative control of MCF-7 cancer cells

Figure 6. *Cont.*

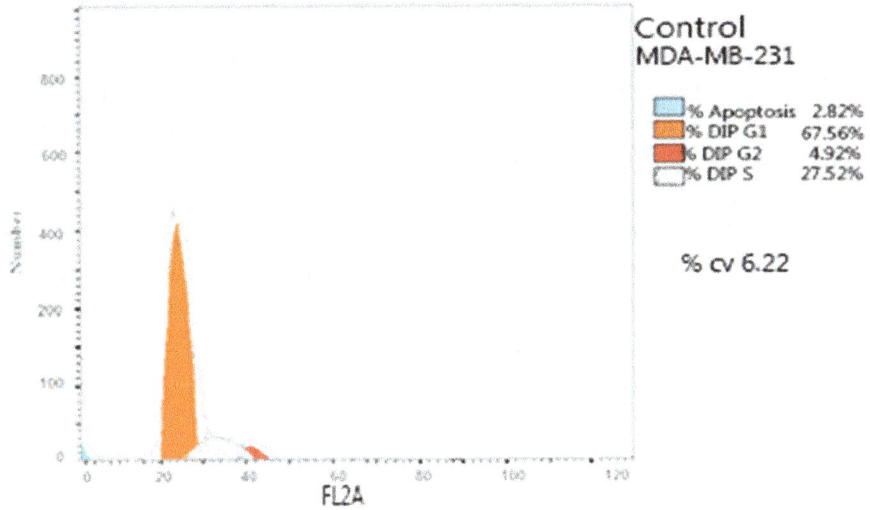

(F): The negative control of MDA-MB-231 cancer cells

Figure 6. Flow cytometric analysis of compound **IV** (**BZP**) and **BZP-NPs** on MCF-7 and MDA-MB-231 cells. The orange color represents G1 phase percentage and red color represents G2/M phase percentage.

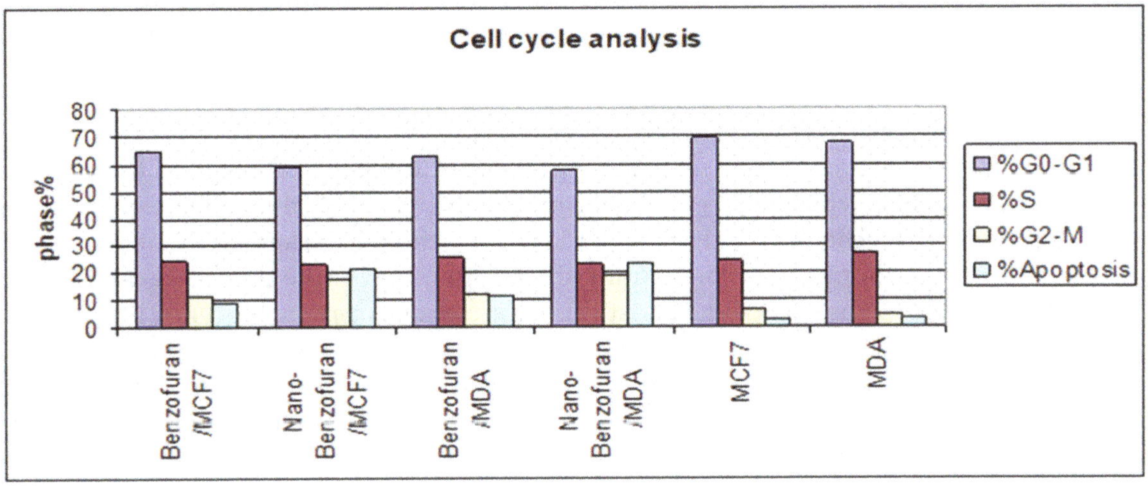

Figure 7. Cycle analysis of compound **IV** (**BZP**) and **BZP-NPs** in MCF-7 and MDA-MB-231 cancer cells.

Table 2. Determination of cell cycle inhibition of MCF-7 and MDA-MB-231 cancer cells by **BZP** and **BZP-NPs**.

Compound Name	Conc. (nM)	%G0-G1	%S	%G2-M	%Pre-G1	Comment
BZP/MCF-7	7	64.52	24.22	11.26	9.18	PreG1apoptosis&Cell growth arrest@ G2/M
BZP-NPs/MCF-7	1	59.47	23.01	17.52	21.54	PreG1apoptosis&Cell growth arrest@ G2/M
BZP/MDA-MB-231	10	62.59	25.3	12.11	11.09	PreG1apoptosis&Cell growth arrest@ G2/M
BZP-NPs/MDA-MB-231	0.6	57.36	23.4	19.24	23.17	PreG1apoptosis&Cell growth arrest@ G2/M
MCF-7		69.55	24.17	6.28	2.64	
MDA-MB-231		67.56	27.52	4.92	2.82	

2.2.3. Effect Compound **IV** (**BZP**) and **BZP-NPs** on the Levels of Caspase-3/p53/Bax/Bcl-2

Caspases are cysteine protease enzymes in humans. Their presence is critical in starting the phase of programmed cell death (apoptosis). Some caspases initiate the intracellular cascade, whereas others (effector caspases) produce their activities downstream by controlling the cellular break via splitting of the structural proteins [19–21]. Caspase-3 displays an important role in the apoptotic process which includes cell shrinkage, chromatin condensation, and DNA fragmentation [22,23]. Enzyme Linked Immuno-Sorbent Assay (ELISA) was used to analyze the apoptotic events of both types of the tested breast cancer cells [16]. Table 3 shows that 24 h treatment of MCF-7 with compound **IV** (**BZP**) and **BZP-NPs** at concentrations of 7 nM and 1 nM and MDA-MB-231 cells at concentrations of 10 nM and 0.6 nM led to significant overexpression of caspase-3 compared to the doxorubicin-treated cells. **BZP** elevated the level of caspase-3 by six and five-fold compared to the untreated cells. A detectable enhancement in the level of caspase-3 occurred upon treatment of the tested cells with **BZP-NPs** by 14 and 17-fold compared to the untreated MCF-7 and MDA-MB-231 cells (Table 3).

Table 3. Determination of caspase-3, p53, Bax, and Bcl-2 levels in the tested cancer cells.

	Results (Fold Change)			
Compound Name	**Caspase-3**	**p53**	**Bax**	**Bcl.2**
BZP/MCF-7	6.383836	7.453852	5.745321	0.272695
BZP-NPs/MCF-7	14.56524	12.51432	9.149760	0.131011
BZP/MDA-MB-231	5.399087	7.792609	7.553853	0.181989
BZP-NPs/MDA-MB-231	17.915	14.60536	13.19230	0.134738
MCF-7	1	1	1	1
MDA-MB-231	1	1	1	1

The tumor suppressor protein p53 serves as a transcription factor. It induces the expression of several downstream targets which are very important in regulation of the cell cycle, apoptosis, and DNA repair, among other mechanisms [24,25]. Cellular stress leads to the activation of the p53 pathway, compromising tumor development and preventing the proliferation of the damaged cells of oncogenic potential. p53 is considered as one of the most relevant tumor suppressor genes [26]. In addition, the B-cell lymphoma protein 2 (Bcl-2) plays a key role in tumor progression via inhibition of the intrinsic apoptotic pathway triggered by mitochondrial dysfunction. Cancer cells can resist apoptosis by modulating the expression of Bcl-2 family proteins which in turn regulate the mitochondrial apoptotic pathway via production Bcl-2 or downregulating pro-apoptotic proteins, such as Bax [26]. Accordingly, in this study, the impact **of IV** (**BZP**) and **BZP-NPs** was assessed on the intrinsic apoptotic pathway via measuring the levels of p53, Bax, and Bcl-2 after treatment of MCF-7 and MDA-MB-231 cells with **BZP** and **BZP-NPs** at their IC_{50} concentrations for 24 h. In comparison to the untreated control, p53 level increased seven-fold in both types of the tested cancer cells upon **BZP** treatment, while the level was doubled to 14-fold by the **BZP-NPs**. On the other hand, **BZP** and **BZP-NPs** elevated the level of the proapoptotic protein Bax by 5.7–13.1-fold with concurrent reduction in the expression levels of the antiapoptotic protein Bcl-2 by four to seven-fold in both tested cancer cell lines in comparison with the untreated control (Table 3).

2.2.4. PARP-1 Cleavage Assay

Breast cancer is among the targets of a new class of drugs known as Poly (ADP-ribose) polymerase-1 (PARP-1) inhibitors. PARP-1 is a nuclear enzyme plays a role in the repair of single-stranded DNA (ss DNA) breaks [26]. The rationale for the therapeutic benefit for the pharmacological inhibition of PARP-1 in breast cancer comes from the following points: (a) sensitization of tumor cells to anticancer therapies such as radiation and cytotoxic agents [27]; (b) certain polymorphisms in PARP-1 can lead to breast cancer and negatively affect the efficacy of the hormone therapies; and (c) breast tumors with deficiencies in DNA-repair genes such as BRCA-1 or BRCA-2 represent acute sensitivity in response to the inhibition of PARP-1. Interestingly, clinical evidence investigates that the usage of PARP-1-inhibiting candidates are not limited to BRCA-1 or BRCA-2 mutated cancers, but they also target non-BRCA mutated breast and ovarian cancers and produce a valuable impact in combination therapy [28,29]. Thus, it was of interest to study the inhibitory effects of **BZP** and **BZP-NPs** against PARP-1 enzyme in MCF-7 and MDA-MB-231 cancer cells using staurosporine as a standard drug. The resulting data were expressed as IC_{50} (nM) values and are summarized in (Table 4). It should be noted that **BZP** produced a slightly weaker inhibitory effect against PARP-than the reference drug, with an IC_{50} of 40 nM vs. 10 nM for staurosporine in MCF-7 cells. A dramatic decrease, about 13-fold, in the sensitivity was noticed in the case of MDA-MB-231 cancer cells against **BZP** which produced an IC_{50} of 60 nM vs. 8 nM for staurosporine. On the other hand, an interesting increase in the inhibitory potency was observed for the **BZP-NPs**, exhibiting an IC_{50} value of 10 nM, which is equal to that obtained by the standard drug in MCF-7 cells. The suppression activity was intensified against PARP-1 in MDA-MB-231 cells, producing an IC_{50} of 6 nM vs. 8 nM for staurosporine.

Table 4. In vitro PARP-1 inhibitory assay of compound **IV (BZP)** and **BZP-NPs**.

Compound Name	IC_{50} (nM)	
	MCF-7	MDA-MB-231
BZP	40 ± 1	60 ±1
BZP-NPs	10 ± 4	6 ± 3
Staurosporine	10 ± 1	8 ± 1

3. Experimental

3.1. *Synthesis of 1-(5-(3-(Benzofuran-2-yl)-1-phenyl-1H-pyrazol-4-yl)-4,5-dihydro-3-(1H-pyrrol-2-yl) pyrazol-1-yl)ethanone* (**IV**).

Compound **IV** was synthesized according to the previously reported procedure [15].

3.2. *Preparation of Nanobenzofuran–Pyrazole* **BZP-NPs**

The nanoparticles were prepared by the nanoprecipitation method [18]. The sizes and morphology of the nanoparticles **BZP-NPs** were examined by transmission electron microscopy (TEM) (H-7600; Hitachi Ltd., Tokyo, Japan). The results exhibited that the nanoparticles were spherical in shape and their average size was 3.8–5.7 nm (Figure 2).

3.3. *Physicochemical Characterization of the Nanobenzofuran–Pyrazole Compound* **BZP-NPs**

3.3.1. Particle Size and Zeta Potential Using Photon Correlation Spectroscopy

Particle size was measured by dynamic light scattering (DLS) using a Zetasizer NANO-ZS (Ver. 7.04, Serial Number: MAL 1074157, Malvern Instruments Ltd., London, United Kingdom) at a wavelength of 633 nm with a 4.0 mW light source for collecting data at a fixed scattering angle of 173°. The electrophoretic mobility (zeta potential) measurements were made using a Zetasizer NANO-ZS (Ver. 7.04, Serial Number: MAL 1074157, Malvern Instruments Ltd., United Kingdom) at 25 °C. **BZP-NPs** morphology was determined using JEOL Transmission Electron Microscope (JEM-1230, Tokyo, Japan) with 500,000 × magnification power, 100 kV acceleration voltage, and 0.5 nm resolving power.

3.3.2. In Vitro Anticancer Activity

In vitro evaluation of the anticancer activity of the **BZP** compound and **BZP-NPs** targeting MCF-7 and MDA-MB-231 cells was performed using MTT assay according to a previously reported method [19]. Each experiment was performed at least three times.

3.4. *Cell Cycle Analysis and Apoptosis Detection*

Cell cycle analysis and apoptosis detection was carried out by flow cytometry (Beckman Coulter, Brea, CA, USA) [19–21]. Apoptosis detection was performed using a FITC Annexin-V/PI commercial kit (Becton Dickenson, Franklin Lakes, NJ, USA) following the manufacturer's protocol.

3.5. *Caspases-3 Assays*

Caspase-3 activity was measured using a Caspase-3 (Active) (human) ELISA kit, Catalog # KHO1091 (96 tests) (Invitrogen Corporation, Carlsbad, CA, USA) according to the manufacturer's instructions [16].

3.6. *In Vitro Determination of p53, Bax, and Bcl-2 Levels*

The levels of p53, Bax, and Bcl-2 markers were assessed using a BIORAD iScript TM One-Step RT-PCR kit with SYBR® Green according to the manufacturer's instructions [26,30].

3.7. *In Vitro PARP-1 Assay*

The procedure was done according to the supplied protocol of ab119690 Cleaved PARP Human ELISA (Enzyme-Linked Immunosorbent Assay) kit for the quantitative measurement of the 89 kDa fragment of Human PARP-1 in cell and tissue lysates [31].

4. Conclusions

This study demonstrates that the conversion of the benzofuran-pyrazole compound **IV** (**BZP**) to nanoparticles **BZP-NPs** greatly intensified its cytotoxic activity against two breast cancer cell lines, MCF-7 and MDA-MB-231, with respective IC_{50} values of 7 nM, 10 nM vs. nanoparticle IC_{50} values of 1 nM, 0.6 nM. The IC_{50} value of DOX was 620 nM. Furthermore, the IC_{50} doses of BZP and BZP-NPs against normal breast cells were >1000-fold greater than those against cancer cells, suggesting acceptable safety profiles in normal cells. The resultant data of cell cycle and apoptosis determination revealed that the tested derivative in both forms induced G2/M phase arrest, accompanied by an increase in apoptosis in the tested cancer cells. Further modes of action of the target compound were also predicted in both types of breast cancer cells. The biological results revealed that **BZP** significantly increased p53, caspase-3, and Bax levels and decreased Bcl-2 levels, and their levels were intensified upon treating the tested cancer cells with (**BZP-NPs**). The PARP1 enzyme assay showed that the efficiency of PARP-1 inhibition by (**BZP**) was slightly less than that of staurosporine, while **BZP-NPs** inhibited the enzyme efficiently as staurosporine in MCF-7 or to a greater extent in case of MDA-MB-231 cancer cells. It has been detected that the nanoparticles were more effective as an anticancer agent against MDA-MB-231 cells than against MCF-7 cancer cells.

Author Contributions: S.S.A.E.-K., M.M.A. performed most of the experiments; A.E.-G.E.A., M.A.A.-O., analyzed the data; A.H.M. the contributed to the anticancer activity assays; All authors read and approved the final manuscript.

Acknowledgments: The authors are grateful to the Deanship of Scientific Research, king Saud University for funding through Vice Deanship of Scientific Research Chairs.

References

1. Giordano, M.C.; Rovitoa, D.; Baroneb, I.; Mancusoc, R.; Bonofigliob, D.; Giordanob, F.; Catalanob, S.; Gabrielec, B.; Andòa, S. Benzofuran-2-acetic ester derivatives induce apoptosis in breastcancer cells by upregulating p21Cip/WAF1gene expression inp53-independent manner. *DNA Repair.* **2017**, *51*, 20–30. [CrossRef] [PubMed]
2. Ferlay, J.; Soerjomataram, I.; Dikshit, R.; Eser, S.; Mathers, C.; Rebelo, M.; Parkin, D.M.; Forman, D.; Bray, F. Cancer incidence and mortality worldwide: sources, methods and majorpatterns in GLOBOCAN. *Int. J. Cancer* **2015**, *136*, 359–386. [CrossRef] [PubMed]
3. Kassab, A.E.; Gedawy, E.M.; El-Nassan, H.B. Synthesis of 4-heteroaryl-quinazoline derivatives as potential anti-breast cancer agents. *J. Heterocycl. Chem.* **2017**, *54*, 624–633. [CrossRef]
4. Amin, K.M.; Syam, Y.M.; Anwar, M.M.; Ali, H.I.; Abdel-Ghani, T.M.; Serry, A.M. Synthesis and molecular docking study of new benzofuran and furo[3,2-*g*]chromone-based cytotoxic agents against breast cancer and p38$^{\alpha}$ MAP kinase inhibitors. *Bioorg. Chem.* **2018**, *76*, 487–500. [CrossRef] [PubMed]
5. Hull, L.C.; Farrell, D.; Grodzinski, P. Highlights of recent developments and trends in cancer nanotechnology research-View from NCI Alliance for Nanotechnology in Cancer. *Biotechnol. Adv.* **2014**, *32*, 666–678. [CrossRef] [PubMed]
6. Zamboni, W.C.; Torchilin, V.; Patri, A.K.; Hrkach, J.; Stern, S.; Lee, R.; Nel, A.; Panaro, N.J.; Grodzinski, P. Best practices in cancer nanotechnology: Perspective from NCI nanotechnology alliance. *Clin. Cancer. Res.* **2012**, *18*, 3229–3241. [CrossRef] [PubMed]
7. Hare, J.I.; Lammers, T.; Ashford, M.B.; Puri, S.; Storm, G.; Barry, S.T. Challenges and strategies in anti-cancer nanomedicine development: An industry perspective. *Adv. Drug Deliv. Rev.* **2017**, *108*, 25–38. [CrossRef] [PubMed]
8. Salata, O.V. Applications of nanoparticles in biology and medicine. *J. Nano Biotechnol.* **2004**, *2*, 1–6.
9. Dyawanapelly, S.; Mehrotra, P.; Ghosh, G.; Jagtap, D.D.; Dandekar, P.; Jain, R. How the surface functionalized nanoparticles affect conformation and activity of proteins: Exploring through protein-nanoparticle interactions. *Bioorg. Chem.* **2019**, *82*, 17–25. [CrossRef]
10. Saraiva, C.; Praça, C.; Ferreira, R.; Santos, T.; Ferreira, L.; Bernardino, L. Nanoparticle-mediated brain drug delivery: Overcoming blood–brain barrier to treat neurodegenerative diseases. *J. Control Release* **2016**, *235*, 34–47. [CrossRef]
11. Popovic, Z.; Liu, W.; Chauhan, V.P.; Lee, J.; Wong, C.; Greytak, A.B.; Insin, N.; Nocera, D.G.; Fukumura, D.; Jain, R.K.; et al. A nanoparticle size series for in vivo fluorescence imaging. *Angew. Chem. Int. Ed. Eng.* **2010**, *49*, 8649–8652. [CrossRef] [PubMed]
12. Cabral, H.; Matsumoto, Y.; Mizuno, K.; Chen, Q.; Murakami, M.; Kimura, M.; Terada, Y.; Kano, M.R.; Miyazono, K.; Uesaka, M.; et al. Accumulation of sub-100 nm polymeric micelles in poorly permeable tumors depends on size. *Nat. Nanotechnol.* **2011**, *6*, 815–823. [CrossRef] [PubMed]
13. Wang, J.; Mao, W.; Lock, L.L.; Tang, J.; Sui, M.; Sun, W.; Cui, H.; Xu, D.; Shen, Y. The role of micelle size in tumor accumulation, penetration, and treatment. *ACS Nano.* **2015**, *9*, 7195–7206. [CrossRef] [PubMed]
14. Thakur, S.; Pramod, K.S.; Malviya, R. Utilization of Polymeric Nanoparticle in Cancer Treatment: A Review. *J. Pharma. Care Health Sys.* **2017**, *4*, 2.
15. Abd El-Karim, S.S.; Anwar, M.M.; Mohamed, N.A.; Nasr, T.; Elseginy, S.A. Design, synthesis, biological evaluation and molecular docking studies of novel benzofuran-pyrazole derivatives as anticancer agents. *Bioorg. Chem.* **2015**, *63*, 1–12. [CrossRef] [PubMed]
16. Amin, K.M.; Syam, Y.M.; Anwar, M.M.; Ali, H.I.; Abdel-Ghani, T.M.; Serry, A.M. Synthesis and molecular docking studies of new furochromone derivatives as p38α MAPK inhibitors targeting human breast cancer MCF-7 cells. *Bioorg. Med. Chem.* **2017**, *25*, 2423–2436. [CrossRef] [PubMed]
17. Abd El-Karim, S.S.; Anwar, M.M.; Zaki, E.R.; Elseginy, S.A.; Nofal, Z.M. Synthesis and molecular modeling of new benzimidazoles as glutathione S-transferase inhibitors and anticancer agents. *Future Med. Chem.* **2018**, *10*, 157–181. [CrossRef]
18. Cherian, A.M.; Snima, K.S.; Kamath, C.R.; Nair, S.V.; Lakshmanan, V.K. Effect of Baliospermummontanumnanomedicine apoptosis induction and anti-migration of prostate cancer cells. *Biomed. Pharm.* **2015**, *71*, 201–209. [CrossRef]

19. Coskun, D.; Erkisa, M.; Ulukaya, E.; Coskun, M.F.; Ari, F. Novel 1-(7-ethoxy-1-benzofuran-2-yl) substituted chalcone derivatives: synthesis, characterization and anticancer activity. *Eur. J. Med. Chem.* **2017**, *136*, 212–222. [CrossRef]
20. Zhang, L.; Ren, W.; Wang, X.; Zhang, J.; Liu, J.; Zhao, L.; Zhang, X. Discovery of novel polycyclic spiro-fused carbocyclicoxindole-based anticancer agents. *Eur. J. Med. Chem.* **2017**, *126*, 1071–1082. [CrossRef]
21. Labib, M.B.; Philoppes, J.N.; Lamie, P.F.; Ahmed, E.R. Azole-hydrazone derivatives: Design, synthesis, in vitro biological evaluation, dual EGFR/HER2 inhibitory activity, cell cycle analysis and molecular docking study as anticancer agents. *Bioorg. Chem.* **2018**, *76*, 67–80. [CrossRef] [PubMed]
22. Van Raam, B.J.; Salvesen, G.S. Handbook of Proteolytic Enzymes, 3rd ed.Elsevier Ltd.: Amsterdam, The Netherlands, 2013; pp. 2252–2255.
23. Ghorab, M.M.; Alsaid, M.S.; Samir, N.; Abdel-Latif, G.A.; Soliman, A.M.; Ragab, F.A.; Abou El Ella, D.A. Aromatase inhibitors and apoptotic inducers: Design, synthesis, anticancer activity and molecular modeling studies of novel phenothiazine derivatives carrying sulfonamide moiety as hybrid molecules. *Eur. J. Med. Chem.* **2017**, *134*, 304–315. [CrossRef] [PubMed]
24. Taguchi, T.; Kato, Y.; Baba, Y.; Nishimura, G.; Tanigaki, Y.; Horiuchi, C.; Mochimatsu, I.; Tsukuda, M. Protein levels of p21, p27, cyclin E and Bax predict sensitivity to cisplatin and paclitaxel in head and neck squamous cell carcinomas. *Oncol. Rep.* **2004**, *11*, 421–426. [CrossRef] [PubMed]
25. Fridman, J.S.; Lowe, S.W. Control of apoptosis by p53. *Oncogene* **2003**, *22*, 9030–9040. [CrossRef] [PubMed]
26. Brandao, P.; Loureiro, J.B.; Carvalho, S.; Hamadou, M.H.; Cravo, S.; Moreira, J.; Pereira, D.; Palmeira, A.; Pinto, M.; Saraiva, L.; et al. Targeting the MDM2-p53 protein-protein interaction with prenylchalcones: Synthesis of a small library and evaluation of potential antitumor activity. *Eur. J. Med. Chem.* **2018**, *156*, 711–721. [CrossRef] [PubMed]
27. Griguolo, G.; Vittoria Dieci, M.; Guarneri, V.; Conte, P.F. Olaparib for the treatment of breast cancer. *Expert Rev. Anticancer Ther.* **2018**, *18*, 519–530. [CrossRef] [PubMed]
28. Amin, K.M.; Anwar, M.M.; Syam, Y.M.; Khedr, M.; Kamel, M.M.; Kassem, E.M.M. A novel class of substituted spiro[quinazoline-2,1′-cyclohexane] derivatives as effective PARP-1 inhibitors: Molecular modeling, synthesis, cytotoxic and enzyme assay evaluation. *Acta Poloni. Pharm. Drug Res.* **2013**, *70*, 687–708.
29. Livraghi, L.J.; Garber, E. PARP inhibitors in the management of breast cancer: Current data and future prospects. *BMC Med.* **2015**, *13*, 188–203. [CrossRef]
30. Abdelhaleem, E.F.; Abdelhameid, M.K.; Kassab, A.E.; Kandeel, M.M. Design and synthesis of thienopyrimidine urea derivatives with potential cytotoxic and proapoptotic activity against breast cancer cell line MCF-7. *Eur. J. Med. Chem.* **2018**, *143*, 1807–1825. [CrossRef]
31. Jagtap, P.G.; Southan, G.J.; Baloglu, E.; Ram, S.; Mabley, J.G.; Marton, A.; Salzman, A.; Szabó, C. The Discovery and Synthesis of Novel Adenosine Substituted 2,3-Dihydro-1H-isoindol-1-ones: Potent Inhibitors of Poly(ADP-ribose) Polymerase-1 (PARP-1). *Bioorg. Med. Chem. Lett.* **2004**, *14*, 81–85. [CrossRef]

13

Synthesis and Antiproliferative Screening of Novel Analogs of Regioselectively Demethylated Colchicine and Thiocolchicine

Dominika Czerwonka [1], Szymon Sobczak [2], Ewa Maj [3], Joanna Wietrzyk [3], Andrzej Katrusiak [2] and Adam Huczyński [1,*]

1 Department of Medical Chemistry, Faculty of Chemistry, Adam Mickiewicz University, Uniwersytetu Poznańskiego 8, 61-614 Poznan, Poland; dominika.czerwonka@amu.edu.pl
2 Department of Materials Chemistry, Faculty of Chemistry Adam Mickiewicz University, Uniwersytetu Poznańskiego 8, 61-614 Poznań, Poland; szymon.sobczak@amu.edu.pl (S.S.); katran@amu.edu.pl (A.K.)
3 Hirszfeld Institute of Immunology and Experimental Therapy, Polish Academy of Sciences, Rudolfa Weigla 12, 53-114 Wrocław, Poland; ewa.maj@hirszfeld.pl (E.M.); joanna.wietrzyk@hirszfeld.pl (J.W.)
* Correspondence: adhucz@amu.edu.pl;

Academic Editor: Qiao-Hong Chen

Abstract: Colchicine, a pseudoalkaloid isolated from *Colchicum autumnale*, has been identified as a potent anticancer agent because of its strong antimitotic activity. It was shown that colchicine modifications by regioselective demethylation affected its biological properties. For demethylated colchicine analogs, 10-demethylcolchicine (colchiceine, **1**) and 1-demethylthiocolchicine (**3**), a series of 12 colchicine derivatives including 5 novel esters (**2b–c** and **4b–d**) and 4 carbonates (**2e–f** and **4e–f**) were synthesized. The antiproliferative activity assay, together with in silico evaluation of physicochemical properties, confirmed attractive biological profiles for all obtained compounds. The substitutions of H-donor and H-acceptor sites at C1 in thiocolchicine position provide an efficient control of the hydration affinity and solubility, as demonstrated for anhydrate **3**, hemihydrate **4e** and monohydrate **4a**.

Keywords: colchicine analogs; thiocolchicine; colchiceine; antimitotic agents; antiproliferative activity; hydrates

---

1. Introduction

Colchicine (Figure 1) is a pseudoalkaloid produced by *Colchicum autumnale* [1]. Its beneficial applications have been known for centuries, as colchicine was used by ancient Greeks and Egyptians to treat swelling and inflammation [2]. Presently, colchicine is considered as the first-line therapy for gout, pericarditis and familial Mediterranean fever [1,3–5]. The most interesting property of colchicine is its high affinity for binding to the tubulin in cancer cells, leading to the inhibition of microtubule polymerization and mitosis arrest [6–8]. These unique properties have attracted great interest to colchicine as an anticancer-drug candidate, however its use is limited by its toxicity towards normal cells [9–11]. For this reason, new derivatives obtained through chemical modifications guided by structure–activity relations are intensively investigated. This research is aimed at reducing the colchicine toxicity and preserving the antimitotic and anticancer properties [12–24]. As it turns out, tubulin interacts with trimethoxyphenyl ring A and tropolone ring C, making the methoxy groups at C1, C2 and C10, as well as the C9-keto group, crucial for colchicine's antimitotic activity [25–27].

Unfortunately, colchicine is also prone to isomerization, resulting in isocolchicine (Figure 1) with 500 times lower affinity for binding to tubulin than colchicine itself [28].

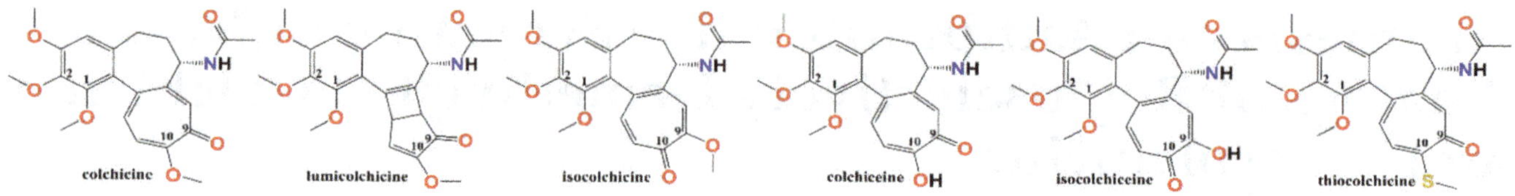

Figure 1. Structures of colchicine, lumicolchicine, isocolchicine, colchiceine, isocolchiceine and thiocolchicine.

Colchiceine (Figure 1) is a C10 demethylated colchicine analog characterized by much lower toxicity [29,30]. It is, next to lumicolchicine (Figure 1), the main product of colchicine degradation and can naturally occur in plant extracts together with colchicine [31]. Elguero et al. [32] have established that colchiceine (as well as its C10-acylated analog) can occur in two tautomeric forms, from which the isoform is slightly more dominant. This equilibrium between colchiceine and isocolchiceine (Figure 1) exists also in the solid state, which has been confirmed by X-ray diffraction studies [33]. The tendency of colchiceine towards tautomerization, in combination with the loss of the C10-methoxy group, may be responsible for its poor antimitotic activity. In contrast, colchiceine shows better bacteriostatic and antifungal activity than colchicine, because its free hydroxyl group may increase its binding affinity towards the cell walls of pathogens [29,33].Interestingly, the replacement of the C10-methoxy group with thiomethyl in a colchicine analog thiocolchicine (Figure 1) decreases its isomerization. Thiocolchicine is more stable, exhibits lower toxicity and has a higher binding affinity to tubulin [34–36]. As could be expected, demethylation of thiocolchicine at C1/C2/C3 positions leads to a lower binding ability to tubulin and lower toxicity [37–39]. As the removal of the methoxy groups from colchicine's structure reduces its toxicity but also lowers its binding affinity to tubulin, we decided to replace these groups with a bigger substituent, such as an ester or carbonate moiety, to investigate an effect of this modification on biological activity [40].

For this reason, we carried out a series of regioselective demethylation reactions of colchicine and thiocolchicine, in order to to obtain colchiceine (**1**) and 1-demethylthiocolchicine (**3**). On the basis of **1** and **3**, we synthesized a series of 12 mono- and double-modified colchicine analogs. Within these analogs, we present 5 novel esters (**2b–c** and **4b–d**) and 4 novel carbonates (**2e–f** and **4e–f**). The pathways used for these syntheses are depicted in Scheme 1.

We also evaluated the antiproliferative activity of these derivatives using three human cancer cell lines, human lung adenocarcinoma (A549), human breast adenocarcinoma (MCF-7) and human colon adenocarcinoma cell line (LoVo), and one normal murine embryonic fibroblast cell line (BALB/3T3). Moreover, on the basis of the in silico calculations, we were able to predict the physicochemical properties of the obtained compounds and check their compliance with Lipiński's rule of 5, permitting evaluation of its drug-likeness.

2. Results and Discussion

2.1. Chemistry

A series of colchicine esters and carbonates substituted at C1 and C10 positions in colchicine were synthesized by performing regioselective demethylation reactions of C1 and C10 methoxy groups, respectively. At first, we performed regioselective demethylation of the colchicine C10 methoxy group by treating colchicine with a mixture of glacial acetic acid and 0.1N hydrochloric acid (i). Reaction resulted in precipitation of yellow solid [41], which was further recrystallized in acetone, leading to growth of good quality, large single crystals. Performed X-ray diffraction analysis proved them to be a colchiceine (**1**, Scheme 1) hemihydrate of the same structure as that reported by Mackay et al. [33], in which the unit-cell accommodates two tautomeric forms: colchiceine and isocolchiceine.

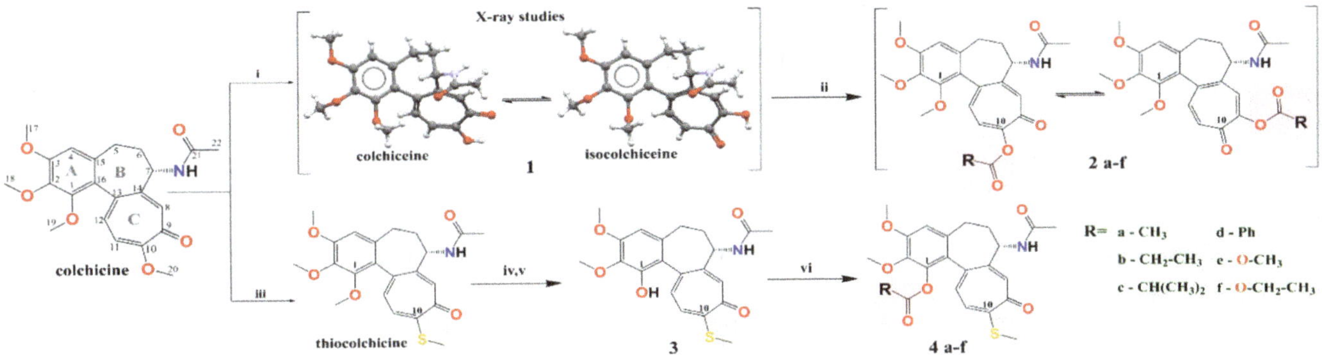

Scheme 1. Synthesis of novel colchicine analogs. The obtained crystal structure of **1** was identical to the one proposed by Mackey et al. [33]. Reagents and conditions: (i) glacial acetic acid, hydrochloric acid, 100 °C, 6h; (iii) MeOH/H_2O, CH_3SNa, RT, 24h; (iv) DCM, acetyl chloride, $SnCl_4$, 0 °C → RT, 48h; (v) MeOH/H_2O, LiOH, RT, 1h; (ii,vi) DCM, Et_3N, respective acyl chloride/chloroformate, 0 °C → RT, 24h.

Colchicine was also treated with sodium methanethiolate (**iii**) to obtain thiocolchicine [42]. By using a slightly modified method proposed by Bladé-Font [43] (**iv,v**), thiocolchicine was regioselectively demethylated at the C1 methoxy group, leading to 1-demethylthiocolchicine (**3**) with 40% yield. This regioselective demethylation was confirmed by X-ray analysis (Figure 2). Finally, compounds **1** and **3** were treated with respective acyl chlorides or chloroformates (**ii, vi**) to give single modified derivatives **2a–f** and double modified derivatives **4a–f** with 38%–58% yields (Scheme 1).

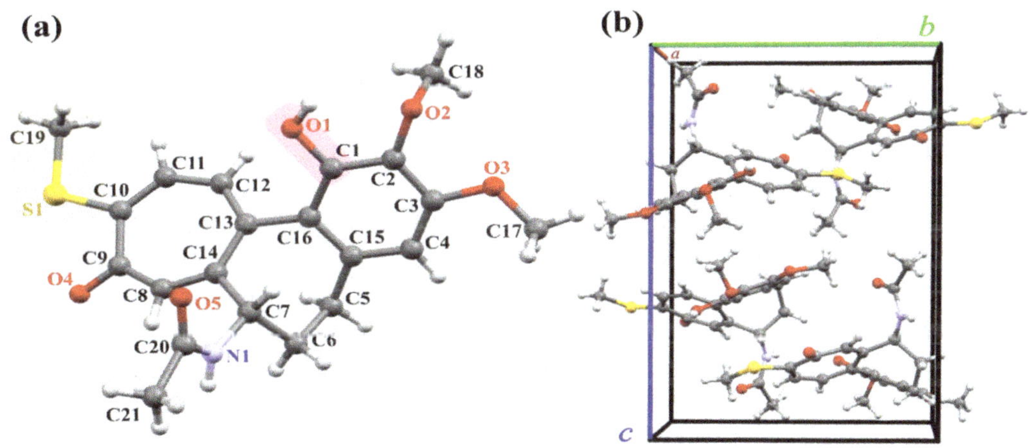

Figure 2. (**a**) Molecule of 1-demethylthiocolchicine (**3**) and (**b**) its crystal structure projected along the crystal direction [100].

The purity and structure of synthesized colchicine derivatives **1**, **2a–f**, **3** and **4a–f** were determined on the basis of ESI-MS, NMR and X-ray analysis. The specific data can be found in Section 3 and in Supplementary Materials. The disappearance of the signal at about 56.5 ppm in the ^{13}C NMR spectrum of colchicine, assigned to the C10 methoxy group, is the evidence of the formation of colchiceine (**1**). Moreover, in the spectra of derivatives **2a–2f**, an additional signal from the carbonyl group can be observed in the range 164.1–174.3 ppm for esters **2a–2d**, and 151.9–152.5 ppm for carbonates **2e–f**. A shift of the signal corresponding to the C10 methoxy group from 56.5 to 15.1 ppm is evidence for the introduction of the thiomethyl group at position C10, and the absence of one of the signals around 61 ppm assigned to the C1 methoxy group is evidence of 1-demethylthiocolchicine (**3**) formation. An additional signal corresponding to the carbonyl carbon atom can be observed in the range 168.3–174.7 ppm for esters **4a–4d** and in the range 152.8–152.9 ppm for carbonates **4e–f**.

2.2. *In Silico Calculations of the Physicochemical Properties*

We used the Molinspiration online database (http://www.molinspiration.com, free of charge) to predict the physicochemical properties of all synthesized compounds and collected them in Table 1 [44].

Table 1. Physicochemical properties of the synthesized compounds based on the Molinspiration database [44].

Compound	MW	clog*P*	tPSA	n(O,N)	N(OH,NH)	Rotb	MV
1	385.42	0.83	94.10	7	2	4	346.63
2a	427.45	0.60	100.18	8	1	6	383.14
2b	441.48	1.27	100.18	8	1	7	399.94
2c	455.51	1.51	100.18	8	1	7	416.53
2d	489.52	2.92	100.18	8	1	7	437.99
2e	443.45	0.95	109.41	9	1	7	392.12
2f	457.48	1.33	109.41	9	1	8	408.93
3	401.48	1.89	84.86	6	2	4	355.77
4a	443.52	1.66	90.94	7	1	6	392.28
4b	457.55	2.33	90.94	7	1	7	409.08
4c	471.57	2.57	90.94	7	1	7	425.67
4d	505.59	3.98	90.94	7	1	7	447.13
4e	459.52	2.02	100.18	8	1	7	401.27
4f	473.55	2.39	100.18	8	1	8	418.07
colchicine	399.44	1.10	83.11	7	1	5	364.15

MW: Molecular weight; clog*P*: calculated log octanol/water partition coefficient; tPSA: total polar surface area; n(O,N): number of hydrogen acceptors; n(OH,NH): number of hydrogen donors; Rotb: rotatable bonds; MV: molecular volume.

According to Lipinski's rule of 5, most "drug-like" molecules should have log$P \leq 5$, molecular weight ≤ 500, number of hydrogen bond acceptors ≤ 10 and number of hydrogen bond donors ≤ 5. Additionally, it was demonstrated that a total polar surface area (tPSA) < 140 and number of rotatable bonds < 10, in combination with log$P < 5$, are crucial for both good bioavailability and permeability through biological membranes [45].

The demethylation of the C1 and C10 position of colchicine, both in **1** and **3**, increases the number of H-donor sites while the substitution of colchicine's C10 methoxy group with thiomethyl results in a decreased number of H-acceptor sites in **3**. Additionally, the demethylation of the C1 and C10 position of colchicine reduces the number of rotatable bonds. Substitution of a hydroxyl group, both in **1** and **3**, with an ester or carbonate substituent, increases the number of H-acceptor sites and reduces the number of H-donor sites to that of colchicine. According to the performed calculations, all synthesized compounds **2a–e** and **4a–e** have a rather lipophilic character, with the clog*P* values between 0.60 and 3.98. Conducted syntheses allowed us to obtain compounds with less lipophilic character than that of colchicine for compounds **1**, **2a** and **2e**, with clog*P* values 0.83, 060 and 0.95, respectively. Interestingly, esters and carbonates in the C10 position (**2a–e**) are in general less lipophilic than corresponding esters and carbonates in the C1 position (**4a–e**). Except for **4d**, whose molecular weight is above 500, the calculations for all colchicine analogs are in agreement with Lipinski's descriptors. Importantly, in order to be active, a drug should not have more than one violation [46]. This, in combination with the number of rotatable bonds between 4 and 8, as well as tPSA between 84.86 and 100.18, confirm good physicochemical profiles of all obtained compounds.

2.3. *X-ray Analysis*

The structures of compounds **3**, **4a** and **4e** were additionally confirmed by X-ray diffraction. Selected crystallographic data are collected in Table 2, and more detailed information can be found in Supplementary Information. The single crystals of **3**, **4a**, **4e** were obtained by slow evaporation from an ethyl acetate mixture. The 1-Demethylthiocolchicine (**3**) crystallizes in the orthorhombic space group $P2_12_12_1$ (Figure 2) while the crystals of **4a** and **4e** are monoclinic, space group $P2_1$. The substitution at the C1 atom with acetyl ester (**4a**) and methyl carbonate (**4e**), and the following change in the ratio between H-bond acceptors and donors, increases the tendency of these colchicine derivatives to co-crystallize with water; hence, monohydrate **4a**·H_2O and hemihydrate **4e**·½H_2O were obtained.

Molecules **4a** and **4e** significantly differ in conformation (Figure 3).The arrangement of the C2 methoxy group, which can be described by the C1-C2-O2-C18 torsion angle, changed from −122.36° to 108.75° in **4a** and **4e**, respectively. Together with increasing mass of the C1 moiety, the twist between the planar phenyl and tropolone rings around the C13-C16 bond increases, altering the C1-C16-C13-C12 angle from 45.43° in **3**, through 58.54° in **4a**, to 60.11° in **4e**.

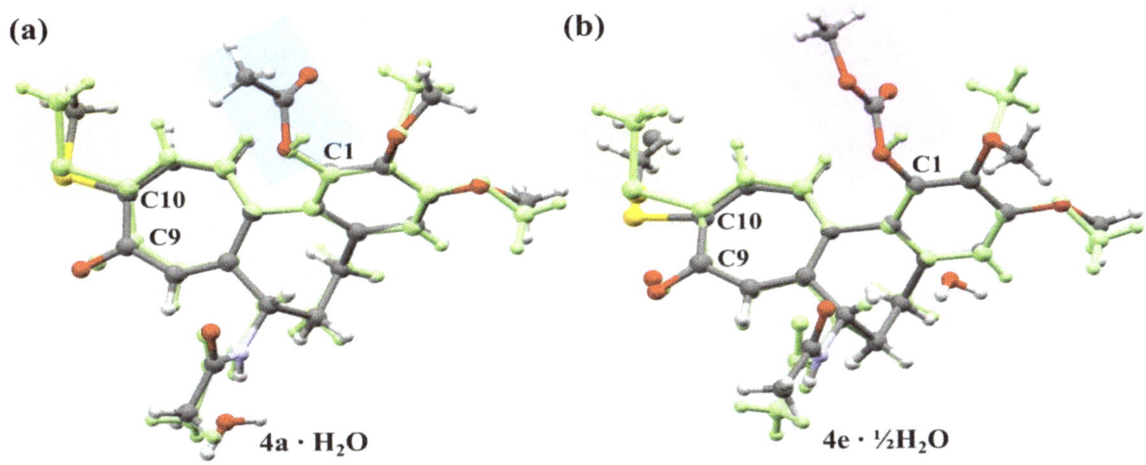

Figure 3. Comparison of the molecular conformation from the X-ray analysis studies between (**a**) molecule **4a** and (**b**) **4e**, superimposed with respect to the benzene ring on the 1-demethylthiocolchicine (molecule 3), highlighted with a light-green color.

Table 2. Selected crystallographic data for compounds **3**, **4a·H_2O** and **4e·½H_2O**.

Label		3	4a·H_2O	4e·1/2H_2O
Formula		$C_{21}H_{22}NO_5S$	$C_{23}H_{25}NO_6S \cdot H_2O$	$C_{23}H_{25}NO_7S \cdot 1/2H_2O$
CCDC number		1966196	1966194	1966195
Crystal system		orthorhombic	monoclinic	monoclinic
Space group		$P2_12_12_1$	$P2_1$	$P2_1$
Unit cell dimensions	a (Å)	9.1005(17)	10.600(2)	10.8835(10)
	b (Å)	11.866(2)	6.9635(11)	9.2158(6)
	c (Å)	17.881(4)	16.712(3)	12.0632(12)
	β (°)	90	107.07(2)	104.613(9)
Volume (Å^3)		1930.8(7)	1179.2(4)	1170.80(18)
Z/Z'		4/1	2/1	2/1
D_x (g/cm^3)		1.378	1.300	1.329

The presence of water significantly alters the pattern of H-bonds between **3** and **4a·H_2O** and **4e·½H_2O**. Although in all structures amide nitrogen participates in the formation of intermolecular contacts, only in **3** are the NH···S, of 2.793(2) Å, and NH···O4, of 2.370(3) Å,bonds formed. In a monohydrate crystal **4a·H_2O**, water interrupts the NH···O4 interaction observed in the crystal structure of **3**, accepting NH amide proton, of 2.086(1) Å and further donating its H-atoms to the HO-H···O4′, of 2.007(3) Å, and HO-H···O5′, of 1.994(3) Å bond. Much weaker H-bonds are present in the crystal structure of **4e·½H_2O**. Despite the presence of a water molecule in the crystal structure of **4e·½H_2O**, the strong NH···O5′ bond, of 2.033(2) Å is present again. The disordered by location at half-occupied sites water molecule is involved in formation of a weak HO-H···O5′′ interaction of 2.538(1) Åand the H-bond at the disordered terminal carbonyl at C9. Due to the HO-H···O4′ of 2.241(1) Å bond, the occupational disorder of H_2O is passed onto the orientation of **4e** molecules as illustrated in Figure 3.

Depending on the presence or absence of this water molecule, its adjacent molecule **4e** is slightly shifted in the crystal structure. This disorder is most apparent for the terminal carbonyl at C9 (dislocated by 0.358 Å) and thiomethyl at C10 (dislocated by 0.625 Å).

2.4. Antiproliferative Activity

The antiproliferative activity of all synthesized colchicine analogs **1**, **2a–f**, **3**, **4a–f** was *tested in vitro* against three human cancer cell lines: human lung adenocarcinoma (A549), human breast adenocarcinoma (MCF-7) and human colon adenocarcinoma cell line (LoVo). For a more accurate evaluation of cytotoxic activity, the effect on normal murine embryonic fibroblast cell line (BALB/3T3) was also tested according to the previously published procedure [12]. Detailed information concerning antiproliferation assay can be found in Supplementary Materials. The mean values of IC_{50} ± SD of the tested compounds are collected in Table 3.

Table 3. Antiproliferative activity (IC_{50}) of 10-demethylcolchicine (colchiceine, **1**), 1-demethylthiocolchicine (**3**) and their derivatives(**2a–f**, **4a–f**) compared to the antiproliferative activity of colchicine and standard anticancer drugs doxorubicin and cisplatin and the calculated values of selectivity index (SI).

Compound	A549	SI	MCF-7	SI	LoVo	SI	BALB/3T3
	IC_{50} (μM)		IC_{50} (μM)		IC_{50} (μM)		IC_{50} (μM)
1	12.99 ± 1.79	0.79	11.23 ± 2.52	0.91	6.00 ± 1.88	1.71	10.25 ± 0.96
2a	12.47 ± 2.77	0.68	10.03 ± 2.18	0.85	6.18 ± 1.48	1.37	8.50 ± 0.50
2b	9.97 ± 0.70	0.75	7.56 ± 2.84	0.99	2.39 ± 1.20	3.13	7.47 ± 0.50
2c	20.39 ± 11.30	0.41	11.95 ± 1.54	0.70	6.47 ± 0.35	1.30	8.42 ± 1.14
2d	8.75 ± 0.33	1.02	8.21 ± 3.35	1.09	4.87 ± 2.17	1.83	8.92 ± 3.93
2e	0.98 ± 0.16	0.84	0.98 ± 0.33	0.84	0.48 ± 0.32	1.70	0.82 ± 0.11
2f	9.67 ± 0.84	0.86	9.07 ± 1.90	0.92	6.41 ± 1.57	1.30	8.36 ± 0.17
3	0.82 ± 0.02	0.74	0.12 ± 0.05	4.92	0.11 ± 0.03	5.38	0.61 ± 0.14
4a	0.48 ± 0.15	1.36	0.10 ± 0.02	6.85	0.11 ± 0.02	5.92	0.65 ± 0.12
4b	0.97 ± 0.04	0.77	0.96 ± 0.13	0.78	0.50 ± 0.19	1.53	0.75 ± 0.10
4c	0.89 ± 0.07	0.80	0.86 ± 0.10	0.83	0.56 ± 0.06	1.27	0.71 ± 0.03
4d	0.60 ± 0.31	0.75	0.78 ± 0.22	0.58	0.10 ± 0.08	4.71	0.45 ± 0.23
4e	0.90 ± 0.09	0.87	1.02 ± 0.10	0.77	0.43 ± 0.19	1.84	0.78 ± 0.06
4f	0.96 ± 0.13	1.08	0.95 ± 0.20	1.09	0.79 ± 0.16	1.31	1.03 ± 0.20
colchicine	0.07 ± 0.01	0.63	0.01 ± 0.01	4.30	0.01 ± 0.01	5.38	0.04 ± 0.01
cisplatin	3.60 ± 0.25	0.81	3.05 ± 0.67	0.95	3.80 ± 0.28	0.77	2.91 ± 1.83
doxorubicin	0.16 ± 0.03	0.25	0.15 ± 0.05	0.26	0.08 ± 0.03	0.49	0.04 ± 0.03

The IC_{50} value is defined as the concentration of a compound at which 50% growth inhibition is observed. Human lung adenocarcinoma (A549), human breast adenocarcinoma (MCF-7), human colon adenocarcinoma cell line (LoVo) and normal murine embryonic fibroblast cell line (BALB/3T3). The SI (Selectivity Index) was calculated for each compound, using the formula SI = IC_{50} for normal cell line BALB/3T3/IC_{50} for the respective cancerous cell line. A beneficial SI > 1.0 indicates a drug with efficacy against tumor cells greater than the toxicity against normal cells.

All colchicine analogs showed stronger antiproliferative activity against all tested cancer cell lines than the conventional chemotherapeutic, cisplatin. In general, the IC_{50} values are better for colchicines doubly modified at C1 and C10 positions (**3**, **4a–f**) than for the analogs singly modified at position C10 only (**1**, **2a–f**). Compound **4a**, with a thiomethyl group at position C10 and an acetyl ester substituent at C1, showed the highest activity against all tested cell lines (IC_{50} = 0.48 ± 0.15, 0.10 ± 0.02, 0.11 ± 0.02 μM for A549, MCF-7, LoVo cancer cell lines, respectively).

All tested colchicine analogs exhibit higher SI values than doxorubicin, which indicates the therapeutic potential of the synthesized compounds. Compound **3**, 1-demethylthiocolchicine, as well as its acylated analog **4a**, showed high SI values against MCF-7 (SI = 4.92, SI = 6.88) as well as LoVo cell lines (SI = 5.36, SI = 5.95). From among analogs modified exclusively at position C10, compound **2b** with propionyl ester substituent revealed a higher SI value towards LoVo cell line (SI = 3.13).

3. Materials and Methods

3.1. General

Information concerning reagents and solvents, as well as equipment used for measurements, can be found in the Supplementary Materials.

3.1.1. Synthesis and Characterization of 10-Demethylcolchicine (colchiceine, 1), Thiocolchicine and 1-Demethylthiocolchicine (3)

Information concerning the synthesis of 10-demethylcolchicine (colchiceine, **1**), thiocolchicine and 1-demethylthiocolchicine (**3**) can be found in Supplementary Materials.

3.1.2. General Route for Synthesis of Compounds 2a–f and 4a–f

To a solution of **1** or **3** (100 mg, 0.25 mmol) in dichloromethane (DCM, 10 mL) cooled to 0 °C, Et_3N (1 mL, 7 mmol) and respective acyl chloride or chloroformate were added (excess). The mixture was first stirred at 0 °C for 30 min and then for the next 24h at RT. Reaction time was determined by TLC. After that time the solution was filtered to remove triethylamine hydrochloride, the DCM was evaporated under reduced pressure and the residue was purified by CombiFlash® (chloroform/acetone, increasing concentration gradient) to give respective compounds as amorphous yellow solids.

3.1.3. Characterization of Acetyl Ester of Colchiceine 2a

Amorphous yellow solid, yield 49%, m.p 120–122 °C; ^{1}H NMR ($CDCl_3$, 400 MHz) δ 7.50 (1H, s), 7.31 (1H, d, *J* = 11.3 Hz), 7.22 (1H, d, *J* = 11.3 Hz), 6.53 (1H, s), 4.60 (1H, dt, *J* = 12.7, 6.5 Hz), 3.91 (3H, s), 3.88 (3H, s), 3.66 (3H, s, 2.50 (1H, dd, J = 13.6, 6.3 Hz), 2.35 (3H, s), 2.26–2.17 (1H, m), 1.96 (3H, s), 1.87 (1H, td, *J* = 12.1, 6.9 Hz). ^{13}C NMR ($CDCl_3$, 101 MHz) δ 169.9, 168.2, 153.9, 151.0, 148.6, 141.8, 141.5, 137.0, 134.5, 131.2, 130.3, 125.2, 107.4, 61.6, 61.3, 56.0, 52.1, 36.8, 29.7, 22.7, 20.7. ESI-MS (m/z): $[M + H]^+$ 428, $[M + Na]^+$ 450, $[M + K]^+$ 466, $[2M + Na]^+$ 877.

3.1.4. Characterization of Propionyl Ester of Colchiceine 2b

Amorphous yellow solid, yield 52%, m.p 133-135 °C; ^{1}H NMR ($CDCl_3$, 400 MHz) δ 7.50 (1H, s), 7.30 (1H, d, *J* = 11.3 Hz), 7.22 (1H, d, *J* = 11.2 Hz), 6.52 (1H, s), 4.66–4.57 (1H, m), 3.91 (3H, s), 3.88 (3H, s), 3.66 (3H, s), 2.66 (2H, q, *J* = 7.4 Hz), 2.50 (1H, dd, *J* = 13.5, 6.3 Hz), 2.35 (1H, ddd, *J* = 12.7, 10.3, 6.0 Hz), 2.24–2.16 (1H, m), 1.97 (3H, s), 1.87 (2H, td, *J* = 12.0, 6.7 Hz), 1.26 (3H, t, *J* = 7.6 Hz). ^{13}C NMR ($CDCl_3$, 101 MHz) δ 171.8, 169.9, 153.9, 151.1, 148.9, 141.7, 141.6, 136.7, 134.5, 130.9, 130.5, 125.2, 107.4, 61.7, 61.4, 56.1, 52.1, 36.9, 29.8, 27.4, 22.8, 9.0. ESI-MS (m/z): $[M + Na]^+$ 464, $[2M + Na]^+$ 905.

3.1.5. Characterization of Isobutyryl Ester of Colchiceine 2c

Yellowish brown oil, yield 55%; ^{1}H NMR ($CDCl_3$, 400 MHz) δ 7.56 (1H, s), 7.28 (1H, d, *J* = 11.0 Hz), 7.23 (1H, d, *J* = 10.6 Hz), 6.52 (1H, s), 4.64 (1H, dt, *J* = 12.2, 6.8 Hz), 3.91 (3H, s), 3.88 (3H, s), 3.65 (3H, s), 2.90–2.82 (1H, m), 2.54–2.47 (1H, m), 2.36 (1H, td, *J* = 13.2, 6.9 Hz), 2.24–2.12 (2H, m), 1.96 (3H, s), 1.92–1.85 (1H, m), 1.35 (3H, d, *J* = 1.4 Hz), 1.33 (3H, d, *J* = 1.3 Hz). ^{13}C NMR ($CDCl_3$, 101 MHz) δ 174.3, 170.0, 153.9, 151.1, 150.3, 142.1, 141.5, 136.0, 134.5, 131.6, 130.1, 125.2, 107.4, 61.7, 61.3, 56.0, 52.1, 36.6, 34.0, 29.8, 26.4, 22.7, 19.0. ESI-MS (m/z): $[M + Na]^+$ 478, $[2M + Na]^+$ 933.

3.1.6. Characterization of Benzyl Ester of Colchiceine 2d

Amorphous yellow solid, yield 41%, m.p 123–125 °C; ^{1}H NMR ($CDCl_3$, 400 MHz) δ 8.18 (2H, d, *J* = 7.4 Hz), 7.65–7.60 (2H, m), 7.49 (1H, ddd, *J* = 4.8, 3.1, 1.1 Hz), 7.34 (2H, s), 6.53 (1H, s), 4.66–4.58 (1H, m), 3.93 (3H, d, *J* = 0.9 Hz,), 3.90 (3H, d, *J* = 0.7 Hz), 3.68 (3H, d, *J* = 1.1 Hz), 2.49 (1H, dd, *J* = 13.4, 4.9 Hz), 2.42–2.32 (1H, m), 2.17–2.06 (1H, m), 1.86 (3H, d, *J* = 4.0 Hz), 1.84–1.78 (1H, m). ^{13}C NMR

($CDCl_3$, 101 MHz) δ 169.9, 164.1, 153.9, 151.1, 142.0, 141.6, 134.5, 133.8, 130.4, 128.9, 128.5, 125.3, 107.4, 61.7, 61.4, 56.1, 52.0, 36.9, 29.8, 22.7. ESI-MS (m/z): $[M + H]^+$ 490, $[M + Na]^+$ 512, $[M + K]^+$ 528.

3.1.7. Characterization of Methyl Carbonate of Colchiceine 2e

Amorphous yellowish brown solid, yield 58%, m.p 115–118 °C; ^{1}H NMR ($CDCl_3$, 400 MHz) δ 7.57 (1H, s), 7.32 (1H, d, *J* = 20.5 Hz), 6.54 (1H, s), 4.62 (1H, dt, *J* = 11.8, 6.0 Hz), 3.92 (3H, s)*, 3.92 (3H, s)*, 3.89 (3H, s), 3.68 (3H, s), 2.52 (1H, dd, *J* = 13.4, 6.1 Hz), 2.37 (1H, td, *J* = 13.0, 6.7 Hz), 2.29–2.18 (1H, m), 1.99 (3H, s), 1.91 (1H, dd, *J* = 19.0, 12.2 Hz). ^{13}C NMR ($CDCl_3$, 101 MHz) δ 169.9, 154.1, 152.5, 151.1, 141.6, 134.5, 125.1, 107.4, 61.7, 61.3, 56.1, 55.8, 52.2, 37.2, 29.8, 22.8. ESI-MS (m/z): $[M + H]^+$ 444, $[M + Na]^+$ 466, $[M + K]^+$ 482, $[2M + Na]^+$ 909.

3.1.8. Characterization of Ethyl Carbonate of Colchiceine 2f

Yellowish brown oil, yield 55%; ^{1}H NMR ($CDCl_3$, 400 MHz) δ 7.46 (1H, s), 7.40–7.32 (1H, m, *J* = 6.2 Hz), 7.30–7.21 (1H, m), 6.55 (1H, s), 4.62 (1H, dt, *J* = 12.6, 6.4 Hz), 4.36 (2H, q, *J* = 7.1 Hz), 3.93 (3H, s, *J* = 2.9 Hz), 3.90 (3H, s), 3.68 (3H, s), 2.54 (1H, dd, *J* = 13.6, 6.4 Hz), 2.41 (1H, td, *J* = 13.1, 7.1 Hz), 2.32–2.21 (1H, m), 2.01 (3H, s), 1.94–1.84 (1H, m), 1.41 (3H, t, *J* = 7.1 Hz). ^{13}C NMR ($CDCl_3$, 101 MHz) δ 169.9, 154.0, 151.9, 151.1, 141.6, 134.5, 125.1, 107.4, 65.4, 61.7, 61.3, 56.1, 52.1, 37.2, 29.8, 22.8, 14.1. ESI-MS (*m/z*): $[M + H]^+$ 458, $[M + Na]^+$ 480, $[M + K]^+$ 496, $[2M + Na]^+$ 937.

3.1.9. Characterization of Acetyl Ester of 1-demethylthiocolchicine 4a

Amorphous yellow solid, yield 45%, m.p 168-172 °C; ^{1}H NMR (DMSO-d_6, 400 MHz) δ 8.51 (1H, d, *J* = 7.7 Hz), 7.23 (1H, d, *J* = 10.8 Hz), 7.02 (1H, s), 6.97 (1H, s), 6.92 (1H, d, *J* = 10.3 Hz), 3.89 (3H, s), 3.74 (3H, s), 2.65 (1H, dd, *J* = 13.5, 6.0 Hz), 2.41 (3H, s), 2.32–2.24 (1H, m), 2.22 (3H, s), 2.12–2.01 (1H, m), 1.85 (3H, s, *J* = 6.3 Hz), 1.84–1.77 (1H, m, *J* = 12.1, 6.8 Hz). ^{13}C NMR (DMSO-d_6, 101 MHz) δ 181.2, 168.9, 168.2, 157.7, 152.8, 150.4, 140.8, 139.3, 136.4, 134.4, 132.7, 128.2, 126.4, 124.6, 109.9, 60.1, 56.0, 50.7, 36.2, 29.1, 22.5, 20.3, 14. ESI-MS (m/z): $[M + Na]^+$ 466, $[2M + Na]^+$ 909.

3.1.10. Characterization of Propionyl Ester of 1-demethylthiocolchicine 4b

Amorphous yellow solid, yield 47%, m.p 136-140 °C; ^{1}H NMR (DMSO-d_6, 400 MHz) δ 8.52 (1H, d, *J* = 7.7 Hz), 7.23 (1H, d, *J* = 10.7 Hz), 7.03 (1H, s), 6.98 (1H, s), 6.92 (1H, d, *J* = 10.2 Hz), 4.34 (1H, dt, *J* = 11.8, 7.1 Hz), 3.90 (3H, s), 3.76–3.71 (3H, m), 2.66 (1H, dd, *J* = 13.2, 6.4 Hz), 2.41 (3H, s), 2.33–2.19 (2H, m), 2.08 (2H, ddd, *J* = 11.4, 9.8, 5.4 Hz), 1.84–1.78 (1H, m), 1.11 (3H, t, *J* = 7.5 Hz). ^{13}C NMR (DMSO-d_6, 101 MHz) δ 181.2, 172.3, 168.3, 157.7, 152.8, 150.5, 140.9, 139.2, 136.4, 134.4, 132.9, 128.3, 126.4, 124.7, 109.9, 60.1, 56.0, 50.7, 36.2, 29.1, 26.7, 22.6, 14.5, 9.2. ESI-MS (m/z): $[M + H]^+$ 458, $[M + Na]^+$ 480, $[M + K]^+$ 496, $[2M + Na]^+$ 937.

3.1.11. Characterization of Isobutyryl Ester of 1-demethylthiocolchicine 4c

Amorphous yellow solid, yield 49%, m.p 165-167 °C; ^{1}H NMR (DMSO-d_6, 101 MHz) δ 8.50 (1H, d, *J* = 7.8 Hz), 7.22 (1H, d, *J* = 10.6 Hz), 7.03 (1H, s), 6.98 (1H, s), 6.91 (1H, d, *J* = 8.8 Hz), 4.35 (1H, dt, *J* = 11.7, 7.3 Hz), 3.90 (3H, s), 3.72 (3H, s), 2.74 (1H, dt, *J* = 13.9, 6.9 Hz), 2.66 (1H, dd, *J* = 13.6, 6.1 Hz), 2.39 (3H, s), 2.34–2.25 (1H, m), 2.09 (1H, td, *J* = 12.7, 5.9 Hz), 1.86 (3H, s), 1.81 (1H, dd, *J* = 12.0, 6.9 Hz, 1.16 (3H, d, *J* = 3.5 Hz), 1.14 (3H, d, *J* = 3.5 Hz). ^{13}C NMR (DMSO-d_6, 101 MHz) δ 181.2, 174.7, 168.3, 157.7, 152.7, 150.4, 140.8, 139.2, 136.4, 134.4, 132.9, 128.3, 126.3, 124.8, 109.9, 60.1, 56.1, 50.7, 36.2, 33.3, 29.1, 22.6, 18.8, 14.6. ESI-MS (m/z): $[M + Na]^+$ 494, $[2M + Na]^+$ 965.

3.1.12. Characterization of Benzyl Ester of 1-demethylthiocolchicine 4d

Amorphous yellow solid, yield 38%, m.p 166-170 °C; ^{1}H NMR (DMSO-d_6, 101 MHz) δ 8.52 (1H, s), 8.07 (2H, d, *J* = 7.3 Hz), 7.77–7.71 (1H, m), 7.63–7.56 (2H, m), 7.22–7.12 (1H, m), 7.06 (1H, s), 7.02 (1H, s), 4.49–4.40 (1H, m), 3.94 (3H, s), 3.74 (3H, s), 2.72 (1H, dd, *J* = 13.0, 5.9 Hz), 2.36 (1H, dd, *J* = 7.4,

5.5 Hz,), 2.31 (3H, s), 2.13 (2H, ddd, J = 19.4, 12.8, 6.9 Hz,), 1.87 (3H, s).^{13}C NMR (DMSO-d$_6$, 101 MHz) δ 181.1, 168.3, 157.7, 152.9, 150.6, 141.0, 139.4, 136.3, 134.6, 134.2, 129.8, 129.1, 128.4, 128.3, 126.2, 124.9, 110.2, 60.3, 56.1, 50.8, 36.3, 29.2, 22.6, 14.5. ESI-MS (m/z): [M + Na]$^+$ 528, [2M + Na]$^+$ 1033.

3.1.13. Characterization of Methyl Carbonate of 1-demethylthiocolchicine 4e

Amorphous yellow solid, yield 53%, m.p 158-162 °C; ^{1}H NMR (DMSO-d$_6$, 101 MHz) δ 8.55 (1H d, J = 7.6 Hz), 7.26 (1H, d, J = 10.6 Hz), 7.05–6.99 (3H, m), 4.34 (1H, dt, J = 11.8, 7.0 Hz), 3.91 (3H, s), 3.82 (3H, s), 3.79 (3H, s), 2.69 (1H, dd, J = 13.5, 6.2 Hz), 2.43 (3H, s), 2.29 (1H, ddd, J = 18.6, 12.3, 5.4 Hz), 2.09 (1H, ddd, J = 18.7, 12.5, 6.2 Hz), 1.88 (3H, s), 1.86–1.80 (1H, m). ^{13}C NMR (DMSO-d$_6$, 101 MHz) δ 181.2, 168.4, 157.9, 152.9, 152.8, 150.5, 140.8, 139.3, 136.0, 134.5, 133.2, 128.2, 126.4, 124.3, 110.2, 60.4, 56.14, 56.07, 50.8, 36.1, 29.1, 22.6, 14.4. ESI-MS (m/z): [M + H]$^+$ 460, [M + Na]$^+$ 482, [M + K]$^+$ 498, [2M + Na]$^+$ 941.

3.1.14. Characterization of Ethyl Carbonate of 1-demethylthiocolchicine 4f

Amorphous yellow solid, yield 48%, m.p 165-167 °C; ^{1}H NMR (DMSO-d$_6$, 400 MHz) δ 8.52 (1H, d, J = 7.6 Hz), 7.23 (1H, d, J = 10.7 Hz), 7.01 (3H, t, J = 10.3 Hz), 4.33 (1H, dt, J = 12.6, 7.5 Hz), 4.27–4.20 (2H, m), 3.90 (3H, s), 3.78 (3H, s), 2.67 (1H, dd, J = 13.2, 6.6 Hz), 2.41 (3H, s), 2.34–2.23 (1H, m), 2.08 (3H, s), 1.87 (3H, s), 1.85–1.78 (1H, m), 1.22 (3H, t, J = 7.1 Hz). ^{13}C NMR (DMSO-d$_6$, 101 MHz) δ 181.2, 168.4, 157.9, 152.8, 152.4, 150.5, 140.8, 139.3, 136.2, 134.5, 133.1, 128.2, 126.3, 124.4, 110.2, 65.1, 60.3, 56.1, 50.8, 36.1, 29.1, 22.6, 14.4, 14.0. ESI-MS (m/z): [M + Na]$^+$ 496, [M + K]$^+$ 512, [2M + Na]$^+$ 969.

3.2. Antiproliferative Activity

Detailed information concerning antiproliferative activity assay is given in Supplementary Materials.

3.3. X-ray Measurements

X-ray measurements and detailed crystallographic data are given in Supplementary Materials.

4. Conclusions

On the basis of regioselectively demethylated colchicine analogs, colchiceine (**1**) and 1-demethylthiocolchicine (**3**), we have designed and synthesized a series of **12** colchicine derivatives bearing ester and carbonate substituents, including **9** entirely novel derivatives (**2b,c,e,f** and **4b,c,d,e,f**). Derivatives **4a·H_2O** and **4e·½H_2O**, with acetyl ester and methyl carbonate moieties, display reduced hydrophilic properties and crystallize as hydrates, which affects their biological activity and increases their solubility. The control over water co-crystallization from monohydrate to hemihydrate has been achieved through the number of H-donor and acceptor sites. These features can be invaluable for the regulation of the bioaccessibility and pharmaceutical processing of this group of compounds [47]. The synthesized derivatives exhibit a considerable in vitro antiproliferative activity against three human cancer cell lines. Compound 4a, carrying the thiomethyl group at position C10 and acetyl ester substituent at C1, showed the highest activity and selectivity index values. The biological evaluation has been supported by prediction of physicochemical properties, which are consistent with Lipinski's rule of five for all synthesized analogs.

Author Contributions: Conceptualization, D.C. and A.H.; methodology, D.C., A.H., S.S. and E.M. validation, A.H., A.K. and J.W.; investigation, D.C, S.S. and E.M. resources, A.H., A.K. and J.W. data curation, D.C., S.S and E.M writing—original draft preparation, D.C. and S.S writing—review and editing, A.H., A.K. and J.W. visualization, D.C.; supervision, A.H.; project administration, A.H.; funding acquisition, A.H. All authors have read and agreed to the published version of the manuscript.

Acknowledgments: D.C. and S.S. acknowledge a scholarship (No. POWR. 03.02.00-00-I026/16 and POWR. 03.02.00-00-I023/17, respectively) co-financed by the European Union through the European Social Fund under the Operational Program Knowledge Education Development.

References

1. Slobodnick, A.; Shah, B.; Pillinger, M.H.; Krasnokutsky, S. Colchicine: Old and New. *Am. J. Med.* **2015**, *128*, 461–470. [CrossRef] [PubMed]
2. Graham, W.; Roberts, J.B. Intravenous colchicine in the management of gouty arthritis. *Ann. Rheum. Dis.* **1953**, *12*, 16–19. [CrossRef] [PubMed]
3. Khanna, D.; Fitzgerald, J.D.; Khanna, P.P.; Bae, S.; Singh, M.K.; Neogi, T.; Pillinger, M.H.; Merill, J.; Lee, S.; Prakash, S.; et al. American college of rheumatology guidelines for management of gout. Part 1: Systematic nonpharmacologic and pharmacologic therapeutic approaches to hyperuricemia. *Arthritis Care Res.* **2012**, *64*, 1431–1446. [CrossRef]
4. Grattagliano, I.; Bonfrate, L.; Ruggiero, V.; Scaccianoce, G.; Palasciano, G.; Portincasa, P. Novel therapeutics for the treatment of familial mediterranean fever: From colchicine to biologics. *Clin. Pharmacol. Ther.* **2014**, *95*, 89–97. [CrossRef]
5. Imazio, M.; Gaita, F.; LeWinter, M. Evaluation and treatment of pericarditis: A systematic review. *J. Am. Med. Assoc.* **2015**, *314*, 1498–1506. [CrossRef]
6. Vindya, N.G.; Sharma, M.; Yadav, M.; Ethiraj, K.R. Tubulins—The Target for Anticancer Therapy. *Curr. Top. Med. Chem.* **2015**, *15*, 73–82. [CrossRef]
7. Seligmann, J.; Twelves, C. Tubulin: An example of targeted chemotherapy. *Future Med. Chem.* **2013**, *5*, 339–352. [CrossRef]
8. Katsetos, C.D.; Draber, P. Tubulins as Therapeutic Targets in Cancer: From Bench to Bedside. *Curr. Pharm. Des.* **2012**, *18*, 2778–2792. [CrossRef]
9. Cocco, G.; Chu, D.C.C.; Pandolfi, S. Colchicine in clinical medicine. A guide for internists. *Eur. J. Intern. Med.* **2010**, *21*, 503–508. [CrossRef]
10. Yang, L.P.H. Oral Colchicine (Colcrys): In the treatment and prophylaxis of gout. *Drugs* **2010**, *70*, 1603–1613. [CrossRef]
11. Avendaño, C.; Menéndez, J.C. *Medicinal Chemistry of Anticancer Drugs*; Elsevier: Amsterdam, The Netherlands, 2008. [CrossRef]
12. Majcher, U.; Klejborowska, G.; Kaik, M.; Maj, E.; Wietrzyk, J.; Moshari, M.; Preto, J.; Tuszynski, J.; Huczyński, A. Synthesis and Biological Evaluation of Novel Triple-Modified Colchicine Derivatives as Potent Tubulin-Targeting Anticancer Agents. *Cells* **2018**, *7*, 216. [CrossRef] [PubMed]
13. Klejborowska, G.; Urbaniak, A.; Preto, J.; Maj, E.; Moshari, M.; Wietrzyk, J.; Tuszynski, J.; Chambers, T.C.; Huczyński, A. Synthesis, biological evaluation and molecular docking studies of new amides of 4-bromothiocolchicine as anticancer agents. *Bioorg. Med. Chem.* **2019**, *23*, 115–144. [CrossRef] [PubMed]
14. Nakagawa-Goto, K.; Chen, C.X.; Hamel, E.; Wu, C.C.; Bastow, K.F.; Brossi, A.; Lee, K.H. Antitumor agents. Part 236: Synthesis of water-soluble colchicine derivatives. *Bioorg. Med. Chem. Lett.* **2015**, *15*, 235–238. [CrossRef]
15. Shchegravina, E.S.; Maleev, A.A.; Ignatov, S.K.; Gracheva, I.A.; Stein, A.; Schmalz, H.G.; Gavryushin, A.E.; Zubareva, A.A.; Svirshchevskaya, E.V.; Fedorov, A.Y. Synthesis and biological evaluation of novel non-racemic indole-containing allocolchicinoids. *Eur. J. Med. Chem.* **2017**, *141*, 51–60. [CrossRef]
16. Yasobu, N.; Kitajima, M.; Kogure, N.; Shishido, Y.; Matsuzaki, T.; Nagaoka, M.; Takayama, H. Design, synthesis, and antitumor activity of 4-halocolchicines and their pro-drugs activated by cathepsin B. *ACS Med. Chem. Lett.* **2011**, *2*, 348–352. [CrossRef]
17. Huczyński, A.; Majcher, U.; Maj, E.; Wietrzyk, J.; Janczak, J.; Moshari, M.; Tuszynski, J.A.; Bartl, F. Synthesis, antiproliferative activity and molecular docking of Colchicine derivatives. *Bioorg. Chem.* **2016**, *64*, 103–112. [CrossRef]
18. Zhang, X.; Kong, Y.; Zhang, J.; Su, M.; Zhou, Y.; Zang, Y.; Li, J.; Chen, Y.; Fang, Y.; Zhang, X.; et al. Design, synthesis and biological evaluation of colchicine derivatives as novel tubulin and histone deacetylase dual inhibitors. *Eur. J. Med. Chem.* **2015**, *95*, 127–135. [CrossRef]

19. Nicolaou, K.C.; Valiulin, R.A.; Pokorski, J.K.; Chang, V.; Chen, J.S. Bio-inspired synthesis and biological evaluation of a colchicine-related compound library. *Bioorg. Med. Chem. Lett.* **2012**, *22*, 3776–3780. [CrossRef]
20. Chang, D.J.; Yoon, E.Y.; Lee, G.B.; Kim, S.O.; Kim, W.J.; Kim, Y.M.; Jung, J.W.; An, H.; Suh, Y.G. Design, synthesis and identification of novel colchicine-derived immunosuppressant. *Bioorg. Med. Chem. Lett.* **2009**, *19*, 4416–4420. [CrossRef]
21. Marzo-Mas, A.; Barbier, P.; Breuzard, G.; Allegro, D.; Falomir, E.; Murga, J.; Carda, M.; Peyrot, V.; Marco, J.A. Interactions of long-chain homologues of colchicine with tubulin. *Eur. J. Med. Chem.* **2017**, *126*, 526–535. [CrossRef] [PubMed]
22. Johnson, L.; Goping, I.S.; Rieger, A.; Mane, J.Y.; Huzil, T.; Banerjee, A.; Luduena, R.; Hassani, B.; Winter, P.; Tuszynski, J.A. Novel Colchicine Derivatives and their Anti-cancer Activity. *Curr. Top. Med. Chem.* **2017**, *17*. [CrossRef] [PubMed]
23. Kumar, A.; Sharma, P.R.; Mondhe, D.M. Potential anticancer role of colchicine-based derivatives: An overview. *Anticancer Drugs* **2016**, *28*, 250–262. [CrossRef]
24. Kozaka, T.; Nakagawa-Goto, K.; Shi, Q.; Lai, C.Y.; Hamel, E.; Bastow, K.F.; Brossi, A.; Lee, K.H. Antitumor agents 273. Design and synthesis of N-alkyl-thiocolchicinoids as potential antitumor agents. *Bioorg. Med. Chem. Lett.* **2010**, *20*, 4091–4094. [CrossRef]
25. Andreu, J.M.; Timasheff, S.N. Tubulin bound to colchicine forms polymers different from microtubules. *Proc. Natl. Acad. Sci. USA* **1982**, *79*, 6753–6756. [CrossRef]
26. Cortese, F.; Bhattacharyya, B.; Wolff, J. Podophyllotoxin as a probe for the colchicine binding site of tubulin. *J. Biol. Chem.* **1977**, *252*, 1134–1140.
27. Chen, J.; Liu, T.; Dong, X.; Hu, Y. Recent Development and SAR Analysis of Colchicine Binding Site Inhibitors. *Mini Rev. Med. Chem.* **2009**, *9*, 1174–1190. [CrossRef]
28. Hastie, S.B.; Williams, R.C.; Puett, D.; Macdonald, T.L. The binding of isocolchicine to tubulin. Mechanisms of ligand association with tubulin. *J. Biol. Chem.* **1989**, *264*, 6682–6688.
29. Gohar, M.A.; Makkawi, M. The Antibacterial Action of Colchicine and Colchiceine. *J. Pharm. Pharmacol.* **1951**, *3*, 415–419. [CrossRef]
30. Boyland, E.; Mawson, E.H. The conversion of colchicine into colchiceine. *Biochem. J.* **1938**, *32*, 1204–1206. [CrossRef]
31. Klein, A.E.; Davis, P.J. Determination of Colchicine and Colchiceine in Microbial Cultures by High-Performance Liquid Chromatography. *Anal. Chem.* **1980**, *52*, 2432–2435. [CrossRef]
32. Elguero, J.; Muller, R.N.; Blade-Font, A.; Faure, R.; Vincent, E.J. Carbon-13 Magnetic Resonance Spectroscopy. A Study Of Colchicine And Related Compounds. *Bull. Soc. Chim. Belges* **1980**, *89*, 193–204. [CrossRef]
33. Mackay, M.F.; Morrison, J.D.; Gulbis, J.M. Crystal Structure of Triclinic Colchiceine Hemihydrate. *Aust. J. Phys.* **1985**, *38*, 413. [CrossRef]
34. Kurek, J.; Barczynski, P. Colchiceine complexes with lithium, sodium and potassium salts-spectroscopic studies. *Croat. Chem. Acta* **2016**, *89*, 297–308. [CrossRef]
35. Shi, Q.; Verdier-Pinard, P.; Brossi, A.; Hamel, E.; Lee, K.H. Antitumor Agents-CLXXV. Anti-tubulin action of (+)-thiocolchicine prepared by partial synthesis. *Bioorg. Med. Chem.* **1997**, *5*, 2277–2282. [CrossRef]
36. Prajapati, P.B.; Bodiwala, K.B.; Marolia, B.P.; Bhingradiya, N.; Shah, S. Oxidative Degradation Kinetic Study of Thiocolchicoside using Stability Indicating High Performance Thin Layer Chromatographic Method. *Pharm. Methods* **2014**, *5*, 69–78. [CrossRef]
37. Banerjee, A.; Kasmala, L.T.; Hamel, E.; Sun, L.; Lee, K.H. Interaction of novel thiocolchicine analogs with the tubulin isoforms from bovine brain. *Biochem. Biophys. Res. Commun.* **1999**, *254*, 334–337. [CrossRef]
38. Kerekes, P.; Sharma, P.N.; Brossi, A.; Chignell, C.F.; Quinn, F.R. Synthesis and Biological Effects of Novel Thiocolchicines. 3. Evaluation of N-Acyldeacetylthiocolchicines, N-(Alkoxycarbonyl)deacetylthiocolchicines, and O-Ethyldemethylthiocolchicines. New Synthesis of Thiodemecolcine and Antileukemic Effects of 2-Demeth. *J. Med. Chem.* **1985**, *28*, 1204–1208. [CrossRef]
39. Alkadi, H.; Khubeiz, M.J. Colchicine: A Review About Chemical Structure and Clinical Using. *Infect. Disord. Drug Targets* **2017**, 17. [CrossRef]
40. Shi, Q.; Chen, K.; Morris-Natschke, S.L.; Lee, K.H. Recent progress in the development of tubulin inhibitors as antimitotic antitumor agents. *Curr. Pharm. Des.* **1998**, *4*, 219–248.

41. Dumont, R.; Brossi, A.; Chignell, C.F.; Quinn, F.R.; Suffness, M. A Novel Synthesis of Colchicide and Analogues from Thiocolchicine and Congeners: Reevaluation of Colchicide as a Potential Antitumor Agent. *J. Med. Chem.* **1987**, *30*, 732–735. [CrossRef] [PubMed]
42. Voitovich, Y.V.; Shegravina, E.S.; Sitnikov, N.S.; Faerman, V.I.; Fokin, V.V.; Schmalz, H.G.; Combes, S.; Allegro, D.; Barbier, P.; Beletskaya, I.P.; et al. Synthesis and biological evaluation of furanoallocolchicinoids. *J. Med. Chem.* **2015**, *58*, 692–704. [CrossRef] [PubMed]
43. Blade-Font, A. New chemistry of colchicine and related compounds IV. Selective demethylation of colchicine with Lewis acids and tge structure of Zeisel's dimethylcolchicinic acid. *Afinidad* **1979**, *36*, 329.
44. Molinspiration Property Calculation Service. Available online: http://www.molinspiration.com (accessed on 15 January 2020).
45. Lipinski, C. Lead-and drug-like compounds: The rule-of-five revolution. *Drug Discov. Today Technol.* **2004**, *4*, 337–341. [CrossRef]
46. Lipinski, C.; Lombardo, F.; Dominy, B.W.; Feeney, P.J. Experimental and Computational Approaches to Estimate Solubility and Permeability in Drug Discovery and Development Settings. *Adv. Drug Deliv. Rev.* **1997**, *23*, 3–25. [CrossRef]
47. Khankari, R.K.; Grant, D.J.W. Pharmaceutical hydrates. *Thermochim. Acta* **1995**, *248*, 61–79. [CrossRef]

Permissions

All chapters in this book were first published by MDPI; hereby published with permission under the Creative Commons Attribution License or equivalent. Every chapter published in this book has been scrutinized by our experts. Their significance has been extensively debated. The topics covered herein carry significant findings which will fuel the growth of the discipline. They may even be implemented as practical applications or may be referred to as a beginning point for another development.

The contributors of this book come from diverse backgrounds, making this book a truly international effort. This book will bring forth new frontiers with its revolutionizing research information and detailed analysis of the nascent developments around the world.

We would like to thank all the contributing authors for lending their expertise to make the book truly unique. They have played a crucial role in the development of this book. Without their invaluable contributions this book wouldn't have been possible. They have made vital efforts to compile up to date information on the varied aspects of this subject to make this book a valuable addition to the collection of many professionals and students.

This book was conceptualized with the vision of imparting up-to-date information and advanced data in this field. To ensure the same, a matchless editorial board was set up. Every individual on the board went through rigorous rounds of assessment to prove their worth. After which they invested a large part of their time researching and compiling the most relevant data for our readers.

The editorial board has been involved in producing this book since its inception. They have spent rigorous hours researching and exploring the diverse topics which have resulted in the successful publishing of this book. They have passed on their knowledge of decades through this book. To expedite this challenging task, the publisher supported the team at every step. A small team of assistant editors was also appointed to further simplify the editing procedure and attain best results for the readers.

Apart from the editorial board, the designing team has also invested a significant amount of their time in understanding the subject and creating the most relevant covers. They scrutinized every image to scout for the most suitable representation of the subject and create an appropriate cover for the book.

The publishing team has been an ardent support to the editorial, designing and production team. Their endless efforts to recruit the best for this project, has resulted in the accomplishment of this book. They are a veteran in the field of academics and their pool of knowledge is as vast as their experience in printing. Their expertise and guidance has proved useful at every step. Their uncompromising quality standards have made this book an exceptional effort. Their encouragement from time to time has been an inspiration for everyone.

The publisher and the editorial board hope that this book will prove to be a valuable piece of knowledge for researchers, students, practitioners and scholars across the globe.

List of Contributors

Aline de Cristo Soares Alves and Silvia Stanisçuaski Guterres
Programa de Pós-Graduação em Ciências Farmacêuticas, Universidade Federal do Rio Grande do Sul, Porto Alegre 90610-000, Brazil

Fabio Sonvico
Food and Drug Department, University of Parma, Parco Area delle Scienze 27/a, 43124 Parma, Italy

Franciele Aline Bruinsmann
Programa de Pós-Graduação em Ciências Farmacêuticas, Universidade Federal do Rio Grande do Sul, Porto Alegre 90610-000, Brazil
Food and Drug Department, University of Parma, Parco Area delle Scienze 27/a, 43124 Parma, Italy

Gustavo Richter Vaz
Food and Drug Department, University of Parma, Parco Area delle Scienze 27/a, 43124 Parma, Italy
Laboratório de Nanotecnologia Aplicada à Saúde, Programa de Pós-Graduação em Ciências da Saúde, Universidade Federal do Rio Grande, Rio Grande, RS 96210-900, Brazil

Tanira Aguirre
Programa de Pós-Graduação em Biociências, Universidade Federal de Ciências da Saúde de Porto Alegre, Porto Alegre, RS 900500-170, Brazil

Adriana Raffin Pohlmann
Programa de Pós-Graduação em Ciências Farmacêuticas, Universidade Federal do Rio Grande do Sul, Porto Alegre 90610-000, Brazil
Departamento de Química Orgânica, Instituto de Química, Universidade Federal do Rio Grande do Sul, Porto Alegre 91501-970, Brazil

Sophie Hoenke, Immo Serbian and René Csuk
Organic Chemistry, Martin-Luther University Halle-Wittenberg, Kurt-Mothes Street 2, D-06120 Halle, Germany

Hans-Peter Deigner
Medical and Life Science Faculty, Institute of Precision Medicine, Furtwangen University, Jakob-Kienzle-Street 17, D-78054 Villigen-Schwenningen, Germany

Ya-Ping Gong, Long-Qian Tang, Tong-Shen Liu and Zhao-Peng Liu
Department of Medicinal Chemistry, Key Laboratory of Chemical Biology (Ministry of Education), School of Pharmaceutical Sciences, Shandong University, Jinan 250012, China

Olga Wesołowska, Krystyna Michalak, Maria Błaszczyk and Kamila Środa-Pomianek
Department of Biophysics and Neuroscience,Wroclaw Medical University, 50-367 Wroclaw, Poland

Joseph Molnár
Institute of Medical Microbiology and Immunobiology, University of Szeged, 6720 Szeged, Hungary

Danielly C. Ferraz da Costa and Ronimara A. Santos
Departamento de Nutrição Básica e Experimental, Instituto de Nutrição, Universidade do Estado do Rio de Janeiro, Rio de Janeiro 20550-013, Brazil

Luciana Pereira Rangel
Faculdade de Farmácia, Universidade Federal do Rio de Janeiro, Rio de Janeiro 21941-902, Brazil

Julia Quarti and Eliane Fialho
Departamento de Nutrição Básica e Experimental, Instituto de Nutrição Josué de Castro, Universidade Federal do Rio de Janeiro, Rio de Janeiro 21941-902, Brazil

Jerson L. Silva
Programa de Biologia Estrutural, Instituto de Bioquímica Médica Leopoldo de Meis, Instituto Nacional de Ciência e Tecnologia de Biologia Estrutural e Bioimagem, Universidade Federal do Rio de Janeiro, Rio de Janeiro 21941-902, Brazil

Zafer Asım Kaplancıklı
Department of Pharmaceutical Chemistry, Faculty of Pharmacy, Anadolu University, Eskisehir 26470, Turkey

Ulviye Acar Çevik, Begüm Nurpelin Sağlık, Derya Osmaniye, Serkan Levent and Yusuf Özkay
Department of Pharmaceutical Chemistry, Faculty of Pharmacy, Anadolu University, Eskisehir 26470, Turkey
Doping and Narcotic Compounds Analysis Laboratory, Faculty of Pharmacy, Anadolu University, Eskisehir 26470, Turkey

Betül Kaya Çavuşoğlu
Department of Pharmaceutical Chemistry, Faculty of Pharmacy, Bülent Ecevit University, Zonguldak 67100, Turkey

Sinem Ilgın
Department of Pharmaceutical Toxicology, Faculty of Pharmacy, Anadolu University, Eskisehir 26470, Turkey

Amy M. Buckley, Margaret R. Dunne, Susan A. Kennedy, Maria B. Davern, Stephen G. Maher and Jacintha O'Sullivan
Department of Surgery, Trinity Translational Medicine Institute, St. James's Hospital, Trinity College Dublin, Dublin 8, Ireland

Becky AS. Bibby
Translational Radiobiology Group, Division of Cancer Sciences, University of Manchester, Manchester Academic Health Science Centre, Christie Hospital, Manchester M20 4BX, UK

Breandán N. Kennedy
UCD Conway Institute & UCD School of Biomolecular and Biomedical Science, University College Dublin, Dublin 4, Ireland

Leticia García-Salguero, José A. Lupiáñez and Eva E. Rufino-Palomares
Department of Biochemistry and Molecular Biology I, Faculty of Sciences, University of Granada, Avenida Fuentenueva, s/n, 18071 Granada, Spain

Khalida Mokhtari
Department of Biochemistry and Molecular Biology I, Faculty of Sciences, University of Granada, Avenida Fuentenueva, s/n, 18071 Granada, Spain
Laboratory of Bioresources, Biotechnologies, Ethnopharmacology and Health, Department of Biology, Faculty of Sciences, Mohammed I University of Oujda, Oujda 60000, Morocco

Amalia Pérez-Jiménez
Department of Zoology, Faculty of Sciences, University of Granada, Avenida Fuentenueva, s/n, 18071 Granada, Spain

Agostinho Lemos and Pedro Brandão
Laboratory of Organic and Pharmaceutical Chemistry, Department of Chemical Sciences, Faculty of Pharmacy, University of Porto, Rua de Jorge Viterbo Ferreira, 228, 4050-313 Porto, Portugal

Ana Sara Gomes, Joana B. Loureiro and Lucília Saraiva
UCIBIO/REQUIMTE, Laboratory of Microbiology, Department of Biological Sciences, Faculty of Pharmacy, University of Porto, Rua de Jorge Viterbo Ferreira, 228, 4050-313 Porto, Portugal

Andreia Palmeira, Madalena M. M. Pinto and Maria Emília Sousa
CIIMAR-Interdisciplinary Centre of Marine and Environmental Research, University of Porto, Novo Edificio do Terminal de Cruzeiros do Porto de Leixões, Avenida General Norton de Matos, S/N, 4450-208 Matosinhos, Portugal

Mariola Napiórkowska
Chair and Department of Biochemistry, Medical University of Warsaw, 1 Banacha Str., 02 097 Warsaw, Poland

Marcin Cieślak, Julia Kaźmierczak-Barańska, Karolina Królewska-Golińska and Barbara Nawrot
Centre of Molecular and Macromolecular Studies, Polish Academy of Sciences, 112 Sienkiewicza Str., 90-363 Łódź, Poland

Joanna Wezgowiec and Mieszko Wieckiewicz
Department of Experimental Dentistry, Wroclaw Medical University, 50-425 Wroclaw, Poland

Roman Gancarz and Kazimiera A. Wilk
Department of Engineering and Technology of Chemical Processes, Wroclaw University of Science and Technology, 50-370 Wroclaw, Poland

Anna Wieczynska
Department of Engineering and Technology of Chemical Processes, Wroclaw University of Science and Technology, 50-370 Wroclaw, Poland
Institute of Genetics and Microbiology, University of Wroclaw, 51-148 Wroclaw, Poland

Wlodzimierz Wieckiewicz
Department of Prosthetic Dentistry, Wroclaw Medical University, 50-425 Wroclaw, Poland

Julita Kulbacka and Jolanta Saczko
Department of Molecular and Cellular Biology, Wroclaw Medical University, 50-556 Wroclaw, Poland

Natalia Pachura
Department of Chemistry, Wroclaw University of Environmental and Life Sciences, 50-375 Wroclaw, Poland

Manal M. Anwar, Somaia S. Abd El-Karim and Ahlam H. Mahmoud
Department of Therapeutic Chemistry, National Research Centre, Dokki, Cairo 12622, Egypt

Mohamed A. Al-Omar
Pharmaceutical Chemistry Department, Drug Exploration & Development Chair (DEDC), College of Pharmacy, King Saud University, Riyadh 11451, Saudi Arabia

Abd El-Galil E. Amr
Pharmaceutical Chemistry Department, Drug Exploration & Development Chair (DEDC), College of Pharmacy, King Saud University, Riyadh 11451, Saudi Arabia
Applied Organic Chemistry Department, National Research Center, Cairo, Dokki 12622, Egypt

Dominika Czerwonka and Adam Huczyński
Department of Medical Chemistry, Faculty of Chemistry, Adam Mickiewicz University, Uniwersytetu Poznańskiego 8, 61-614 Poznan, Poland

Szymon Sobczak and Andrzej Katrusiak
Department of Materials Chemistry, Faculty of Chemistry Adam Mickiewicz University, Uniwersytetu Poznańskiego 8, 61-614 Poznań, Poland

Ewa Maj and Joanna Wietrzyk
Hirszfeld Institute of Immunology and Experimental Therapy, Polish Academy of Sciences, Rudolfa Weigla 12, 53-114 Wrocław, Poland

Index